Gastrointestinal Imaging: THE REQUISITES

SERIES EDITOR

James H. Thrall, MD
Radiologist-in-Chief
Massachusetts General Hospital
Juan M. Taveras Professor of Radiology
Harvard Medical School
Boston, Massachusetts

OTHER VOLUMES IN THE REQUISITES IN RADIOLOGY SERIES

Breast Imaging

Cardiac Imaging

Genitourinary Radiology

Musculoskeletal Imaging

Neuroradiology

Nuclear Medicine

Pediatric Radiology

Ultrasound

Thoracic Radiology

Vascular & Interventional Radiology

Gastrointestinal Imaging

THE REQUISITES

THIRD EDITION

Robert D. Halpert, MD, FACR
Professor of Radiology
University of Mississippi Medical Center
Jackson, Mississippi

with 748 illustrations

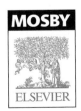

MOSBY
ELSEVIER

MOSBY
ELSEVIER

1600 John F. Kennedy Blvd.
Ste 1800
Philadelphia, PA 19103

THE REQUISITES™
THE REQUISITES
THE REQUISITES
THE REQUISITES
THE REQUISITES

GASTROINTESTINAL IMAGING: THE REQUISITES ISBN-13: 978-0-323-03221-6
ISBN-10: 0-323-03221-4

Library of Congress Cataloging-in-Publication Data

Halpert, Robert D., M.D.
Gastrointestinal imaging / Robert D. Halpert. — 3rd ed.
p. ; cm. — (The requisites)
Includes bibliographical references and index.
ISBN-13: 978-0-323-03221-6 ISBN-10: 0-323-03221-4
1. Gastrointestinal system—Radiography. I. Title. II. Requisites series.
[DNLM: 1. Digestive System—radiography. 2. Digestive System Diseases—diagnosis.
WI 100 H195g 2006]
RC804.R6H27 2005
616.3'307572—dc22 2005051085

ISBN-13: 978-0-323-03221-6
ISBN-10: 0-323-03221-4

Editor: Meghan McAteer
Developmental Editor: Karen Lynn Carter
Publishing Services Manager: Tina Rebane
Project Manager: Jodi Kaye
Design Direction: Karen O'Keefe Owens
Marketing Manager: Emily M. Christie

Printed in the United States of America

Last digit is the print number: 9 8 7 6 5 4 3 2

Foreword

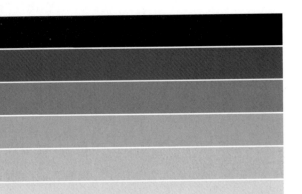

The textbooks encompassing THE REQUISITES in Radiology series have flourished in the series' first decade because of the diligence and success of the authors in producing such high quality works. *Gastrointestinal Imaging: THE REQUISITES* again exemplifies this high standard as it now appears in its third edition through the authorship of Robert D. Halpert, MD.

The organizational plan for *Gastrointestinal Imaging: THE REQUISITES* remains logically structured in chapters devoted to each major organ. Indeed, the first edition (published under the title of *Gastrointestinal Radiology: THE REQUISITES*) and the third edition share the same table of contents. This, of course, belies the enormous changes that have taken place in the clinical practice of gastrointestinal imaging. Advances in ultrasound, magnetic resonance imaging, and computed tomography make it challenging to keep any text up to date and reflective of current practices. Dr. Halpert has captured the important advances in his book. Indeed, gastrointestinal radiology was once dominated by studies using barium, fluoroscopy, and conventional radiography and is now an area of radiology sharing heavily in new cross-sectional imaging methods. Throughout the book, Dr. Halpert has added new and updated illustrations to support the text, although it is arguably becoming more difficult in print medium to illustrate functional and multidimensional images or methods such as fly-through virtual colonoscopy.

Perhaps an even bigger challenge than incorporating new information on new imaging methods is to keep the thread of knowledge intact regarding older methods, most importantly gastrointestinal fluoroscopy. While this imaging method is used far less frequently in current practice than it was historically, there are still important clinical applications and it is still vital to the practice of gastrointestinal radiology that a level of expertise with fluoroscopy be maintained. Dr. Halpert is a nationally and internationally recognized authority in fluoroscopic methods and ably describes them in *Gastrointestinal Imaging*: *THE REQUISITES.*

The cross-sectional era has given radiologists unprecedented ability to study the solid organs of the gastrointestinal tract as well as paraluminal and mesenteric structures. These abilities have positioned imaging studies as important methods for diagnosing, staging, and following the response of tumors to therapy at a level of detail simply not possible using historical imaging methods. Likewise, imaging now plays a leading role in studying the acute abdomen and has improved outcomes for patients with suspected appendicitis, diverticulitis, and innumerable other conditions. Taken together, these and other new applications have transformed both the specialty area of gastrointestinal radiology and the practice of medicine.

THE REQUISITES in Radiology have now become old friends to a generation of radiologists. The original intent of the series was to provide the resident or fellow with a text that might be reasonably read within several days at the beginning of each subspecialty rotation and perhaps reread several times during subsequent rotations or for board preparation.

The books in THE REQUISITES series are not intended to be exhaustive but rather to provide basic conceptual, factual, and interpretive material required for clinical practice. Each book is written by a nationally recognized authority in the different subspecialty areas of radiology, and each author is challenged to present material in a concise and efficient way for the benefit of the reader.

Dr. Halpert has once again done an outstanding job in sustaining the philosophy of THE REQUISITES in Radiology series and has produced another truly contemporary text for gastrointestinal imaging. I believe that *Gastrointestinal Imaging: THE REQUISITES* will serve residents in radiology as a very efficient, concise introduction to the subject and will also serve as a very manageable text for review by fellows and practicing radiologists.

James H. Thrall, MD
Radiologist-in-Chief
Massachusetts General Hospital
Juan M. Taveras Professor of Radiology
Harvard Medical School
Boston, Massachusetts

Preface

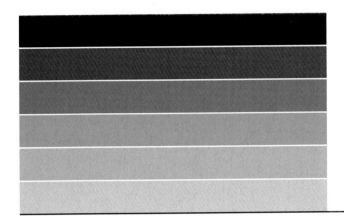

The advent of the third edition of *Gastrointestinal Radiology*, now renamed *Gastrointestinal Imaging* to reflect the inclusion of the newer imaging modalities, as part of the REQUISITES series is a gratifying experience, partly because I did not anticipate the success of the first and second editions, and partly because it has kept my head and mind in gastrointestinal disease and its imaging while at the same time having a considerable amount of my time taken up in administrative responsibilities.

Once again I must both lose and acknowledge co-authors who collaborated with me in the past on the first and second editions. Dr. Peter Feczko has chosen to bow out of the series after wonderful contributions to both the second edition of this text and the Gastrointestinal Case Review, a series of case review books spawned by the REQUISITES. Both his contribution and that of Dr. Philip Goodman, who co-authored the first edition, are still evident in the third edition, and I thank both of these former co-workers for their contributions.

This edition again strives to be concise and readable. Additional images have been added, some removed or replaced, and then some text updated to reflect the rapidly moving changes in our specialty. There is little doubt in my mind that imaging and image-assisted therapy will be the most important and robust aspects of medicine in the twenty-first century. If properly utilized, they will address issues of cost containment and improved patient care and safety.

We are a relatively young specialty. It has been little over 105 years since x-ray was first inadvertently discovered by Wilhelm Konrad Roentgen. Today we stand on the surge of a great tide of a new era in medicine where technology will take us places we have never been before. With that tide comes great responsibility: responsibility to handle our resources in the most cost-effective manner; responsibility to remember that at the center of the glitter, the technologic wonders, and the mystique of medicine is the patient, the very basis of who and what we are. Radiology is no longer the choice of senior medical students seeking to evade patient care. The world has changed.

Robert D. Halpert, MD

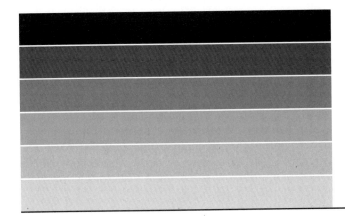

Preface
to the First Edition

In August of 1879, while attending the Annual Meeting of the American Association for the Advancement of Science in Saratoga, New York, the renowned physician Sir William Osler chanced to meet the inventor, Thomas Edison. Edison, having a passing interest in the medical applications of his inventions, suggested to Osler that it might be possible to "illumine the interior of the body by passing a small electric burner into the stomach." Sir William's response is not recorded, but his account of the encounter suggests some degree of amusement at the prospect of passing a tube with a light on the end into the stomach.

Nevertheless, Edison's words were prophetic and 114 years later, endoscopic direct visualization of the mucosal surface has established itself as the standard of gastrointestinal (GI) diagnosis, following several decades of virtual domination of this field by radiologists. However, the expected demise of radiological imaging of the gastrointestinal tract has not occurred. Instead, a collaborative, complementary relationship between endoscopy and radiological imaging of the gut has evolved, spurred on and encouraged by the profound effect of cost constraint and the increasing diagnostic sensitivity and relatively low cost of the radiological procedures.

Barium studies have decreased but not disappeared since the advent of widely available endoscopy. Moreover, the technical refinement of low-cost barium examinations may, in all likelihood, carve out a well-defined niche as a screening examination for many patients.

In addition, the development of other imaging methods has tremendously enhanced the role of imaging in GI diagnosis. Without doubt, the use of helical computer-assisted tomography, real-time ultrasound, and to an increasing extent, magnetic resonance imaging has greatly impacted gastrointestinal imaging. Indeed, modern cross-sectional multiplanar imaging has opened the abdomen for radiological inspection in a way that had been hitherto unattainable. Enhanced liver diagnosis and evaluation of the spleen, pancreas, lymphatics, and the structures surrounding the gut are now possible and signal the beginning of yet a new era in abdominal imaging and diagnosis.

In recent decades, our clinical colleagues have developed what they refer to as the *problem-oriented approach* to patient care and patient records. This refers to an orderly approach to patient diagnosis and management wherein the problems of greatest concern are appropriately weighted, while diagnoses of lesser importance are not lost sight of or neglected in the process. The goal is to establish a global perspective of patient care. Moreover, it should also facilitate a more readable and organized medical record.

In a similar fashion, we have tried to view the "radiological terrain" through the eyes of a first-year resident, a resident preparing for boards, or possibly a radiologist desiring to acquire a concise and abbreviated review of the specialty of gastrointestinal imaging. It would seem appropriate, from our view, to develop a problem-oriented approach to radiology to best address all of these demands and to attempt to present radiological problem solving (diagnosis) in an organized prioritized fashion.

This is generally referred to in radiology as the pattern approach. However, in keeping with a patient-oriented perspective on the practice of radiology, I would prefer to call these radiological patterns of disease "problems." The irregular thickened gastric fold, from the referring physician's point of view (and especially the patient's perspective) is not a pattern, but a problem! For the attending radiologist, the issue is one of problem solving. Although some may see this as nothing more than hair splitting and semantics (and they may be correct), it is, nevertheless, an accurate reflection of a philosophical perspective on the practice of radiology, no doubt left over from my days as a family practitioner.

The advantage of this approach, as opposed to the disease-oriented method, is to allow a closer paralleling of the real day-to-day world of radiology, and as a result, be of more practical value. The disadvantage is in the complexities of presenting material. In terms of writing a textbook, it is easier to describe a disease and all its radiological presentations, than to start with the radiological problem and work backward toward a reasonable differential diagnosis. The former is the organizational basis of almost all reference texts, while the latter is the daily experience of most radiologists. However, in the problem-oriented clinical management of a patient, problems often overlap, or the same disease may result in several very different problems. In the same way, a disease may have several radiological presentations. Gastric carcinoma, for example, may present as a problem of gastric folds, gastric mass, or ulceration. Hence, the inherent weakness in such a presentation of material.

Accordingly, we have tried to avoid undue redundancy while at the same time overlapping wherever necessary. Usually, the more in depth discussion will be reserved for the most common radiological problem posed by the disease entity.

Robert D. Halpert, MD

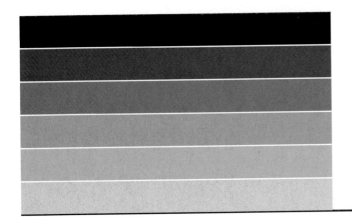

Acknowledgements

This third edition of *Gastrointestinal Imaging: THE REQUISITES* would not be possible without the invaluable assistance of several of the faculty and residents of the University of Mississippi Medical Center. These include faculty members Drs. Ottis Ball, Ron Gray, Joseph Navoy, Ramesh Patel, Michael Doherty, and Jay Faust. My thanks also for the contributions of residents and fellows, including Drs. Tim Zinkus, Joe Oliver, Greg Verville, Jeff Howard, Jim Massie, and Srinivas Potturi. I would also like to acknowledge Dr. Danny Meyers, head of abdominal imaging at the Henry Ford Hospital in Detroit, for his contribution, as well as Dr. Duane Mezwa of the William Beaumont Hospital in Royal Oak, Michigan.

Additionally, I must say a special word of thanks to Renea Hays, who patiently put up with my changes and rewrites in manuscript development and who did wonderful work in helping me with production of the images. I should be remiss if I did not mention Karen Carter at Elsevier for her patience, suggestions, and encouragement. The occasional, encouraging, and judiciously timed e-mail from Karen helped me to get this project back on track several times.

Robert D. Halpert, MD,

Jackson, Mississippi, April, 2005

Contents

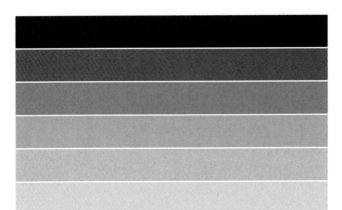

CHAPTER 1

Esophagus and Gastroesophageal Junction

EXAMINATION TECHNIQUES

Radiographic examination of the esophagus encompasses conventional fluoroscopic studies and various cross-sectional imaging methods. The esophagram (or barium swallow) is most often performed as a biphasic examination in which double-contrast and single-contrast techniques are employed (Box 1-1). In the upright position, the patient ingests an effervescent agent followed by a cup of high-density barium. Films obtained during this time, in the upright position, show the esophageal lumen distended with gas and the mucosal surface coated with barium (Fig. 1-1). The most common error seen in this procedure is the failure to rotate the patient sufficiently to the left to project the esophagus off the spine. This double-contrast phase of the examination is especially useful for showing fine mucosal detail, such as superficial nodules or ulcerations. When pooling of barium prevents visualization of the distal esophagus,

Box 1-1 Components of the Esophagram

Oropharyngeal function
Morphology of the esophageal tube
Esophageal motility
Esophageal mucosal surface
Appearance of the gastroesophageal junction
Presence or absence of spontaneous gastroesophageal reflux and efficiency of secondary wave clearance

a tube esophagram may be performed by injecting air directly into the esophageal lumen through a tube placed in the esophagus. This technique is not frequently used; it is associated with considerable patient discomfort and requires considerable operator skill and good patient communication skills. It is a highly effective and sensitive method, however, of showing subtle strictures in patients with a history of dysphagia. Probably as useful, and less traumatic to the patient, is

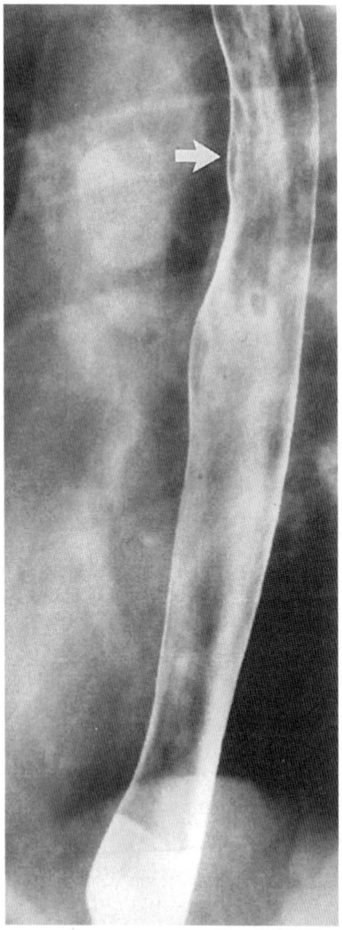

Figure 1-1 Double-contrast film of the thoracic esophagus. Note mild marginal nodularity *(arrow)* at the impression of the left main bronchus. This is a normal finding and should not be confused with disease.

fluoroscopically following the course of a 12.5-mm barium tablet taken with water. This is an excellent alternative, used to show the presence of a subtle stricture. Some radiologists give every patient with a solid dysphagia history a barium tablet at the conclusion of the examination.

If the esophagram is performed as part of an upper gastrointestinal (UGI) series, double-contrast films of the stomach and duodenum are obtained after double-contrast films of the esophagus. Single-contrast examination of the esophagus is usually performed with the patient in the right anterior oblique prone position. Esophageal peristalsis is observed fluoroscopically after the patient has taken a *single swallow* of low-density barium. The next swallow obliterates the previous primary wave and potentially causes the evaluation of primary wave function to be faulty; this is a protective mechanism that allows people to take successive swallows without aspiration. If you have ever watched a football game and wondered how some fans can "chug-a-lug" large quantities of beer without taking a breath, you understand how efficient and important this protective mechanism is. It certainly protects the lungs from drowning in beer.

Keeping the aforementioned issues in mind, the presence and function of primary wave activity should be noted at this time. Primary waves or "stripping" waves of the esophagus are triggered by the swallowing reflex (but are extinguished by the following swallow). Films are obtained as the patient continues to drink the cup of low-density barium (Fig. 1-2). This single-contrast phase of the examination is especially useful for evaluating esophageal motility and distensibility and for detecting extrinsic processes and certain abnormalities of the distal esophagus, including sliding hiatal hernia and mucosal ring (B-ring).

Spontaneous gastroesophageal reflux also may be observed fluoroscopically during the single-contrast phase of the examination. Provocative maneuvers to increase intraabdominal pressure and elicit reflux are sometimes performed, but the significance of reflux induced by these maneuvers is controversial and of questionable value. Spontaneous reflux observed while rolling the patient, especially to the right, is a significant finding. The demonstration of reflux should be grossly quantified and reported (mild reflux, barium refluxes and fills the lower esophagus; moderate reflux, barium is seen to fill at least the lower half of the esophagus; severe reflux, barium fills the entire esophagus up to the level of the pharyngoesophageal junction). Of even more importance is what the esophagus does with refluxed material. In normal circumstances, the refluxed material is rapidly cleared by secondary wave activity. Secondary waves are triggered by luminal distention of the esophagus, such as occurs with gastroesophageal reflux, and is the body's natural protective mechanism to protect sensitive esophageal mucosa from prolonged

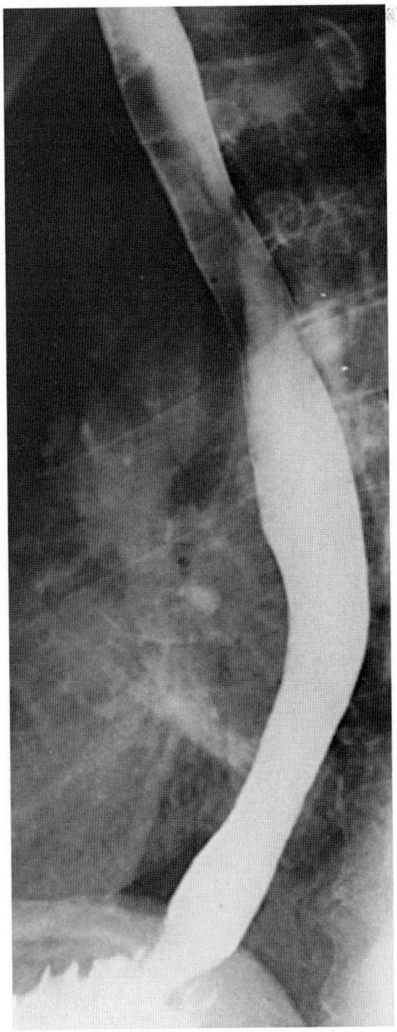

Figure 1-2 Single-contrast film of the thoracic esophagus.

exposure to highly acidic refluxed gastric content. Because all individuals have reflux in varying degrees, the health and function of the secondary wave is worthy of serious interest and evaluation. Impaired secondary wave activity may mean slow or prolonged clearing of reflux, and this constitutes the most important finding of all with respect to gastroesophageal reflux.

Mucosal-relief views of the collapsed esophagus show the longitudinal fold pattern and may be useful for showing esophageal varices. Although the esophagram is usually performed as part of a complete UGI series, it is sometimes requested as an isolated examination in patients with dysphagia or other complaints localized to the esophagus. All esophagrams should include evaluation of the proximal stomach, however, because proximal stomach lesions may cause dysphagia, chest or left shoulder pain, or other symptoms suggesting esophageal disease and sometimes lead to a cardiac workup.

Detailed examination of the pharynx and cervical esophagus may be incorporated into the routine esophagram in patients with cervical dysphagia or other symptoms localized to the neck. This examination is performed during the double-contrast phase with the patient in an upright position. Rapid-sequence films (three exposures per second) may be used on older fluoroscopic units. More advantageous would be a videotape recording obtained in frontal and lateral projections while the patient drinks high-density barium. In newer digital units, dynamic images may be stored, along with static images, on the PACS system and replayed anywhere on the system. This capability allows dynamic evaluation of swallowing function, detection of physiologic abnormalities such as incomplete cricopharyngeal relaxation and dynamic dysfunctions of the pharynx, hypopharynx, soft palate, and epiglottis, and evaluation for airway protection and possible aspiration to be seen by multiple viewers at multiple sites. Frontal and lateral spot films are obtained while the patient phonates (phonation of the letter "E" seems to get the best result) to distend the hypopharynx. The distention and mucosal coating seen on these spot films provide detailed anatomical information that might be obscured by barium on dynamic recording.

In cases of suspected esophageal perforation, water-soluble contrast material is recommended because leakage of barium into the mediastinum may induce mediastinitis, although this is rare. If water-soluble contrast material does not show an esophageal perforation, the study may be repeated using barium, in that a small leak using water-soluble contrast material can be difficult to visualize. Water-soluble contrast material is hyperosmolar; it can induce chemical pneumonitis or even pulmonary edema when introduced into the respiratory tract, either by aspiration from the hypopharynx or by extension through an esophagorespiratory fistula. Low-osmolality, water-soluble contrast material does not cause pulmonary edema, however, and can be used safely in patients with suspected esophageal perforation who are at risk of aspirating or who are known to have an esophagorespiratory fistula. Nevertheless, its palatability leaves much to be desired.

Computed tomography (CT) is the most commonly used cross-sectional technique for evaluating the esophagus (Fig. 1-3). CT is most helpful for showing the extraluminal components of esophageal disease; this includes staging of esophageal carcinoma (wall thickening, invasion of adjacent structures, and distant metastases), evaluating esophageal trauma (perforation and extension to mediastinum or pleural cavity), and assessing for free air or contrast material in the submucosa or periesophageal space. Additionally, multiplanar CT is becoming routine and adds considerably to the examination. Magnetic resonance imaging (MRI) at this time offers cross-sectional evaluation, also with the advantages of high-quality multiplanar capabilities but without the use

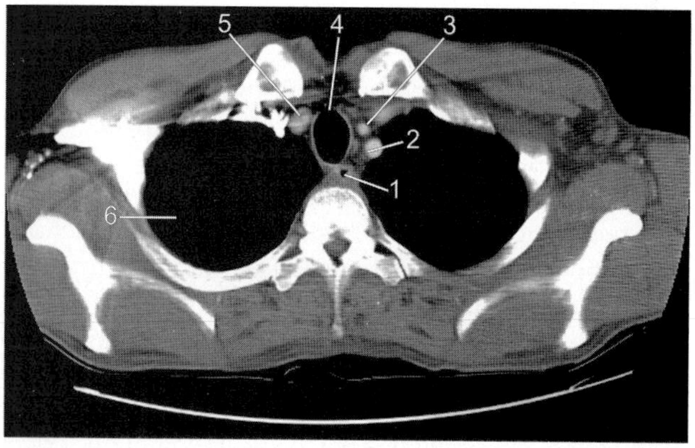

Figure 1-3 Normal computed tomographic anatomy of the upper thorax: 1, esophagus; 2, left subclavian artery; 3, left common carotid artery; 4, trachea; 5, innominate artery; 6, lung apex.

of ionizing radiation. Although MRI has been of limited usefulness because of motion artifact and long imaging times, image quality is improving with the use of cardiorespiratory gating techniques and newer imaging sequences requiring less time. Endoscopic ultrasound, in which a transducer is placed endoscopically into the esophageal lumen, can differentiate the individual layers of the esophageal wall and has been especially useful in evaluating the depth of esophageal tumors (resulting in more precise staging) or muscular thickening, such as seen in achalasia (Fig. 1-4).

SOLITARY MUCOSAL MASSES

Nonneoplastic

Inflammatory Esophagogastric Polyp/Fold

Inflammatory esophagogastric polyp/fold is a prominent fold extending from the gastric cardia into the distal esophagus. This fold often has a distal protuberant tip that may simulate an esophageal polyp (Fig. 1-5). This polyp/fold complex (sometimes referred to as a "sentinel polyp") is almost always associated with gastroesophageal reflux disease and inflammation of the mucosa of the lower esophagus. If the polypoid tip is larger than 2.5 cm in diameter or appears irregular, a biopsy is indicated to exclude an adenocarcinoma at or near the gastroesophageal junction.

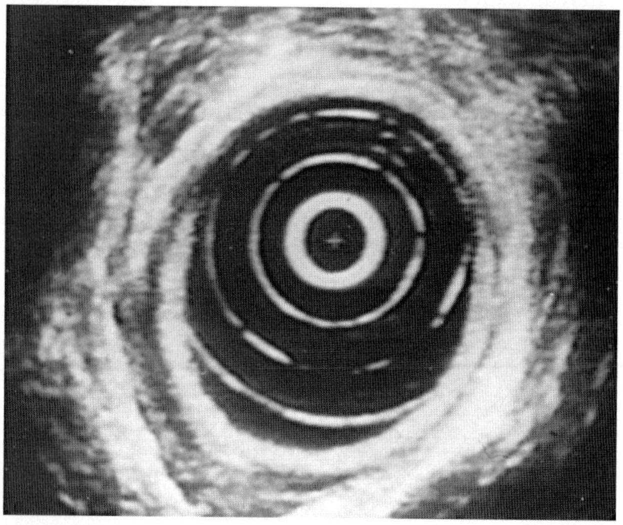

Figure 1-4 Endoscopic ultrasonogram shows a hypoechoic mural mass, representing esophageal carcinoma.

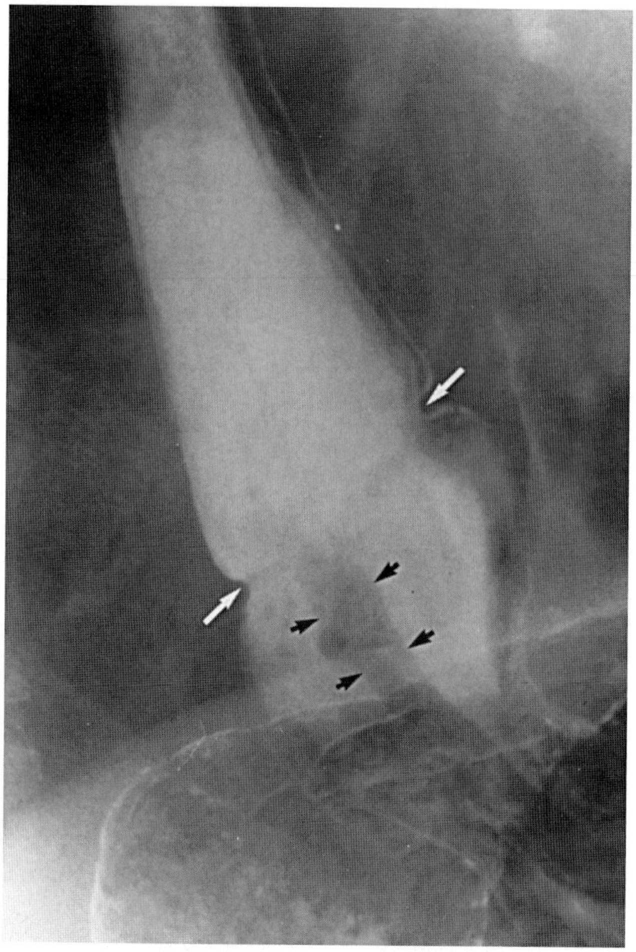

Figure 1-5 Inflammatory esophagogastric polyp/fold *(black arrows)* in a small hiatal hernia. A nonobstructing B-ring *(white arrows)* is also present.

Neoplastic

Carcinomas

A carcinoma of the esophagus can look like almost anything—from stricture to ulcer, mass, plaque, mural infiltrating process to irregular nodules seen focally in the esophagus. Primary squamous cell carcinoma of the hypopharynx or esophagus can present as a solitary mucosal mass, either small and plaquelike or large and polypoid (Figs. 1-6 and 1-7). Ulceration of the mass can occur in small and large lesions.

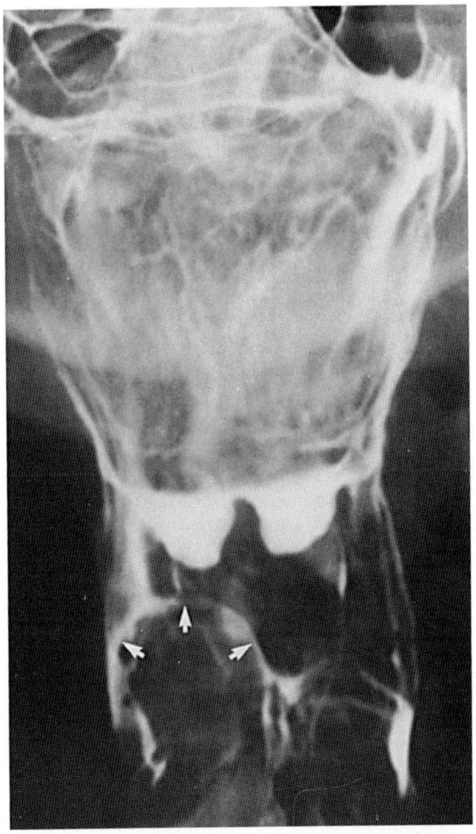

A

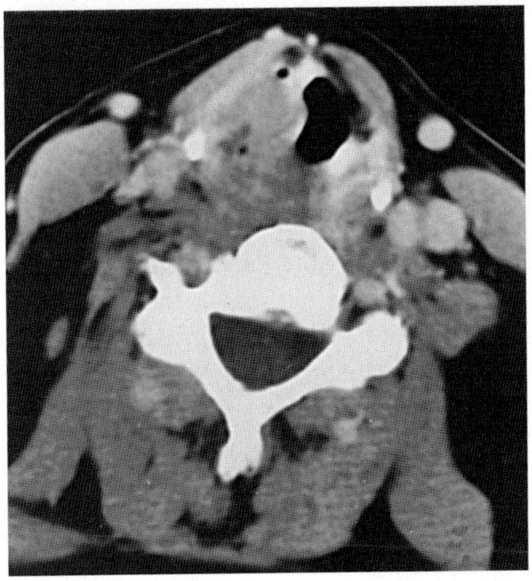

B

Figure 1-6 **A,** Frontal film of the pharynx shows a large mass in the right pyriform sinus *(arrows)* representing squamous cell carcinoma. **B,** CT shows the soft tissue mass obliterating the right pyriform sinus.

Squamous cell carcinoma was said to represent 95% of esophageal carcinomas until the 1970s, when an increase in the incidence of adenocarcinoma began that has not abated. Most lesions at the distal esophagus and gastroesophageal junction are adenocarcinoma, whereas most lesions in the proximal esophagus are usually squamous and have a much poorer prognosis. The most common

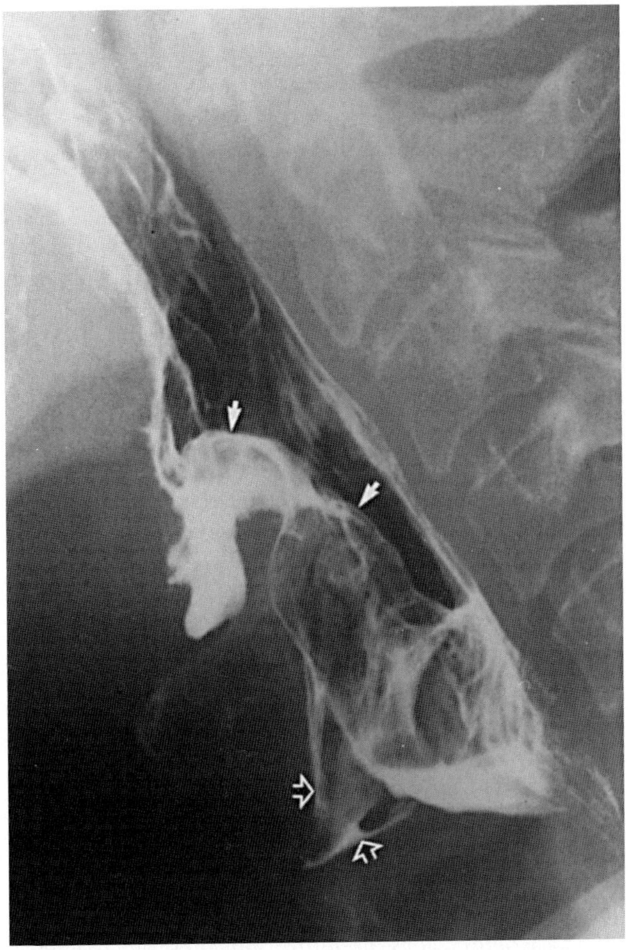

Figure 1-7 Lateral film of the hypopharynx reveals a large mass involving the epiglottis and aryepiglottic fold *(arrows)*, representing squamous cell carcinoma. Barium also is seen in the larynx and supraglottic portion of the airway *(open arrows)*.

risk factors (Box 1-2) for development of squamous cell carcinoma of the esophagus are cigarette smoking and alcohol ingestion. Other risk factors include the following:

- Chronic food stasis (achalasia or scleroderma)
- Chronic inflammation and scarring (lye stricture or radiation) usually 2 to 4 decades after the initial injury

Box 1-2 Risk Factors for Esophageal Cancer

Chronic reflux/Barrett's metaplasia
Lye stricture
Achalasia
Head and neck cancers
Plantar and palmar hyperkeratosis
Plummer-Vinson syndrome
Sprue
Tobacco
Alcohol

- Tylosis (a rare genetic disease of the skin characterized by palmar and plantar hyperkeratosis and an almost 100% incidence of squamous cell carcinoma of the esophagus by age 65)
- Plummer-Vinson syndrome (also called Patterson-Kelly syndrome in the United Kingdom), an association of cervical esophageal webs, nail deformities, iron deficiency anemia, and dysphagia)
- Sprue; there seems to be an increased incidence of esophageal malignancy associated with gluten enteropathy
- Certain skin disorders, such as pemphigoid and epidermolysis bullosa
- Squamous cell carcinomas of the head and neck also are associated with an increased incidence of subsequent squamous cell carcinoma of the esophagus, resulting from either common risk factors (e.g., cigarettes and alcohol) or radiation used to treat the original tumor.

Adenocarcinoma of the esophagus and the gastroesophageal junction has been increasing at an alarming rate in recent decades. At this time, esophageal adenocarcinoma seems to account for most esophageal cancers seen in the United States and Western Europe. It is estimated that 8000 new cases are diagnosed each year in the United States. Some cases may represent superior extension of gastric adenocarcinoma or, more likely, malignant transformation of gastric/intestinal-type epithelium in Barrett's metaplasia of the esophagus. The gastroenterology literature indicates that Barrett's metaplasia is common, being seen in 10% to 15% of all patients undergoing UGI endoscopy. Adenocarcinoma develops in approximately 2% to 5% of patients with Barrett's esophagus, suggesting the need for regular surveillance of this condition.

The treatment for serious gastroesophageal reflux disease (GERD) traditionally has involved medication or antireflux surgery (fundal plication), with the Nissen type being the most common, or both. More recently, gastroenterologists have begun to treat these patients with an endoscopic antireflux procedure using radiofrequency power to create a series of rings (Stretta therapy) around the lower esophageal sphincter. Initial results seem promising. Radiological evaluation of these patients conceivably could be confusing, however, and the radiologist should be aware of the patient's history of endoscopic procedures.

What is the cause of this dramatic increase in adenocarcinoma of the esophagus? There are several theories, the most obvious being the increased incidence of acid reflux (GERD) in some individuals, leading to increased Barrett's metaplasia and increased cancer risk. In the past, the treatment of Barrett's metaplasia was indirect (i.e., stop or reduce GERD using medications or antireflux surgery). The assumption historically has been held that the metaplastic changes may be arrested by treatment, but not cured, the only definitive cure being esosphagectomy. In recent years, gastroenterologists have been treating Barrett's metaplasia and dysplastic changes using photodynamic therapy, with varying degrees of success. There is now an attempt to treat superficial metaplastic/dysplastic, or even very superficial neoplastic conversion, by laser thermal ablation. Argon plasma coagulation therapy can be applied through a standard endoscope.

The epidemic proportions of obesity in the United States and its multiple problems are well documented and have been observed over approximately the same period as the increase in Barrett's metaplasia and adenocarcinoma of the esophagus. If general obesity is associated with increased amounts of intramesenteric fat, might this increased mesenteric fat lead to elevation of the stomach, alterations in the angle of the lower esophageal sphincter, and increased incidence in reflux, such as is well documented in the latter stages of pregnancy (hormonal issues aside) when the enlarged uterus impresses and elevates the stomach?

The puzzle becomes even more confusing and interesting, as there is some evidence to suggest an unusual inverse relationship between the presence of gastric *Helicobacter pylori* and the conversion of the esophageal metaplastic changes to cancer; that is, the presence of gastric *Helicobacter* confers some sort of protection.

It is possible that a few adenocarcinomas of the esophagus may arise from the sparse adenomatous elements known to be present in the squamous mucosa of the esophagus. Spindle cell carcinoma (or verrucous carcinoma) represents an uncommon variant of squamous cell carcinoma that has undergone focal mesenchymal metaplasia. This carcinoma typically appears as a bulky, polypoid intraluminal mass. Carcinosarcoma (spindle cell elements in a slow-growing squamous cell carcinoma) and primary malignant melanoma of the esophagus are rare epithelial malignancies that appear morphologically similar to spindle cell carcinoma.

Adenomas and Papillomas

Adenomas and papillomas are uncommon, benign tumors of the esophagus that arise from columnar and squamous epithelium.

MULTIPLE MUCOSAL MASSES

Nonneoplastic

Candida Esophagitis

Fungal esophagitis caused by *Candida albicans* is most commonly seen in patients with acquired immunodeficiency syndrome (AIDS) or in patients with other

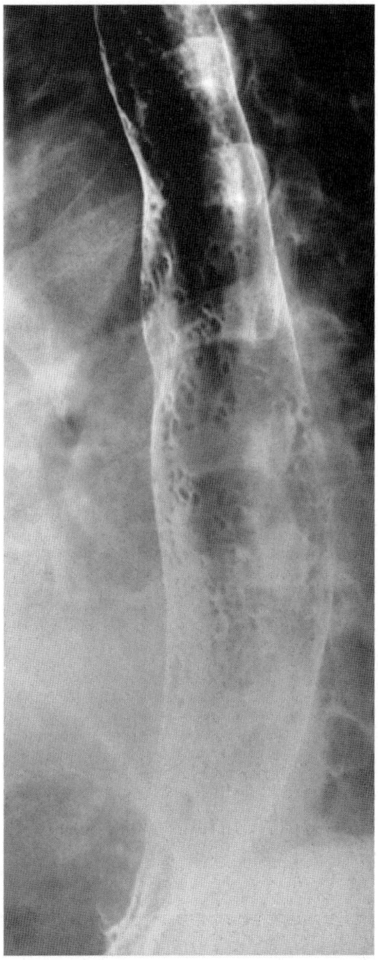

Figure 1-8 Early findings of monilial esophagitis (colonization stage). Note the well-developed, rounded plaques without ulceration.

immunocompromising diseases. This fungus causes whitish, slightly raised plaques that may also involve the pharynx or tongue (oral thrush). In the esophagus, these plaques resemble small mucosal nodules that often occur in longitudinal columns (Figs. 1-8 and 1-9). Patients with esophageal stasis, such as those with achalasia or scleroderma, are also at risk for the development of *Candida* esophagitis.

Reflux Esophagitis

All individuals experience gastroesophageal reflux to varying degrees. Most refluxed acidic stomach content is easily dealt with by secondary esophageal wave activity, which clears the gastric content quickly back into the stomach. Reflux esophagitis occurs in patients with gastroesophageal reflux as a result of sensitivity of the esophageal squamous mucosa to the harsh acidic gastric fluid and failure of the secondary wave to function properly. It can be a perpetuating cycle, as acid reflux may overwhelm the ability of the esophagus to generate the needed secondary wave, leaving the esophagus yet more vulnerable to the damage of gastric acid. Because reflux usually does not extend beyond the distal esophagus, esophagitis is most commonly confined to this area. Abnormal esophageal motility and mucosal edema are early signs of reflux esophagitis, with erosions, ulcerations, and stricture formation occurring with prolonged or severe reflux.

Glycogenic Acanthosis

Glycogenic acanthosis is a benign degenerative condition of the esophagus seen in middle-aged and elderly people. Focal deposits of glycogen form discrete plaques that appear as small mucosal nodules of varying size and shape on contrast studies (Fig. 1-10). This condition does not cause dysphagia and is usually an incidental finding.

Crohn's Disease

Filiform polyps are a rare manifestation of Crohn's disease of the esophagus. These thin, tubular or branching mucosal polyps resemble the polyps seen in the colon or ileum in the healing stage of inflammatory bowel

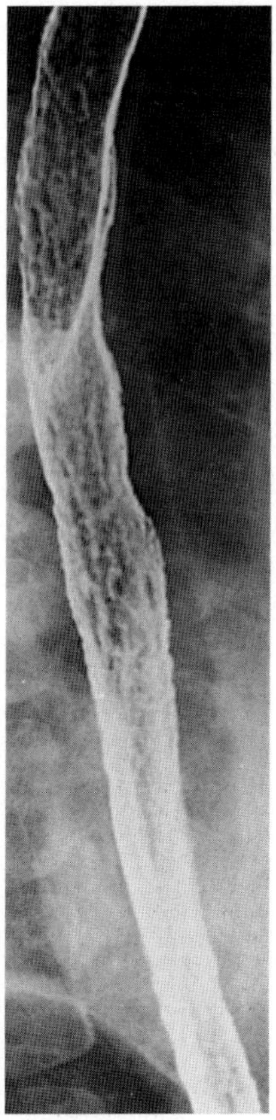

Figure 1-9 Diffuse mucosal nodularity and ulceration represents advanced esophageal candidiasis in a patient with AIDS.

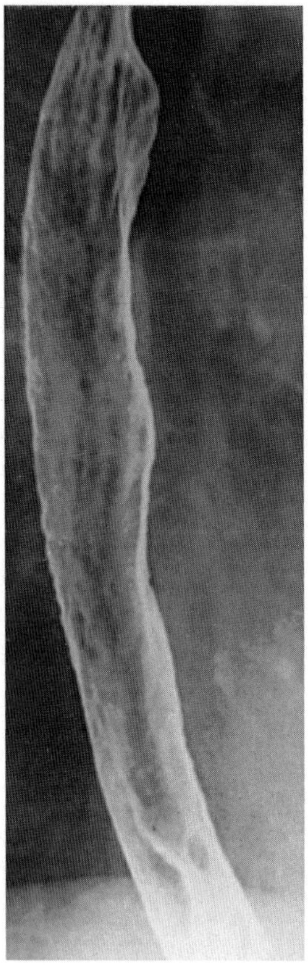

Figure 1-10 Diffuse mucosal nodularity represents glycogenic acanthosis.

disease. Ulceration in the esophagus may be seen as an early presentation, however.

Pemphigoid and Epidermolysis Bullosa

Subepidermal bullae, or blebs, in the esophagus may be associated with cutaneous lesions in benign mucous membrane pemphigoid and epidermolysis bullosa. These appear initially as small mucosal nodules, but subsequently undergo inflammation, ulceration, and fibrosis with stricture formation.

"Hairy" Esophagus

After certain types of pharyngoesophageal reconstructive surgery, hair follicles from the skin graft may appear as multiple, small mucosal masses ("hairy" or hirsute esophagus).

Neoplastic

Papillomatosis

Papillomatosis is a rare condition characterized by multiple esophageal papillomas. These benign epithelial growths are usually solitary, but they can be multiple in squamous papillomatosis, an unusual genetic disease, or in acanthosis nigricans, a disease in which esophageal papillomas occur in association with focal thickening and hyperpigmentation of the skin.

Superficial Spreading Carcinoma

Superficial spreading carcinoma is an unusual form of squamous cell carcinoma characterized by small mucosal nodules. These tumors are limited to the mucosal and submucosal layers of the esophagus, but metastasis to adjacent lymph nodes may be present.

Cowden's Syndrome

Cowden's syndrome (multiple hamartoma syndrome) is a rare genetic disease in which tiny hamartomas may cause diffuse mucosal nodularity of the gastrointestinal tract, including the esophagus. This disorder is often associated with various tumors of the skin, breast, and thyroid gland.

Leukoplakia

Leukoplakia represents small, whitish plaques resulting from hyperplasia of squamous epithelium. This rare cause of esophageal nodularity has an uncertain malignant potential, although it appears histologically identical to the more common premalignant leukoplakia of the oropharynx.

SUBMUCOSAL MASSES

Nonneoplastic

Varices

Esophageal varices represent dilated veins in the submucosal layer of the esophageal wall (Box 1-3). The more common uphill varices involve the distal esophagus and result from elevated portal venous pressure, usually secondary to cirrhosis of the liver. The elevated portal venous pressure causes increased blood flow through the coronary (left gastric) veins into the distal esophageal venous plexus, which then empties via the azygos system

Box 1-3 Esophageal Varices: Direction Matters

Uphill varices are related to portal hypertension with resultant ascending varices.

Downhill varices result from obstruction of the superior vena cava with varicoid collateral veins descending along the upper esophagus toward the right heart.

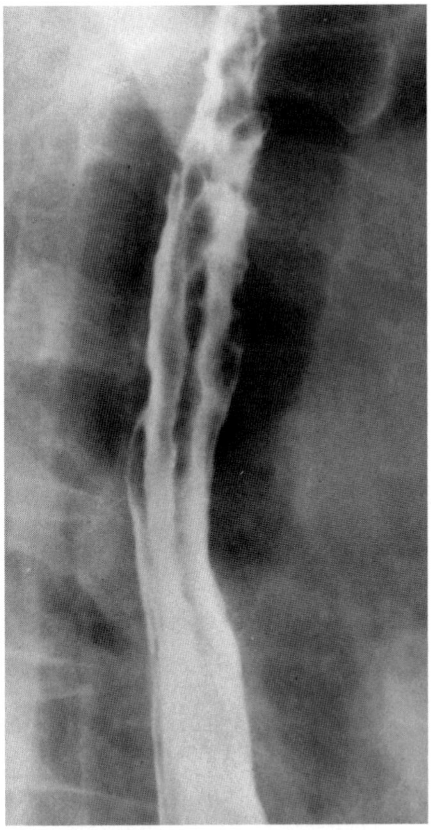

Figure 1-11 Downhill varices. A 61-year-old patient with upper mediastinal mass, occluded superior vena cava, and venous congestion (superior vena cava syndrome).

into the superior vena cava. Gastric fundal varices are sometimes associated with distal esophageal varices.

The less common downhill varices involve the proximal thoracic esophagus and result from obstruction of the superior vena cava, manifesting in the superior vena cava syndrome. Collateral blood flow bypasses the obstruction and enters the superior vena cava through the azygos system, sparing the distal esophageal veins (Fig. 1-11). An obstruction involving either the azygos system or the superior vena cava inferior to its junction with the azygos vein may lead, however, to collateral blood flow through the coronary and portal veins into the inferior vena cava. This flow results in varices involving the entire length of the thoracic esophagus.

On contrast studies, esophageal varices are best shown with the patient in the prone or supine position because in the upright position, gravity decreases distention of esophageal veins and can render varices less visible. The optimal technique for detecting varices is to have the patient take a single swallow of high-density barium. Continuous drinking may overcompress the varices; a single swallow usually shows the smooth, serpentine submucosal masses typical of varices. Mucosal relief views of the collapsed esophagus are also useful for showing this appearance (Fig. 1-12). Varices usually change with position. Any varicoid pattern that appears rigid or fails to change in the upright position should be viewed with suspicion, and "varicoid" appearance of a carcinoma should be considered.

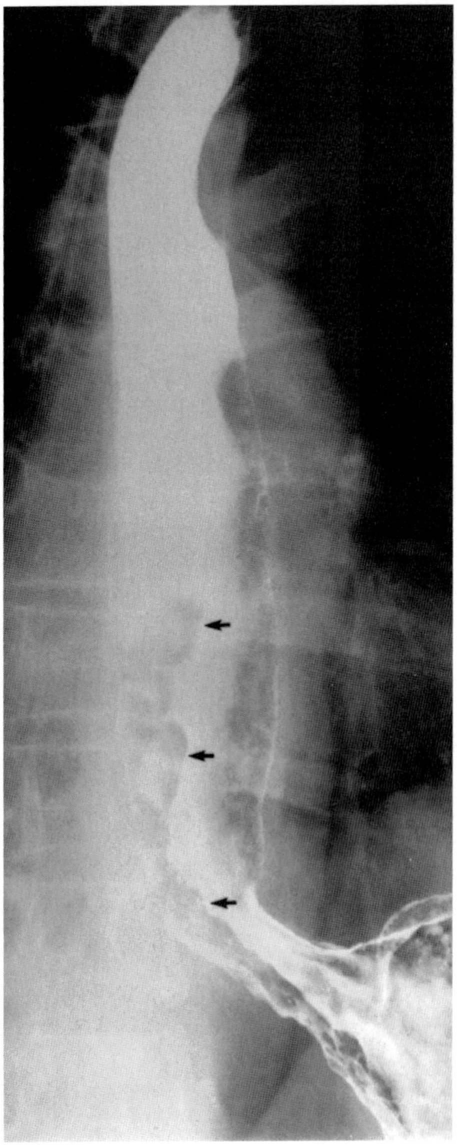

Figure 1-12 Uphill varices. Typical serpiginous filling defects in distal esophagus *(arrows)* in a patient with portal hypertension.

On CT, varices can appear as thickening of the esophageal wall or as adjacent lobulated soft tissue masses in the gastrohepatic ligament. Intravenous boluses of contrast material may be necessary to differentiate enhancing varices from nonenhancing neoplastic or inflammatory disease (Fig. 1-13). Angiography also is useful for showing esophageal varices and may be combined with interventional techniques for treating acute variceal bleeding.

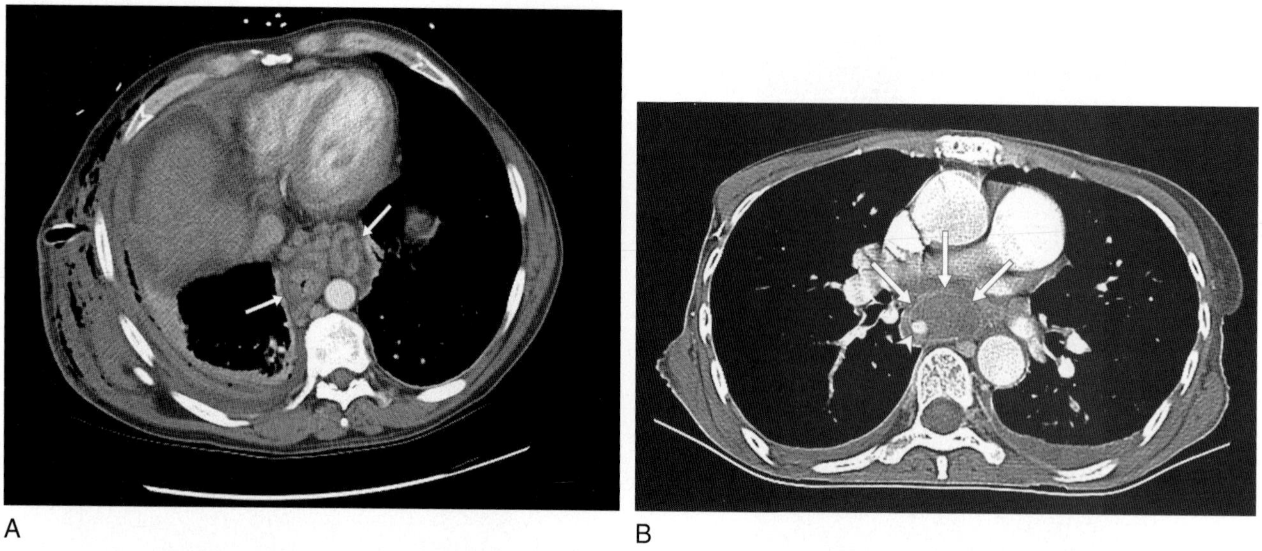

Figure 1-13 **A,** Bulky, serpiginous contrast-enhanced esophageal varices *(arrows)* around the gastroesophageal junction. **B,** Bleeding varices *(arrowhead)* filling and distending the esophagus with hematoma.

Cysts

Esophageal cysts may be congenital (foregut duplication cysts) or acquired (retention cysts). Duplication cysts are usually asymptomatic and, although usually discovered in childhood, are first noted in adults in 30% of cases (Fig. 1-14). They appear as a round or ovoid, soft tissue density, mediastinal mass on chest films and as a submucosal or extrinsic mass on esophagrams. Retention cysts, rare lesions that arise from dilated mucous glands in the distal esophagus, have a similar radiographic appearance.

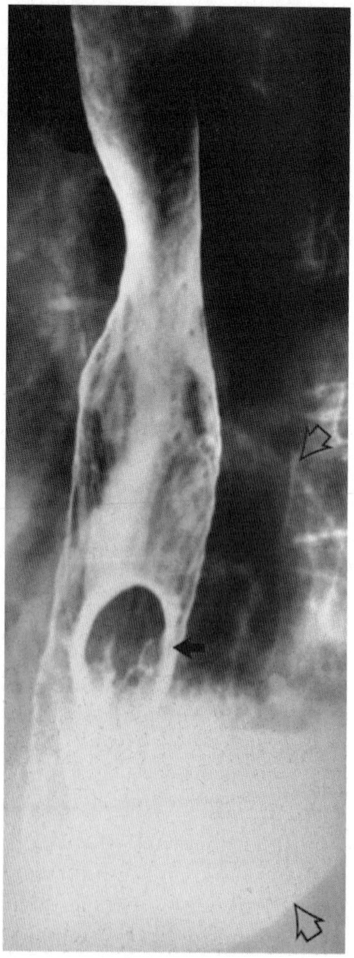

Fgure 1-14 Duplication cyst. Note communicating mouth of cyst *(arrow)* and the outer contours of the cyst *(open arrows)* showing its size.

Neoplastic

Mesenchymal Tumors

Benign stromal cell tumor, or leiomyoma, is the most common benign neoplasm of the esophagus. This smooth muscle tumor produces a focal rounded impression (Fig. 1-15). Although usually solitary, multiple benign stromal cell tumors of the esophagus occur in 3% of cases. Stromal cell tumors occasionally contain mottled calcifications.

Other benign submucosal tumors of the esophagus are uncommon. Similar to stromal cell tumors, they arise from mesenchymal tissues and appear radiographically as smooth, rounded masses. These tumors include hemangiomas, lipomas, and neurofibromas.

Kaposi's Sarcoma

Kaposi's sarcoma is a vascular tumor that originally was described as a rare cutaneous lesion affecting elderly men of Mediterranean descent. It is now recognized as a common lesion involving the skin, gastrointestinal tract,

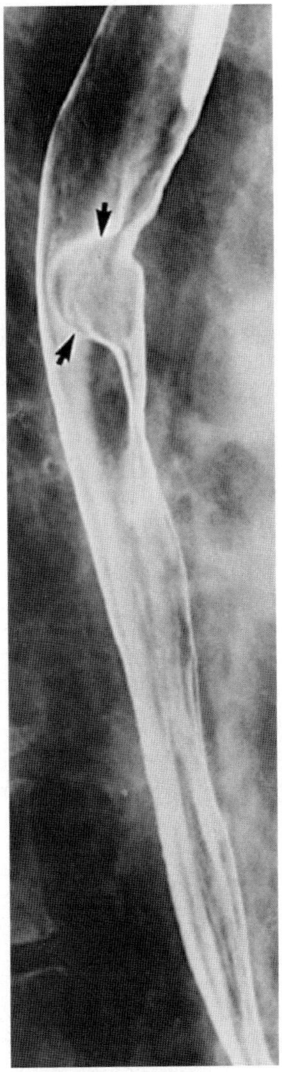

Figure 1-15 Smooth submucosal mass *(arrows)* in the upper thoracic esophagus represents a leiomyoma.

and respiratory tract of patients with AIDS. The esophageal lesion is a mesenchymal sarcomatous lesion that is seen in both solitary and multiple presentations.

Fibrovascular Polyp

Fibrovascular polyp, an unusual benign tumor, originates in the wall of the proximal esophagus and elongates to form a smooth intraluminal mass. This mass may extend inferiorly to occupy the entire esophageal lumen or may be regurgitated into the pharynx and out the mouth and put patients at risk for asphyxiation.

Granular Cell Tumors

Granular cell tumors are rare submucosal tumors thought to have a neural origin, possibly Schwann cells. About 10% occur in the gastrointestinal tract as solitary small submucosal lesions usually involving the esophagus, although they have been reported in the stomach and colon. Radiologically, they are identical in appearance to any small submucosal mass (Fig. 1-16).

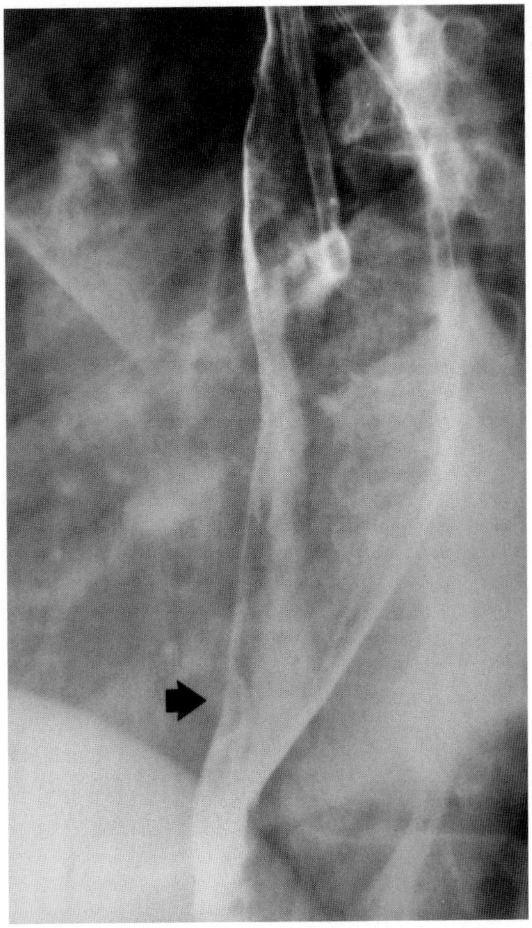

Figure 1-16 Granular cell tumor of the distal esophagus *(arrow)*.

Lymphoma and Metastases

Primary malignant neoplasms (sarcomas) and secondary malignancies (lymphoma, leukemia, and hematogenous metastases) are rare causes of discrete submucosal masses in the esophagus.

EXTRINSIC PROCESSES

Box 1-4 lists extrinsic abnormalities affecting the esophagus.

Cervical Esophagus

The postcricoid defect is a normal indentation on the anterior aspect of the hypopharynx at approximately the level of the C4 vertebra. This indentation was originally thought to represent a venous plexus, but is now

Box 1-4 Problems in the Neighborhood: Extrinsic Abnormalities Affecting the Esophagus

- Cricopharyngeal spasm
- Vertebral osteophytes
- Thyroid enlargement
- Mediastinal masses
- Abnormal vessels, e.g., aberrant right subclavian artery, pulmonary sling
- Cardiac enlargement
- Ectatic thoracic aorta

considered to result from redundant mucosa. This incidental finding may simulate a superficial neoplasm.

Incomplete relaxation of the cricopharyngeal muscle can cause transient extrinsic impression on the posterior aspect of the cervical esophagus at the level of the C5 or C6 vertebra. This localized esophageal striated muscle spasm can cause significant dysphagia when the amount of luminal occlusion exceeds 50%.

Anterior osteophytes of the cervical spine and, rarely, anterior herniation of an intervertebral disk may cause focal impressions on the posterior wall of the cervical esophagus. Osteophytes resulting from chronic osteoarthritis never cause dysphagia, and other causes should be sought. Osteophytes resulting from diffuse idiopathic skeletal hyperostosis, posttraumatic osteophytes, or post anterior cervical spine fusion, especially in the midcervical region, may cause dysphagia symptoms. Focal or diffuse enlargement of the thyroid gland can deviate and compress the esophagus, but infrequently causes dysphagia. Retropharyngeal tumor, hematoma, or abscess may displace the hypopharynx and cervical esophagus anteriorly. Cervical adenopathy and parathyroid enlargement also may lead to extrinsic compression of the cervical esophagus (Fig. 1-17).

Thoracic Esophagus

The most commonly seen normal extrinsic impressions on the thoracic esophagus are the aortic arch and left main bronchus (Fig. 1-18). Abnormal vessels, such as a right aortic arch, aortic aneurysm, ectasia of the thoracic aorta, and aberrant right subclavian artery, may also compress or displace the esophagus (Figs. 1-19 and 1-20). Rarely an aberrant left pulmonary artery arising from the right pulmonary artery and crossing the mediastinum to

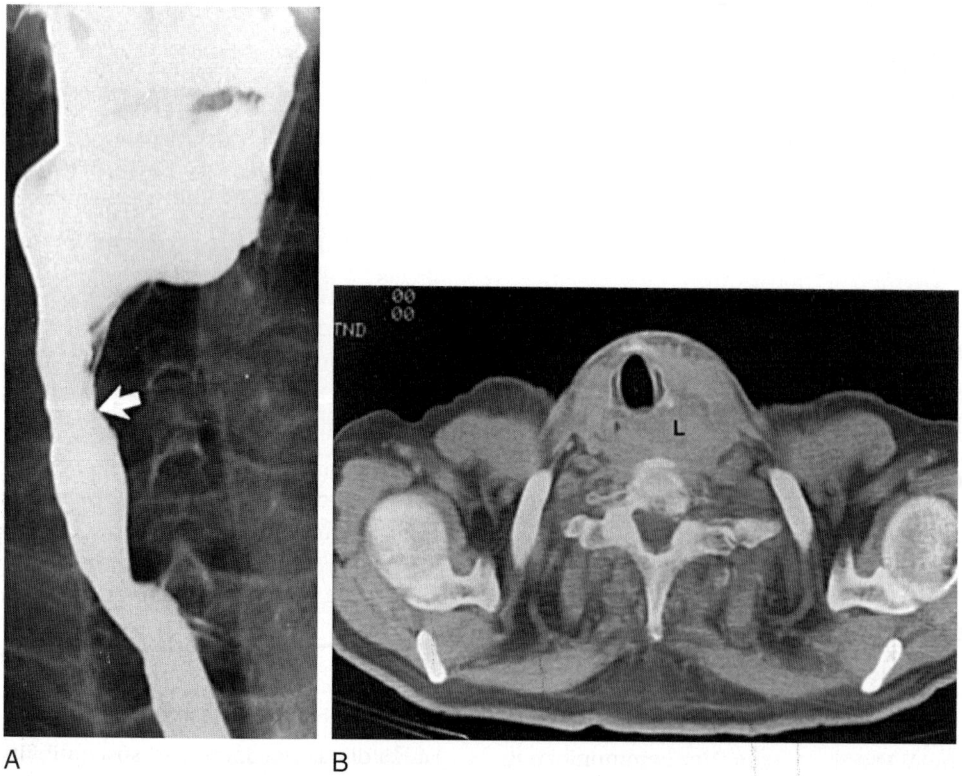

Figure 1-17 **A,** Compression and deviation of the upper esophagus to the right *(arrow)*. **B,** CT shows a large soft tissue mass *(L)* in the left neck, representing lymphoma.

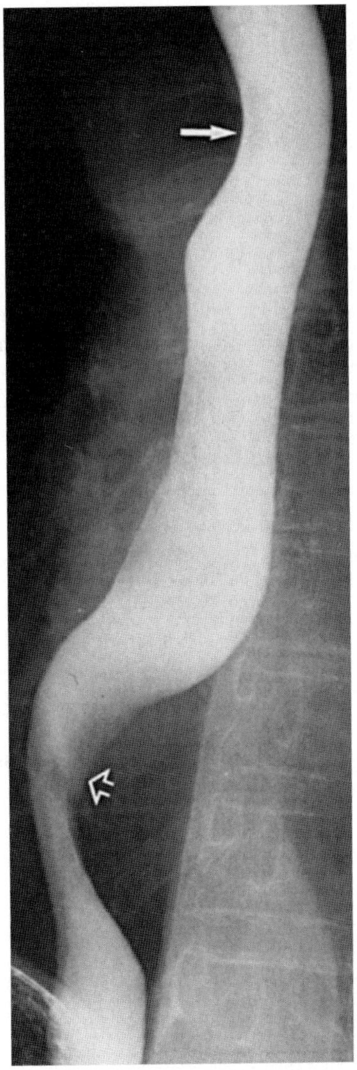

Figure 1-18 Esophageal compression by the aortic arch *(arrow)* and tortuous descending thoracic aorta *(open arrow)*.

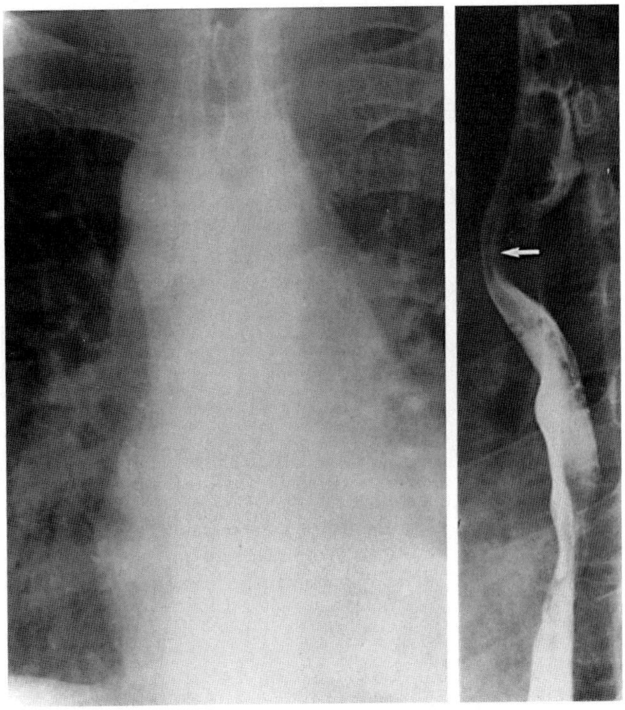

A B

Figure 1-19 **A,** Chest film shows a right aortic arch. **B,** Lateral view from esophagram shows smooth posterior compression of the upper thoracic esophagus *(arrow)* by an aberrant left subclavian artery.

the left lung can produce an anterior focal impression on the esophagus at about the level of the carina; this is known as the "pulmonary sling."

Mediastinal adenopathy causes impressions along the anterior aspect of the midesophagus, and spinous osteophytes result in one or more focal impressions on the posterior esophageal wall. Cardiac impressions on the esophagus can be focal (left atrial enlargement) or more diffuse (generalized cardiomegaly and pericardial effusion) (Fig. 1-21). An adjacent lung tumor or mediastinal mass may compress and deviate the esophagus; pulmonary volume loss as a result of fibrosis typically causes ipsilateral traction of the esophagus. Noncommunicating duplication cysts can be seen as mediastinal masses impressing the esophageal lumen (Fig. 1-22).

ULCERATIONS AND FISTULAS

Nonneoplastic

Infections

Infectious causes of esophageal ulceration include viruses, fungi, and bacteria. Viral esophagitis most often affects immunocompromised patients, particularly patients with AIDS. Herpes simplex virus and cytomegalovirus cause solitary or multiple discrete shallow ulcers on a normal esophageal mucosal background (Fig. 1-23). The ulcers of cytomegalovirus may be quite large. Human immunodeficiency virus has been reported to produce giant esophageal ulcers identical to the ulcers caused by cytomegalovirus. All of these conditions result in painful dysphagia.

Tuberculous esophagitis usually occurs in patients with pulmonary or mediastinal tuberculosis and may result from contiguous extension of disease or from swallowing infected sputum. Additionally, there has been an increase in active *Mycobacterium* infections as a result of the AIDS epidemic and reactivation of latent disease or increased susceptibility owing to compromised immunological status. Esophageal ulcerations, sinus tracts, and nodularity are typically noted (Fig. 1-24).

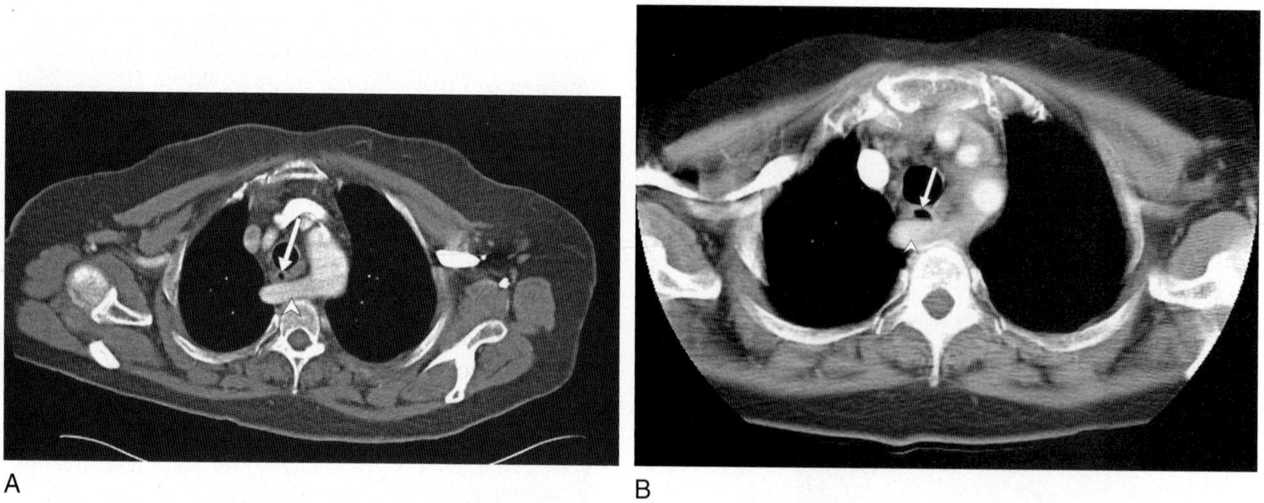

Figure 1-20 **A,** Aberrant right subclavian artery. Note right subclavian artery *(arrowhead)* swinging posterior to the esophagus *(arrow)*. **B,** More inferior computed tomographic section shows impression of the right subclavian artery *(arrowhead)* on the posterior wall of the esophagus *(arrow)*.

These esophageal findings are being reported with increasing frequency in patients with AIDS and may result in esophagorespiratory fistulas. Esophageal ulceration caused by atypical mycobacteria also has been described in AIDS patients.

In *Candida* esophagitis, the presentation initially may be small, round, smooth plaques (colonization stage) with minimal symptoms. Confluence and elongation of fungal plaques, allowing barium to penetrate between the plaques, follows, resulting in pseudoulceration. True ulceration occurs as the infection progresses to severe esophageal candidiasis, and rhizoid extensions into the submucosa result in diffuse and severe ulceration (the "shaggy esophagus").

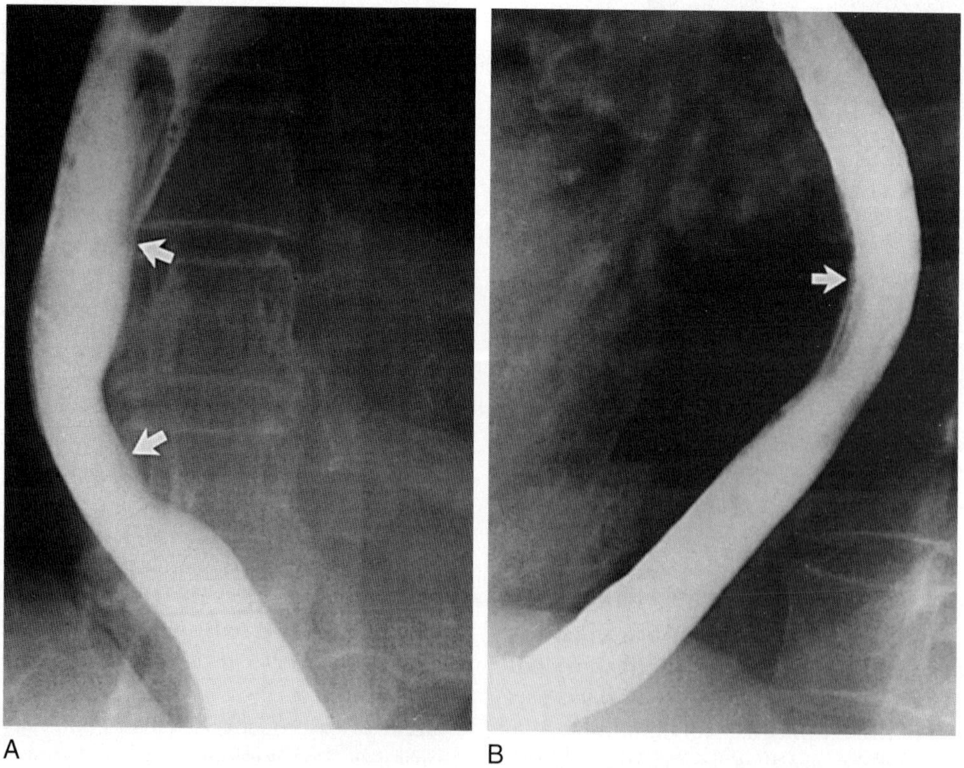

Figure 1-21 Frontal **(A)** and lateral **(B)** films show extrinsic compression of the distal esophagus *(arrows)* by an enlarged left atrium.

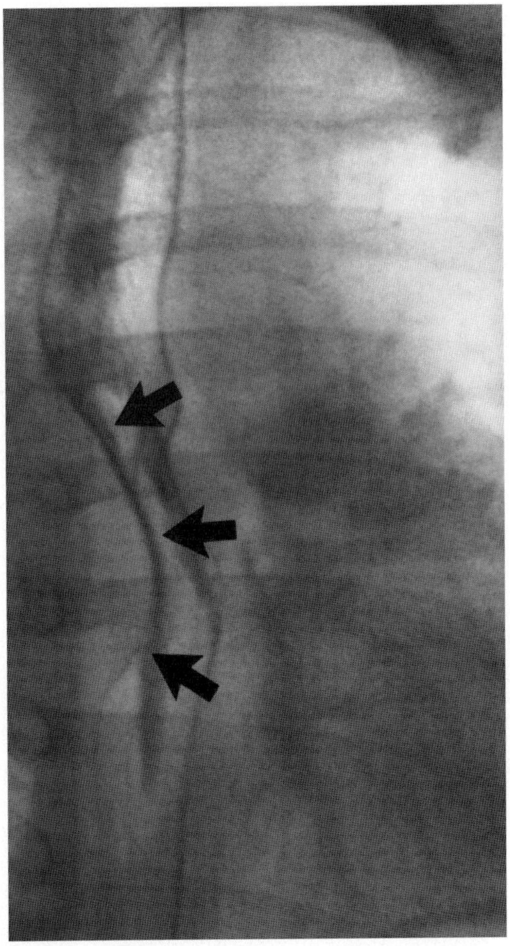

Figure 1-22 Extrinsic compression of the midesophagus by a mediastinal mass *(arrows)*. At surgery, the mass proved to be a noncommunicating duplication cyst.

Inflammation (Noninfectious)

Reflux esophagitis (GERD) (Box 1-5) is a common disease, with at least 10% to 15% of the population experiencing heartburn daily. It becomes more severe and can cause erosions or ulcerations in the distal esophagus as a result of irritation of the esophageal mucosa by gastric acid (Figs. 1-25 and 1-26). Conditions predisposing to development of severe reflux esophagitis include hiatal hernia, incompetence in the lower esophageal sphincter, and lack of integrity of the phrenoesophageal ligament. Dysfunction of the esophageal secondary stripping wave is commonly seen in severe GERD. It is not clear, however, whether this function is an etiological basis of GERD or the result of chronic esophageal inflammation. Increased incidence of GERD has been described in Zollinger-Ellison syndrome, prolonged nasogastric intubation, scleroderma, and pregnancy. Reflux esophagitis is commonly seen in patients with almost any type of gastric procedure, even gastroenterostomies. In patients with previous partial or complete gastric resection, alkaline bile from the proximal small bowel refluxes into the stomach and quickly into the distal esophagus. This reflux of alkaline bile may also lead to esophageal ulceration and stricturing. This complication can be avoided by surgically diverting the flow of bile away from the gastric remnant or esophagus (revision of gastroduodenostomy or creation of Roux-en-Y enteroenterostomy).

Prolonged nasogastric intubation, by not allowing complete closure of the lower esophageal sphincter around the indwelling tube, permits continuous gastric reflux to occur. The tube also alters esophageal peristalsis, preventing rapid clearance of the refluxed material from the esophagus; this may eventually result in diffuse esophageal narrowing. In scleroderma, GERD is a result of aperistalsis of the esophagus and a patulous gastroesophageal junction. The increasing size of the uterus in pregnancy causes compression of the stomach, causing the lower esophageal sphincter pressure to be reduced with resultant reflux.

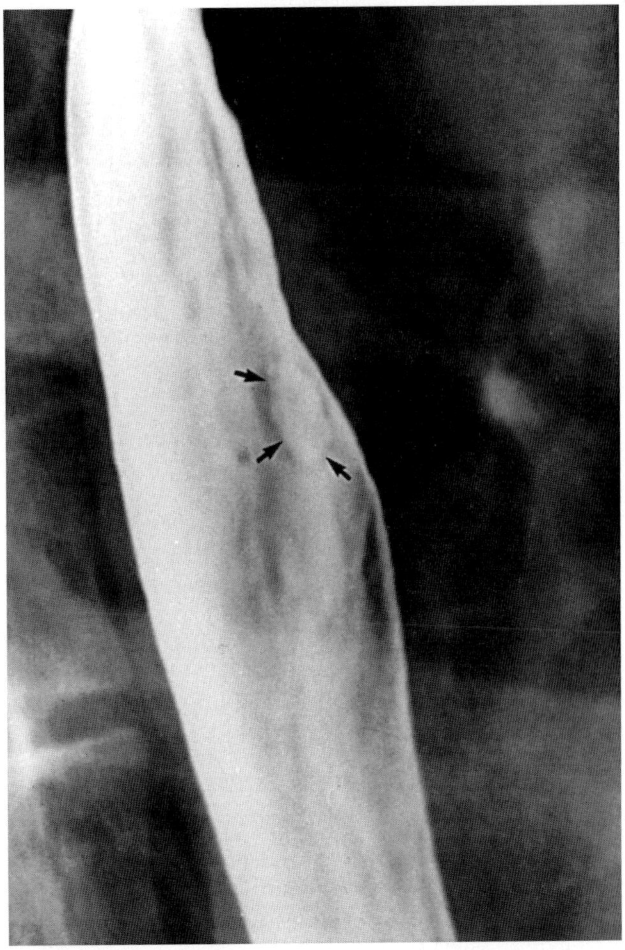

Figure 1-23 Focal ulceration in the midesophagus *(arrows)* represents cytomegalovirus esophagitis in a patient with AIDS.

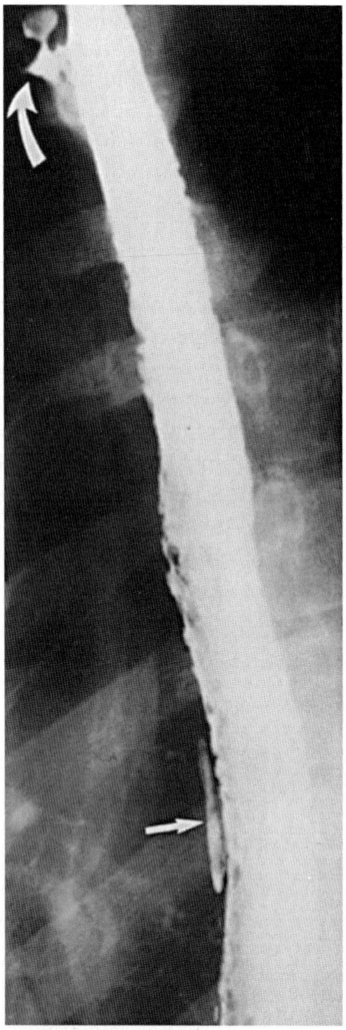

Figure 1-24 Sinus tract *(curved arrow)* and longitudinal ulceration *(straight arrow)* in a patient with AIDS and mycobacterial esophagitis. (From Goodman P, Pinero SS, Rance RM, et al: Mycobacterial esophagitis in AIDS. Gastrointest Radiol 14:103, 1989.)

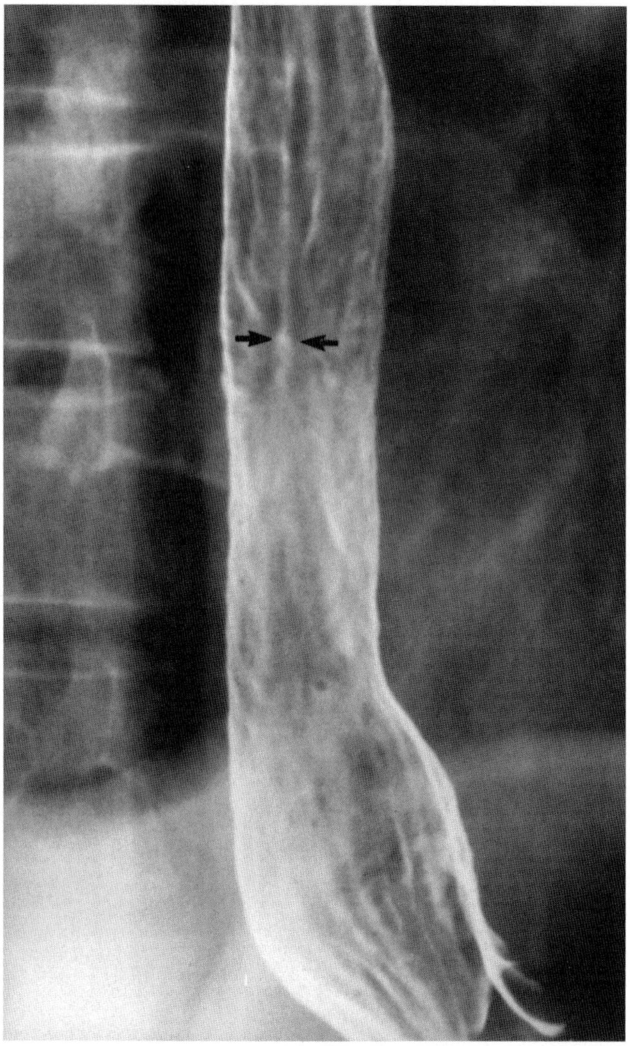

Figure 1-25 Severe reflux esophagitis with diffuse nodularity, granularity, and linear longitudinal ulceration *(arrows)*.

Barrett's esophagus is a condition in which esophageal squamous epithelium undergoes metaplasia to a gastric-intestinal-type columnar epithelium (Box 1-6). This condition occurs in about 2% to 5% of patients with reflux esophagitis and is thought to be directly related to chronic GERD. Although Barrett's esophagus is usually seen in the distal esophagus (where reflux most often affects the esophagus), it also may involve the midesophagus or upper third of the esophagus, with areas of intervening normal esophageal mucosa. Radiographic manifestations of Barrett's esophagus are nonspecific and include mucosal nodularity, a reticular mucosal pattern (on double-contrast films), focal ulceration, and focal narrowing or stricture formation.

Certain oral medications may cause focal irritation and ulceration of the esophagus by prolonged contact with the esophageal mucosa (Fig. 1-27). Patients universally experience severe odynophagia. This condition is most often seen with tetracycline and its derivatives and has been reported with quinidine, potassium chloride, some nonsteroidal antiinflammatory drugs, and several

Box 1-5 Radiological Signs of Reflux Esophagitis

- Thickened distal folds, e.g., esophagogastric polyp
- Benign strictures
- Ulcers, usually linear and located distally
- Hiatal hernias with spontaneous gastroesophageal reflux commonly seen, but not absolutely necessary for diagnosis

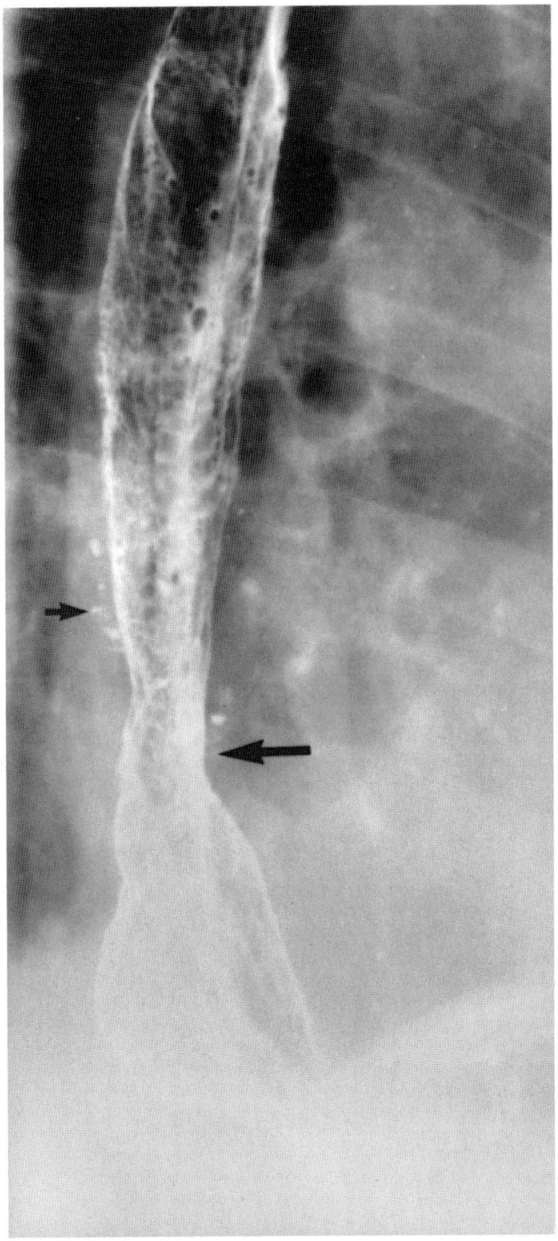

Figure 1-26 Severe chronic reflux esophagitis. Note stricture *(large arrow)* and multiple pseudodiverticula *(small arrow)*, commonly associated with chronic reflux disease.

Box 1-6 What We Know About Barrett's Metaplasia

Caused by chronic reflux esophagitis (GERD)
Chronic corrosive effect of acid on esophageal mucosa damages squamous epithelium resulting in metaplastic changes (the patchy development of gastric and intestinal mucosa in the distal esophagus)
Thought to occur in 2%-5% of patients with GERD
Is premalignant, and dysplastic changes can lead to adenocarcinoma; the process can be arrested by treatment

other medications including aspirin and vitamin C. A capsule or tablet, especially when taken at bedtime with a small amount of water, may lodge in the esophagus at the level of the aortic arch or distal esophagus, spilling its contents locally on the esophagus. The focal esophagitis usually heals promptly after discontinuation of the offending medication.

Corrosive esophagitis resulting from the ingestion of lye or other caustic substances often leads to severe edema and ulceration of the esophagus in the acute stage, followed by stricture formation after healing occurs. Contrast studies are not usually performed in the acute stage of a severe corrosive esophagitis.

In acute alcoholic esophagitis, superficial ulcerations are seen in the midesophagus and distal esophagus shortly after alcoholic binges; these ulcerations were first suggested by Beaumont in his 1836 treatise regarding in vivo studies of the human stomach. His subject, a young French-Canadian fur trapper, had sustained a gunshot wound to the flank and abdomen that had left him with a permanent anterior gastrocutaneous

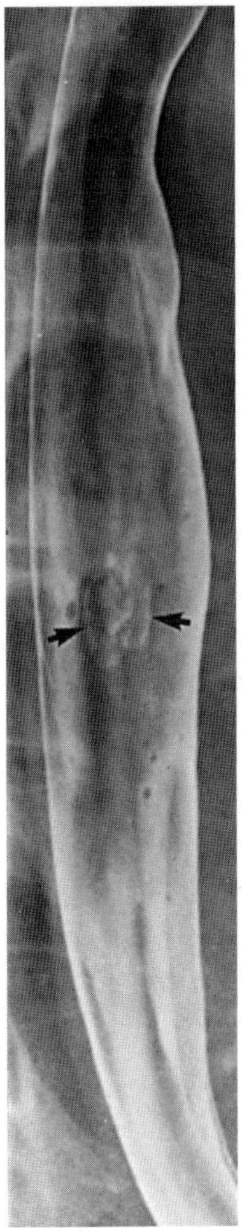

Figure 1-27 Discrete ulcerations *(arrows)* in the midesophagus caused by the ingestion of antibiotic capsules.

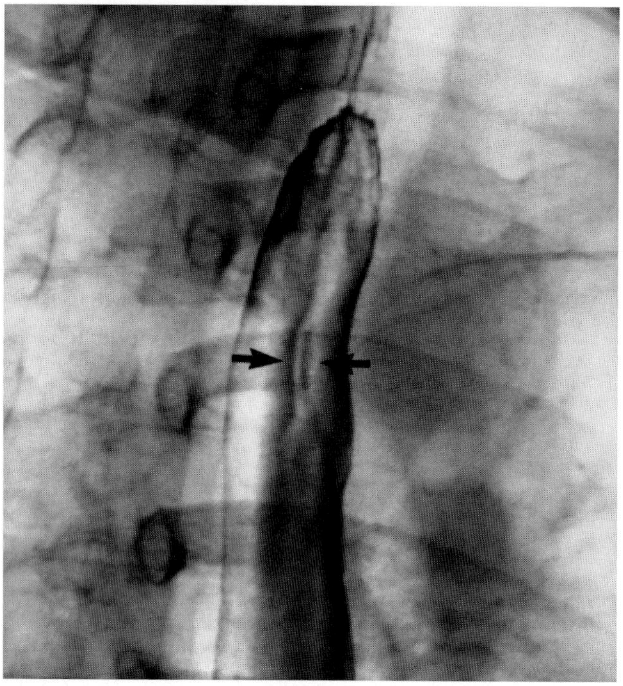

Figure 1-28 Esophageal Crohn's ulcer. A 26-year-old patient with known small bowel Crohn's disease presents with odynophagia. Processed digital images from esophagram show to advantage a solitary linear Crohn's ulcer *(arrows)* of proximal esophagus.

fistula. After several especially "rousing" weekends involving alcoholic binges, reddened, inflamed tissue and superficial ulcers over the entire stomach and lower esophagus of the fur trapper were seen by Beaumont.

Although the esophagus is relatively radioresistant, radiation therapy to the mediastinum may cause esophagitis and esophageal ulcerations. This condition occurs in the acute stage and may lead to stricture formation after healing. The location of inflammatory changes conforms to the radiation port used.

Changes associated with radiation esophagitis are typically seen after doses of 4500 to 6000 cGy over a 6- to 8-week period and are even more common after combination radiation therapy and chemotherapy. After radiation therapy, esophagorespiratory fistulas may develop in patients with mediastinal adenopathy compressing the esophagus, presumably as a result of tumor necrosis induced by radiation. Similarly, patients who undergo external beam or intracavitary radiation therapy for primary esophageal carcinoma may develop necrosis of the tumor with subsequent ulceration or formation of an esophagorespiratory fistula.

Esophageal involvement occurs in approximately 3% of patients with Crohn's disease of the ileum or colon and may be seen as aphthous or longitudinal ulcers (Fig. 1-28). Crohn's disease of the esophagus rarely occurs in the absence of ileal or colonic disease.

Behçet's disease (the Silk Route disease) is an unusual condition of unknown etiology that is characterized by oral and genital ulcerations, ocular inflammation, and vascular thrombosis. Focal ulcerations have been reported mostly in the colon, but esophageal and small bowel lesions are not unknown.

Benign mucous membrane pemphigoid and epidermolysis bullosa are rare skin diseases that may be associated with ulcerations, webs, and strictures in the pharynx and esophagus (Fig. 1-29). The initial finding in these conditions is multiple mucosal nodules.

Eosinophilic esophagitis is a rare cause of esophageal ulcerations. This disease, similar to eosinophilic gastroenteritis, is associated with eosinophilic infiltration, peripheral eosinophilia, and a history of allergies. In addition to ulcerations, esophageal nodularity and stricture formation may occur in this disease.

Aortoesophageal Fistula

Aortoesophageal fistula is an unusual complication of thoracic aortic aneurysms or aortic grafts. Erosion into the esophagus causes hematemesis, usually followed

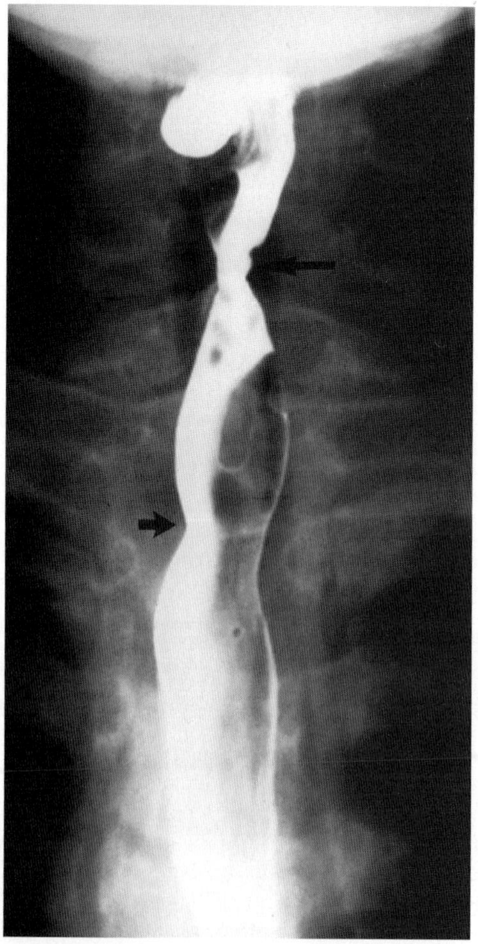

Figure 1-29 Epidermolysis bullosa. At least two proximal esophageal strictures are identified *(arrows)*.

within hours to days by massive bleeding and potential exsanguination.

Trauma

Trauma may lead to ulceration, laceration, or perforation of the esophagus. This includes iatrogenic causes, such as instrumentation, endoscopic perforation of an esophageal diverticulum, and sclerotherapy of esophageal varices with resultant ulceration (Fig. 1-30). Endoscopic complications vary with the procedure, with variceal sclerotherapy having the highest complication rate (about 8%). Taco chips or corn chips may lacerate the esophagus, and impacted foreign bodies may cause focal irritation and ulceration. Vomiting can lead to mucosal disruption (Mallory-Weiss tear) (Fig. 1-31) or transmural perforation (Boerhaave's syndrome) of the distal esophagus.

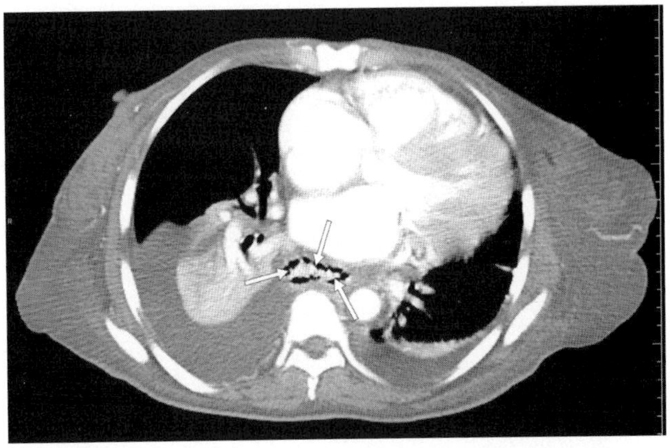

Figure 1-31 Intramural air in the distal esophagus *(arrows)*.

Neoplastic

Carcinoma, Metastases, and Lymphoma

Focal necrosis and ulceration are not unusual in primary squamous cell carcinoma of the esophagus. Extensive ulceration (in which the tumor is almost completely ulcerated) is uncommonly seen radiographically, however. Primary esophageal adenocarcinoma arising in Barrett's epithelium also may undergo focal ulceration. Other malignant lesions that may appear ulcerated include metastases and lymphoma. Additionally, fistulous communication between squamous cell carcinoma of the esophagus and the bronchial or tracheal airway occasionally can be seen with midesophageal lesions (Fig. 1-32).

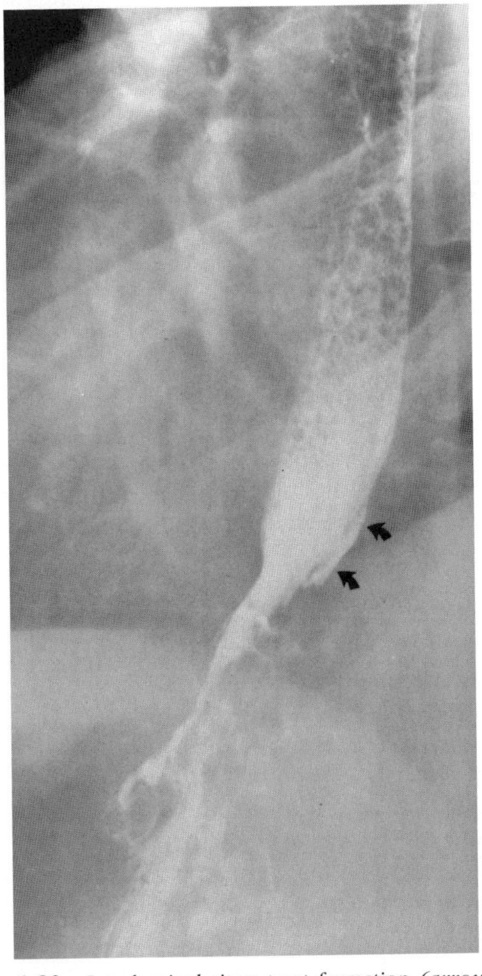

Figure 1-30 Intraluminal sinus tract formation *(arrows)* after sclerotherapy treatment for varices.

DYSMOTILITY

Normal esophageal motility or peristalsis refers to the coordinated propulsion of a bolus from the pharynx to the stomach. This process is regulated by complex neuromuscular interactions and appears radiographically as a continuous, smooth, wavelike contraction. A primary wave is initiated by the act of swallowing, whereas a secondary wave is produced in response to distention of the esophagus caused by refluxed stomach content. Tertiary noncontractile waves occasionally may be seen in older patients. In the presence of an adequate primary wave, however, this finding is of no consequence. The presence of tertiary waves with no primary wave indicates esophageal dysmotility

Cervical Esophagus

Neuromuscular Abnormalities

Diseases of striated muscle, such as dermatomyositis and muscular dystrophy, can affect motility of the cervical esophagus because this portion of the esophagus is composed of striated muscle rather than smooth muscle. Various neuromuscular abnormalities, including brainstem infarction, multiple sclerosis, and pseudobulbar palsy, can cause dysmotility of the cervical esophagus because swallowing function is controlled by the central

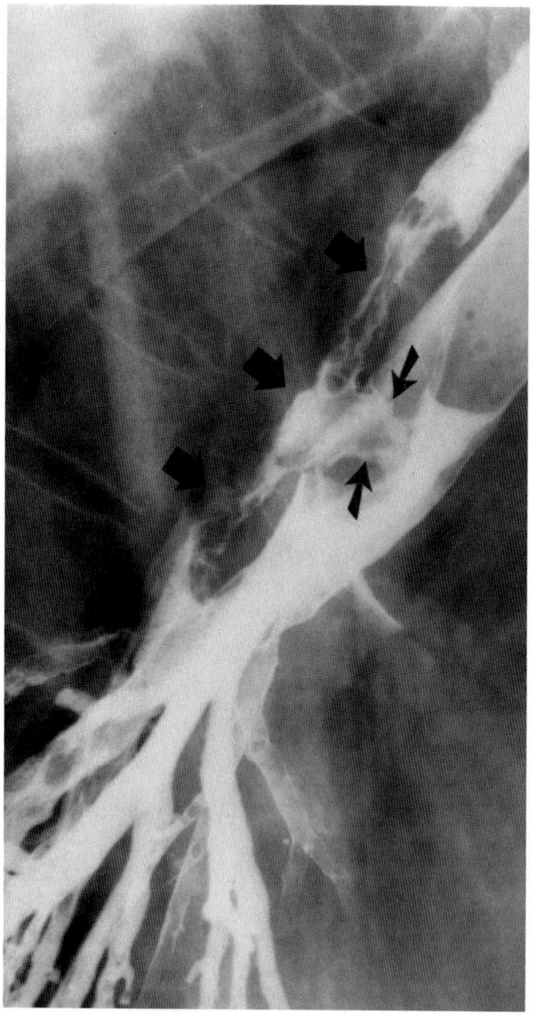

Figure 1-32 Tracheoesophageal fistula in a 59-year-old man with a long, destructive malignant lesion of the midesophagus *(large arrows)* and a wide fistulous communication *(small arrows)* with the trachea.

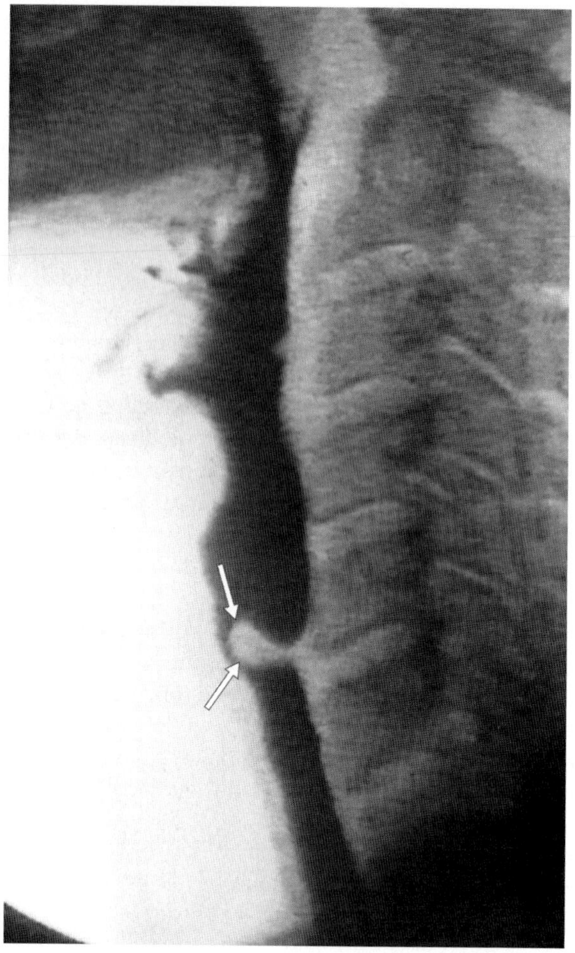

Figure 1-33 Lateral image of the cervical esophagus obtained during fluoroscopic examination shows prominence of the cricopharyngeus muscle *(arrows)*.

nervous system, cranial nerves, and peripheral autonomic nerves. Myasthenia gravis, a disorder involving the neuromuscular junction, also can affect cervical esophageal motility.

Incomplete Cricopharyngeal Relaxation

The cricopharyngeal muscle, as the lower portion of the inferior constrictor muscle, forms the posterior wall of the pharyngoesophageal junction. During swallowing, the cricopharyngeus muscle normally relaxes to allow the food bolus to pass from the pharynx into the esophagus. If this muscle remains contracted during swallowing, it causes a smooth, rounded impression at the level of the C5-C6 disk space that may persist for a variable length of time (Fig. 1-33). This is an important cause of dysphagia and may lead to the formation of a Zenker's diverticulum by creating increased intraluminal pressure in the hypopharynx. Incomplete cricopharyngeal relaxation may develop as a protective mechanism in patients with gastroesophageal reflux to prevent aspiration of gastric contents. Prominence of the cricopharyngeal muscle also can be seen after laryngectomy.

Thoracic Esophagus

Scleroderma is a systemic disorder of connective tissue in which smooth muscle is replaced by fibrous tissue. In the esophagus, the proximal third that is composed of striated muscle is unaffected, whereas the distal two thirds, composed of smooth muscle, displays abnormal motility. Typically the esophagus appears dilated, and the gastroesophageal junction is widely patent. Gastroesophageal reflux is common and may be marked. Because of the long-standing reflux and the delayed clearance of refluxed material by the flaccid esophagus, reflux esophagitis usually develops. This reflux esophagitis may be severe, with resultant stricture

Box 1-7 Two Faces of Achalasia

Idiopathic achalasia—a neuromuscular abnormality of the lower esophageal sphincter of unknown cause
Secondary achalasia—a neuromuscular abnormality of the lower esophageal sphincter caused by subtle malignant infiltration of the region of the gastroesophageal junction; can be easily confused with idiopathic type

formation or development of Barrett's esophagus. Mixed connective tissue diseases that often include scleroderma also may show these findings.

Achalasia (Box 1-7) is a disease of the myenteric plexus of the esophagus of unknown origin (although an autoimmune process is suspected), in which peristalsis is diffusely decreased or absent, and the lower esophageal sphincter fails to relax. The esophagus is often dilated and may appear on frontal chest films as an air-filled or fluid-filled tubular structure in the medial right hemithorax (with an air-fluid level present on upright films). Contrast studies show dilution of barium by retained fluid in the esophagus. Peristaltic contractions appear disordered in the early stage of the disease and diminished or absent in later stages. The distal esophagus shows smooth, tapered narrowing caused by the contracted lower esophageal sphincter (Fig. 1-34). In the upright position, gravity may partially overcome the decreased peristalsis and the tightened sphincter to allow intermittent passage of small amounts of contrast material into the stomach. In the horizontal position, little, if any, contrast material passes into the stomach.

Primary or idiopathic achalasia usually has its onset in early adulthood and results in dysphagia, regurgitation, and other complications of esophageal stasis, including bad breath, aspiration pneumonia, and esophageal candidiasis (Fig. 1-35). In cases of long-standing achalasia, there is an increased incidence of squamous cell carcinoma of the esophagus, probably secondary to chronic mucosal irritation by retained food (Fig. 1-36). Diagnosis of superimposed carcinoma in achalasia is rarely made before the tumor has become large and invasive. Early radiological detection is limited by the patient's underlying chronic dysphagia, the markedly dilated esophageal lumen, and the presence of food and debris within the esophagus.

Secondary achalasia simulates primary achalasia, but results from malignancy and usually has an abrupt onset later in life (Fig. 1-37). The decreased peristalsis and smooth tapering of the distal esophagus in secondary achalasia typically result from tumor infiltrating the myenteric plexus of the distal esophagus. This infiltration can occur in invasive gastric carcinoma, lymphoma, and metastatic

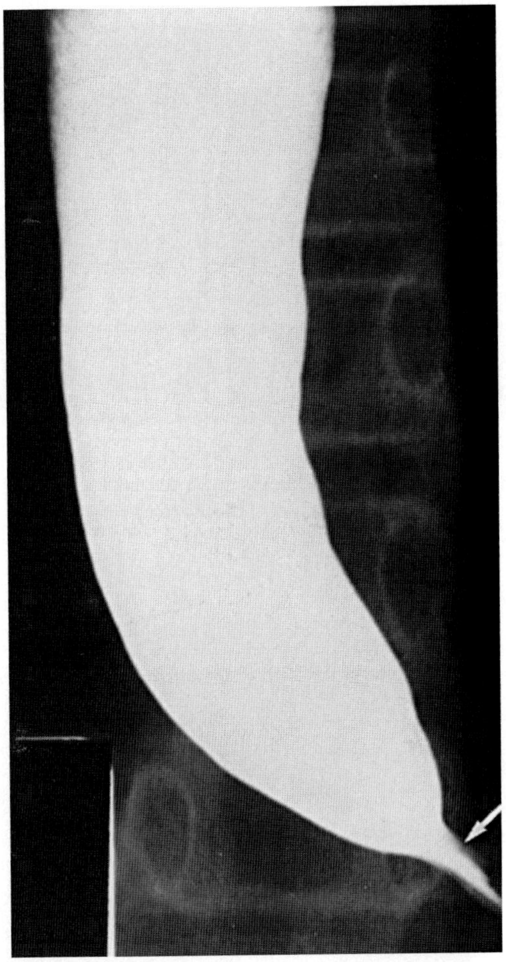

Figure 1-34 Esophageal dilatation with smooth distal tapering at the gastroesophageal junction *(arrow)* represents achalasia.

disease involving the gastroesophageal junction. Other suggested pathogenetic mechanisms in secondary achalasia include paraneoplastic syndrome and central nervous system lesions affecting the vagal nerve nuclei.

Chagas' disease, an infectious disease seen in Brazil and other tropical areas, also mimics idiopathic achalasia. Chagas' disease is caused by *Trypanosoma cruzi,* a protozoan transmitted to humans by the reduviid bug, and affects the esophagus, duodenum, colon, and heart.

Diffuse esophageal spasm and related disorders (e.g., presbyesophagus and corkscrew esophagus) cause a spectrum of esophageal dysmotility. Disordered peristalsis is often reflected by the presence of tertiary waves (Fig. 1-38). These nonpropulsive, sometimes bizarre-appearing contractions may be associated with significant dysphagia.

Abnormal esophageal motility is one of the earliest findings in reflux esophagitis and in other inflammatory causes of esophagitis, such as radiation and caustic ingestion. Systemic diseases that may cause esophageal dysmotility include myxedema, thyrotoxicosis, amyloidosis, and

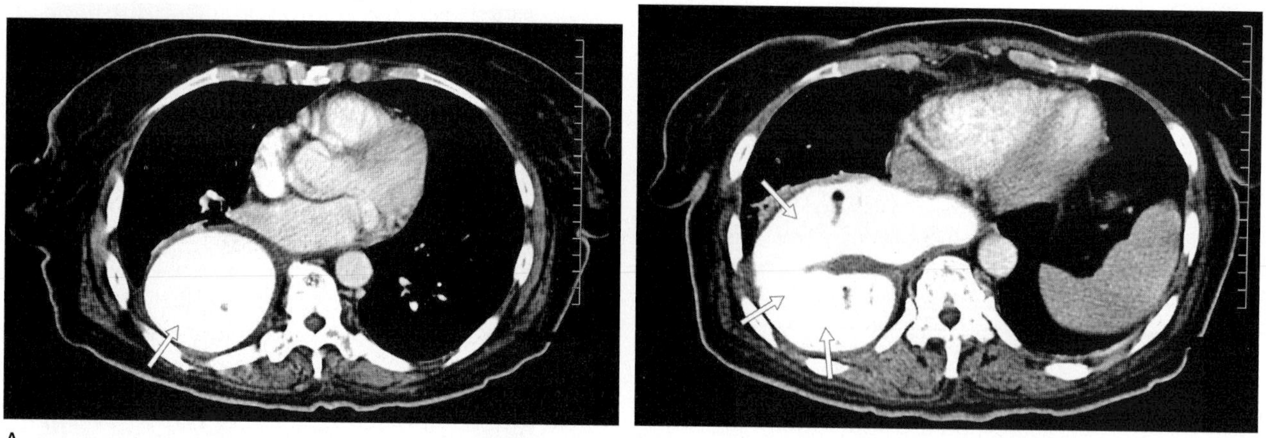

A B

Figure 1-35 **A,** A markedly dilated thoracic esophagus *(arrow)* in a patient with long-standing primary achalasia. **B,** In the lower esophagus, the "sigmoid" configuration *(arrows)* of long-standing achalasia can be seen.

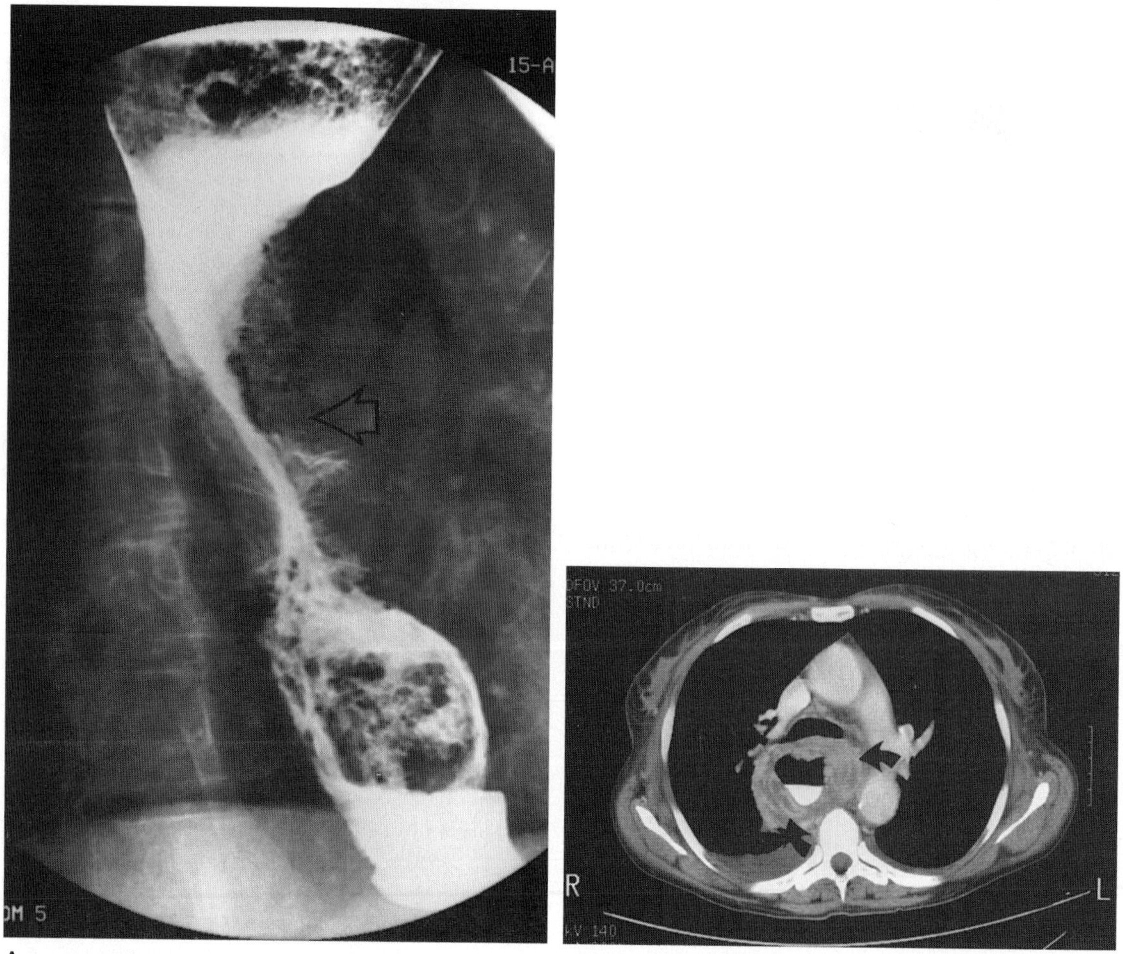

A B

Figure 1-36 Achalasia with complicating carcinoma. **A,** Esophagram of patient with long-standing achalasia showing dilated atonic esophagus with midesophageal irregular stricture. **B,** CT of the same patient shows thickened infiltrated esophageal wall *(curved arrows)* at the level of the carina. Note air-fluid level in the esophagus.

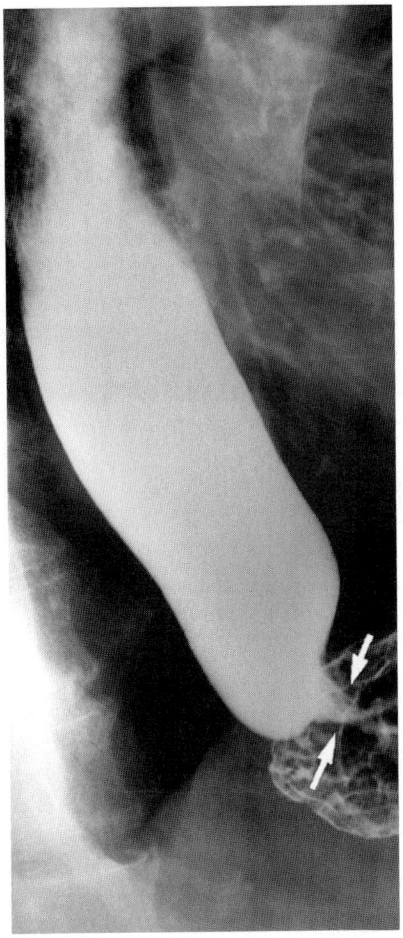

Figure 1-37 Secondary achalasia. A 70-year-old man with recent history of dysphagia and weight loss. Esophagram shows tapered narrowing of distal esophagus *(arrows)*. The "beak" lacks a pointed tip and has some mild irregularity that, along with the history, makes it suspicious. A biopsy specimen showed infiltrating carcinoma.

diabetes mellitus. Drugs, particularly atropine and other anticholinergics, can also cause esophageal dysmotility.

NARROWED ESOPHAGUS

Narrowing of the esophagus may result from intrinsic or extrinsic causes. Narrowing can be characterized further as focal or diffuse, mild or severe, and smooth or irregular.

Neoplasms

Esophageal neoplasms, especially squamous cell carcinoma, are common causes of focal esophageal narrowing. The most typical appearance of esophageal squamous cell carcinoma on contrast studies is an abrupt, irregular narrowing by an annular mass (Fig. 1-39). CT is used to evaluate the primary lesion and to determine depth of invasion and presence of regional adenopathy and distant metastases (Figs. 1-40 to 1-42). Contiguous extension of tumor may involve the tracheobronchial tree, aorta, pleura, or pericardium and is shown by infiltration of paraesophageal fat planes. This extension may be overestimated, however, in the absence of fat planes secondary to cachexia or fibrosis. Lymphatic extension of tumors, although usually present when adjacent lymph nodes appear enlarged, may be underestimated (if malignant nodes do not appear enlarged) or, less commonly, overestimated (if nodes are enlarged because of benign disease).

The role of MRI has been limited in the evaluation of esophageal carcinoma because of motion artifact, but is beginning to play a more important role with the development of cardiorespiratory gating techniques.

Esophageal adenocarcinoma arising in Barrett's epithelium can cause irregular luminal narrowing similar to that seen in squamous cell carcinoma (Fig. 1-43).

Metastatic disease to the esophagus occurs through contiguous or hematogenous spread of tumor. Direct invasion can involve the cervical esophagus (laryngeal carcinoma and thyroid carcinoma), midesophagus

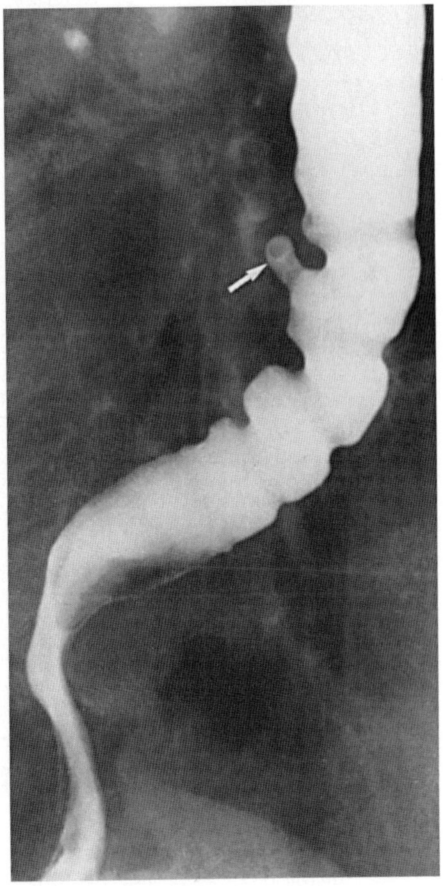

Figure 1-38 Tertiary contractions and a pulsion diverticulum *(arrow)* in the distal esophagus.

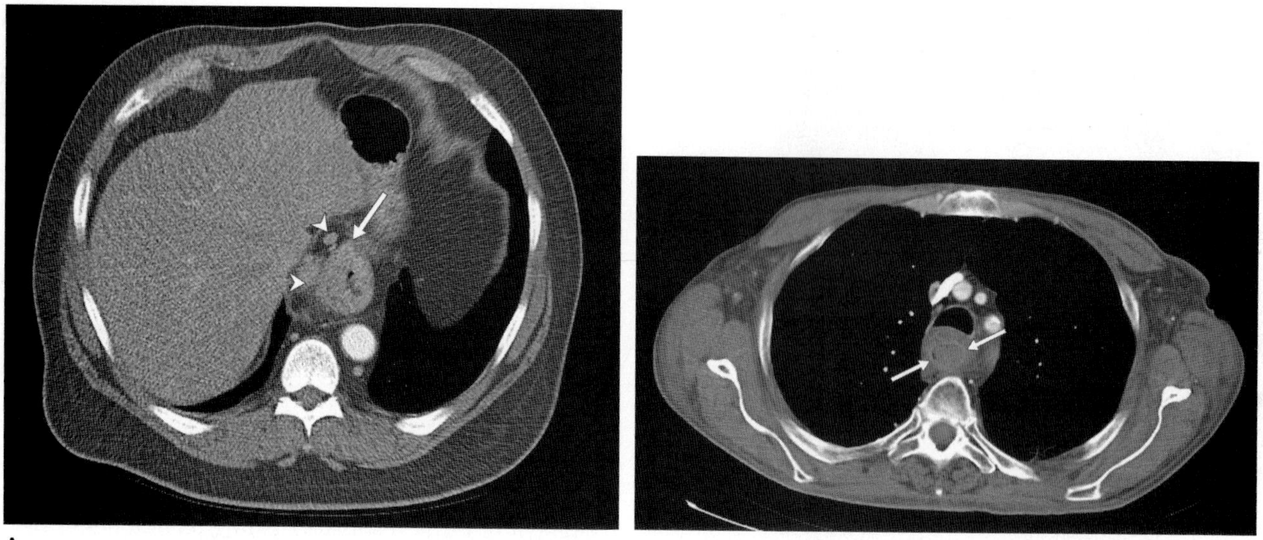

A B

Figure 1-39 **A,** Irregular narrowing in the upper thoracic esophagus represents squamous cell carcinoma. **B,** CT shows marked circumferential wall thickening *(arrows)* as a result of tumor infiltration.

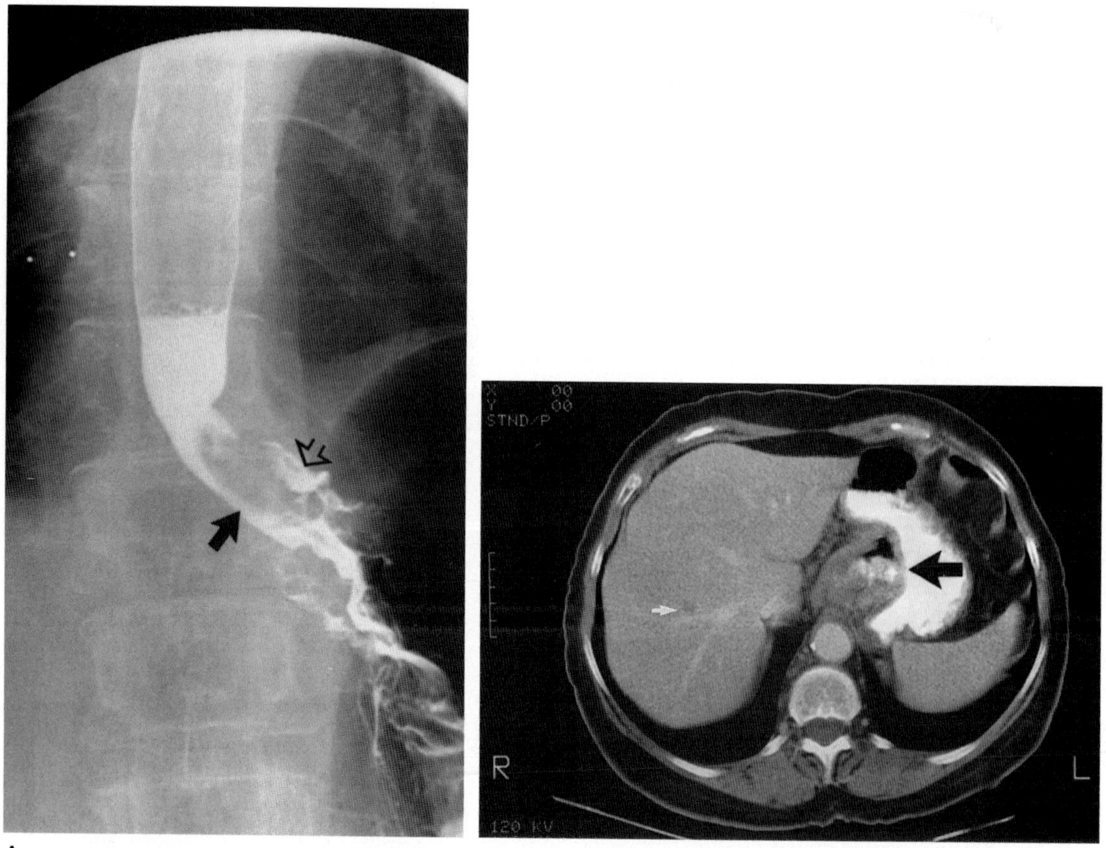

A B

Figure 1-40 A 22-year-old with dysphagia. **A,** Esophagram shows an ulcerated malignant lesion of the distal esophagus involving the gastroesophageal junction. The *solid arrow* indicates the lesion, and the *open arrow* identifies the large ulceration. **B,** CT shows mass with a large ulceration *(arrow)* in the distal esophagus.

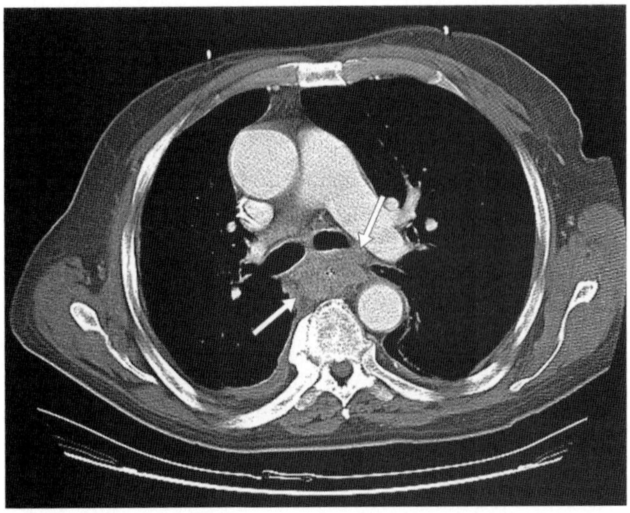

Figure 1-41 Patient with midesophageal carcinoma *(arrows)* with spread to the mediastinum. Note the hazy density in the mediastinum and the poor definition of the outer margins of the thickened esophagus.

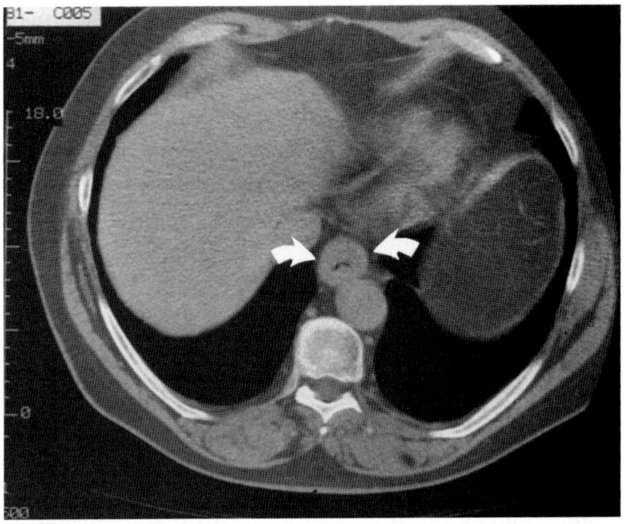

Figure 1-42 Carcinoma of the distal esophagus. Note subtle computed tomographic appearance of lesion. Findings consist of wall thickening *(arrows)* and luminal narrowing.

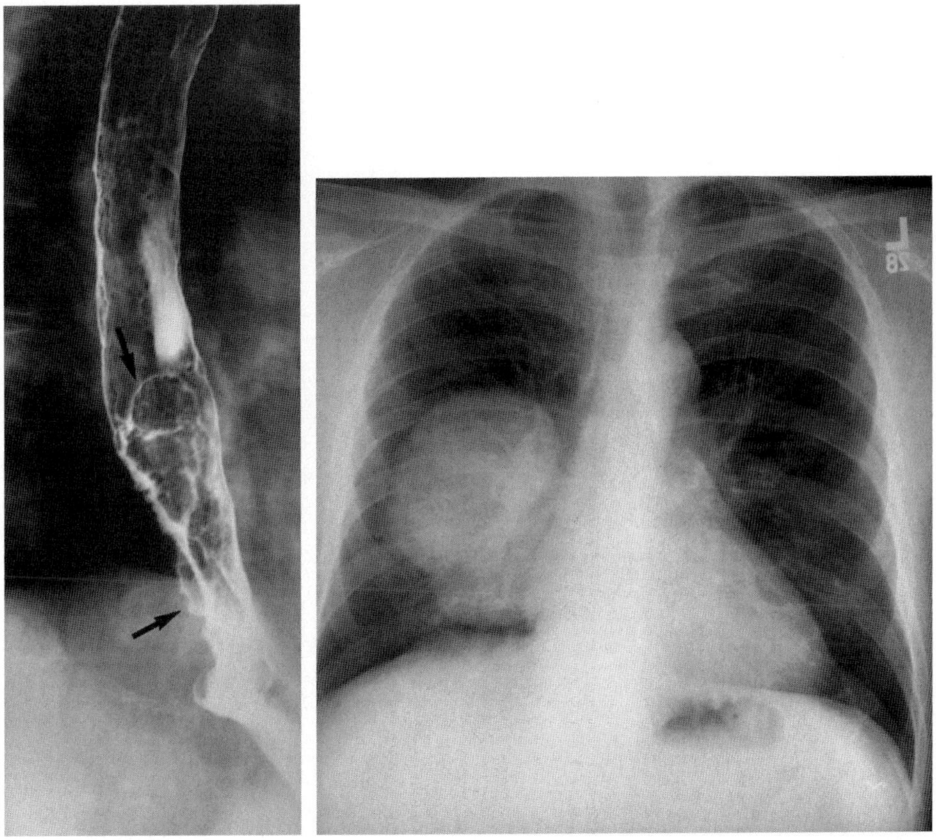

A B

Figure 1-43 Barrett's metaplasia complicated by adenocarcinoma. **A,** A 60-year-old patient with known scleroderma presents with dysphagia, weight loss, and fatigue. Esophagram shows ulcerated mass lesion *(arrows)* of distal esophagus. Biopsy confirmed malignant lesion and evidence of Barrett's metaplasia. **B,** Admission chest film shows large pulmonary metastatic lesion.

(lung carcinoma and mediastinal adenopathy), or distal esophagus (superior extension of gastric carcinoma). Radiographic findings include esophageal obstruction, displacement, narrowing, ulceration, and fistula formation. Hematogenous metastasis to the esophagus (breast carcinoma and malignant melanoma) is less common than contiguous spread, but may also produce a variety of radiographic findings, including focal narrowing and submucosal masses.

Lymphoma (Fig. 1-44) affects the esophagus in less than 1% of cases and is more often a result of extrinsic compression by mediastinal adenopathy than of intrinsic esophageal involvement. Esophageal lymphoma has many different radiographic appearances and may simulate achalasia, varices, contiguous extension of gastric carcinoma, and hematogenous metastases (Fig. 1-45). It also may cause luminal narrowing or a polypoid mass, either of which may be associated with ulceration. Leiomyomas or other benign esophageal neoplasms, when of sufficient size, can cause smooth compression and narrowing of the esophageal lumen.

Infection

Another intrinsic cause of esophageal narrowing is inflammatory stricture formation (Fig. 1-46). Infectious

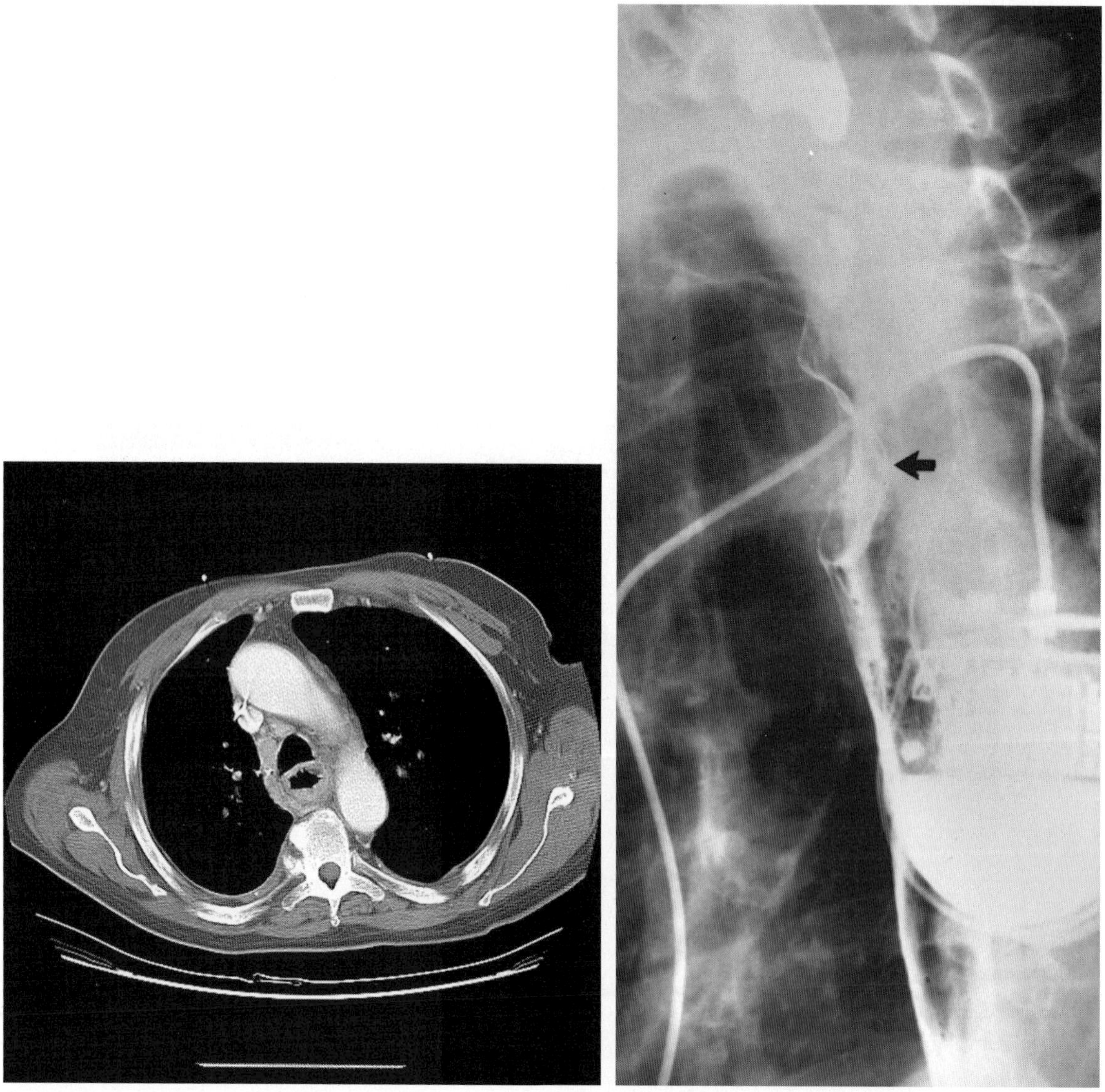

A B

Figure 1-44 **A,** Lymphoma of midesophagus with extraesophageal spread of disease. **B,** It could be a mucosal or submucosal lesion *(arrow)*.

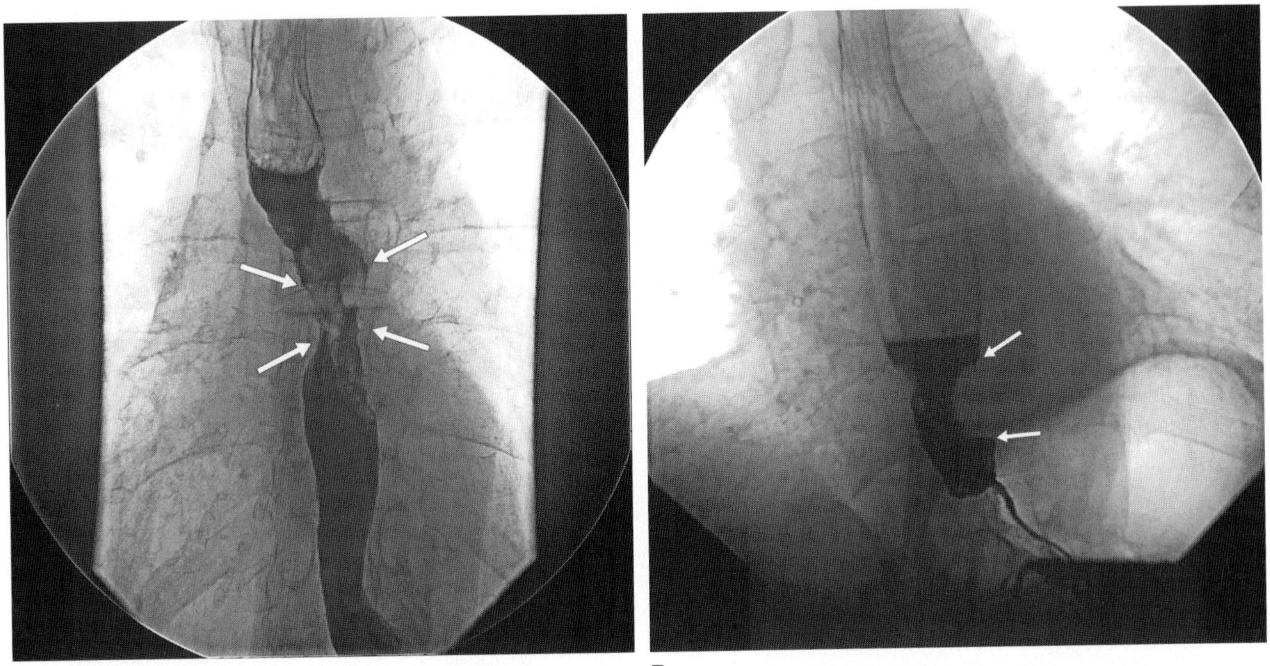

A B

Figure 1-45 Metastatic lesion to lower esophagus in a patient with widespread colonic carcinoma. **A,** CT shows irregular wall thickening *(arrow)* and some adjacent satellite lesions *(arrowheads)*. **B,** Barium esophagram shows irregular polypoid lesion in distal esophagus *(arrows)*.

causes of stricturing include tuberculosis, candidiasis, and, rarely, syphilis.

Inflammation (Noninfectious)

Noninfectious inflammatory strictures may result from gastroesophageal reflux (and disorders associated with reflux), Barrett's esophagus, corrosive ingestion, and radiation (Figs. 1-47 to 1-51). Less common causes include Crohn's disease, benign mucous membrane pemphigoid, epidermolysis bullosa (Fig. 1-52), eosinophilic esophagitis, graft-versus-host disease, and prior sclerotherapy for varices.

Motility Abnormalities, Hematoma, and Extrinsic Compression

Motility abnormalities may focally narrow the esophagus by causing tertiary contractions (diffuse esophageal spasm) or incomplete relaxation of the distal esophageal sphincter (achalasia). Traumatic intramural hematoma of the distal esophagus also can cause focal narrowing. Extrinsic compression by adjacent benign or malignant processes typically causes smooth, eccentric narrowing.

DILATED ESOPHAGUS

Esophageal Distention, Mechanical Obstruction

Dilatation of the esophagus most often occurs proximal to a mechanical obstruction, either a neoplasm or an inflammatory stricture. Extrinsic compression or intraluminal obstruction (food impaction) also can result in esophageal dilatation proximally.

Esophageal Distention, No Obstruction

In the absence of mechanical obstruction, the esophagus may appear diffusely dilated secondary to motility disorders (achalasia and scleroderma), drugs (anticholinergics), and systemic diseases (myxedema, thyrotoxicosis, amyloidosis, and diabetes mellitus). Saccular dilatations of the esophagus are an uncommon manifestation of scleroderma and other connective tissue diseases. Saccular dilatations of the esophagus appear similar to the saccular dilatation more typically seen in the small bowel and colon in these disorders.

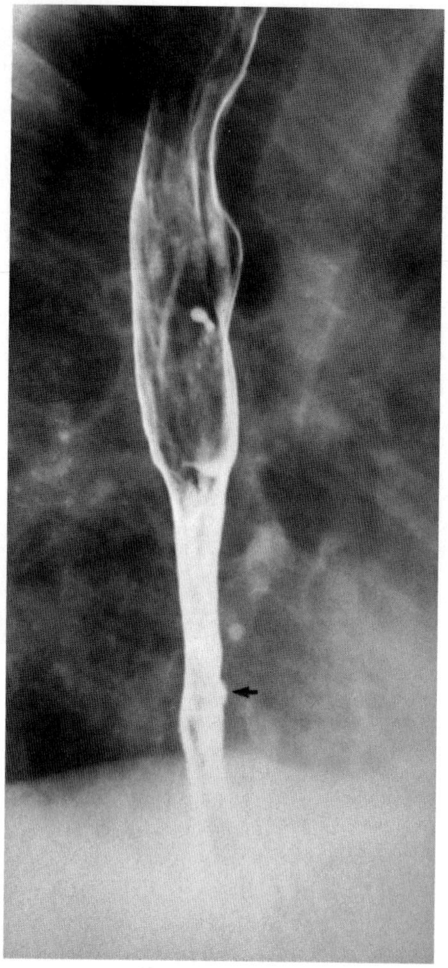

Figure 1-46 Long esophageal stricture. A 47-year-old patient with a long history of chronic reflux esophagitis. Barium esophagram shows a long, benign stricture with ulceration *(arrow)*.

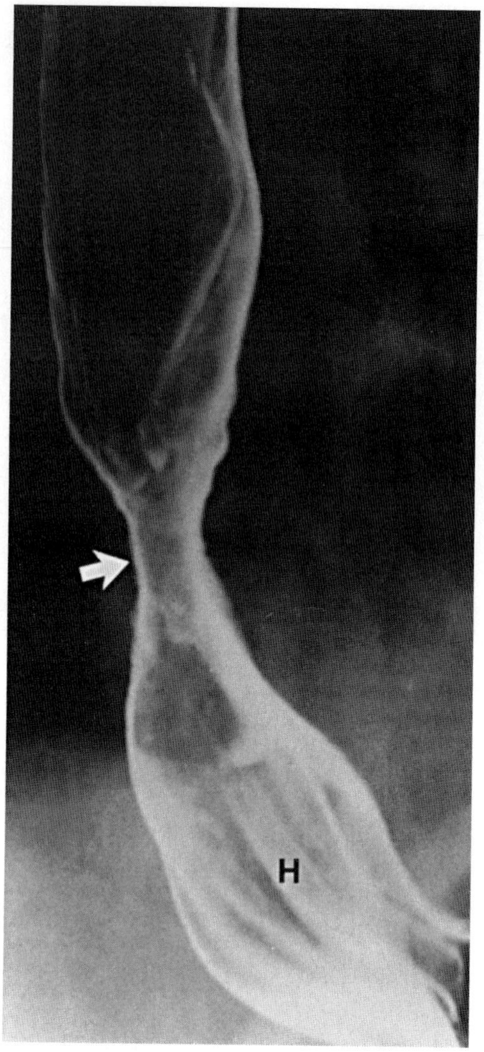

Figure 1-47 Narrowing of the distal esophagus *(arrow)* proximal to an axial hiatal hernia *(H)* represents a reflux stricture.

Esophageal Distention, Focal

Focal dilatation of the esophagus can result from expansion around a bulky, intraluminal neoplasm, such as a mesenchymal sarcoma or spindle cell carcinoma. It can also occur after various operations, including Heller's myotomy (distal esophagus) and resection of esophageal duplication cyst (midesophagus). Retraction of the esophagus secondary to pulmonary scarring typically results in focal esophageal dilatation.

DIVERTICULA

Box 1-8 lists differential diagnostic considerations for diverticula.

Zenker's Diverticula

Zenker's diverticulum is a herniation of mucosa and submucosa through a defect in the posterior aspect of

Box 1-8 Esophageal Diverticulum: Not All Contrast Collections Outside the Lumen Are Ulcers or Perforations

Zenker's diverticulum—motility disorder, possibly associated with chronic GERD
Pulsion diverticulum—motility disorder
Traction diverticulum—related to inflammation in the mediastinum, traditionally tuberculosis
Epiphrenic diverticulum—motility disorder
Pseudodiverticulum—dilated esophageal mucous gland related to chronic inflammation and possible increased risk of cancer

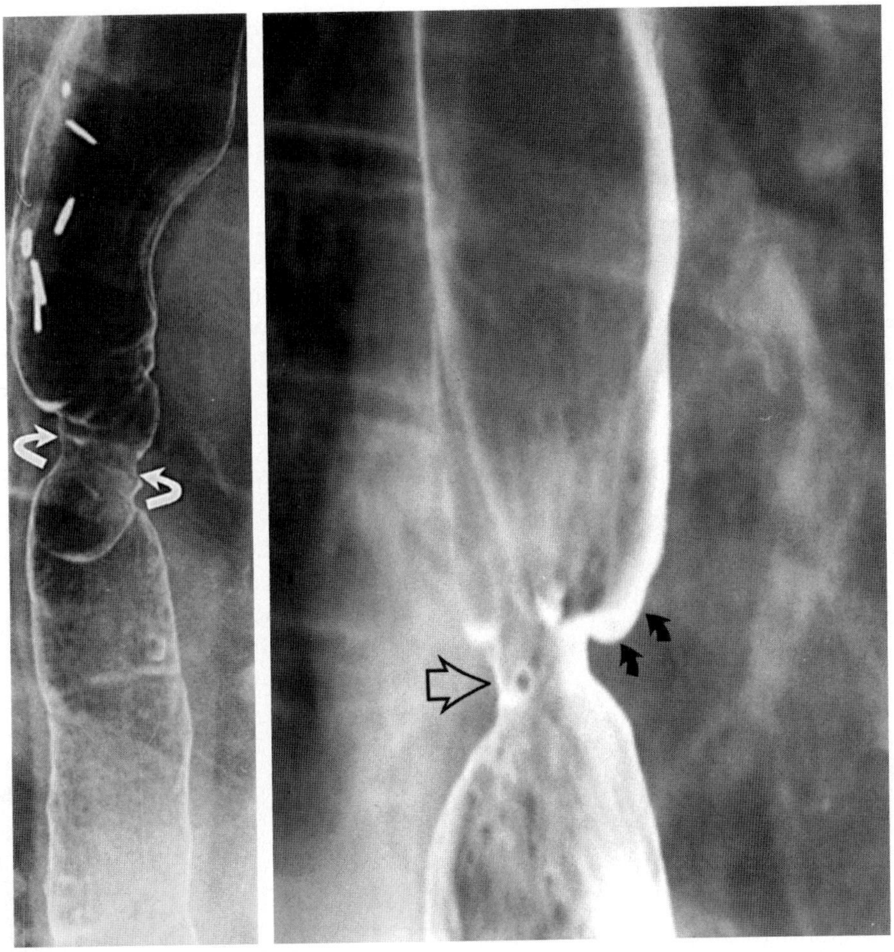

Figure 1-48 Inflammatory strictures. **A,** Short narrowing in the midthoracic esophagus *(arrows)* represents a Barrett's stricture in a patient with long-standing scleroderma. The surgical clips are from a previous sympathectomy. **B,** Patient with chronic benign esophageal stricture *(open arrow)* with "overhanging edge" *(solid arrows)*. This radiological sign, in which a cul-de-sac of the prestrictured esophagus is projected below the level of the stricture, indicates benign and chronic nature of the lesion. It is the reverse of the "shoulder" sign seen in malignant lesions.

the pharyngoesophageal junction. This defect occurs in an area of potential weakness (Killian's dehiscence) in the midline between horizontal and oblique fibers of the inferior constrictor muscle (Fig. 1-53). Zenker's diverticulum most likely results from increased intraluminal pressure in the hypopharynx and may be associated with incomplete relaxation of the cricopharyngeal muscle. When small, Zenker's diverticulum extends directly posteriorly and is best visualized in the lateral projection on contrast examination (Fig. 1-54). With continued increased pressure, the diverticulum may enlarge and extend laterally. Complications associated with Zenker's diverticulum include dysphagia, bad breath, and aspiration pneumonia, and iatrogenic perforation of the diverticulum at endoscopy is a recognized danger. Less commonly, diverticula can arise from the lateral aspects of the pharyngoesophageal junction.

Midesophageal Diverticula

Midesophageal diverticula often occur at the anterior aspect of the esophagus at the level of the carina (Fig. 1-55). They may represent traction diverticula resulting from retraction of the esophageal wall by healed granulomatous disease of the mediastinum. More recent studies suggest, however, that most midesophageal diverticula are caused by increased intraluminal pressure and represent pulsion diverticula. On contrast examination, traction diverticula, which contain a muscular wall, typically have an angular contour and can contract, whereas pulsion

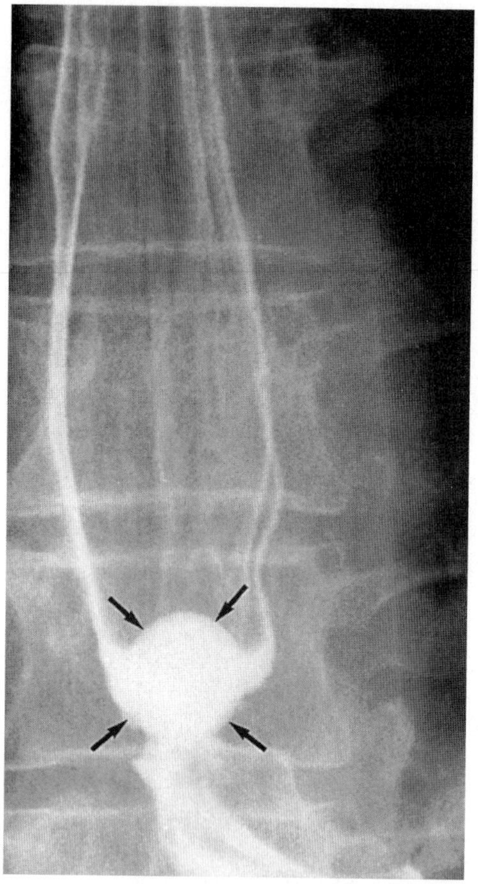

Figure 1-49 A 13-mm barium tablet *(arrows)* lodges above a distal esophageal stricture with the patient in the upright position.

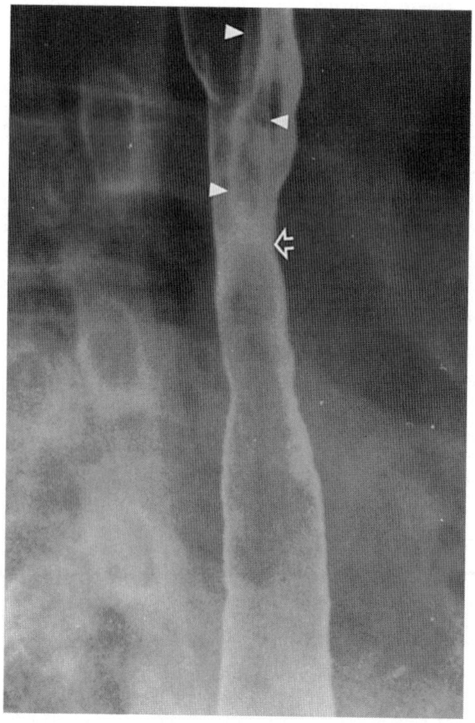

Figure 1-50 Tube esophagram shows a midesophageal lye stricture *(open arrow)*. The tube *(arrowheads)* lies proximal to the stricture.

diverticula, which lack a muscular wall, have a rounded configuration and do not contract.

Epiphrenic Diverticula

Epiphrenic diverticula are located in the distal esophagus near the gastroesophageal junction (Fig. 1-56). These pulsion diverticula result from abnormal intraluminal pressure and may be associated with tertiary contractions of the esophagus. Accidental entry of the endoscope into an epiphrenic diverticulum may lead to perforation.

Intramural Pseudodiverticula

Esophageal intramural pseudodiverticulosis is an unusual condition in which dilated mucous glands in the esophageal wall may simulate true diverticula on contrast studies (Fig. 1-57). The pseudodiverticula are usually flask shaped and of uniform depth. They may be solitary or multiple, and distribution may be segmental

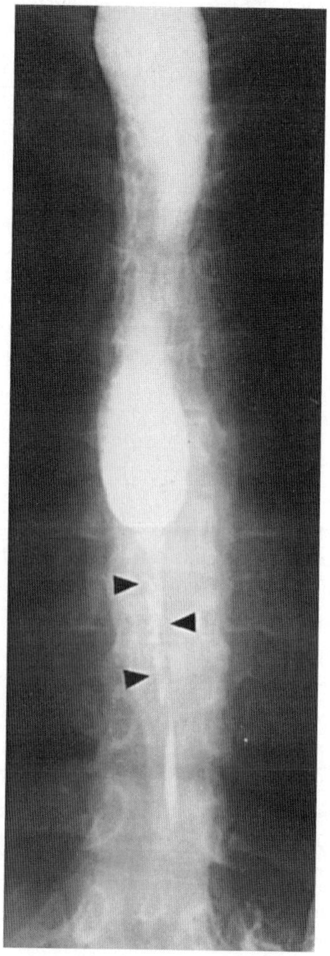

Figure 1-51 Long, irregular narrowing of the distal esophagus *(arrowheads)* resulting from lye ingestion.

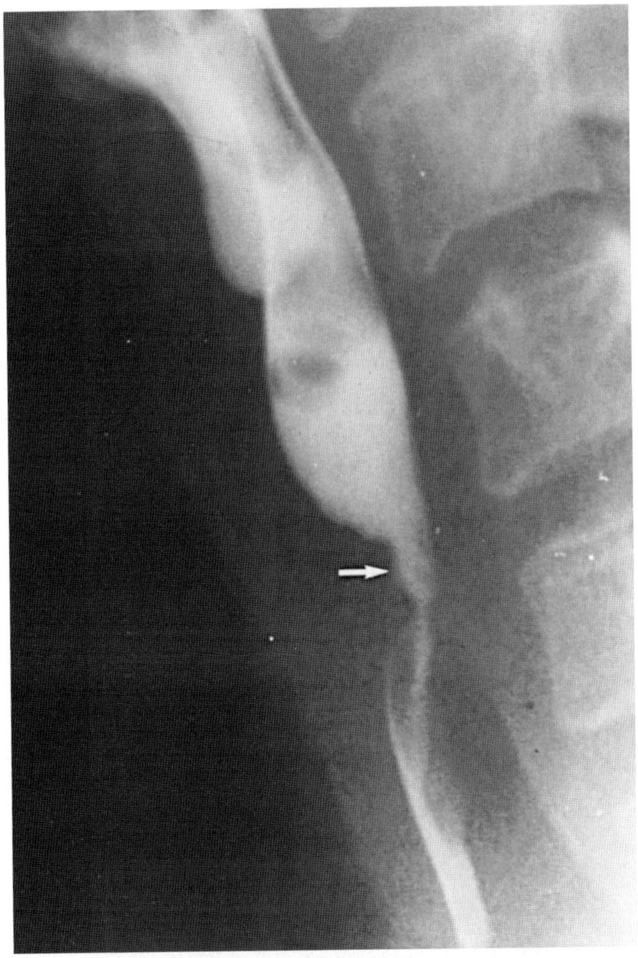

Figure 1-52 Lateral view of the cervical esophagus shows a focal stricture *(arrow)* in a patient with epidermolysis bullosa.

or diffuse. This condition is most often associated with esophageal strictures, although the diverticula may be located proximal or distal to the stricture site. Intramural pseudodiverticulosis usually occurs as a rare sequela of esophagitis. There may be an association between this process and esophageal malignancies.

Intraluminal (Artifactual) Diverticula

Intraluminal esophageal diverticulum represents a transient artifact that results from barium mixing with retained fluid or debris in the esophagus. This artifact appears similar to an intraluminal duodenal diverticulum ("windsock") on contrast examination, but is not associated with an intraluminal membrane.

FOLDS

Normal

Longitudinal folds extend along the entire length of the esophagus and are best shown on collapsed views.

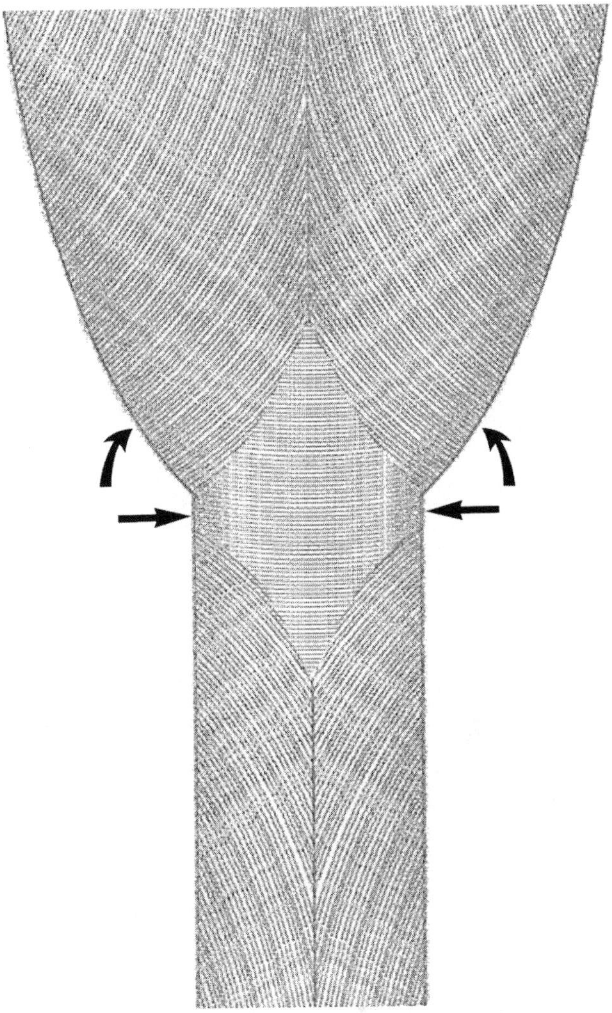

Figure 1-53 Diagram of the posterior wall of the hypopharynx and cervical esophagus illustrates the horizontal fibers *(arrows)* and oblique fibers *(curved arrows)* of the inferior constrictor muscle.

Transverse folds also occur normally, although they are seen less frequently than longitudinal folds. These thin, transient folds represent contraction of the muscularis mucosa of the esophageal wall (Fig. 1-58). This is sometimes referred to as a "feline esophagus" because the transverse folds resemble those seen normally in the esophagus of a cat.

Thickened

Thickening of longitudinal and transverse folds as a result of edema and inflammation has been described as an early finding in reflux esophagitis and may occur in other forms of esophagitis as well. Esophageal varices may appear as thickened folds, but are differentiated by their tortuosity and changeability with position and esophageal distention.

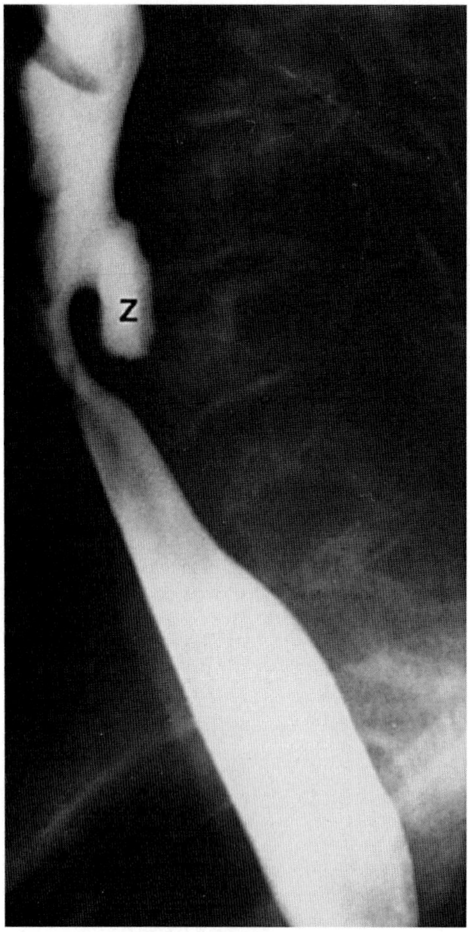

Figure 1-54 Lateral view of the cervical esophagus shows a Zenker's diverticulum *(Z)*.

Varicoid carcinoma is a form of squamous cell esophageal carcinoma in which submucosal spread of tumor causes esophageal folds to appear thickened (Fig. 1-59 on p. 34). Esophageal lymphoma is a rare neoplasm that also may produce thickening of esophageal folds because of submucosal spread of tumor. In contrast to varices, the deformity seen in varicoid carcinoma and esophageal lymphoma is fixed.

WEBS, HERNIAS, AND RINGS

Webs

Webs are incomplete membranes that appear as thin, transverse filling defects on contrast studies (Fig. 1-60). They most often occur at the anterior aspect of the proximal cervical esophagus and are less often circumferential. Webs can occur spontaneously or secondary to scarring from benign mucous membrane pemphigoid and epidermolysis bullosa. They also can develop in graft-versus-host disease, a complication of bone marrow transplantation in which host tissues are attacked by donor lymphocytes. In Plummer-Vinson syndrome, cervical esophageal webs are associated with iron deficiency anemia and dysphagia (Fig. 1-61). Distal esophageal webs may result from reflux esophagitis.

Hernias

A hiatal hernia represents an extension of the stomach into the chest through the esophageal hiatus. In the more common axial or sliding hiatal hernia, the gastroesophageal junction lies more than 2 cm above the diaphragm, and at least three gastric folds can be recognized within the hernia. One of the most common errors in diagnosing a small hiatal hernia is confusing it with

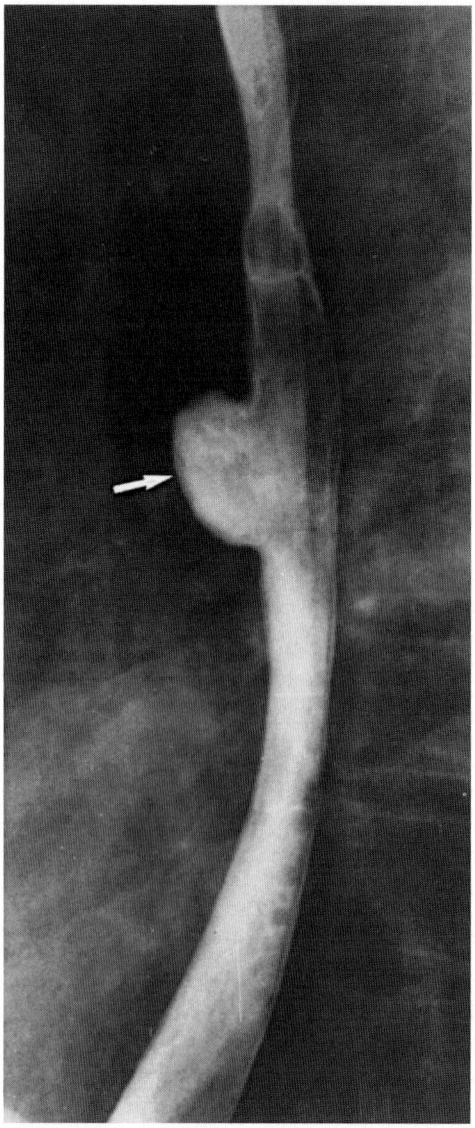

Figure 1-55 Anterior midesophageal diverticulum *(arrow)*.

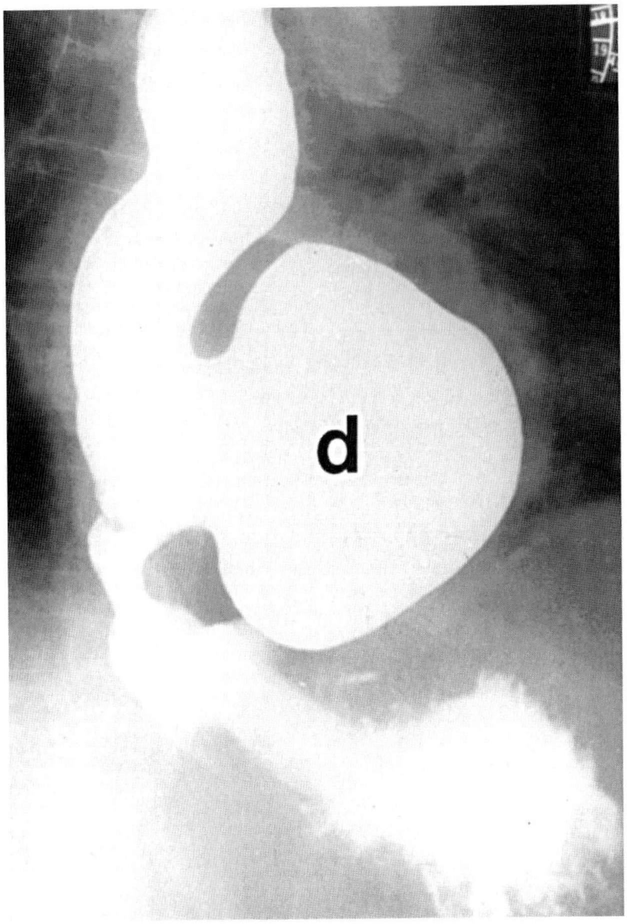

Figure 1-56 Large epiphrenic diverticulum *(d)*.

a prominent vestibular portion of the distal esophagus, in which no gastric fold and no evidence of a B-ring can be seen (Fig. 1-62). Sliding type of hiatal hernia is frequently associated with gastroesophageal reflux.

Although hiatal hernias usually involve only the proximal portion of the stomach, the entire stomach may herniate into the chest, resulting in an intrathoracic stomach (Fig. 1-63). The stomach assumes an inverted position in the chest, with the greater curvature located superiorly and the lesser curvature inferiorly. Subsequently, the proximal portion of the stomach may return through the esophageal hiatus to its normal position below the diaphragm, leaving the distal portion within the chest. These giant intrathoracic hiatal hernias may be asymptomatic in some patients. It is important to convey these findings to the referring physician, however, because the patient is at a much higher risk for obstruction, volvulus (compromise of the gastric blood supply), and perforation.

Paraesophageal hernias account for less than 5% of all hiatal hernias and are not associated with gastroesophageal reflux. In this type of hernia, the gastroesophageal junction is located below the diaphragm, but the gastric fundus partially extends upward through the esophageal hiatus or a diaphragmatic defect to the left of the distal esophagus (Figs. 1-64 and 1-65).

A large hiatal hernia may seemingly show features of the sliding and paraesophageal types. The radiologist should take careful note of the location of the gastroesophageal junction, however. As a sliding-type hernia gets bigger over time, the gastroesophageal junction rotates counterclockwise toward the diaphragm. A carefully performed examination shows that the gastroesophageal junction remains above the diaphragm despite its downward migration.

Rings

Rings represent areas of narrowing in the region of the esophageal vestibule, which is the distal end of the esophagus that normally appears slightly distended (see Fig. 1-62). The muscular ring (A-ring) is a variable, smooth,

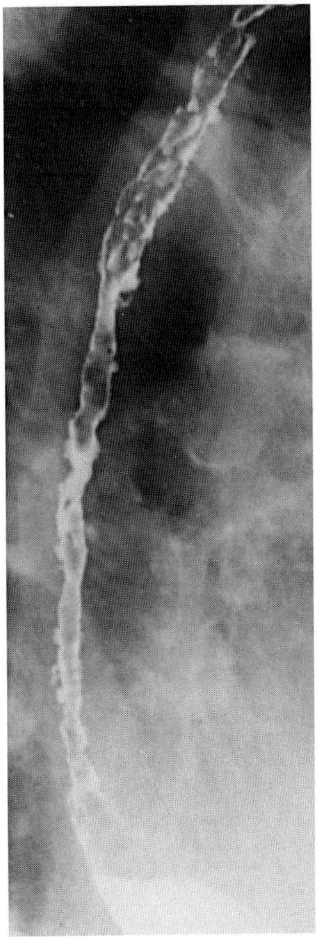

Figure 1-57 Long stricture of the thoracic esophagus with numerous intramural pseudodiverticula.

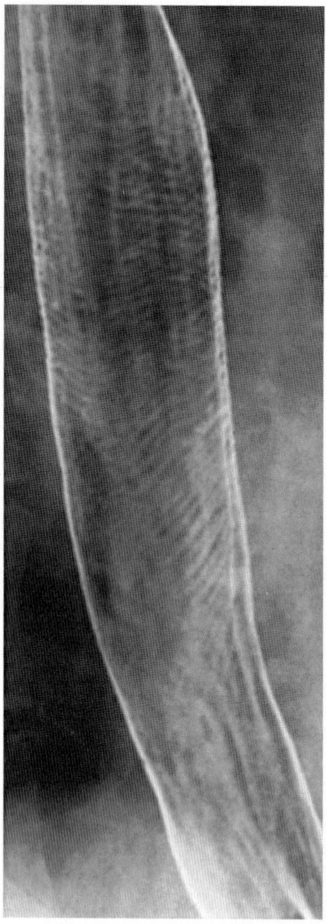

Figure 1-58 Thin transverse folds (feline esophagus).

broad narrowing at the superior aspect of the vestibule. This ring rarely causes dysphagia and most likely results from transient muscle contractions.

The more commonly noted mucosal ring (B-ring) is a persistent, thin, transverse constriction at the inferior aspect of the esophageal vestibule in the region of the gastroesophageal junction. The mucosal ring is smooth and symmetrical and rarely causes dysphagia unless it measures less than 13 mm in diameter (this is a generally accepted number, although exceptions are seen). A narrowed mucosal ring that actually causes dysphagia is known as Schatzki's ring. Mucosal rings are commonly associated with hiatal hernias and are most easily visualized when the esophagogastric junction is distended during contrast examination in the horizontal position (Fig. 1-66). The maximal diameter of the ring can best be determined by having the patient swallow, with water, a 12.5-mm barium tablet while standing. The tablet lodges above Schatzki's ring, but passes through a nonstenotic mucosal ring into the stomach.

Although the mucosal ring occurs at the gastroesophageal junction, it does not correspond to the histological squamocolumnar junction (Z line) (Fig. 1-67). This is true in Barrett's esophagus, in which metaplasia of the distal esophageal epithelium may cause the Z line to be located more proximal to the esophagogastric junction. The Z line is sometimes seen on double-contrast films as a thin, serrated line in the distal esophagus at the gastroesophageal junction. Artificially induced webs, such as caused by Stretta therapy for GERD, also may be seen as ringlike indentations on the mucosa around the gastroesophageal junction.

TRAUMA AND FOREIGN BODIES

Mallory-Weiss Tear

Mallory-Weiss tear represents a mucosal disruption in the distal esophagus, usually resulting from prolonged or severe vomiting. This disruption causes hematemesis and is sometimes identified on double-contrast films as a thin linear collection of barium in the distal esophagus.

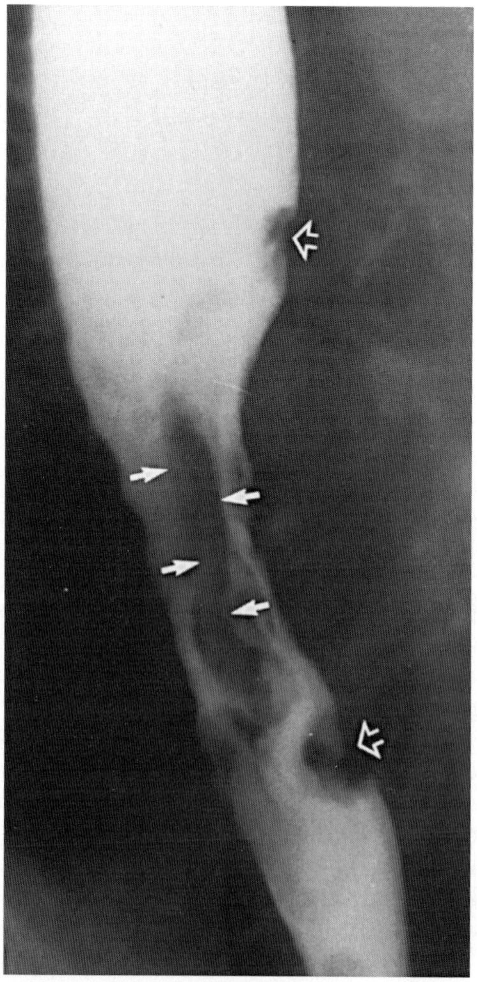

Figure 1-59 Thickened longitudinal fold *(arrows)* and mural masses *(open arrows)* in the distal esophagus represent varicoid carcinoma.

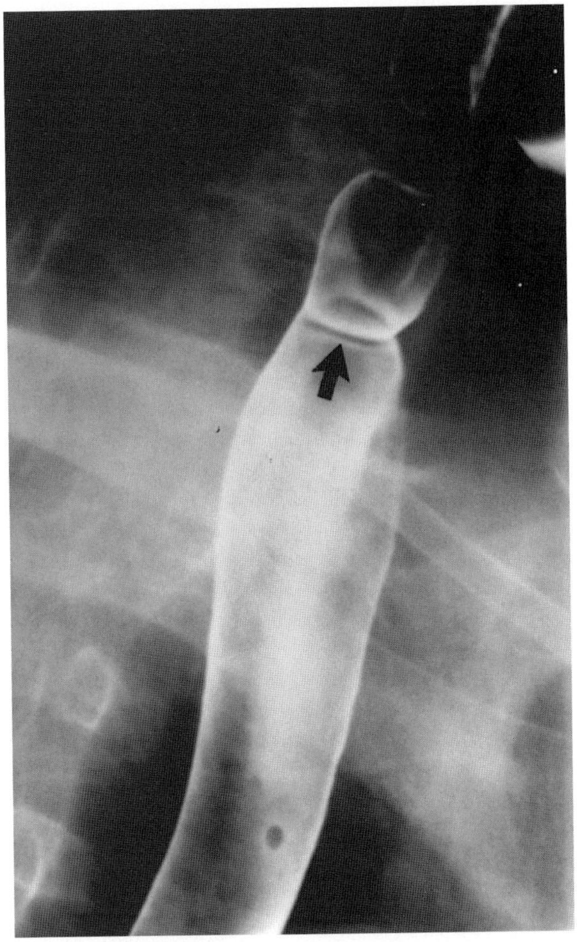

Figure 1-60 Esophageal web. This 40-year-old patient complained of "pills sticking." Esophagram shows circumferential web in proximal esophagus *(arrow)*.

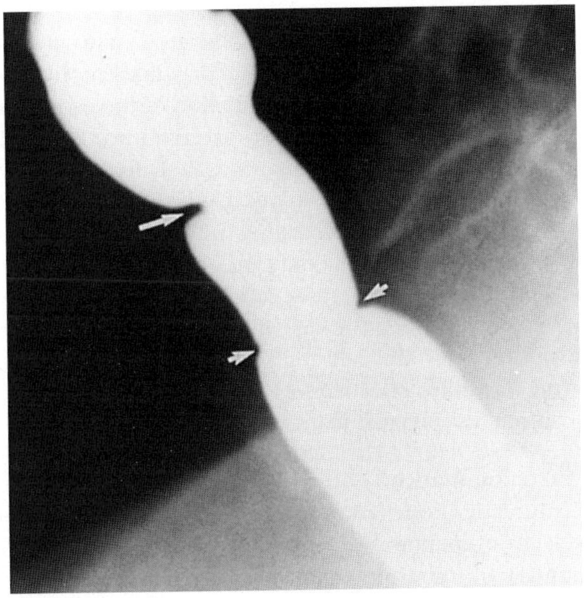

Figure 1-61 Lateral view of the cervical esophagus shows an anterior web *(arrow)* and a circumferential web *(short arrows)* in a patient with dysphagia and microcytic anemia.

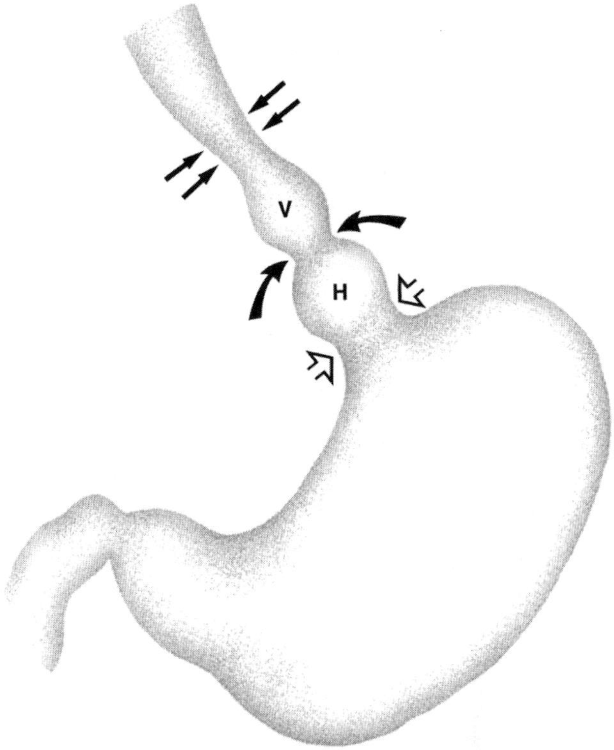

Figure 1-62 Diagram of the distal esophagus and stomach illustrates esophageal vestibule *(V)*, axial hiatal hernia *(H)*, A-ring *(arrows)*, B-ring *(curved arrows)*, and diaphragmatic impressions *(open arrows)*.

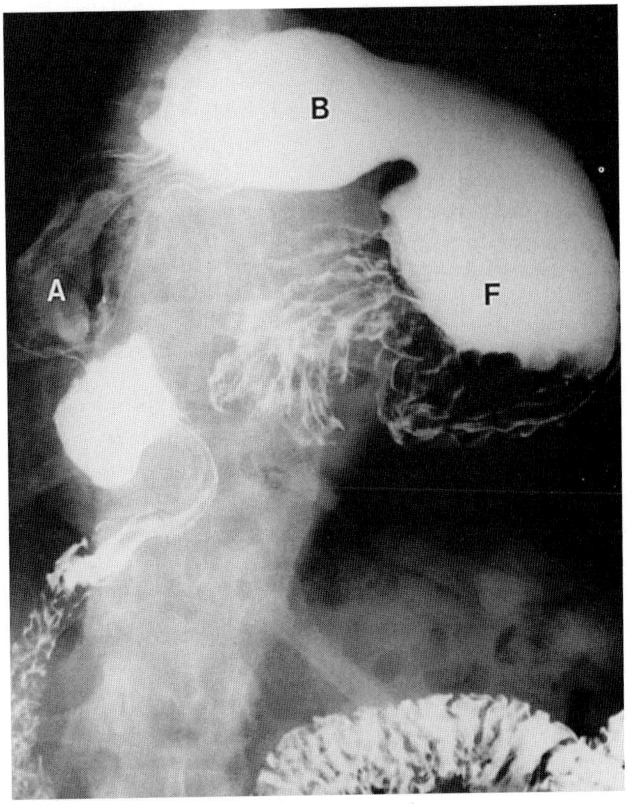

Figure 1-63 Large hiatal hernia contains the fundus *(F)*, body *(B)*, and antrum *(A)* of the stomach.

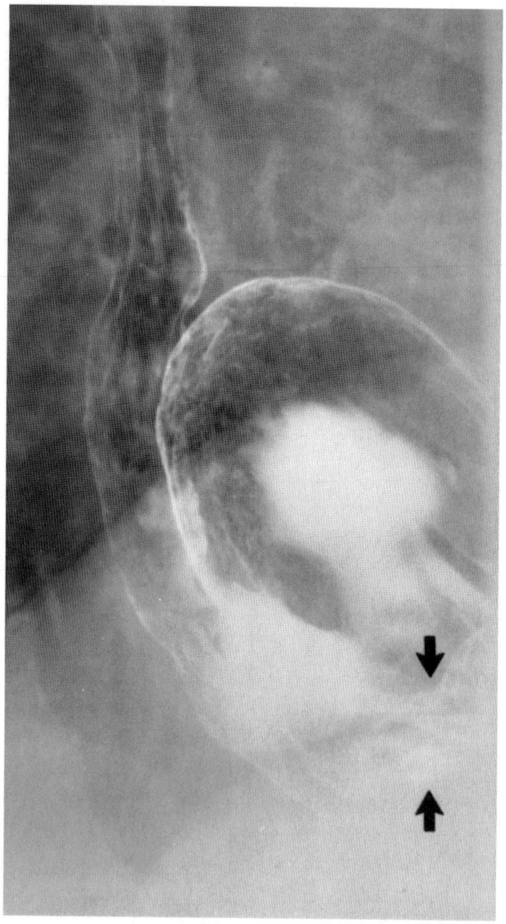

Figure 1-64 Paraesophageal hiatal hernia. The herniated portion of the stomach protruding upward through the diaphragmatic hiatus next to the gastroesophageal junction *(arrows)*.

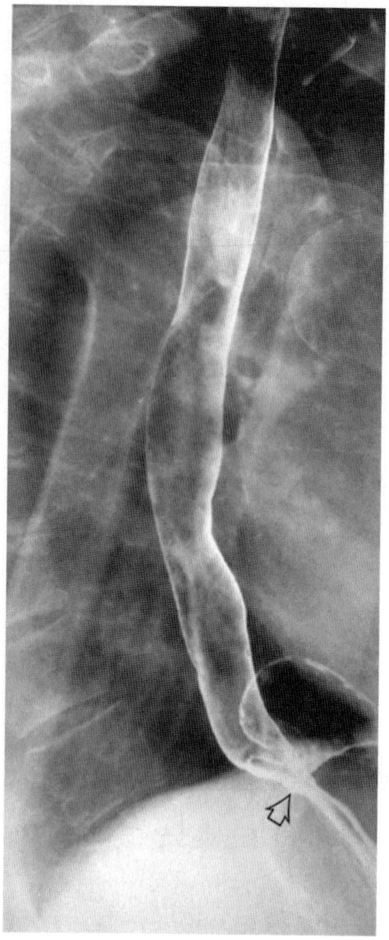

Figure 1-65 Paraesophageal hernia. The herniated segment of the stomach protrudes upward in a diaphragmatic defect near the hiatus.

Mallory-Weiss tear usually heals spontaneously within several days. Contrast studies of the esophagus often are normal. Occasionally one can see intramural air of the esophagus in an asymptomatic patient (Fig. 1-68).

Intramural Hematoma

Esophageal intramural hematoma represents hemorrhage in the submucosal layer of the esophageal wall (see Fig. 1-13B). This hemorrhage usually occurs by extension of a mucosal tear and appears on contrast examination as a smooth submucosal mass.

Perforation

Boerhaave's syndrome

Boerhaave's syndrome also is usually caused by persistent or severe vomiting, but represents transmural perforation of the distal esophagus. This perforation causes mediastinitis and requires immediate surgical repair of the esophageal perforation. Delay in surgical treatment of Boerhaave's syndrome is associated with a high mortality rate. Chest films show mediastinal emphysema, and water-soluble contrast examination of the esophagus shows extravasation of contrast material into the mediastinum (Fig. 1-69). Boerhaave was a Dutch physician called to attend a retired admiral who indulged in the old Roman custom of vomiting up a meal, emptying the stomach so another could be enjoyed immediately. The admiral experienced severe chest pain and died. Boerhaave described the case in the literature, including the contents of the admiral's last meal discovered in his mediastinum. His name has been attached to any transmural esophageal tear ever since.

Instrumentation

Traumatic perforation of the esophagus also may result from penetrating injuries (e.g., knife or bullet wounds) and instrumentation, either surgical (inadvertent laceration during intrathoracic surgery) or nonsurgical (routine endoscopy, dilatation procedures, and stent placements) (Figs. 1-70 and 1-71).

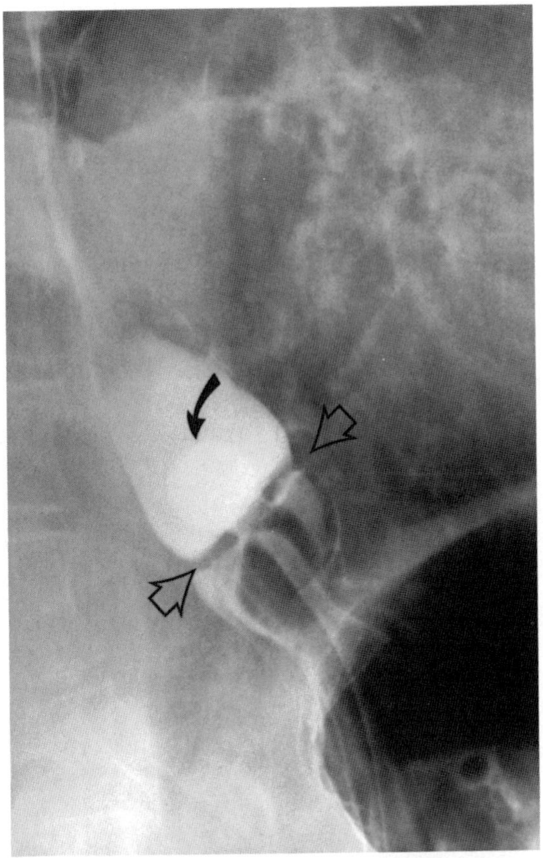

Figure 1-66 Small hiatal hernia with obstructing B-ring (Schatzki ring) *(open arrows)* and luminal narrowing. Note the 12.5-mm barium tablet held up above the obstruction *(curved arrow)*.

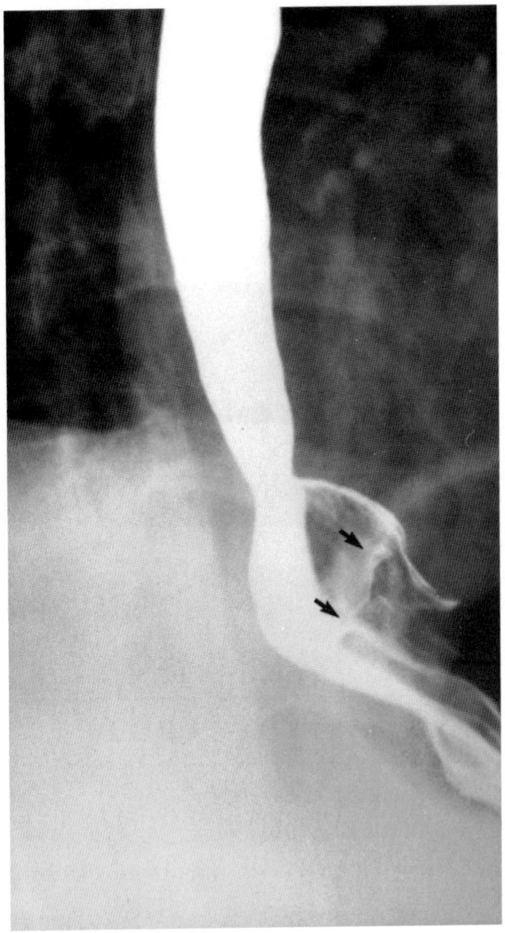

Figure 1-67 Z line. Occasionally a fortuitous finding on a double-contrast esophagram, the Z line *(arrows)* represents the squamocolumnar junction.

Foreign Bodies

Ingested foreign bodies, such as chicken bones or fish bones, may lodge in the cervical or thoracic portions of the esophagus and cause focal irritation or perforation (Fig. 1-72). Taco chips and corn chips have been reported to cause mucosal laceration of the esophagus. Ingestion of sharp metallic objects, such as pins or nails, also may cause laceration or perforation of the esophagus.

Food Impaction

Food impaction (Box 1-9) usually occurs when a poorly chewed piece of meat lodges in the esophagus. Although the underlying esophagus may be normal on very rare occasions, strictures or other causes of esophageal narrowing usually can be implicated in the predisposition to the development of a food impaction, and any case of food impaction should arouse suspicion for underlying pathology. Contrast studies in cases of food impaction usually show a completely or partially obstructing intraluminal mass (Figs. 1-73 and 1-74). Glucagon, anticholinergic medications, and ingestion of effervescent granules have been used with varying success to dislodge impacted food boluses from the esophagus. Ingestion of enzymes or other meat tenderizers is no longer recommended because of complications, including esophageal perforation.

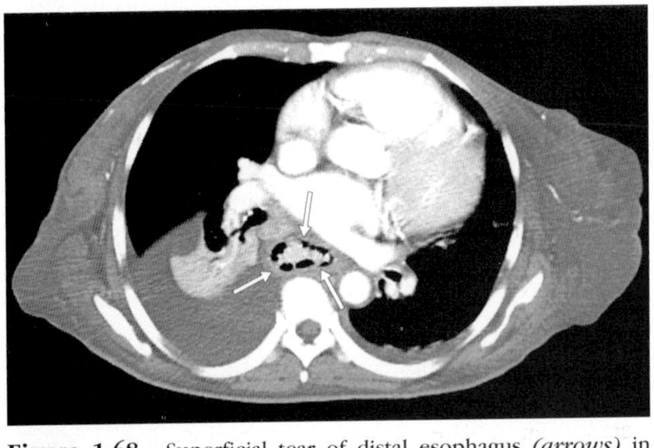

Figure 1-68 Superficial tear of distal esophagus *(arrows)* in a patient with no history of endoscopy or instrumentation or nasogastric tube placement.

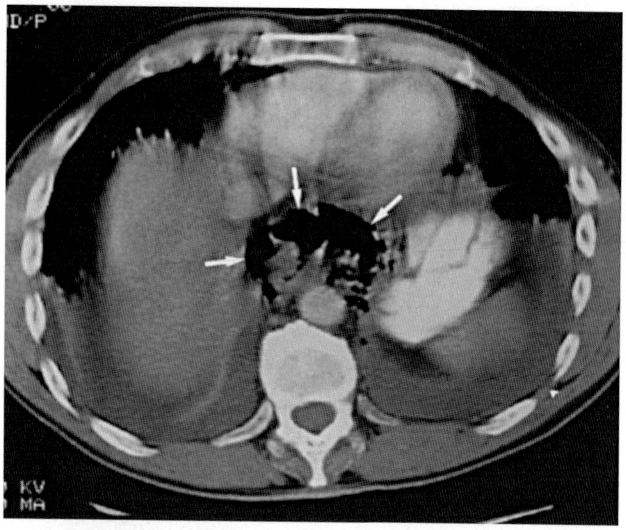

Figure 1-69 CT shows a large amorphous air collection *(arrows)* in the posterior mediastinum in a patient with esophageal rupture.

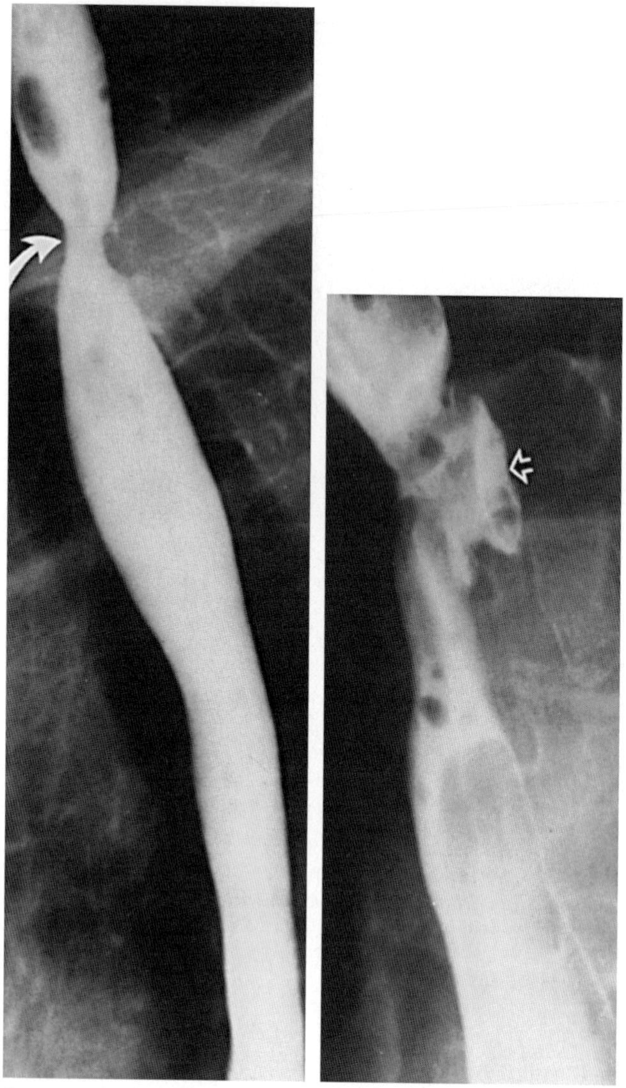

A B

Figure 1-70 **A,** Short stricture *(curved arrow)* after radiation and chemotherapy for squamous cell carcinoma of the lower cervical esophagus. **B,** Focal collection of contrast material *(open arrow)* at the site of previous stricture represents perforation secondary to endoscopic dilatation procedure.

POSTOPERATIVE ESOPHAGUS

Nonsurgical Procedures

A variety of surgical and nonsurgical procedures have been developed for the treatment of esophageal diseases.

Bougienage and Balloon Dilatation

Bougienage consists of passage of a graded series of dilators into the esophagus to distend a benign stricture. Balloon or pneumatic dilators are much more commonly used and contain a segment that can be placed directly at the site of narrowing and then inflated. In achalasia, pneumatic dilation is used to tear some of the contracted muscle fibers of the lower esophageal sphincter, similar to, but not as invasive as, the effect of a surgical myotomy. The most important complication of these procedures is esophageal perforation.

Stent Placement

Endoscopically guided stent placement is often used to maintain patency of the esophagus in patients with esophageal carcinoma (Fig. 1-75). Obstruction and migration of the tube and esophageal perforation are recognized complications of this palliative procedure.

Laser Therapy

Laser therapy is another endoscopic palliative procedure, in which a laser beam (neodymium: yttrium-aluminum-garnet laser) is used to destroy tumor tissue and widen an obstructed esophageal lumen. This procedure can lead to esophageal perforation or

Box 1-9 Food Impaction: A Sign/ Symptom, Not a Disease

Food impaction occurs in most cases in the distal esophagus at the gastroesophageal junction.
Consider the cause of food impaction. Almost all cases of food impaction have some underlying esophageal abnormality, such as inflammatory strictures or obstructing B-rings. It is rare for esophageal cancer to present with food impaction.

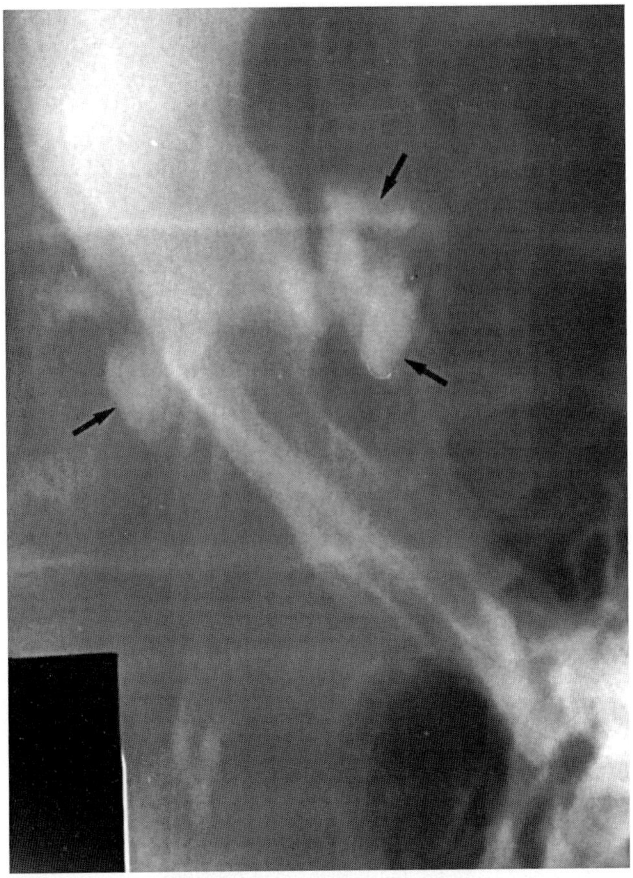

Figure 1-71 Water-soluble contrast examination shows two focal collections of contrast material *(arrows)* adjacent to the distal esophagus. They represent perforations after endoscopic dilatation for achalasia.

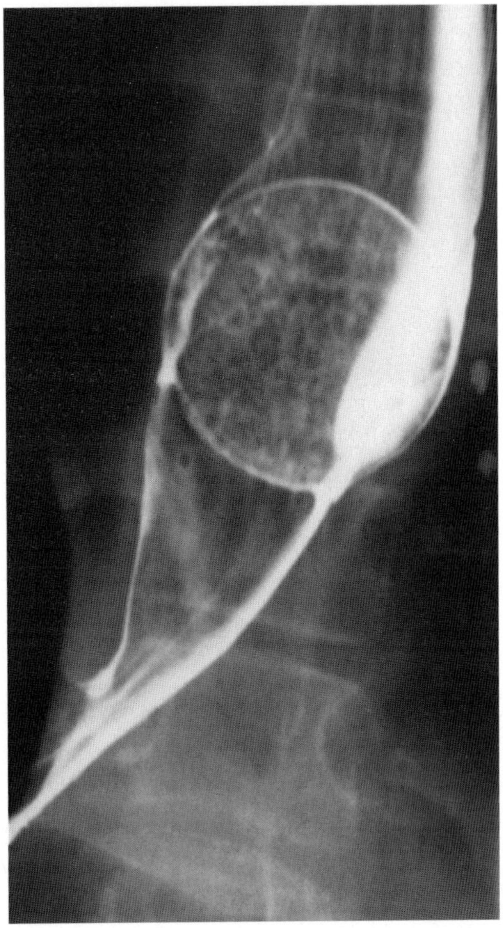

Figure 1-72 Esophageal foreign body. This 19-year-old mentally retarded patient swallowed a Ping-Pong ball that partially occludes the distal esophagus.

esophagorespiratory fistula. More recently, there have been reports of microscopic endoscopic laser mucosal surgery to treat dysplastic foci or early superficial malignancies in patients with Barrett's esophagus. These particular types of superficial laser treatments are rarely associated with perforation.

Sclerotherapy

Sclerotherapy is sometimes used in the treatment of esophageal varices. Sclerosing agents are injected directly into the varices, causing fibrosis and obliteration of the varices. Complications of sclerotherapy include inflammation, ulceration, stricturing, fistula formation, and perforation.

Gastric Balloon

Placement of a balloon into the gastric fundus (Sengstaken-Blakemore tube) is used to control variceal bleeding through a tamponading effect. Incorrect placement of the tube with inflation of the balloon in the distal esophagus may cause esophageal perforation, however.

Surgical Procedures

Myotomy

Surgical esophageal myotomy has been used to treat idiopathic achalasia (Heller's myotomy) and incomplete cricopharyngeal relaxation (cricopharyngeal myotomy). Extensive myotomy of the thoracic esophagus is sometimes performed in severe diffuse esophageal spasm that is unresponsive to other treatments and in idiopathic muscular hypertrophy of the esophagus, a rare condition characterized by diffuse marked thickening of the esophageal musculature. In these procedures, the abnormally contracted or thickened muscle is surgically incised.

Interposition

Various types of surgical interpositions can be performed in conjunction with esophageal carcinoma or extensive stricture formation. Stomach, colon, or jejunum can be used for this purpose. Contrast studies and CT are useful for showing postoperative

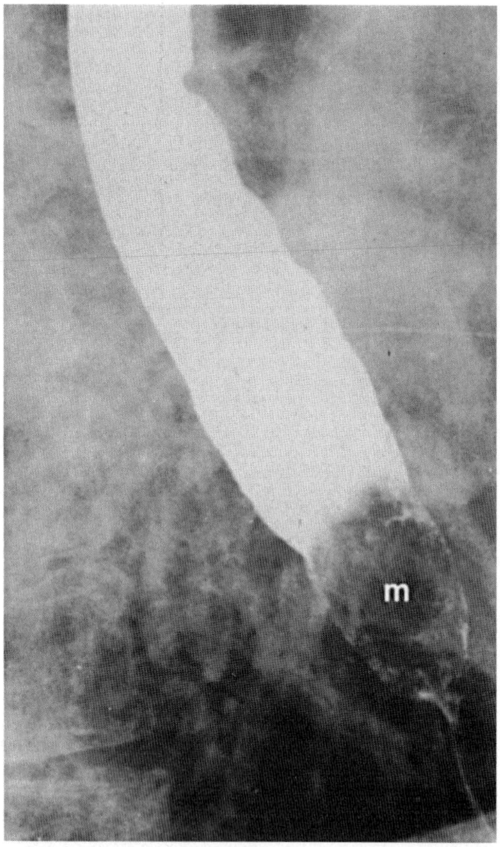

Figure 1-73 Large piece of meat *(m)* in the distal esophagus causes almost complete obstruction.

complications: early (anastomotic leak, perforation, obstruction as a result of edema) and late (anastomotic stricture and recurrent tumor).

Fundoplication

Fundoplication and related surgical procedures can be used to reduce hiatal hernias and prevent associated gastroesophageal reflux. In fundoplication (Nissen, Mark IV [Belsey], and Hill types), a portion of the gastric fundus is wrapped around the distal esophagus (Fig. 1-76). This fundal wrap prevents reflux by compressing the distal esophagus and may appear as a pseudotumor on routine contrast studies and CT. Complications include obstruction if the wrap is too tight and persistent reflux if it is too loose. The Angelchik device, a ringlike structure filled with silicone, can be used in place of a fundal wrap, but is associated with additional complications, including migration of the device into the abdominal or thoracic cavity and erosion into the gastric lumen.

Sugiura Procedure

The Sugiura procedure is a complex surgical procedure used for treating esophageal varices. This extensive operation includes esophageal transection with devascularization of the distal esophagus and proximal stomach. Postoperative contrast studies typically reveal indentation at the distal esophageal suture line.

RADIOLOGICAL EVALUATION OF DYSPHAGIA

Dysphagia (Box 1-10) is a serious symptom and should be evaluated thoroughly. There are few instances in radiology in which history-taking skills are as necessary as in the workup of these patients. The radiologist must be prepared to take time and elicit the history of the dysphagic symptom for two reasons. The first reason is to confirm the dysphagia. Patients commonly complain of a sensation in the throat during or even after swallowing, but they have no difficulty in swallowing solids or liquids. In other instances, coughing episodes, postnasal drip, or heartburn is presented to the radiologist

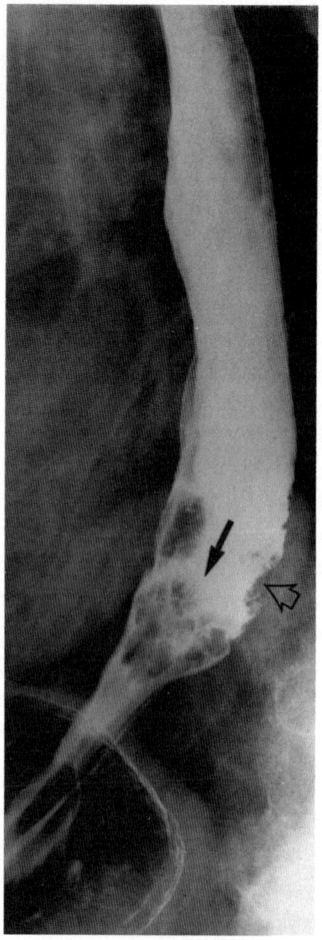

Figure 1-74 Patient with carcinoma of distal esophagus. An esophagram has the appearance of food impaction *(arrow)*, which is actually a tumor. Note destroyed mucosa *(open arrow)*.

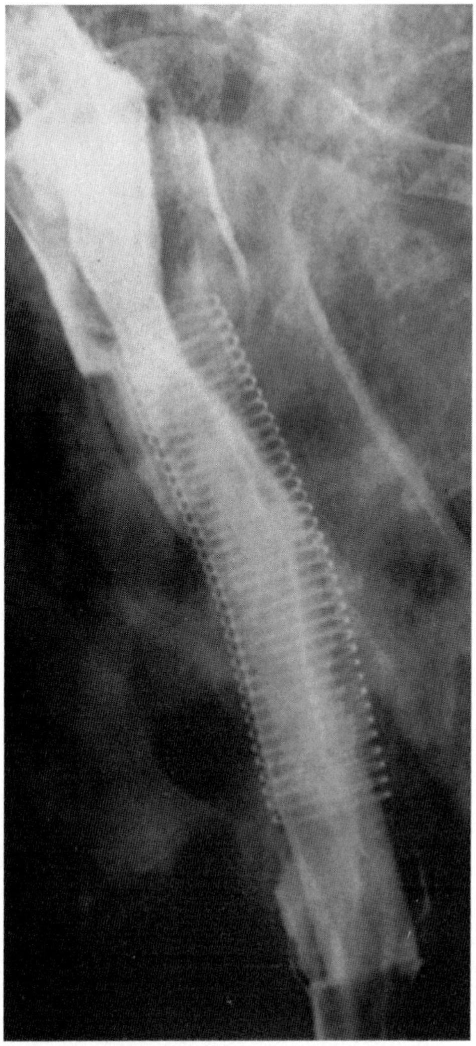

Figure 1-75 Esophageal stent in a patient with advanced esophageal carcinoma.

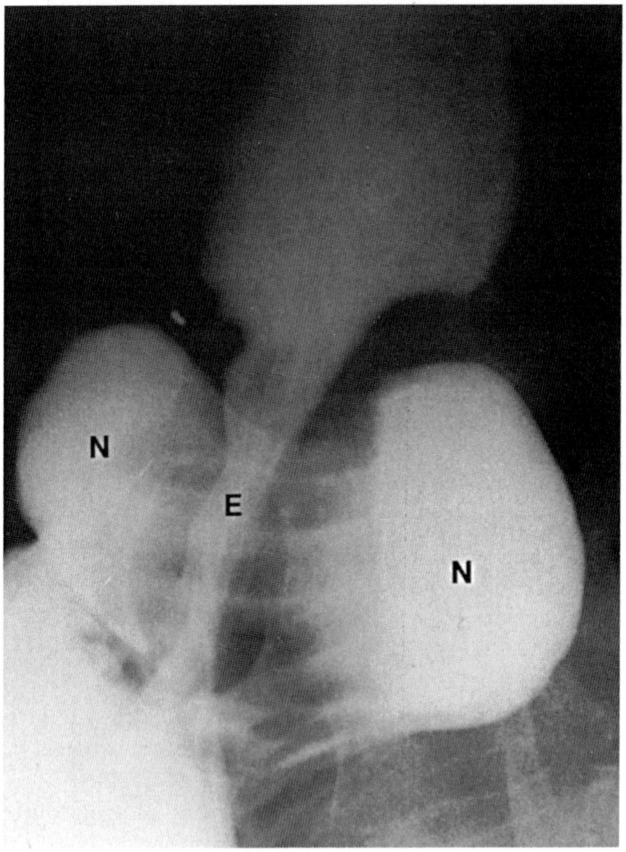

Figure 1-76 Distal esophagus *(E)* is compressed by Nissen's fundoplication *(N)*.

as a clinical history of dysphagia. These are potentially important symptoms; however, it is important that the radiologist establish by history the presence or absence of true dysphagia (the inability or difficulty in passing the food bolus from mouth to stomach) or odynophagia (painful swallowing).

The second reason for eliciting the history of the dysphagic symptom is to determine a suitable radiological examination. Although the radiological evaluation of dysphagia requires basic evaluation of the morphology and function of the oropharynx, esophagus, gastroesophageal junction, and proximal stomach, it is often necessary to tailor the examination to fit the diagnostic problem. Additionally the radiologist does not want to do anything that might harm the patient or increase patient discomfort. A patient presenting with weight loss or dysphagia to solids may not require the full biphasic examination with carbon dioxide granules and highly dense barium, which could potentially be aspirated. Patients with moderate to severe odynophagia experience considerable aggravation of their pain when carbon dioxide granules are used. A thorough history might suggest the problem to be of oropharyngeal origin, in which a videotape recording or rapid digital image acquisition, if available, should be used. After taking the history and performing the clinical evaluation, the radiologist can plan the form that the radiological

Box 1-10 Dysphagia: The Radiologist's Dilemma

Always consider dysphagia to be a serious problem. Assume and look for a mechanical or dynamic basis for the symptom.

An appropriate clinical swallowing history and constitutional history are essential.

For purposes of evaluation, the swallowing function begins at the lips and terminates at the stomach.

study will take to optimize diagnostic opportunity and diminish complications.

If there is any question as to what might be encountered, I recommend a "test swallow" of approximately 5 mL of thin barium. Patients with possible high-grade mechanical obstruction, esophageal-airway fistula, or history suggestive of significant aspirations might be candidates for a test swallow. This test swallow would not seriously degrade the routine study that might follow and may prevent the occurrence of massive aspiration.

A concise but complete swallowing history allows the radiologist to tailor the examination, and in most instances allows the experienced radiologist to predict the nature of the abnormality before the study.

History

The following should be considered:

1. Is it truly dysphagia? Does food "get stuck"? Does the patient have to work at getting the food down (e.g., require fluids to force it down)?
2. What type of dysphagia is it? Is it dysphagia to liquids, solids, or both? In general, liquid dysphagia may suggest motility abnormalities, whereas dysphagia to solids tends to point to mechanical difficulties.
3. What are the duration and constancy of symptoms? Persistent dysphagia is more worrisome than symptoms that are intermittent. Are the symptoms progressive? Progressive solid dysphagia is a serious concern. This is particularly true when it is associated with constitutional changes, such as weight loss, decreased energy, and decreased appetite.
4. Are there accompanying constitutional changes? Has the patient experienced weight change? Has appetite been affected? Has eating pattern been altered? Potentially serious problems are suggested in patients who experience a slow progression of dysphagia that requires them to avoid certain foods (e.g., meat) or puree their food. One should be cautious, however, when inquiring about eating habits. Many patients with chronic benign esophageal strictures have come to terms with their swallowing limitations and have altered their eating habits accordingly. They may consider their eating patterns perfectly normal and unchanged. One occasionally has to put very specific questions to the patient. Consider the following real-life exchange between a radiology resident before an examination and a 62-year-old patient with a prior history of a chest tumor who is currently complaining of intermittent heartburn for approximately 1 year's duration.

Resident: Do you ever notice food getting stuck while eating?

Patient: No.

Resident: Do you ever have any problems swallowing?

Patient: No.

Resident: Do you ever notice the feeling of food getting stuck in your neck or upper abdomen?

Patient: No.

Resident: Do you have any pain when you swallow?

Patient: No.

The subsequent UGI examination disclosed a moderate lower esophageal stricture that had a benign appearance. The radiology resident was encouraged to question the patient in more detail. After the radiological examination, the interview proceeded as follows:

Resident: So, you never notice any problems with swallowing?

Patient: No.

Resident: Food never seems to get stuck when you swallow?

Patient: No.

Resident: Any problems with swallowing, say, steak?

Patient: Actually, steak seems to get stuck.

Resident: What about other meats?

Patient: Usually. I seem to have problems whenever I swallow meat or bread because it usually gets stuck, so I avoid those foods. Sometimes when I take my vitamins in the morning, they seem to get stuck. Apart from that, I don't have any problems.

A conversation such as this would not be unique. There is no suggestion that the patient was deliberately intending to mislead or deceive the resident. Some patients are anxious or frightened about the procedures and may find the questions confusing. Some patients reach the point that their nonprogressive dysphagia is compensated by avoiding certain types and consistencies of food, and their swallowing assumes normalcy in their own mind. The skills of history taking, which are learned and, it is hoped, mastered in medical school, should be retained and frequently used by radiologists.

Radiological Evaluation

The radiological evaluation consists of five parts. Clinical history may emphasize one part over another; however, all parts of the examination should be included to some extent in every radiological dysphagia workup.

Oropharyngeal Airway

In this part of the examination, the following observations are to be made:

1. Morphology:
   - Size of the oropharyngeal airway. Is the airway dilated?
   - Shape and size of the epiglottis.
2. Bolus organization in transit in the mouth and on the tongue:
   - Is the bolus well organized on the tongue?
   - Is there spillage into the buccal cavity?
   - Is there spillage of contrast material into the oral pharynx before the initiation of swallow?
3. Normal triggering of the autonomic swallowing reflex:
   - Is there a prompt and rapid triggering of the swallowing reflex when the bolus touches the posterior pharyngeal wall?
   - Delays of the triggering of the swallowing reflex should be noted.
4. Contraction, elevation of the soft palate, and exclusion of the nasopharynx:
   - Does the soft palate effectively occlude the nasopharynx during swallowing?
   - Is there any nasopharyngeal reflux?
5. Pharyngeal contraction:
   - Is the pharyngeal contraction symmetrical? Is there weakness in the contraction? Is the weakness unilateral or bilateral? Contrast material tends to flow to the weak side in situations in which the pharyngeal contraction is asymmetrically weak.
6. Excursion of the laryngeal-hyoid complex and the posterior-inferior tipping of the epiglottis. These are the mechanisms of airway protection, the former being especially important:
   - Is swallowing accompanied by the normal upward and outward movement of the laryngeal hyoid complex?
   - Does the epiglottis tilt posteriorly and inferiorly with the bolus?
7. Relaxation of the cricopharyngeal muscle. The cricopharyngeal constitutes the upper esophageal sphincter:
   - During maximal bolus distention, does this area completely open?

Some patients show a mild cricopharyngeal impression during maximum bolus transit. If the luminal compromise is less than 25% during maximum distention, however, it is always asymptomatic and of no clinical consequence.

Posterior impressions caused by cervical spine osteophyte formation are also a common finding, but almost never result in dysphagia and should be ignored. The only exceptions might be the large bridging osteophytes of diffuse idiopathic skeletal hyperostosis, large posttraumatic osteophytes, or possibly anterior cervical spine fusion.

8. Postswallow residual:
   - Is there residual barium in the hypopharynx following the swallow?
   - If so, estimate the amount (small, moderate, or large).
9. Aspiration. This is defined as contrast material that is inhaled into the airway and descends below the laryngeal vestibule and the cords. Contrast material that does not pass the vestibule is referred to as penetration:
   - If aspiration is present, record type and amount present. Is there a spontaneous cough reflex with aspiration?

   Three types of aspiration can be identified:
   - *Preswallow aspiration.* When patients spill barium over the posterior tongue into the oropharynx or into the valleculae before the initiation of swallowing and immediately aspirate the bolus, it is referred to as preswallow aspiration. This is the most serious type of aspiration, and most examinations are terminated at this point.
   - *Swallowing aspiration.* This is the most common form of aspiration. Failure to protect the airway completely may result in some aspiration during swallowing. This type of aspiration can be transient (e.g., in patients following stroke) and may be treated by the speech pathologist with varying therapeutic maneuvers.
   - *Aspiration after swallowing.* This occurs when the pharyngeal contraction is incomplete or incompetent if the cricopharyngeal muscle fails to relax fully. The resultant residual material can be aspirated as the multifunctional oropharynx (eating, breathing, and phonation) switches to breathing mode, and contrast material is subsequently aspirated.

Esophagus: Tube Morphology

With the biphasic examination, one evaluates structure, filling defects, barium collections suggesting ulcers or diverticula, and extrinsic impressions.

Esophageal Dynamics

The presence and gross evaluation of the primary wave is observed. The presence of secondary or tertiary waves also is noted.

Primary waves are stripping waves triggered by the swallowing reflex, whereas secondary waves are triggered by luminal distention or presence of acid and relate to refluxed contrast material from the stomach or poorly cleared contrast material from the esophagus. Tertiary waves are nonpropulsive contractions of the esophagus, frequently seen in elderly individuals with otherwise normal esophageal dynamics. The condition is referred to as presbyesophagus. This is not a pathologic condition. The presence of tertiary waves as the *only* form of esophageal contraction is abnormal.

Esophageal dynamics are best evaluated with gravity eliminated as a factor and with the patient in the recumbent position (right anterior oblique being the optimal position). The primary wave must be evaluated with a single swallow. Multiple swallows obliterate the primary wave ahead of it. This is a normal protective mechanism, but it could be misinterpreted as dynamic abnormality.

Gastroesophageal Junction

This is the most common site of esophageal disease and requires careful attention. One should never make judgments about the gastroesophageal junction based on air-contrast upright views. Invariably the gastroesophageal junction is pulled downward by gravity and by the weight of the stomach and its contents (especially if that content is barium). The need for single-contrast evaluation of the esophagus in the recumbent position is best shown at the gastroesophageal junction. Occasionally, small hiatal hernias, B-rings, ulcers, thickened folds, and even small neoplastic lesions may be subtle or not seen on upright air-contrast views but effectively shown on single-contrast recumbent views (Fig. 1-77).

Additionally, it is important to note the absence or presence of gastroesophageal reflux and to quantify it to some extent. It is natural to reflux acidic stomach content into the esophagus occasionally. The protective mechanisms are (1) the secondary wave stripping the acid back into the stomach and (2) the cricopharyngeus, which protects the oropharynx from refluxed

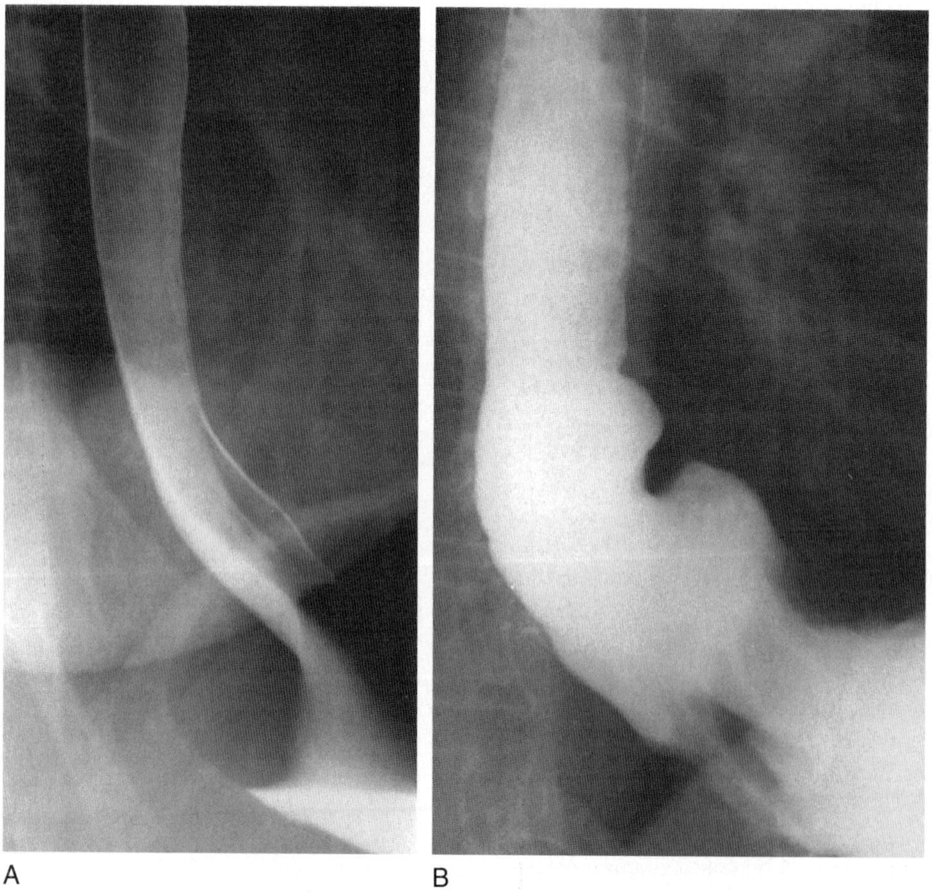

Figure 1-77 The gastroesophageal junction. **A,** Gastroesophageal junction during upright double-contrast views in a patient with a complaint of heartburn. The junction looks normal. **B,** The same patient recumbent during single-contrast phase of the biphasic examination. Note hiatal hernia is not seen on the upright view.

gastric content. Failure of the secondary wave to clear the esophagus rapidly and completely increases the risk of reflux esophagitis. Failure of the cricopharyngeus to bar the way of refluxed acid into the oropharynx can result in confusing and occasionally deadly consequences. Patients may complain of sore throat or hoarseness in the morning or awake with alarming coughing fits during the night as reflux and aspiration occur. Sometimes the aspiration amount is tiny and silent and continuous, which can result in either pneumonia or bronchospasm. These patients may be treated with antibiotics or anti-asthma medication,or both, when in fact the underlying problem is gastroesophageal reflux. Quantifying gastroesophageal reflux is subjective. In the lower third of the esophagus, it may be called "small." Reflux to the midesophagus can be termed "moderate," whereas reflux up the entire esophageal column to the level of the cricopharyngeus can be considered "large." It is not the presence of reflux, however, that is important, but the effectiveness of the protective mechanisms—the clearing function of the secondary wave and the protective function of the cricopharyngeus muscle.

Cardiofundal Region of the Stomach

The cardia and fundus of the stomach should be included as part of the dysphagia workup. Neoplastic lesions in these areas not directly affecting the gastroesophageal junction have been seen in patients presenting with dysphagia, for which no other cause of dysphagia is evident.

Conclusion

Two additional issues require attention in the radiological workup of dysphagia. The first issue to consider is the type of contrast agent. Barium is always the contrast agent of choice for any patient who presents with a dysphagia history and in whom there is no suspicion of an esophageal tear, leak, or possible aspiration.

Water-soluble contrast material has little or no role in this radiological examination. Because many of these patients may aspirate, it is preferable that barium be the aspirated agent rather than a water-soluble iodine-based contrast agent. The latter can cause chemical pneumonitis and even pulmonary edema in patients whose pulmonary function is already compromised.

In patients with relatively healthy lungs, barium aspiration is relatively harmless. It was only 4 to 5 decades ago that radiological bronchography was performed using barium as the contrast agent. In patients with chronic lung disease, barium may be seen for a protracted period in the lungs, but it is still unquestionably preferable to water-soluble contrast material and its complications.

The second issue to consider is the modified barium swallow. This is sometimes referred to as a dynamic swallowing study and is performed in the radiology department in conjunction with a speech pathologist. Because swallowing is a function that starts at the lips and tongue and ceases in the stomach, it is necessary for the radiologist to be completely involved in these types of examinations. This involvement is important not only to provide professional fluoroscopic imaging and management of radiation safety issues but also to ensure that whenever possible a lesion of the esophagus, gastroesophageal junction, or proximal stomach is not missed because only the oropharynx is evaluated.

The speech pathologist's role in the examination is to evaluate the patient's capacity for oral feeding and to plan strategies relative to that issue. These examinations should not be performed to evaluate for dysphagia unrelated to central nervous system incidents, degenerative muscle diseases, or neurological diseases. If they are, it is the radiologist's responsibility to do what is necessary for a proper radiological evaluation. This is particularly true if the oropharyngeal phase of the evaluation is normal.

SUGGESTED READINGS

Balthazar EJ, Naidich DP, Megibow AJ, et al: CT evaluation of esophageal varices. AJR Am J Roentgenol 148:131-135, 1987.

Bleshman MH, Banner MP, Johnson RC, et al: The inflammatory esophagogastric polyp and fold. Radiology 128:589-593, 1978.

Bova JG, Dutton NE, Goldstein HM, et al: Medication-induced esophagitis: diagnosis by double-contrast esophagography. AJR Am J Roentgenol 148:731-732, 1987.

Buchholz D: Neurologic causes of dysphagia. Dysphagia 1:152-156, 1987.

Buecker A, Wein BB, Neuerburg JM, et al: Esophageal perforation: comparison of use of aqueous and barium-containing contrast agents. Radiology 202:683-686, 1997.

Callahan MJ, Taylor GA: CT of pediatric esophagus. AJR Am J Roentgenol 181:1391-1396, 2003.

Carter MM, Kulkarni MV: Giant fibrovascular polyp of the esophagus, Gastrointest Radiol 9:301-303. 1984.

Chasen MH, Rugh KS, Shelton DK: Mediastinal impressions on the dilated esophagus, Radiol Clin North Am 22:591-605, 1984.

Curtis DJ: Radiographic anatomy of the pharynx. Dysphagia 1:51-62, 1986.

Desai RK, Tagiabue JR, Wegryn SAY, et al: CT evaluation of wall thickening in the alimentary tract. Radiographics 11:771-783, 1991.

Donner MW, Bosma JF, Robertson DL: Anatomy and physiology of the pharynx. Gastrointest Radiol 10:196-212, 1985.

Donner MW, Saba GP, Martinez CR: Diffuse diseases of the esophagus: a practical approach. Semin Roentgenol 16:198-213, 1981.

Ekberg O, Nylander G: Dysfunction of the cricopharyngeal muscle: a cineradiographic study of patients with dysphagia. Radiology 143:481-486, 1982.

Fadoo F, Ruiz DE, Dawn SK, et al: Helical CT esophagography for the evaluation of suspected esophageal perforation or rupture. AJR Am J Roentgenol 182:1177-1179, 2004.

Freeny PC, Marks WM: Adenocarcinoma of the gastroesophageal junction: barium and CT examination. AJR Am J Roentgenol 138:1077-1084, 1982.

Gedgaudas-McClees RK, Torres WE, Colvin RS, et al: Thoracic findings in gastrointestinal pathology. Radiol Clin North Am 22:563-589, 1984.

Ghahremani GG, Rushovich AM: Glycogenic acanthosis of the esophagus: radiographic and pathologic features. Gastrointest Radiol 9:93-98, 1984.

Gilchrist AM, Levine MS, Carr RF, et al: Barrett's esophagus: diagnosis by double-contrast esophagography. AJR Am J Roentgenol 150:97-102, 1988.

Goldstein HM, Zornoza J, Hopens T: Intrinsic diseases of the adult esophagus: benign and malignant tumors. Semin Roentgenol 16:183-197, 1981.

Gore RM: Esophageal cancer: clinical and pathological features. Radiol Clin North Am 35:243-263, 1997.

Grishaw EK, Ott DJ, Frederick MG, et al: Functional abnormalities of the esophagus: a prospective analysis of the radiographic findings relative to age and symptoms. AJR Am J Roentgenol 167:719-723, 1996.

Halvorsen RA Jr, Thompson WM: CT of esophageal neoplasms. Radiol Clin North Am 27:667-685, 1989.

Heiken JP, Balfe DM, Roper CL: CT evaluation after esophagogastrectomy. AJR Am J Roentgenol 143:555-560, 1984.

Jones B, Kramer SS, Donner MW: Dynamic imaging of the pharynx. Gastrointest Radiol 10:213-224, 1985.

Kawamoto K, Yamada Y, Utsunomiya T, et al: Gastrointestinal submucosal tumors: evaluation with endoscopic US. Radiology 205:733-740, 1997.

Lepke RA, Libshitz HI: Radiation-induced injury of the esophagus. Radiology 148:375-378, 1983.

Levine MS, Caroline DF, Thompson JJ, et al: Adenocarcinoma of the esophagus: relationship to Barrett mucosa. Radiology 150:305-309, 1984.

Levine MS, Chu P, Furth EE, et al: Carcinoma of the esophagogastric junction: sensitivity of radiographic diagnosis. AJR Am J Roentgenol 168:1423-1426, 1997.

Levine MS, Moolten DN, Herlinger H, et al: Esophageal intramural pseudodiverticulosis: a reevaluation. AJR Am J Roentgenol 147:1165-1170, 1986.

Levine MS, Rubesin SE, Herlinger H, et al: Double-contrast upper gastrointestinal examination: technique and interpretation. Radiology 168:593-602, 1988.

Lowe GM, Donaldson JS, Backer CL: Vascular rings: 10 year review of imaging. Radiographics 11:637-646, 1991.

Marx MV, Balfe DM: Computed tomography of the esophagus. Semin Ultrasound CT MR 8:316-348, 1987.

Mauro MA, Parker LA, Hartley WS, et al: Epidermolysis bullosa: radiographic findings in 16 cases. AJR Am J Roentgenol 149:925-927, 1987.

Newcomer MK, Brazer SR: Complications of upper gastrointestinal endoscopy and their management. Gastrointest Endosc Clin N Am 4:551, 1994.

Olmsted WW, Lichtenstein JE, Hyams VJ: Polypoid epithelial malignancies of the esophagus. AJR Am J Roentgenol 140:921-925, 1983.

Ott DJ, Gelfand DW, Wu WC, et al: Esophagogastric region and its rings. AJR Am J Roentgenol 142:281-287, 1984.

Owen JW, Balfe DM, Koehler RE, et al: Radiologic evaluation of complications after esophagogastrectomy. AJR Am J Roentgenol 140:1163-1169, 1983.

Phillips LG, Cunningham J: Esophageal perforation. Radiol Clin North Am 22:607-613, 1984.

Rubesin S, Herlinger H, Sigal H: Granular cell tumors of the esophagus. Gastrointest Radiol 10:11-15, 1985.

Rubesin SE, Glick SN: The tailored double-contrast pharyngogram. Crit Rev Diagn Imaging 28:133-179, 1988.

Seaman WB: Pathophysiology of the esophagus. Semin Roentgenol 16:214-227, 1981.

Triadafilpoulos G: Stretta: an effective minimally invasive treatment for gastroesophgeal reflux disease. Am J Med 115:192-200, 2003.

CHAPTER 2 Stomach and Duodenum

EXAMINATION TECHNIQUES

The biphasic-contrast examination of the stomach is considered to be the radiological examination of choice at present. This technique consists of examining the stomach using double-contrast and single-contrast techniques (Box 2-1).

In most cases, the stomach examination is combined with the esophagus study. After the ingestion of effervescent granules and high-density barium and the double-contrast evaluation of the esophagus in the upright position, the patient is quickly lowered into a supine recumbent position. To avoid excessive spillage of contrast material into the small bowel, this repositioning should be done promptly after the last esophageal film has been obtained. With the patient in the supine position, a quick fluoroscopic evaluation of the stomach indicates to the fluoroscopist whether gastric distention is adequate and if a sufficient amount of barium is retained within the stomach to continue with the examination or whether remedial measures may be necessary at this time.

If the stomach is adequately distended and contains sufficient barium, the patient is rotated one or two times to achieve gastric coating. By rotating patients to the left, it is thought that less barium is spilled into the small bowel. The gastric mucosa is covered by a surface layer of mucus that must be washed away by the barium to achieve optimal mucosal coating and detail. Inadequate washing of the barium over the mucosal surface or residual food and secretions degrade mucosal coating and cause the examination to be limited. After rotation of the patient, the stomach is fluoroscopically evaluated again for the quality of the mucosal coating.

The menu of spot images obtained varies among different institutions. Generally, a supine image of the stomach is obtained when adequate coating has been achieved.

Box 2-1 Biphasic Upper Gastrointestinal Examination: The Best of Both Worlds

Air-contrast view to display and evaluate the mucosal surfaces of the esophagus, stomach, and duodenum.

Single-contrast component to study esophageal motility, the gastrointestinal junction, contrast distention, and contour of the bowel wall.

Box 2-2 Importance of Being Superficial: Flow Technique in the Stomach

Barium coating of the gut is normally an amorphous layer in which superficial lesions are difficult to recognize.

A thin coating of barium (flow technique) flowing across the antrum (where most disease occurs) results in a very thin superficial barium layer that nicely shows lesions such as erosions and superficial neoplasms.

This thin superficial layer of flow technique persists for 5 to 7 seconds.

The patient is turned sharply to the right into a steep right posterior oblique or right lateral position in which air-contrast views of the cardia and fundus are obtained. Under fluoroscopic control, the patient is turned back into the supine position and slightly to the left to thin out the barium pool in the antrum. As the barium flows from the antrum into the proximal stomach, a thin layer of barium is left in the antrum, achieving the "flow technique" (Box 2-2), which is an excellent method for showing subtle mucosal findings, such as tiny nodules and linear or punctate erosions (Fig. 2-1). A spot film is obtained at this point. The patient is turned to the left again, and air-contrast views of the antrum and duodenum are obtained. This series of maneuvers basically represents the double-contrast portion of the stomach examination. Additional films and maneuvers may be necessary to show completely all areas within the stomach and the duodenal bulb and sweep.

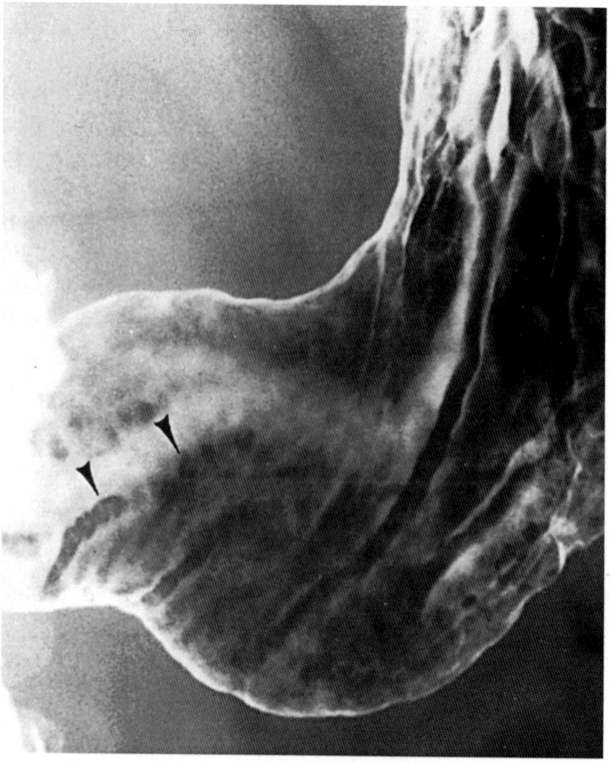

Figure 2-1 Using flow technique, tiny superficial erosions are seen along one of the folds of the distal stomach. Edema around the erosions results in a beaded appearance of the fold *(arrows)*.

At this point, the patient is turned to a recumbent right anterior oblique position and ingests low-density barium. A limited evaluation of oropharyngeal function may be obtained during this phase. Esophageal dynamics also are studied, and barium-distended views of the gastroesophageal junction are obtained. The latter constitutes an important part of the stomach evaluation. With sufficient barium within the stomach and antrum and duodenal bulb, right anterior oblique or prone compression views of the antrum and duodenal bulb are obtained. This maneuver is as important in the upper gastrointestinal (UGI) series today as it was in the early years of gastrointestinal imaging of the stomach. Occasionally, ulcers that are either unfilled during the earlier part of the examination or not well shown can be seen easily with compression views of the antrum and duodenal bulb.

Occasionally, the duodenal bulb and possibly the distal antrum are in a posterior position. In some cases, the bulb lies almost directly behind the distal antrum; this makes compression of the area difficult. It also makes air-contrast views of the bulb and antropyloric region difficult. In such an instance, the fluoroscopist may use angulation of the tube, if this is available. Most fluoroscopic suites have a tableside type of fluoroscopy, however, without the benefit of angulation. In such a situation, the fluoroscopist can turn the patient onto the left side and firmly position a bolster, which may be an inflated compression paddle or a balloon against the left costochondral margin. The patient, under fluoroscopy, is moved down into a left anterior oblique position, compressing the abdomen as the patient rolls to the left and toward the table. This movement is often sufficient compression to push away the antrum of the stomach and allow the duodenal bulb and pyloric channel to be shown (Fig. 2-2).

The use of glucagon in UGI studies has been advocated and practiced since the 1980s. Small doses of glucagon have been shown to be effective in improving the visibility of the antrum and duodenal bulb. Many centers have now ceased this practice, however, and no intravenous injection is given before the examination; no objective evidence shows that this results in any decreased sensitivity in the detection of disease in these areas. Without the use of an antiperistaltic agent, such as glucagon, gastric contractions may be observed and evaluated.

The last part of the examination consists of rotating the patient again to evaluate for the possibility of spontaneous gastroesophageal reflux. I tend not to use any extraordinary methods for inducing reflux. Valsalva maneuvers,

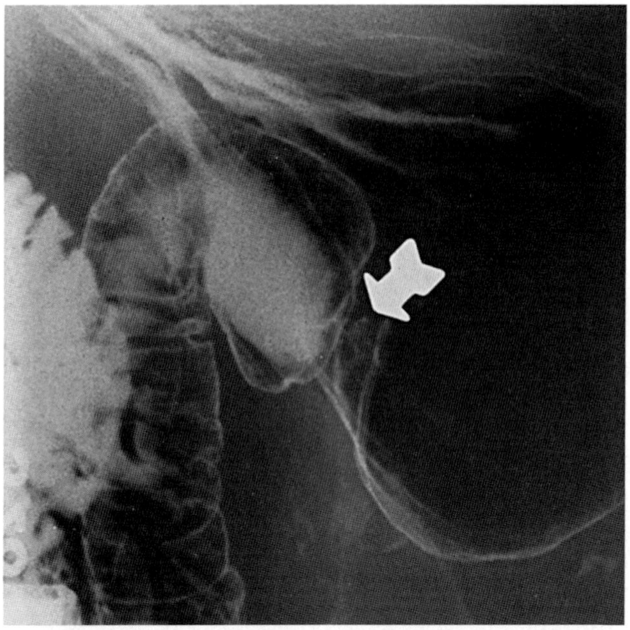

Figure 2-2 Left anterior oblique view with compression shows the profiled pyloric channel and duodenal bulb. A small pyloric channel ulcer, not seen on other views, is shown *(arrow)*.

abdominal compression, and bolstering all have been described. Reflux can be produced in virtually any patient with sufficient effort. The significance of this reflux is doubtful. The rotation of a patient that results in a spontaneous and significant amount of reflux is probably important, however. Rotation often simulates what happens when the patient rolls over in bed at night and experiences gastric reflux and associated symptoms. The lack of demonstrated reflux may not rule out gastroesophageal reflux as the cause of the patient's symptoms.

In many instances, instead of the standard biphasic examination, a single-contrast study using low-density barium is performed. Although this situation should represent a minority of cases, there are acceptable indications for a single-contrast examination. In elderly or debilitated patients who are unable to stand or who cannot roll or provide the compliance necessary for a double-contrast evaluation of the stomach, a single-contrast examination is an alternative. In patients with suspected gastric outlet obstruction, a single-contrast examination suffices. In patients who have had surgery or procedures involving use of instrumentation and in whom there is any question of perforation or leakage, a water-soluble, single-contrast examination is indicated. When faced with the decision as to whether a single-contrast or biphasic examination should be undertaken, the radiologist should be guided by the same axiom that applies to the radiological evaluation of the colon—a limited single-contrast evaluation is better than a limited double-contrast evaluation of the organ.

Multitrack computed tomography (CT) is extremely useful in evaluating for known or suspected malignant lesions of the stomach. The extent of perigastric involvement and spread to adjacent organs can usually be shown with this type of imaging. Of great importance in the newest generation of CT scanners is the ability to perform multiplanar imaging and three-dimensional reconstruction of sites of interest (Fig. 2-3). Endoscopic ultrasound with a rotating transducer placed on the tip of a specially prepared endoscope has been useful in the evaluation of malignant diseases of the stomach. It is shown to be superior to CT in evaluating the extent of gastric wall involvement and limited perigastric spread and adenopathy, which may not be evident on CT. For evaluation of metastatic involvement of the liver, however, three-phase multitrack CT of the liver using arterial, portal, and venous phase scanning remains the examination of choice. Occasionally, delayed or "equilibrium" images may be obtained. CT also is invaluable for the demonstration of distal metastatic disease or spread to lymph nodes in the retroperitoneum.

Magnetic resonance imaging (MRI) has had a limited role in the imaging evaluation of the stomach to date. The possibility of a selective MRI contrast agent taken up only by the various layers of the mucosa holds some promise. This modality remains in the experimental stage, however.

The old barium examination, refined over the years with better barium products and better imaging equipment, is still an inexpensive and relatively reliable way of examining the stomach. Although the number of barium procedures has diminished over the last 2 decades, the cost of health care has dramatically increased. There are numerous reasons for this increase, but one is the developing, and almost routine, choice of clinicians who go immediately to much more costly examinations, such as endoscopy. When there is a good gastrointestinal radiologist, the quality and accuracy of a barium study approaches that of endoscopy at a fraction of the price.

The following sections approach the differential diagnosis of gastric disease, based on the dominant radiological problems seen on barium examinations. It closely reflects the way cases are encountered in a daily clinical practice. The same condition may be discussed under several categories, however, reflecting the different manifestations or stages of the same disease process.

STOMACH

Gastric Outlet Obstruction Resulting in Gastric Distention

Peptic Ulcer Disease

The most common cause of gastric outlet obstruction in adults before 1980 was peptic ulcer disease involving the gastric antrum, the pyloric channel of the stomach,

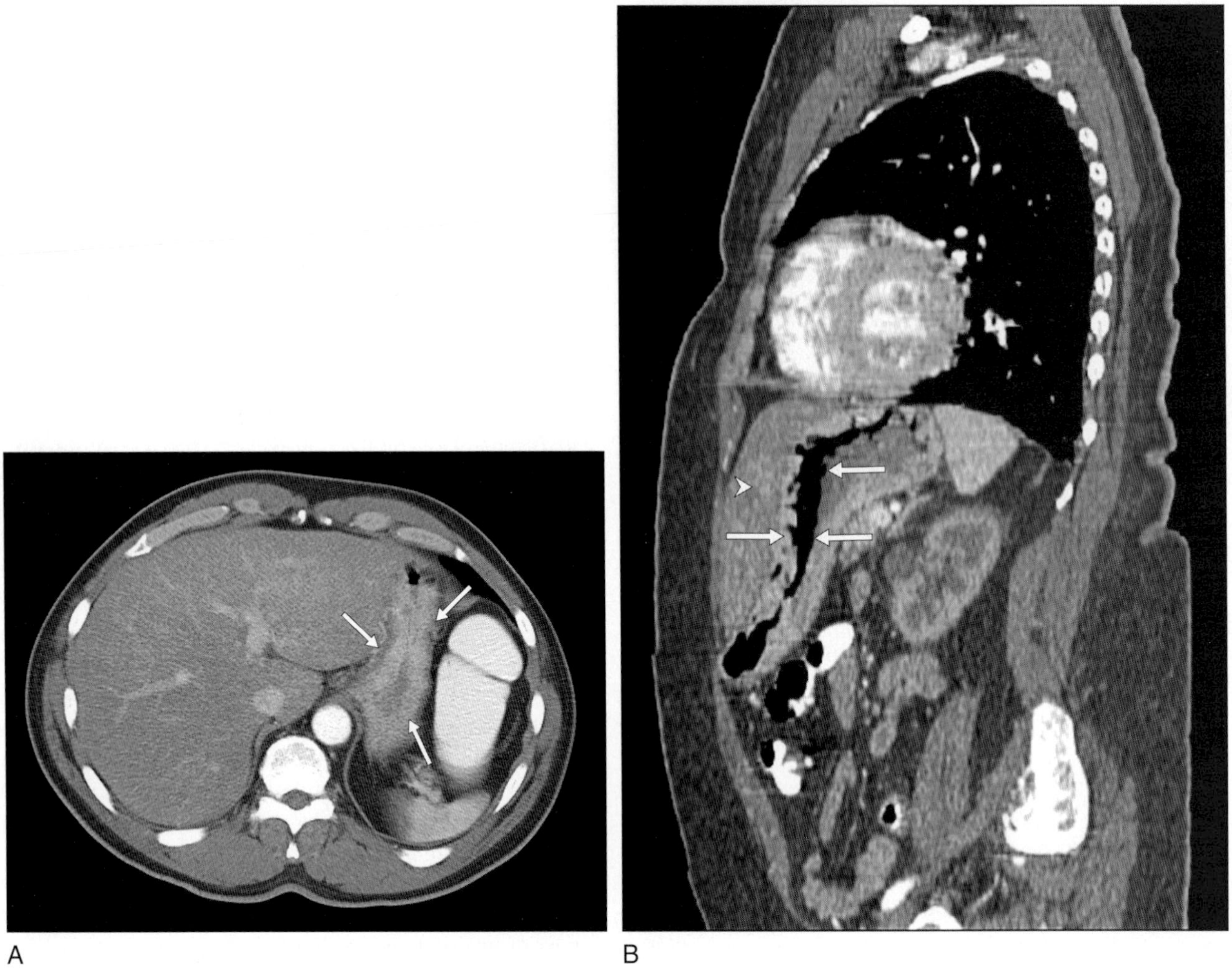

Figure 2-3 **A,** Normal collapsed stomach axial view *(arrows)*. **B,** Demonstration of sagittal view of collapsed stomach *(arrows)* and liver *(arrowhead)*.

and the first portion of the duodenum. Even before 1980, this complication was seen in only 5% of patients with peptic ulcer disease. With newer medications and more prompt treatment of peptic ulcer disease, it is more common today to see malignancy as a cause for gastric outlet obstruction. Gastric outlet obstruction secondary to ulcer and inflammation is still encountered, with duodenal bulb and pyloric channel ulcers responsible for greater than 80% of the cases. Luminal narrowing usually results from the combined changes of chronic and acute inflammation and ulceration. These patients commonly have a long history of peptic ulcer disease and recurrent peptic ulcers. It is unusual for gastric outlet obstruction to be the presenting complaint in a patient without a history of peptic ulcer disease. In such an instance, other possibilities, particularly malignancy, should be strongly considered.

The most common presenting symptoms are vomiting, abdominal pain, and upper abdominal distention. Less prominent findings include weight loss and anorexia. Distention of the stomach in patients with chronic peptic ulcer disease is a gradual process in which symptoms can be present for several months or years before diagnosis. As a result, the size of the stomach, when seen on plain films of the abdomen, can be surprisingly large. Over time, the capability of the stomach to distend is remarkable (Fig. 2-4). It may appear on plain films as a huge, confusing, mottled, soft tissue mass in the upper abdomen. At other times, the amount of distention can be less, and a discernible dilated stomach can be identified. The mottled appearance of the dilated stomach is the result of the accumulation of secretions and the residue of numerous meals (Fig. 2-5). There may be diminished gas distally, although complete obstruction is unusual, and air is generally seen in the small bowel and colon. These organs may have a normal appearance except for depression of the transverse colon. Upright films show an air-fluid level within the stomach. In general, the presence of significant outlet obstruction with a huge distended stomach is almost always benign.

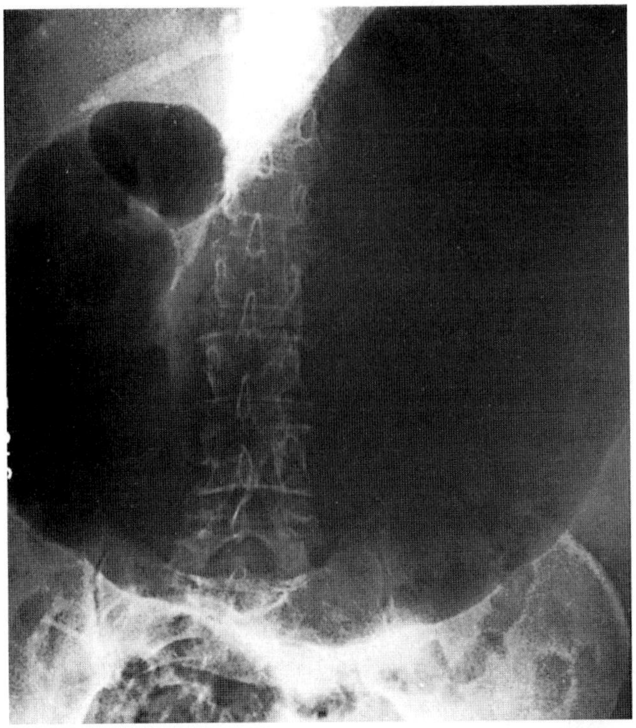

Figure 2-4 A large, air-filled stomach occupying the entire upper abdomen and displacing air-filled loops of bowel laterally and inferiorly represents a grossly distended stomach resulting from chronic peptic ulcer disease.

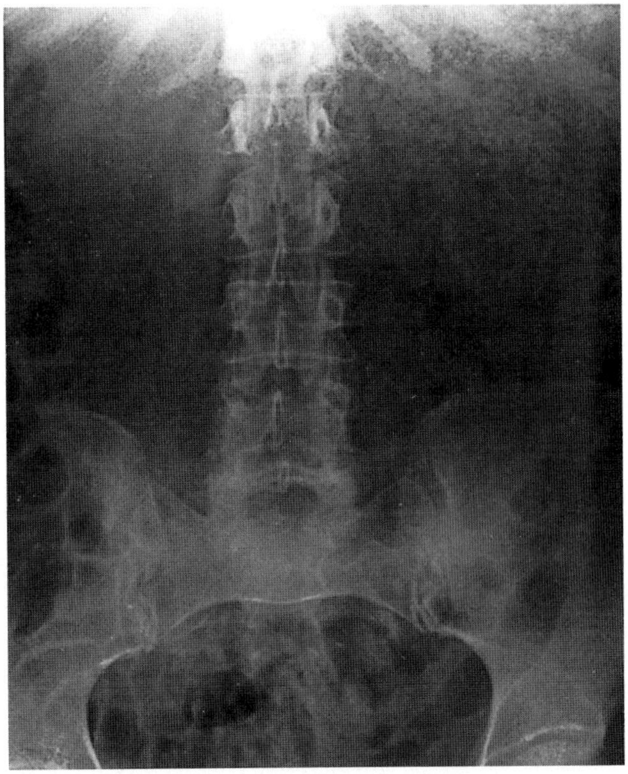

Figure 2-5 A large, mottled mass occupying the entire upper abdomen and displacing air-filled loops of bowel laterally and inferiorly represents a grossly distended stomach filled with food debris and secretions.

The presence of an air-fluid level within the duodenum is helpful in distinguishing between pyloric and duodenal obstruction.

Plain films are often diagnostic, and barium studies can be undertaken, not to confirm outlet obstruction but rather to attempt to identify the site (duodenal or gastric) and the nature of the obstructing process (Fig. 2-6). Gastric dilatation and delayed flow into the small bowel are the major findings. Ulcers may or may not be seen. Residual food generally limits the examination. The contrast agent of choice in the absence of free intraperitoneal air is barium. The large amount of residual fluid within the stomach of most of these patients, along with the propensity for frequent vomiting, makes the use of water-soluble contrast material relatively contraindicated.

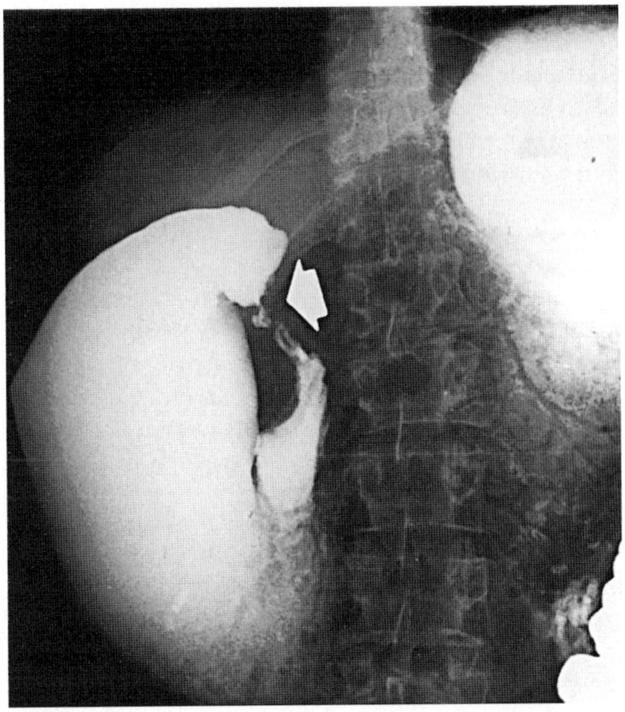

Figure 2-6 UGI examination in a patient presenting with chronic abdominal pain and distention shows a grossly distended stomach with ulceration in the pyloric channel *(arrow)* and the duodenal bulb.

Other Inflammatory Causes

Crohn's Disease

In various studies, gastric involvement with Crohn's disease has been identified in 0.5% to 10% of patients. The classic pattern of severe gastric involvement with Crohn's disease is a narrowed *(ram's horn stomach)*, rigid stomach (Fig. 2-7). Rarely, involvement of the distal antrum, in particular the pyloric channel, can result in gastric obstruction. The disease almost always manifests at the same time as involvement of other parts of the

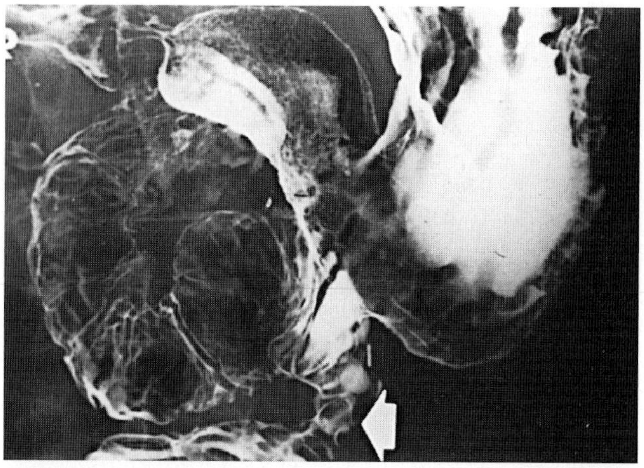

Figure 2-7 UGI examination shows a contracted stomach and a gastrojejunostomy. There is also fold thickening and narrowing of the efferent loop below the anastomosis *(arrow)*. All the observed inflammatory changes in the stomach and adjacent small bowel are due to Crohn's disease.

intestinal tract, especially the ileum. In the stomach, the distal stomach seems to be more commonly involved, and the radiological findings are similar to the findings seen in the usual sites of involvement. This includes granulomatous inflammation with superficial or linear ulcerations.

Pancreatitis

Patients with severe pancreatitis may present with degrees of gastric outlet obstruction. This obstruction is generally secondary to contiguous involvement of the adjacent structures with the inflammatory changes. In the stomach, wall thickening, edema, and spasm can lead to luminal compromise.

Corrosive Ingestion

Patients ingesting corrosive materials, particularly acids, can present with severe inflammatory changes in the distal antrum, especially along the lesser curvature, and luminal stricturing can occur acutely or chronically. The radiological features of such a lesion may be indistinguishable from malignancy. Rarely it can lead to outlet obstruction.

Other Causes

Other unusual inflammatory causes of gastric outlet obstruction include radiation gastritis, tuberculosis, and syphilis. The changing pattern of disease prevalence and the more recent increased incidence of both of these latter diseases in the population conceivably could result in an increased incidence of gastric involvement. Because modern treatment regimens usually limit the severity of these diseases commonly seen in previous decades, the number of cases with severe involvement of the stomach and potential gastric outlet obstruction probably will not increase and will remain extremely rare.

Malignancy

Carcinoma, especially of the scirrhous variety, involving the antrum or pyloric region commonly results in gastric outlet obstruction (Fig. 2-8). In addition, carcinoma of the head of the pancreas with adjacent spread involving the gastric antrum can compromise gastric outflow. These two tumors are probably the most common causes of gastric outlet obstruction resulting from neoplastic diseases. Rarely, lymphoma can result in outlet obstruction. Lymphomas, especially non-Hodgkin's lymphomas, tend to be pliable tumors, however, and infrequently cause obstruction, even when the tumor traverses the pyloric channel and involves the duodenal bulb. Rarely a polypoid mass involving the distal stomach and pyloric channel can result in mechanical obstruction by the presence of its sheer bulk in the most anatomically narrowed region of the stomach.

Gastric Bezoars

Generally, gastric bezoars (Box 2-3) do not obstruct. They may be asymptomatic for long periods (Fig. 2-9). Occasionally, the bezoar may act as an occluding agent, however, in a ball-valve type of obstructive process within the stomach. Postgastrectomy patients are most susceptible to bezoar formation and gastric distention. Although a few patients may show degrees of outlet obstruction, distention of the stomach or gastric remnant is often a result of the increasing size of the bezoar.

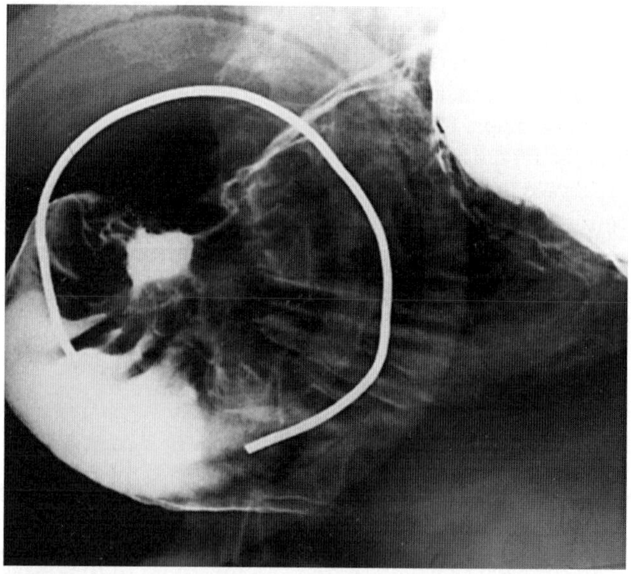

Figure 2-8 Ulcerating mass with a central barium collection occupies the distal prepyloric region of the stomach resulting in gastric outlet obstruction. The lesion was found to be adenocarcinoma of the stomach.

Box 2-3 Epicurean Oddities: Gastric Bezoars

Phytobezoars, the most common type of bezoar, are composed of vegetable matter, primarily fiber.
Trichobezoars result from the ingestion of hair.
Bezoars cause chronic gastritis and occasionally early satiety. Phytobezoars are a complication of Billroth II gastric resection.

The most common bezoar encountered is the phytobezoar, composed of fiber, plant matter, leaves, and roots. These are usually smaller and more compact than hair bezoars (trichobezoars). They also are more abrasive, and the incidence of associated peptic ulcer is higher with phytobezoars. They are the most common type of bezoar encountered after gastric surgery. Occasionally, a bezoar representing an overgrowth of fungi and yeast is encountered in postoperative patients. The susceptibility of postoperative patients to bezoar formation probably relates to the accompanying vagotomy and diminished ability of the stomach to empty.

Trichobezoars, or hairballs, are the second most commonly occurring gastric bezoar. They represent a congealed collection of hair enmeshed with mucus and decaying food material. They are always black in appearance and have a characteristic odor. They can be asymptomatic and can attain great size, with resultant gastric dilatation. Trichobezoars tend to be found in younger female patients. Incidences are higher in institutionalized patients and patients with psychiatric disturbances.

A type of bezoar commonly encountered in medical literature is the persimmon bezoar. This bezoar is generally unrelated to gastric surgery and is named for the native American persimmon tree. The fruit of the persimmon tree, although possessing little fiber, has considerable pulp quantity. Unripe persimmon fruit has a well-known astringent property. The interaction of the astringent and the stomach acid results in a coagulum or gelatinous pulpy mass within the stomach and occasionally results in acute gastric outlet obstruction. Other uncommon types of bezoars that have been reported include food bezoars, representing variations of phytobezoars. Some cases of bezoar formation in the stomach relating to the ingestion of vegetable fiber powder and psyllium have been reported. These cases no doubt are related to postoperative patients, abnormal gastric emptying, and inadequate amounts of fluids ingested with the vegetable powders.

Foreign body bezoars, although previously uncommon and seen almost exclusively in children or emotionally disturbed individuals, are being brought to the public's notice as individuals attempting to smuggle illegal drugs into the United States have discovered new and lucrative uses for condoms. In such individuals, however, the problem of gastric outlet obstruction fades into insignificance in the light of the relatively high incidence of condom leakage or rupture.

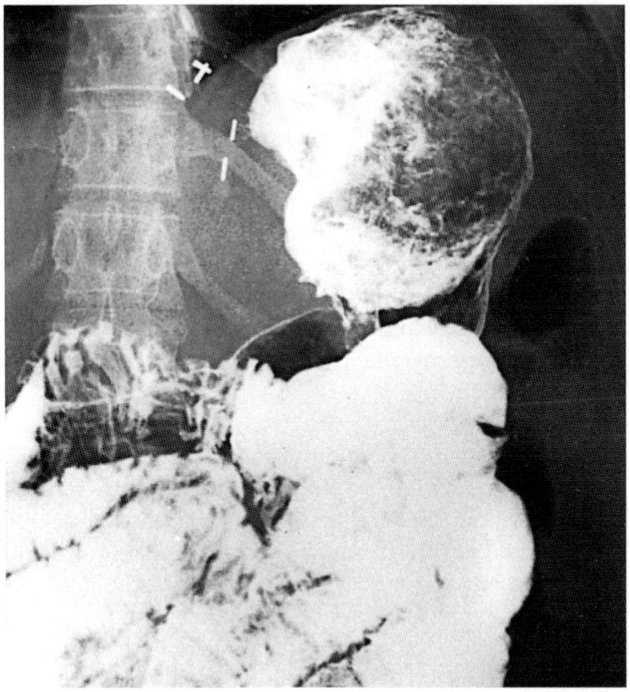

Figure 2-9 Gastric bezoar is shown in a stomach postoperatively.

Antral Diaphragms

Antral diaphragms are thin, well-defined, symmetrical mucosal webs seen in the distal portion of the antrum, compromising the antral lumen to varying degrees. Many authors believe they are congenital because of the lack of histological evidence of scarring in some patients. The origins of the antral web or diaphragm remain unclear, however. Not all antral diaphragms are congenital in nature. The history of chronic peptic inflammatory disease in many of these patients seriously suggests the possibility that some of these antral diaphragms may be narrowed, well-defined bands of scarring. The circumferential healing of gastric ulcers is well known.

Most antral diaphragms are not associated with obstruction. When the lumen is sufficiently compromised, however, degrees of gastric obstruction may be encountered. Generally, luminal narrowing of 1.5 cm or less is symptomatic. Careful fluoroscopic evaluation of the motility through this region and the use of a 12.5-mm barium tablet are helpful in establishing the degree of luminal compromise.

Fluoroscopically, antral diaphragms must be shown as fixed, weblike areas of narrowing in the antral portion of

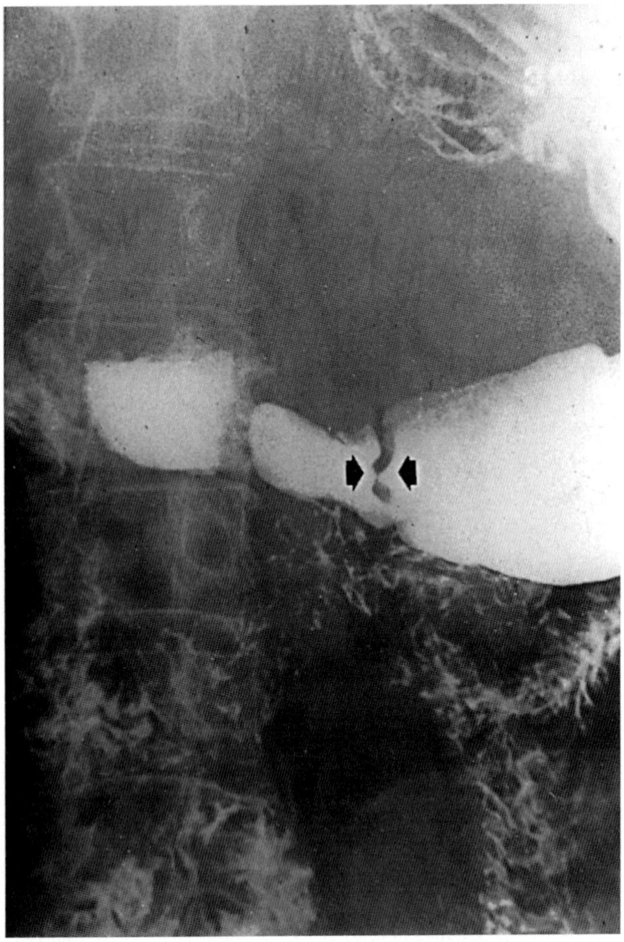

Figure 2-10 UGI study shows a thin, incomplete, weblike structure in the antrum of the stomach representing an antral web *(arrows)*.

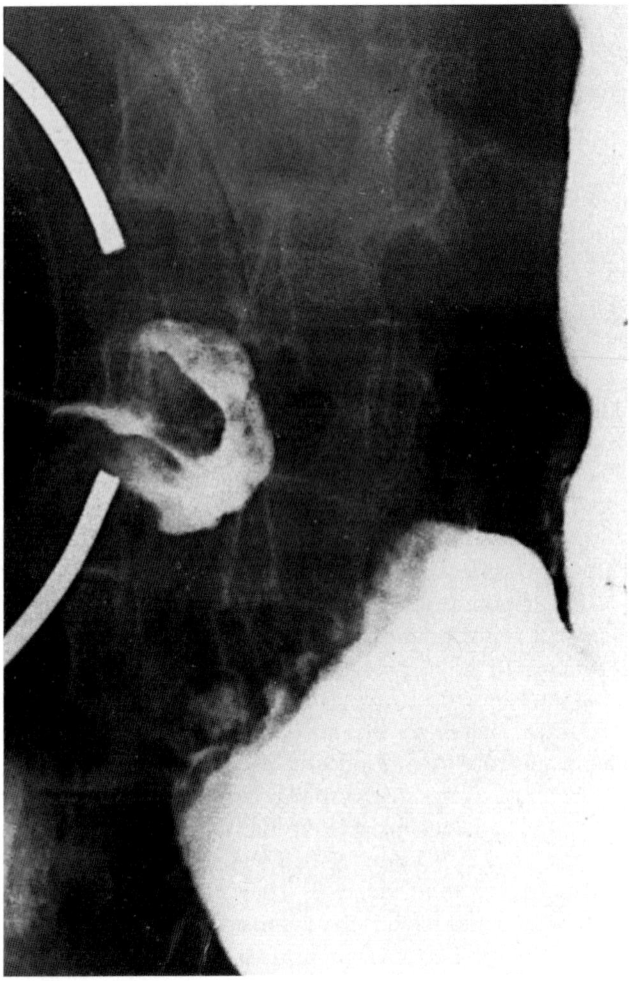

Figure 2-11 UGI examination in a patient with gastric outlet obstruction shows mass effect in the pyloric region with elongated pyloric channel and possible ulceration along the course of the channel.

the stomach (Fig. 2-10). The degree of circumferential involvement may or may not be complete.

Pyloric Stenosis

In an adult, pyloric stenosis is a confusing and rare entity. Whether it represents a true congenital pyloric stenosis or is an unusual sequela of peptic inflammatory disease is unclear. Most patients with the radiological findings of adult hypertrophic pyloric stenosis have concomitant peptic inflammatory disease and are men. Presentation with significant gastric outlet obstruction is unusual. The radiological findings have been described as mass effect in the pyloric region with an elongated pyloric channel measuring two to three times its normal length. A bulging mass in the base of the duodenum or antrum is commonly seen with this process (Fig. 2-11). *This condition should not be confused with prolapsed gastric mucosa, which is a transient finding in patients with antral gastritis* (Fig. 2-12). Prolapsing gastric mucosa is rarely, if ever, associated with gastric outlet obstruction.

A few patients show a small triangular outpouching of the antrum along the greater curvature, just proximal to the pyloric channel, called "Twining's recess." This outpouching represents a protrusion of mucosa between the hypertrophied circular torus muscles of the distal antrum. Twining's recess has been frequently associated with adult hypertrophic pyloric stenosis.

Gastric Volvulus

Gastric volvulus is an unusual condition in which the stomach undergoes a torsion abnormality as a result of twisting on itself. This twisting can occur around the luminal axis of the stomach (organoaxial) or around its mesentery on a plane perpendicular to its luminal axis (mesenteroaxial). These configurations almost always occur as a result of large hiatal hernias with migration of a large amount, if not all, of the stomach into an intrathoracic location (Fig. 2-13).

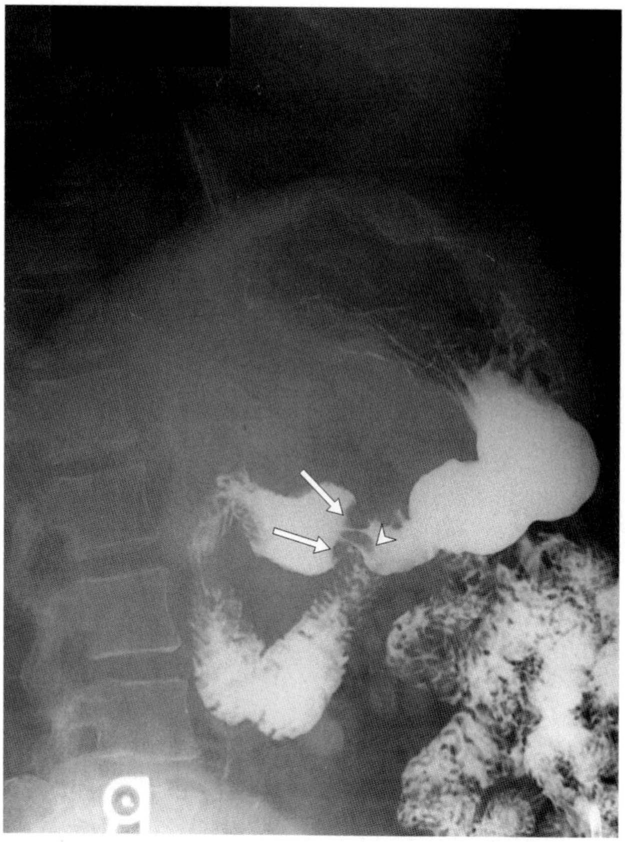

Figure 2-12 Gastric folds *(arrows)* prolapsed into base of mucosa. This occurs only with antral gastritis. Note thickened antral folds *(arrowhead)*.

Unless the degree of torsion is significant enough to result in luminal obstruction, these patients exhibit few symptoms. When obstruction does occur, it becomes a surgical emergency as a result of compromise of the blood supply (Fig. 2-14). Patients present with severe upper abdominal pain, severe chest pain, constant vomiting, and obstructive interference in attempts to pass a nasogastric tube.

Plain films of the abdomen and chest reveal findings typical of dilated air-filled proximal segments of the stomach either in the chest or in the upper abdomen. Barium studies show the abnormal positioning of the stomach as a result of the torsion abnormality. Attempts should be made to identify the relative positions of the lesser and greater curvature.

Duodenal Obstruction Resulting in Gastric Distention

Gastric distention and impaired outflow resulting from obstructive disease in the proximal duodenum are probably more common than those resulting from primary gastric disease. The most common of the duodenal processes resulting in a gastric outlet obstruction is peptic ulcer disease. Severe pancreatitis and pseudocysts with secondary involvement of the duodenum can also result in obstruction. In addition, pancreatic malignancy commonly invades the duodenum. Primary duodenal malignancy is rare, but does commonly present as obstruction with gastric distention. Other processes, such as lymphoma, duodenal adenoma, annular pancreas (Fig. 2-15), superior mesenteric artery syndrome, and intraluminal diverticulum, can also result in obstruction. These entities are covered in more detail in the duodenal section of this chapter.

Bouveret's Syndrome

The potential of erosion of gallstones into the gastrointestinal tract is well known. Most commonly, the erosion is into the duodenum, setting up the scenario of the so-called gallstone ileus, which is a mechanical obstruction (if the stone is large enough) in the most narrow part of the small bowel, the distal ileum. Occasionally, the stone may erode into the hepatic flexure of the colon. Even more rare is gallstone erosion into the distal stomach and obstruction at the pyloric channel and gastric outlet obstruction. This condition was first described by a French physician, Bouveret, in 1896 and bears his name.

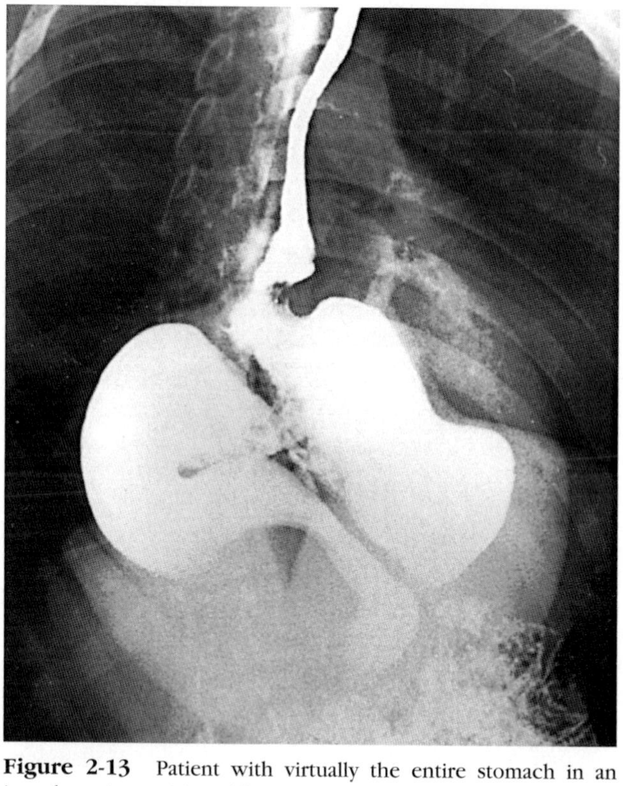

Figure 2-13 Patient with virtually the entire stomach in an intrathoracic position. There is an organoaxial configuration, although the stomach is not obstructed at this time.

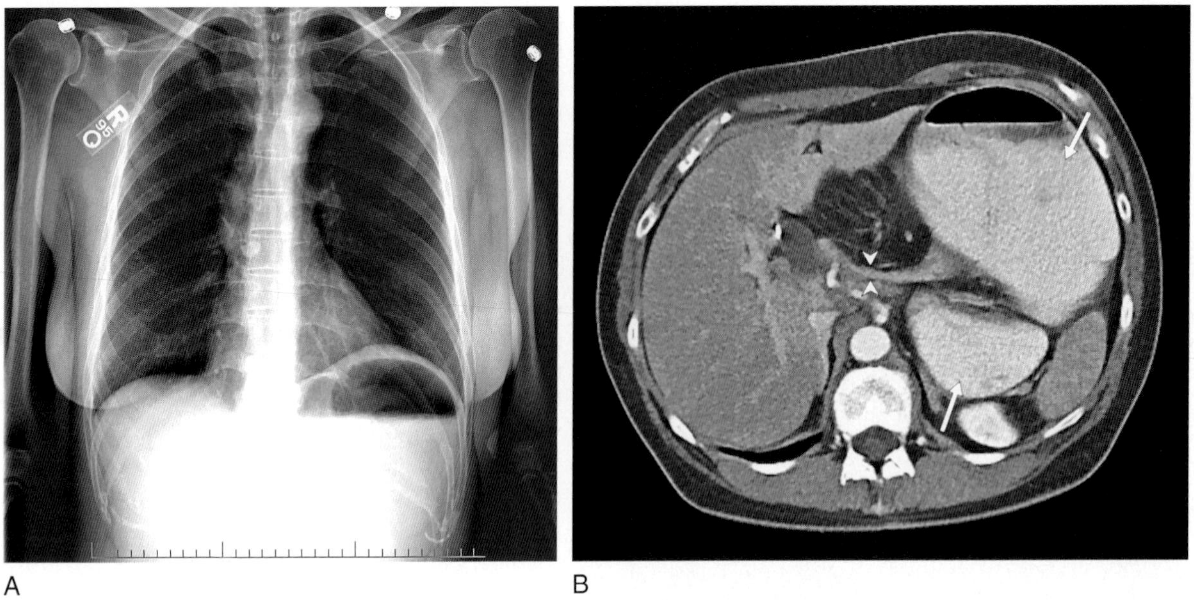

Figure 2-14 **A,** Upright chest film in a patient with gastric volvulus and obstruction shows volvulus to be under the diaphragm. **B,** Organoaxial volvulus of the stomach. Axial CT shows obstructed stomach *(arrows)* and torsion abnormality *(arrowheads)*.

Gastric Atony without Obstruction

Neuromuscular Abnormalities

In scleroderma (progressive systemic sclerosis), the entire bowel can be involved with the neuromuscular degenerative processes, resulting in diminished gut motility and subsequent stasis. As a result, it is possible for gastric distention to be observed in some of these patients. More commonly, distention of the esophagus, colon, and duodenum is encountered.

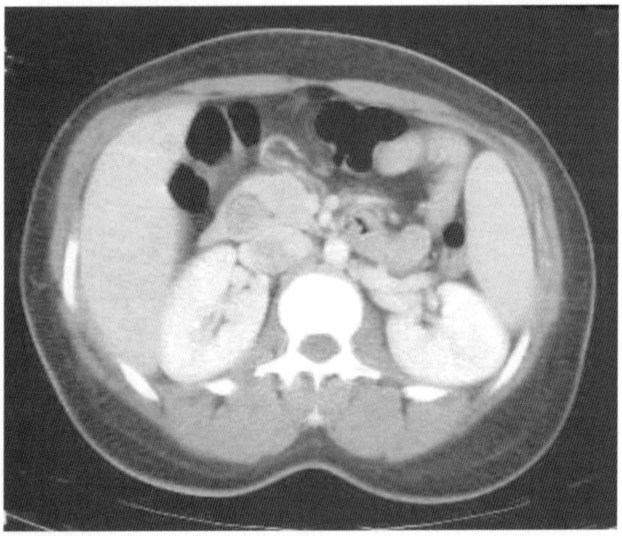

Figure 2-15 Incidental finding of annular pancreas in a patient with dilated common bile duct.

Chronic Idiopathic Intestinal Pseudoobstruction

For similar reasons thought to relate to diffuse neuromuscular dysfunction throughout the gut, chronic idiopathic intestinal pseudoobstruction also can result in abnormal gut motility, stasis, and distended portions of the gut. Although the small bowel and colon would predominate in this disorder, a few patients may manifest gastric distention as well.

Central Nervous System and Electrolyte Abnormalities

Patients with more central neurological abnormalities, such as tabes dorsalis or bulbar poliomyelitis, may develop degrees of gastric distention. Significant electrolyte and acid-base imbalances commonly can produce a transient distention of the colon and stomach with the impairment of contractility of the smooth muscle of the gut, probably secondary to hypokalemia.

Drug-Induced Atony

Gastric atony also can be drug induced and is often associated with atropine-like anticholinergic medications. Elderly and bedridden patients are particularly susceptible to drug-induced gastric atony. The use of glucagon rarely may induce acute gastric atony. This condition has been reported in a few patients receiving glucagon for routine UGI examinations. Patients with diabetes mellitus and significant degrees of diabetic peripheral neuropathy may manifest prominent gastric atony as a result of diminished neuromuscular function.

Agonal Atony

Acute massive gastric distention can be seen on abdominal radiographs of patients who are dying. The presence of this finding carries a bleak prognosis for survival beyond the next 48 hours. The exact cause of this finding is unclear. It may relate to severe and irreversible electrolyte imbalance or may be associated with major cardiovascular collapse. These patients are severely ill and are almost always unconscious. Clinical findings are limited to a distended tympanic upper abdomen. Nasogastric decompression does not alter the outcome. The radiological finding is a reflection of catastrophic systemic events that are occurring simultaneously.

Other Considerations

Another diagnostic consideration when one is faced with the radiological finding of gastric atony is aerophagia, which is not an unusual occurrence in patients undergoing acute severe emotional stress. Patients who have recently ingested large amounts of carbonated drinks may show gas in a distended stomach on plain films of the abdomen. The gas also should be well distributed throughout the remainder of the gut, however. Other considerations include porphyria and lead poisoning, both of which can result in degrees of gastric distention. In addition, degrees of gastric atony may be encountered in pregnant patients.

In patients with severe spinal deformity, chronic gastric distention has been described. The exact cause is not clear.

Contracted or Narrowed Stomach

A contracted, narrow stomach (Box 2-4) historically has been referred to as the "linitis plastica (leather bottle) stomach." This name generally implies that all or a large part of the stomach is involved by the pathological process, which results in a rigid, narrowed, contracted lumen. When not all of the stomach is involved, the proximal portion of the stomach is generally spared.

Box 2-4 Case of the Tapering Tube: The Contracted or Narrowed Stomach

Carcinoma, scirrhous type
Metastatic disease (especially breast and lung)
Chronic gastritis
Corrosive gastritis
Crohn's disease (ram's horn sign)
Zollinger-Ellison syndrome
Eosinophilic gastritis
Radiation
Sarcoidosis
Syphilis

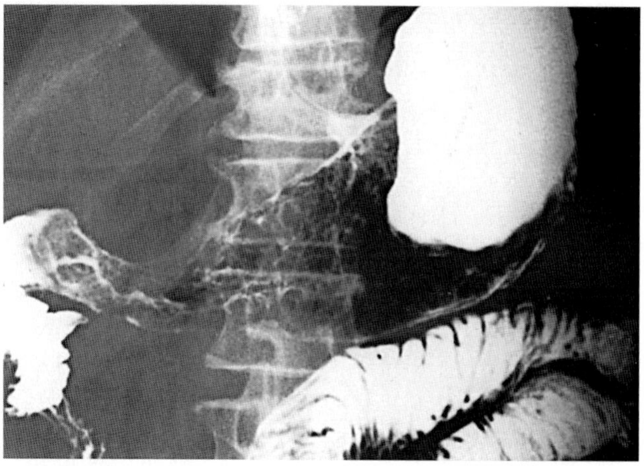

Figure 2-16 Gastric carcinoma involving the distal half of the stomach with narrowing, irregularity, and rigidity as a result of the desmoplastic changes induced by the neoplasm.

The problem of a contracted, narrowed stomach gives rise to the consideration of diffuse infiltrative changes in which the normal pliability and peristaltic activity of the stomach wall are impaired or absent. Any process that can excite a desmoplastic or fibrotic reaction within the gastric tissues, whether it be neoplastic or inflammatory in nature, can result in such a radiological appearance.

Scirrhous Carcinoma

The original description of the linitis plastica stomach was associated with an infiltrating scirrhous (desmoplastic) type of primary malignancy of the stomach. Although there are varied presentations of gastric carcinoma, the most common seems to be focal gastric wall thickening with or without ulceration. Diffuse infiltrative wall thickening, which results in a contracted, narrow stomach, is common, however, and generally has been identified in patients with less differentiated tumors and poorer prognoses (Fig. 2-16). There is also some evidence to suggest that this form may be more common in younger patients (Fig. 2-17).

The mortality rate and incidence of gastric cancer has declined steadily in the United States since the 1940s. Environmental factors that have been implicated in an increased incidence of gastric carcinoma in some parts of the world include an increase in salt consumption and an increase in ingestion of smoked meat and fish products and nitrosamines. There is a questionable increase in the incidence of gastric cancer in patients on long-term cimetidine therapy and in patients with chronic *Helicobacter pylori* gastritis. An unusual subset of *H. pylori* that may lead to achlorhydric states, atrophic gastritis, and

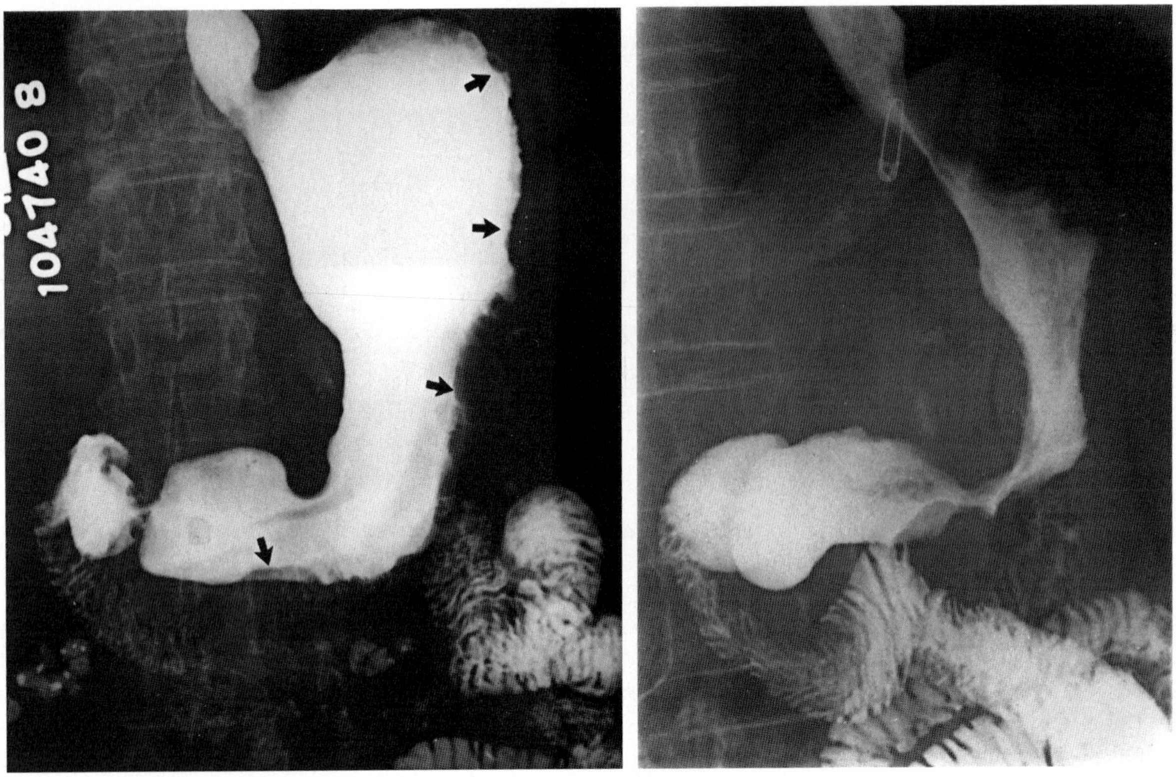

A B

Figure 2-17 Linitis plastica. **A,** Patient presents with abdominal pain and weight loss. UGI shows irregularity and rigidity of stomach wall along greater curve *(arrows)*. Patient refused treatment. **B,** Follow-up examination 11 months later discloses progression of the disease and typical appearance of linitis plastica with narrowing and rigidity of almost the entire stomach.

increased risk for gastric cancer has been described. Because of this subset, the World Health Organization designated *H. pylori* a type I carcinogen in the mid-1990s. Traditionally, precancerous conditions included pernicious anemia, chronic atrophic gastritis (which may be a reflection of chronic *H. pylori* infection), gastric adenomas, and possibly long-term postgastrectomy patients. Genetic disposition also is thought to account for approximately a third of all gastric cancers. First-degree relatives of index cases have a higher than normal risk for the disease. This risk is a part of the polyposis syndromes, which carry a higher risk of stomach cancer and a well-known risk of colon cancer. Patients with hereditary nonpolyposis colorectal cancer have an approximately 10% increased risk of gastric cancer.

The infiltrative form of gastric carcinoma results in diffuse thickening and rigidity of the stomach wall. The involved stomach has a tubular appearance, and a normal fold pattern is not discernible. At fluoroscopy, no peristaltic activity can be detected in the involved area. The infiltrating process usually starts in the pyloric antral region and extends proximally. It is unusual for the tumor to cross the pyloric channel into the duodenum.

Barium studies reveal the expected narrow, tubular, rigid, aperistaltic appearance of the involved portion of the stomach. Ulcerations may be present. A fold pattern is either absent or clearly abnormal. Multitrack CT is particularly helpful in the evaluation of gastric carcinoma and shows extension beyond the gastric wall and involvement of the adjacent perigastric, peripancreatic, and retroperitoneal lymph nodes, in addition to aiding in the evaluation of liver metastatic lesions (Fig. 2-18).

Metastatic Disease

Metastatic lesions of the stomach have a varied appearance. A common appearance is diffuse infiltrative scirrhous involvement of the stomach, which is indistinguishable from primary scirrhous carcinoma. The two major primary sites that result in infliltrative spread in the stomach are breast and lung. Metastatic disease from the breast involving the stomach has been described in 10% to 15% of patients. In more than half of these patients, the appearance of gastric involvement is of linitis plastica.

Involvement of the stomach by carcinoma of the pancreas as a result of contiguous spread, especially when it involves the distal stomach, also can give an appearance

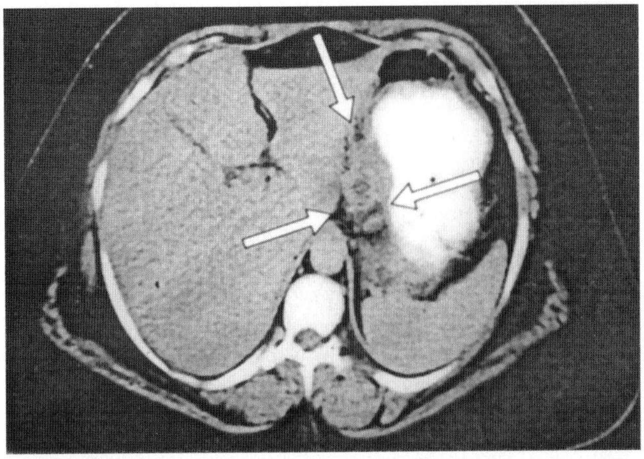

Figure 2-18 Axial computed tomographic scan through the distal stomach shows marked focal wall thickening *(arrows)* as a result of lymphomatous infiltration of the stomach.

of a narrow, rigid antrum. These changes are usually regional and are not widespread throughout the stomach, such as may be found in the primary or secondary hematogenous scirrhous lesions of the stomach.

Corrosive Gastritis

Patients who ingest strong corrosive materials, such as alkaline caustic agents, tend to have more esophageal damage than stomach damage. The ingestion of strong acids seems to involve the stomach to a greater extent; this is particularly true in the distal antrum and along the lesser curvature. The antrum and body can be involved circumferentially, however, giving a narrowed, rigid appearance. This involvement can be seen in the acute and chronic stages, with accompanying ulceration and mass effect. After healing, permanent stricturing and rigidity of the distal stomach are common findings, indistinguishable from infiltrating gastric carcinoma.

Extrinsic Compression of the Stomach

A retrogastric or retroperitoneal process causing sufficient compression or invasion of the stomach to result in a narrowed or contracted stomach is unusual. A large retroperitoneal tumor, such as leiomyosarcoma or liposarcoma, could result in such an appearance, however. In addition, significant splenomegaly associated with hepatomegaly could compress the stomach sufficiently to give a narrowed appearance (Fig. 2-19). A large left upper quadrant mass, such as a subphrenic abscess, could result in a similar appearance, with the gastric spasm resulting from adjacent inflammation. A large pancreatic mass, such as a pseudocyst, can compress the stomach posteriorly and give the impression of a narrowed lumen (Fig. 2-20). Other pancreatic lesions that could result in such an appearance include nonfunctioning islet cell tumors of the pancreas,

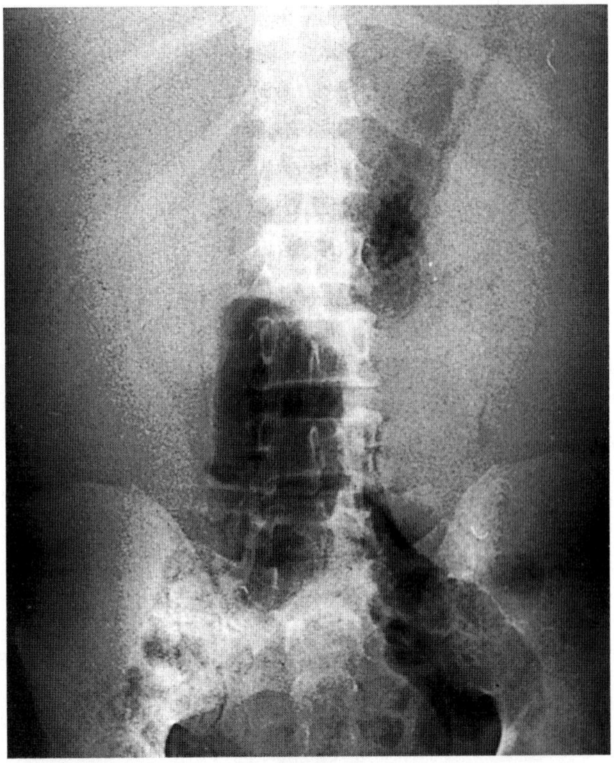

Figure 2-19 Patient with massive hepatosplenomegaly. Central compression of air-filled stomach is seen on plain film of the abdomen.

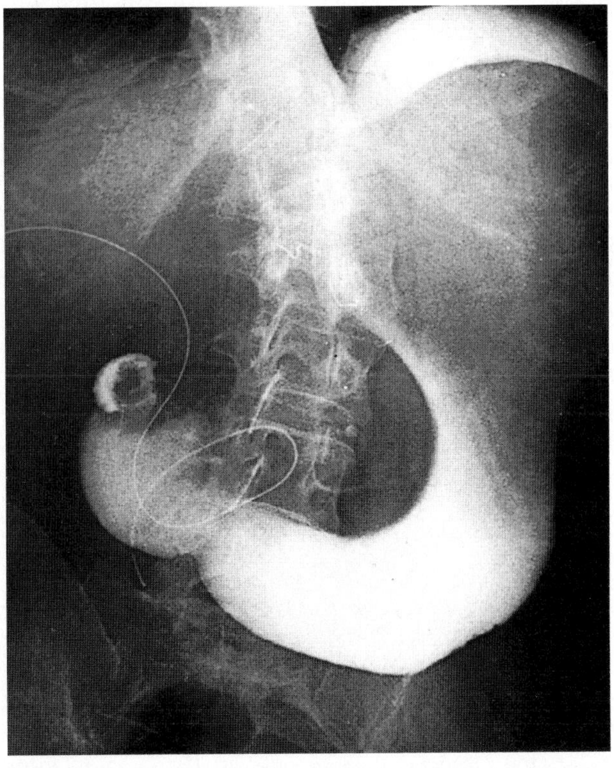

Figure 2-20 UGI examination shows large extrinsic impression on the fundus and proximal body of the stomach from huge pancreatic pseudocyst.

which can grow to great size; acute or chronic pancreatitis; and cystadenomas of the pancreas.

Lymphoma

Although the common appearance of lymphoma is generally wall thickening, mass effect, and ulceration, the occasional lymphomatous lesion of the stomach can be diffusely infiltrative and result in a severe desmoplastic reaction so that the radiological appearance is identical to that of scirrhous adenocarcinoma (Fig. 2-21). This appearance is seen especially in Hodgkin's-type lesions. Computed tomographic scanning for lymphoma has become the imaging mainstay for this lesion and is particularly useful for evaluation of wall thickening, perigastric nodal disease, and liver, spleen, and renal involvement (Fig. 2-22). There is some evidence that intraluminal endoscopic ultrasound may be more sensitive in detecting intramural and perigastric disease.

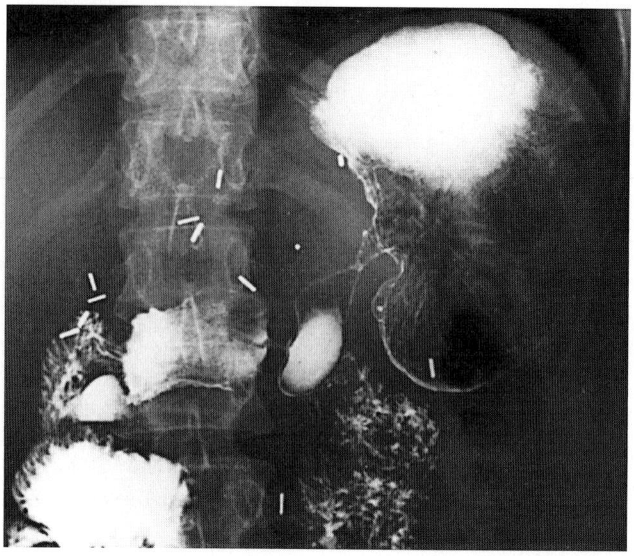

Figure 2-21 UGI examination in a patient with Hodgkin's disease of the stomach. Note the marked narrowing and irregularity of the distal stomach.

Crohn's Disease

Severe involvement of the stomach with Crohn's disease causing narrowing and rigidity of the stomach is unusual. The classic appearance of the narrow distal stomach and widened normal proximal stomach has given rise to the historical description of the "ram's horn" stomach of Crohn's disease. This stenotic involvement of severe disease in the distal stomach may or may not result in gastric outlet obstruction. The presence of Crohn's disease in the stomach is almost always associated with involvement of the small bowel or colon. Involvement of the stomach in patients with Crohn's disease should be differentiated from *H. pylori*-negative peptic ulcer disease, which has been shown to be increased in patients with proximal Crohn's disease. Proximal disease also is thought to present earlier than distal disease with UGI-type symptoms.

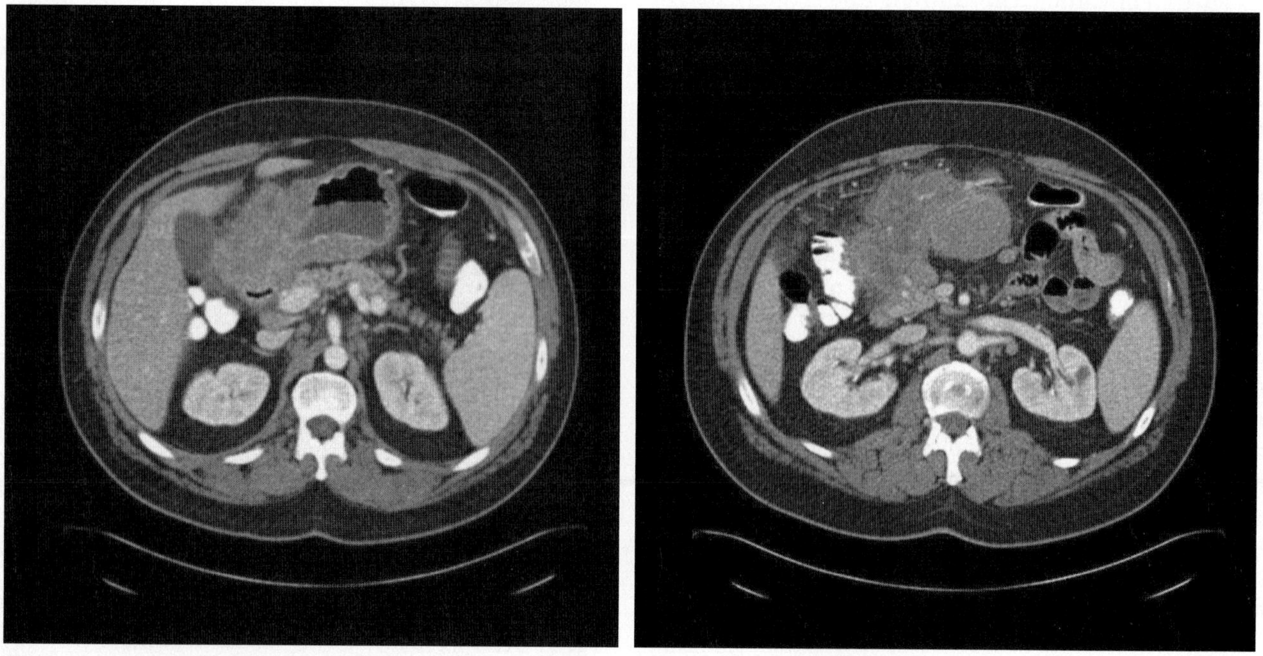

A B

Figure 2-22 **A,** Large nonobstructing gastric lymphoma involving distal stomach. **B,** Same patient. Axial CT reveals significant amount of extragastric disease.

Zollinger-Ellison Syndrome

Zollinger-Ellison syndrome results from the presence of a non–beta islet cell (gastrinoma) tumor of the head of the pancreas or (less commonly) ectopic pancreatic tissue in the proximal duodenum that continuously secretes gastrin. The high levels of this hormone result in an increased stimulus of the gastric parietal cells to form and secrete hydrochloric acid, resulting in marked hyperacidity of the stomach and proximal small bowel. The severe inflammatory changes involving the stomach are usually manifested by multiple ulcerations, thickened folds, and hypersecretion. The presence of chronic inflammation throughout the stomach, particularly in the distal stomach, can result in a narrowed, contracted appearance. Additional radiological findings that may suggest the diagnosis include proximal small bowel ulcerations and history of recurrent intractable ulcer disease.

Of the islet cell lesions, 50% are malignant, with metastatic disease present within the liver at the time of presentation. About a third of patients with Zollinger-Ellison syndrome fall within the multiple endocrine neoplasia type I syndrome, also known as Wermer's syndrome. In addition, the primary neoplasms are often small (most <2 cm), and many of these were not detectable on routine computed tomographic scanning until more recently. Advances in multiple-track detectors (multitrack CT) and better and more efficient imaging in the arterial phase have resulted in improved detection with CT. In general, the larger the gastrinoma, the more likely it is to have metastasized to the liver. In approximately 60% of cases, the lesions are multiple. The lesions also may be detected on angiographic studies of the pancreaticoduodenal region as a result of their hypervascularity. This same vascularity is making multitrack CT more efficient, however, to the point that angiographic studies are expected to diminish as a diagnostic tool in the workup of these patients in the future. Additionally, since it was discovered that gastrinomas possess somatostatin receptor sites, radiolabeled somatostatin for the detection of gastrinoma (Fig. 2-23) has been used as a cellular target–specific substance to identify the lesion on nuclear studies. The method has shown sensitivity in detection of gastrinomas exceeding 75%. This method also holds out the hope of being able to use the same approach for delivering therapeutic agents to the same site on the tumor at some point in the future. In the past, the procedure of choice was to remove the entire target organ, which is represented by the parietal cell–containing portions of the stomach. As pharmaceutical advances in gastric acid suppression have occurred, however, the number of gastric surgeries has decreased, and surgical management has been directed to the resection of the gastrinoma, if possible.

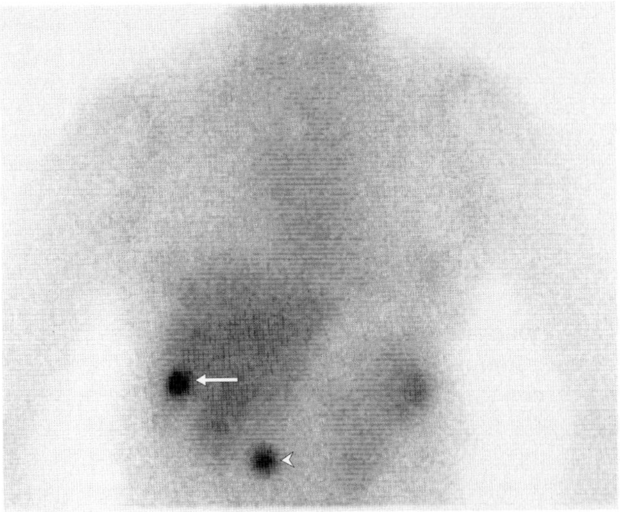

Figure 2-23 Indium-111 octreotide (somatostatin) images. A 55-year-old woman with a several-month history of abdominal pain and recent weight loss. Laboratory studies were suggestive of gastrinoma. After a 6-mCi dose of indium-111 pentetreotide, 4-hour and 24-hour delayed planar images were obtained. Primary lesion shows primary gastrinoma in pancreas *(arrow)* and gastrinoma liver metastatic lesion *(arrowhead)*.

Eosinophilic Gastritis

Eosinophilic infiltration of the muscular layers of the distal stomach can result in a narrowed, contracted antrum and body (Fig. 2-24). The appearance can be similar to that of malignancy. Patients usually have an associated peripheral eosinophilia and a history of food allergies. The infiltration can result in erosions, ulceration, and subsequent anemia. Affected patients also may show elevated IgE levels. Proximal small bowel involvement may be present, although isolated gastric involvement is not unusual. The disorder usually responds well to daily doses of steroids.

Radiation Injury

A narrowed, contracted stomach may be the sequela of radiation injury to the stomach. Radiation doses greater than 5000 cGy involving the stomach result in an acute inflammatory response, with resultant healing that may include ulceration and extensive fibrosis.

Sarcoidosis

Although involvement of the gastrointestinal tract in sarcoidosis is unusual, the stomach is the most commonly affected site. Often, patients are asymptomatic. In chronic severe involvement, the possibility of contracture and narrowing of the stomach increases (Fig. 2-25), and it may be indistinguishable from linitus plastica, gastric tuberculosis, Crohn's disease, or secondary syphilis.

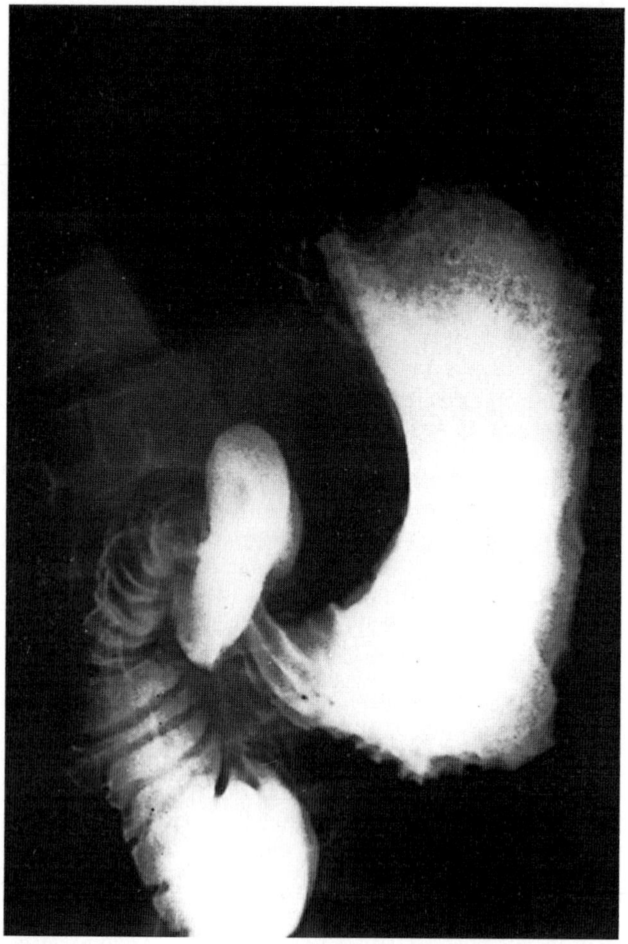

Figure 2-24 UGI study in patient with eosinophilic gastroenteritis shows a contracted and rigid stomach with some irregularity along the greater curvature. The findings could easily be interpreted as malignant infiltration.

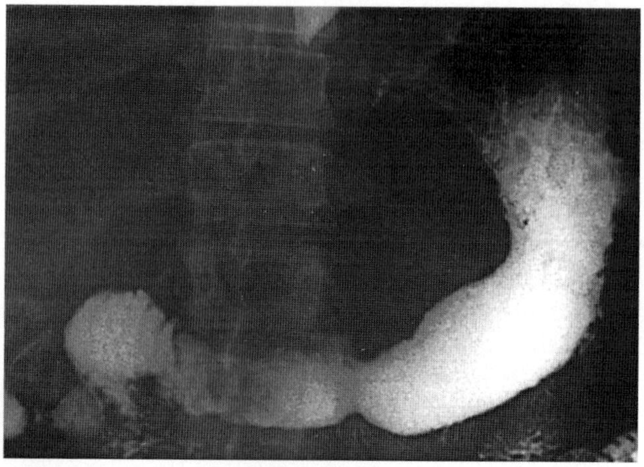

Figure 2-25 UGI study in patient with diffuse involvement of the stomach with sarcoidosis, resulting in a tubular, narrowed stomach.

Hepatic Artery Infusion Chemotherapy

The increasing use of hepatic artery infusion of chemotherapeutic and cytotoxic agents has resulted in increased incidence of resultant inflammatory changes within the stomach. Despite attempts to control the flow of the chemotherapeutic agents and to reduce deleterious flow to the stomach, the vascular arterial anatomy in the region of the celiac axis can be quite variable, and occasionally some of the agent is delivered to the gastric wall, with resultant marked inflammatory changes. The inflammatory changes tend to regress with the termination of the therapy.

Phlegmonous Gastritis

Phlegmonous gastritis, although common in the early part of the 20th century, is rare today. It is a suppurative bacterial infection and invasion of the stomach that results in marked thickening of the stomach wall and mucosa. Most reported cases are associated with alpha-hemolytic streptococci, although other organisms, including staphylococci, pneumococci, and some of the more common gram-negative organisms, also have been shown to be involved. Often, when there is associated emphysematous gastritis, clostridial organisms or gram-negative bacteria have been implicated. Ulceration and instrumentation can also result in intramural air in the stomach wall (Fig. 2-26). The exact underlying cause of this condition is unclear, although many causes have been suggested, including ischemia, ulceration, gastric malignancy, and ingestion of corrosive material or large amounts of concentrated alcohol. The treatment consists of

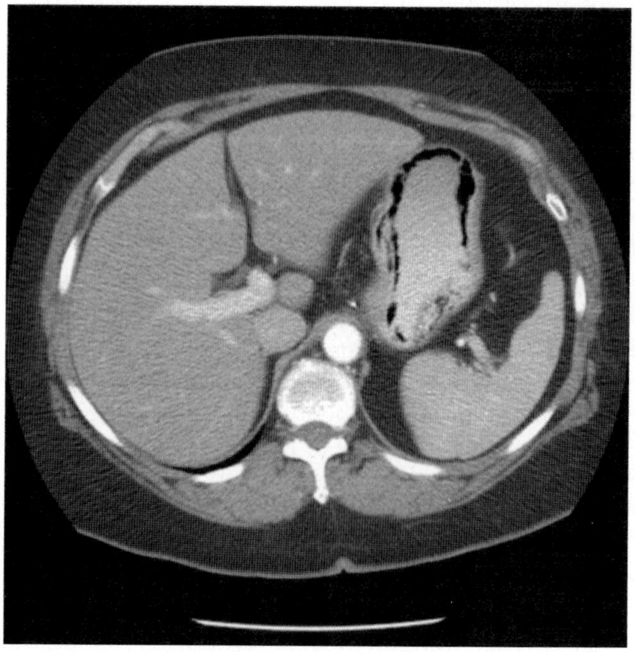

Figure 2-26 Air in gastric wall.

vigorous antibiotic therapy and prompt surgical intervention; the mortality approaches 60% when treated appropriately.

Tuberculosis

Involvement of the stomach with tuberculosis is rare, but can occur, particularly in the pyloric antral region. Wall thickening, rigidity, and a contracted lumen may be seen.

Syphilis

Involvement of the stomach with syphilis is rare, although this manifestation is seen occasionally. Involvement may be identical to that of peptic ulcer disease with erosive changes, ulceration, and thickened folds. Additionally, a contracted, narrowed, deformed stomach has been described in chronic involvement.

Thickened Gastric Folds

In the normal, adequately distended stomach, the folds in the fundal region usually measure approximately 1 cm or less in thickness. As they descend toward the body and antrum of the stomach, the folds become increasingly narrow and ribbon-like, until the prepyloric antral folds are found to be 5 mm or less in diameter. The folds should be symmetrical without nodularity, focal thickening, or areas of discontinuity. The fold pattern in the region of the gastric cardia and along the greater curvature of the body can be complex and at times difficult to evaluate.

Focal Thickening

Peptic Gastritis

Peptic gastritis can present as widespread diffuse thickening of the gastric folds, although the much more common presentation is fold thickening in the antrum and possibly the distal body (Fig. 2-27). The folds can be nodular. There may or may not be ulceration or evidence of erosions. Folds that are beaded in appearance generally have small erosions along their course (Fig. 2-28). The beading process is secondary to the focal edematous changes around the erosions. These erosions commonly may be seen on double-contrast study. Meticulous attention to detail and use of flow technique often show the erosions (Fig. 2-29). When the involvement is throughout the stomach, some consideration should be given to Zollinger-Ellison syndrome, particularly if there is duodenal and proximal small bowel involvement (Fig. 2-30).

Aspirin-Induced and Nonsteroidal Antiinflammatory Drug-Induced Gastritis

The increasing use of aspirin and the availability of over-the-counter nonsteroidal antiinflammatory drugs (NSAIDs) are expected to increase the frequency of aspirin-induced and NSAID-induced gastritis (Fig. 2-31). These changes tend to be localized in the antral and body region, although diffuse involvement is possible. Although most of the damage caused by these drugs relates to local mucosal irritation and erosions, the process seems to be more complicated. Alterations, as a result of aspirin-induced changes in the gastric mucosal barrier, have been described, along with loss of blood across the barrier unrelated to ulcer or erosion formation. There also seem to be higher incidences of peptic mucosal erosions and ulcer disease. Patients with chronic rheumatic disease taking significant doses of aspirin have a 50% increased incidence of gastric erosions and a 20% increase in gastric ulcers (Fig. 2-32). The use of enteric-coated forms of aspirin is helpful in dealing with the local and erosive effects. It probably has little impact, however, on the systemic effect of the drug on the stomach wall. Aside from the emergence of *H. pylori* as the major factor in the development of gastritis and peptic ulcer disease, NSAIDs and aspirin are probably the next most important factor. Of patients routinely taking over-the-counter NSAIDs, 2% to 4% experience bleeding from silent gastric erosions. If one considers the availability of over-the-counter NSAIDs and the millions of individuals who routinely use them in the United States, this probably accounts for many

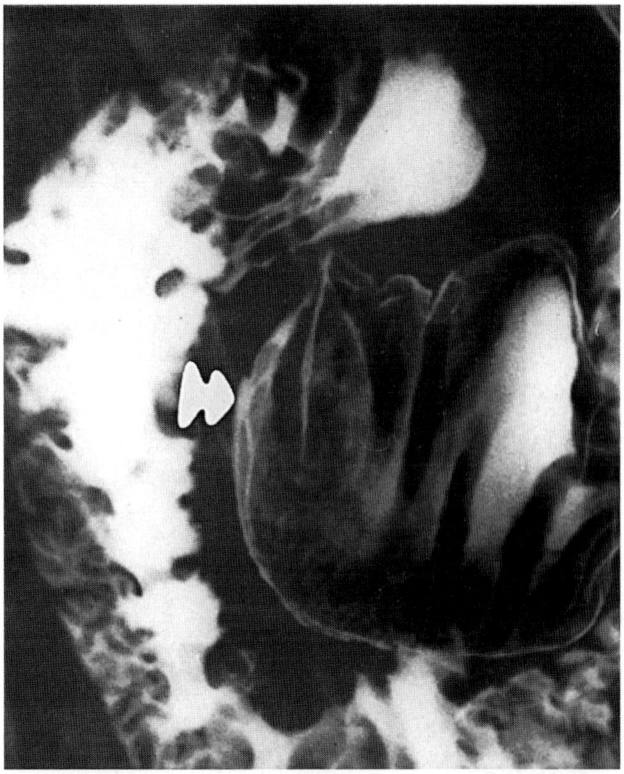

Figure 2-27 Spot film from gastric antrum shows transverse thickened gastric folds representing peptic gastritis. A tiny shallow ulcer is seen along the greater curvature *(arrow)*.

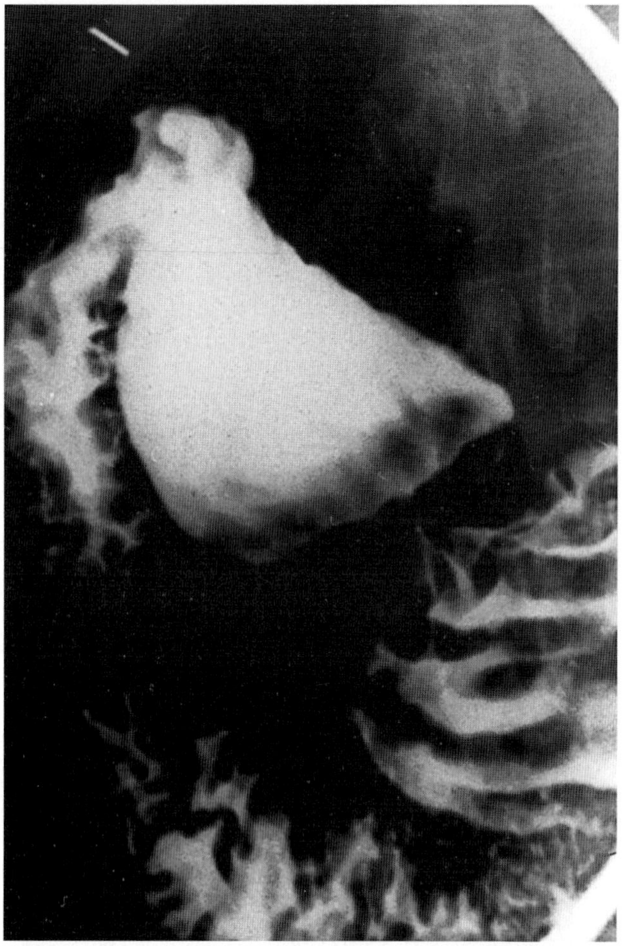

Figure 2-28 Spot film from the gastric antrum and duodenum shows thickened, beaded appearance of the folds in the gastric antrum, almost always associated with tiny erosions along the folds.

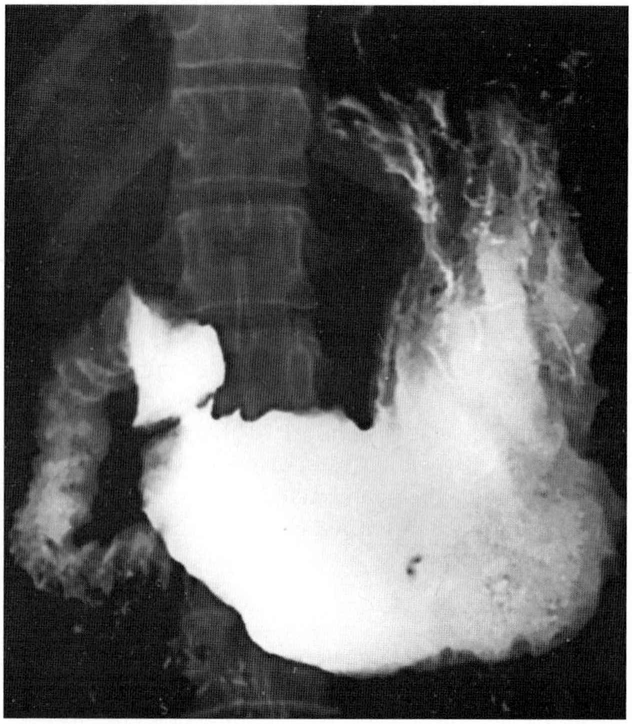

Figure 2-30 Patient with Zollinger-Ellison syndrome shows abnormalities of the stomach in UGI study with diffuse fold thickening, hypersecretion, and multiple small ulcers.

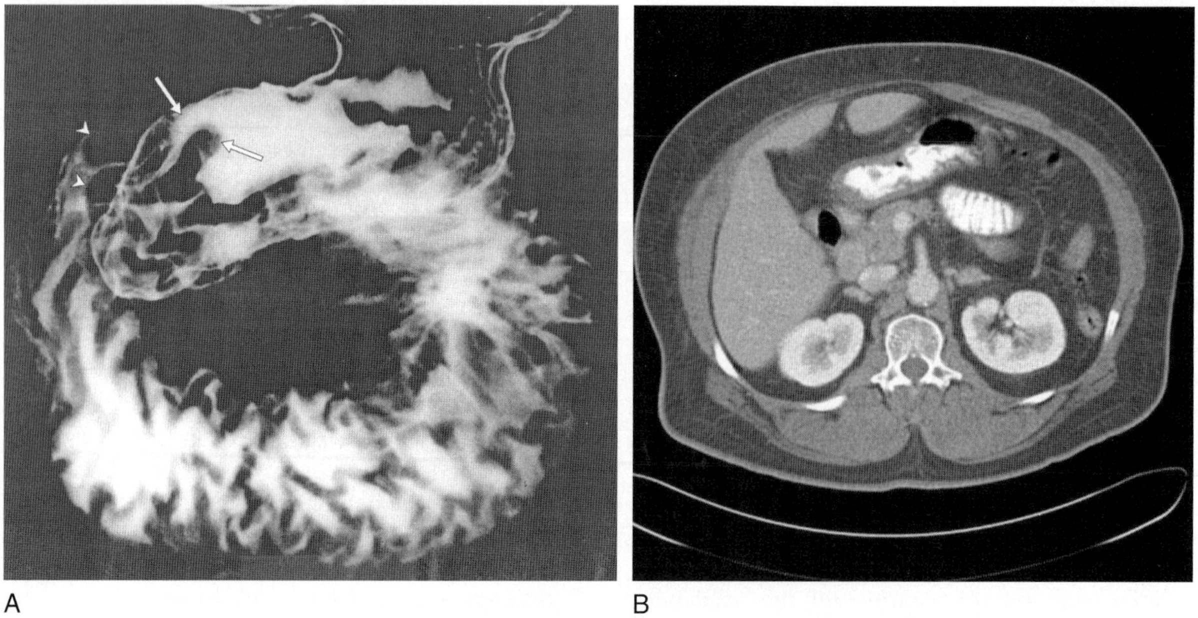

Figure 2-29 **A,** Prominent thickened antral folds in a patient with antral gastritis. **B,** Axial CT in this patient shows thickened antral wall secondary to inflammation.

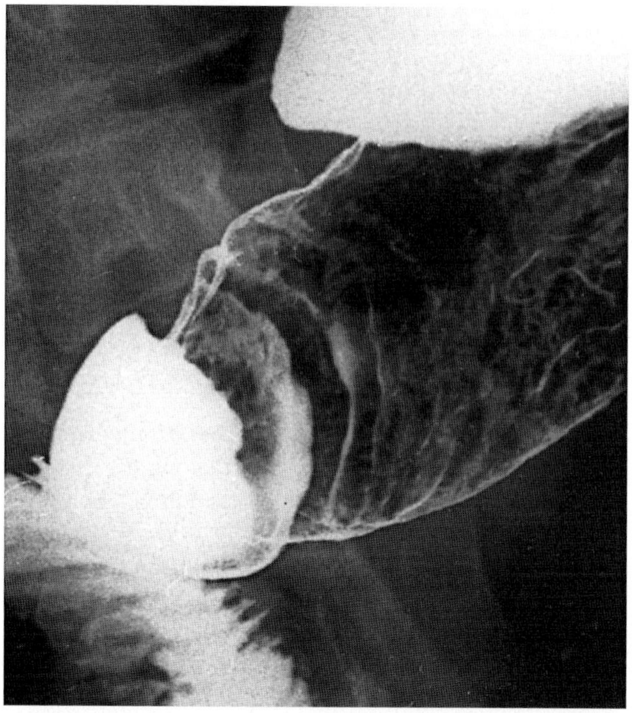

Figure 2-31 Patient taking high doses of NSAIDs complained of abdominal pain. UGI study shows transverse thickened folds in the antrum of the stomach.

of the Hemoccult-positive patients worked up for colorectal cancer who turn out to have false-positive Hemoccult tests.

Corrosive Gastritis

Ingestion of acid-corrosive materials can give rise to focal inflammatory changes within the distal stomach. The appearance can vary, but focal fold thickening is one manifestation. This condition is often associated with ulceration.

Hypertrophic Gastritis

Hypertrophic gastritis is thought to represent a widening of the folds secondary to mucosal hyperplastic changes of the epithelial cells (Fig. 2-33). The cause and prevalence of this entity are controversial, and the changes are thought to relate to chronic inflammation. It may be focal or diffuse and tends to be chronic in nature. In a patient with thickened gastric folds, possibly associated with hyperacidity and without a significant history of alcohol ingestion, hypertrophic gastritis is a differential consideration. Other types of gastritis can present with focal thickening of the fold pattern and include entities such as herpetic gastritis and gastric candidiasis.

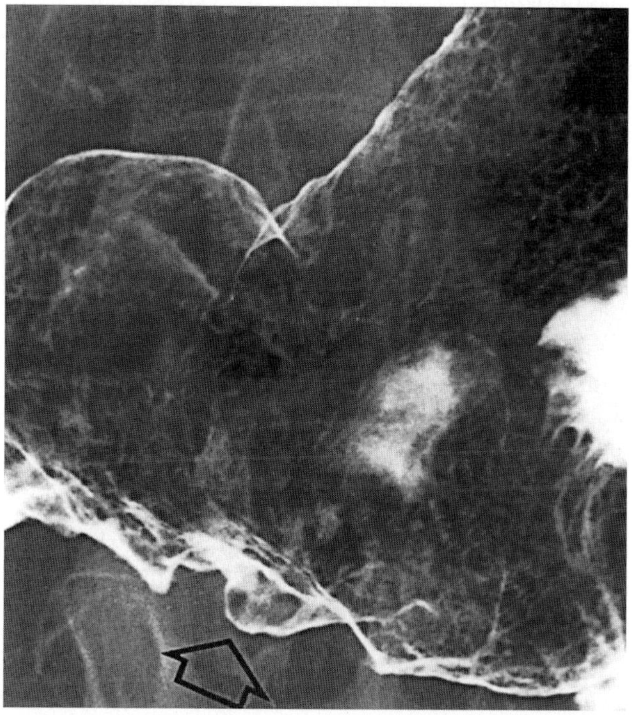

Figure 2-32 UGI study in patient with abdominal pain and bleeding being treated with high doses of aspirin for arthritic disease. An area of mass, with irregularity and ulceration, is seen along the greater curvature of the stomach *(arrow)*. The ulcer does not project beyond the confines and is extremely suspicious. The biopsy specimen was entirely benign. The patient improved rapidly with withdrawal of the medication.

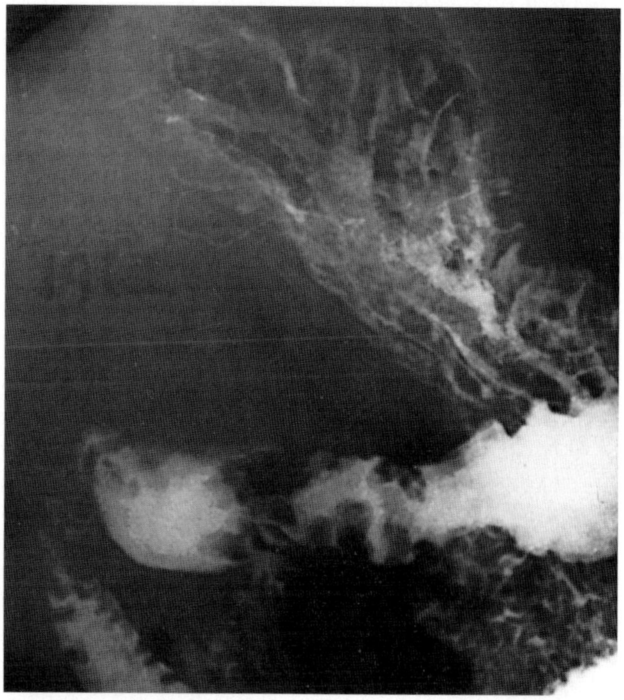

Figure 2-33 UGI study in patient with history of chronic abdominal pain shows diffuse fold thickening throughout the stomach. Biopsy specimen showed epithelial hyperplastic changes of hypertrophic gastritis.

Helicobacter ***Gastritis***

In the early 1980s, researchers in Australia isolated *H. pylori* from the stomach and suggested the possibility of a relationship among the bacteria, gastritis, and peptic ulcer disease. Since then, the literature has abounded with additional research regarding the role of *H. pylori* in an array of gastrointestinal diseases. The isolation of the bacteria and the exploration of its potential role in the pathogenesis of disease have been among the most important developments in gastroenterology in the past 2 decades. Today, there is general consensus that *H. pylori* is linked etiologically to the development of certain types of gastritis and most peptic ulcer disease. The inoculation of volunteers' stomachs with the organism and the subsequent development of mucosal inflammation and the resolution of disease after the eradication of the organism have provided fundamental scientific evidence of the etiological relationship. Some interesting questions remain, however. The prevalence of the organism is widespread, and it can be found in the stomachs of many asymptomatic individuals. In most instances, there may be evidence of some mucosal inflammation, but only a few individuals develop symptomatic peptic ulcer disease. Although before the 1980s the stomach was thought to be a sterile environment, the presence of this organism in the human stomach has been known since the early days of microbiology and bacteriology in the late 19th century. In patients with the organism in the stomach, there is no evidence of bacterial proliferation or invasiveness common to most bacterial infections. Is *H. pylori* the one and only issue in peptic disease, or is it a major factor in a multifactorial pathological process? It has been shown that the incidence of gastroesophageal reflux disease increases with the eradication of *H. pylori* from the stomach: Could this be a factor in the increasing incidence of Barrett's metaplasia and adenocarcinoma of the esophagus (see Chapter 1)? Despite fulfilling Koch's criteria of being a pathogen, there are still many puzzling questions surrounding the oraganism.

How does *H. pylori* cause mucosal damage? Research in this area has suggested three possible mechanisms (Box 2-5):

- *Local tissue injury.* The bacteria produce several toxins that may cause local mucosal damage. Among these is urea, which is the basis for the current breath test for the presence of the organism.
- *Elevated gastrin levels with resultant increased acid secretion. H. pylori* may contribute to elevated gastrin levels by interfering with the cellular process that limits the amount of gastrin being produced. Although the research in this area has been interesting, it is currently inconclusive and contradictory because there is also evidence that *H. pylori* decreases gastric acid.
- *Focal mucosal immune response. H. pylori* seems to recruit white blood cells to the mucosa, possibly resulting in the inflammatory response.

Box 2-5 *Helicobacter pylori*: Theories on Mechanisms of Mucosal Tissue Damage

May cause focal tissue injury owing to bacteria-produced toxins
May cause elevated gastrin levels and resultant increased acid secretion
May cause local mucosal inflammation by increasing presence of white blood cells focally

H. pylori has been implicated in more than peptic inflammatory disease. It is now considered an important risk factor in the development of gastric carcinoma. The organism is frequently seen with gastric carcinoma and is most prevalent in geographical locations and ethnic groups that have known high incidences of gastric carcinoma. Some authors have suggested that harboring the bacteria in the upper gut from an early age is an important factor in determining the risk for malignancy. As previously indicated, the World Health Organization has designated *H. pylori* as a class 1 carcinogen.

H. pylori also has been determined to be the cause of the rare low-grade gastric mucosa–associated lymphoid tissue lymphoma. It has been reported that the eradication of the bacteria alone, without any other treatments, can lead to regression of gastric mucosa–associated lymphoid tissue lymphoma in most patients.

H. pylori can be diagnosed by a variety of means, of which the gold standard is considered to be endoscopic biopsy of the stomach. This diagnosis can be achieved either by staging the specimen with Giemsa, silver, or Genta stains to show the organism or by "rapid urease tests," which indicate the presence of the bacteria through color change when exposed to the biopsy specimen. The diagnosis also can be made through serological testing or the urea breath test. The latter is about 95% sensitive and can be read in 10 to 30 minutes.

What is the role of radiology in the diagnosis of *H. pylori* gastritis or ulcer disease? On the surface, the UGI examination—even the high-quality, double-contrast technique—seems to offer little and is of no value with respect to the presence or absence of the bacteria. In the ever-accelerating era of cost containment and capitated health care, however, the UGI examination may make a significant contribution to the diagnosis and treatment of *H. pylori* disease of the stomach and duodenum. As mentioned earlier, the UGI examination cannot detect the presence of the bacteria, but if quality double-contrast imaging is undertaken, it is good in detecting erosive and

Box 2-6 *Helicobacter pylori*: What We Know/What We Do Not Know

High incidence in gastric ulcers
Low incidence in duodenal ulceration
Does not invade gastric mucosa, is found in mucous layer
Eradication leads to improvement of symptoms
Infection of uninfected stomach results in inflammatory disease
Some carriers of *H. pylori* are asymptomatic
Eradication may lead to increased incidence of gastroesophageal reflux disease
Detection can be by biopsy, blood serum test, or breath test

nonerosive gastritis. Enlarged gastric folds or nodular folds are a common finding on the double-contrast UGI examination. Although these findings cannot establish the absence or presence of *H. pylori,* the bacteria have been found in approximately 50% of patients with enlarged folds (Box 2-6). The radiological examination has a place in a diagnostic algorithm that can provide effective diagnosis and treatment of *H. pylori* infection of the stomach in a less costly and less invasive manner than an endoscopic survey on potential multitudes of patients. Thickened or nodular folds in the gastric antrum seem to be the best indicators of the possible presence of *H. pylori*. A test for *H. pylori* can be undertaken in such patients who have no symptoms or signs that might suggest malignancy. If positive, eradication therapy can be started, and a repeat UGI examination may be undertaken to assess for change. If folds have returned to normal, no further workup or treatment is indicated. If folds remain enlarged or are increasing in size, endoscopy in indicated. In such an algorithm, much refinement is possible. Nevertheless, the potential exists for considerable savings. The very low risk of carcinoma and its decline with the eradication of the bacteria have not resulted in the need for widespread endoscopic screening. Unless double-contrast UGI examinations are of consistently high quality, however, the resurgence of the radiological examination as an important factor in the workup of *H. pylori* will not occur. It may happen only sporadically in areas where gastrointestinal radiology is practiced with consistent excellence. The radiological community would be well advised to note the exceptional opportunity and act accordingly.

The most widely used treatment for the eradication of *H. pylori* consists of a bismuth-based triple therapy. This therapy usually consists of a 2-week course of colloidal bismuth, metronidazole, and tetracycline or amoxicillin and cessation of NSAIDs if possible.

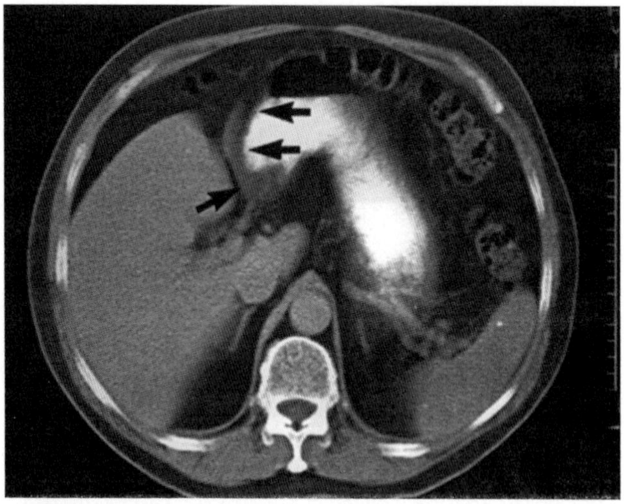

Figure 2-34 Patient with weight loss and decreased appetite. Computed tomographic scan of upper abdomen shows focal wall thickening along the greater curvature of the distal stomach *(arrows)*. Biopsy specimen showed adenocarcinoma of the stomach.

Carcinoma

Irregular focal thickening is an unusual presentation of carcinoma of the stomach (Fig. 2-34). The most common presentation tends to be a mass with ulceration. Thickened irregular folds, usually limited to one portion of the stomach and indistinguishable from gastric lymphoma, are not a rare finding, however, in gastric carcinoma (Fig. 2-35).

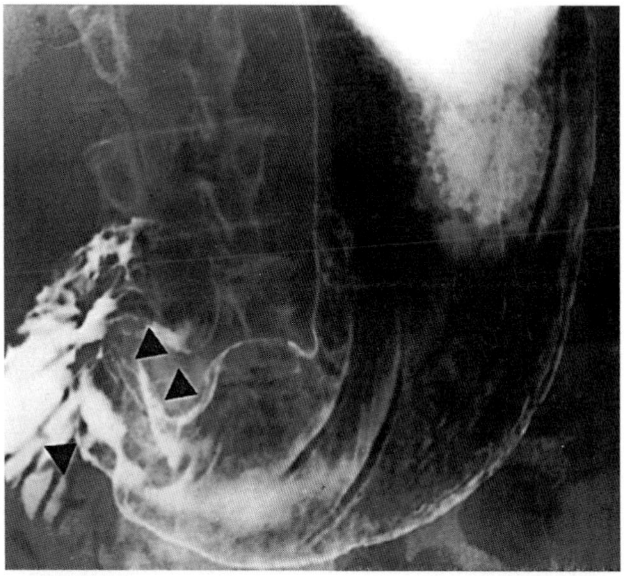

Figure 2-35 UGI study in patient with abdominal pain and weight loss shows some slight narrowing of the distal stomach with thickened nodular folds through the area *(arrowheads)*. Biopsy specimen confirmed the diagnosis of gastric carcinoma.

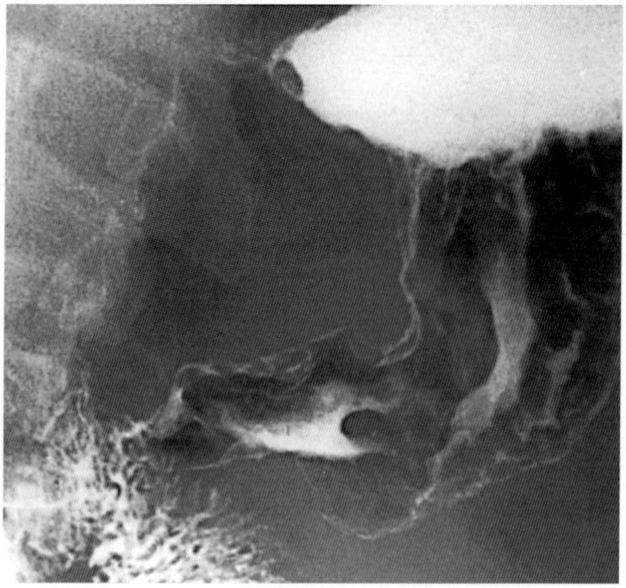

Figure 2-36 Patient with diffuse lymphomatous involvement of the stomach. Marked thickening and nodularity and distortion of the folds throughout the distal two thirds of the stomach are seen.

Lymphoma

The most common presentation of lymphoma is a thickened, distorted, nodular gastric fold pattern (Fig. 2-36). This pattern may or may not be associated with a mass effect or ulceration. There may be a degree of residual distensibility and pliability that may help distinguish lymphoma from carcinoma. The definitive diagnosis requires biopsy, however. Extension across the pyloric channel into the duodenal bulb tends to be more common with lymphoma than with carcinoma, although one should bear in mind that lymphoma represents 5% or less of gastric malignancies. In actuality, most lesions that cross the pylorus are adenocarcinomas. Associated findings that may be seen with lymphoma include extrinsic masses associated with aggregates of lymphomatous nodes or an enlarged spleen.

Pseudolymphoma

Lymphoreticular hyperplasia of the stomach (pseudolymphoma or lymphoreticular gastritis) can present with findings of focal fold thickening. These benign lesions almost always have the radiological appearance of malignancy, with most common findings being mass and ulceration. Cases of infiltrative lesions with associated focal fold thickening have been reported, however. Anemia is a common finding, and the average age of the patient is slightly younger than seen in gastric carcinoma.

Metastatic Disease

Metastatic disease presenting with focal fold thickening is unusual but does occur (Fig. 2-37). Focal fold thickening may be seen in the early metastatic involvement of the stomach with breast or lung lesions. Leukemic involvement of the stomach may result in a focal or diffuse thickening of gastric folds. Direct contiguous spread of carcinoma of the pancreas to the stomach also can produce a radiological pattern of focal gastric fold thickening along the greater curvature.

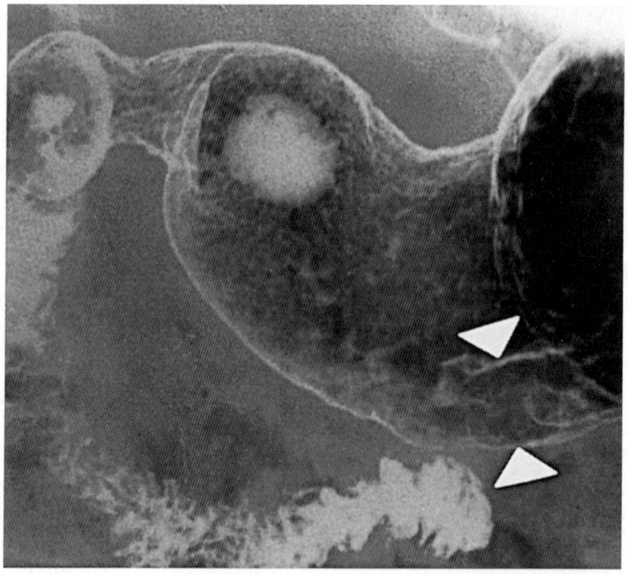

Figure 2-37 UGI examination in patient with history of breast cancer. There are chronic changes seen in the distal stomach. There is an area of focal fold thickening and nodularity *(arrowheads)*; however, that proved to be a focal metastatic lesion.

Crohn's Disease

Crohn's involvement of the stomach may manifest as fold thickening in the antral region. Superficial erosions also may be detected.

Pancreatitis

A relatively common cause of fold thickening within the distal stomach relates to inflammatory disease in the adjacent pancreas. Folds along the greater curvature of the body and in the antrum may be enlarged and nodular, as a result of contiguous inflammatory changes. More severe disease may result in more widespread gastric changes (Fig. 2-38).

Ménétrier's disease

Ménétrier's disease is a relatively rare condition of unknown cause. It is characterized by prominence and tortuosity of the gastric mucosal fold pattern. At one time, this disease was thought to be an antral-sparing process, although more recently degrees of antral involvement have been shown. The preponderance of changes seems to be in the proximal stomach, however. The process is associated with increased protein loss from the stomach and diminished gastric acid production. The disease is generally detected in individuals between 30 and 60 years of age and tends to be more common in men. Presenting complaints include epigastric pain, anorexia, and weight loss. The radiological pattern shows a large, tortuous fold pattern predominantly proximally and with sparing of the antrum in most cases. There also is some evidence of hypersecretion within the stomach.

Gastric Varices

Gastric varices can readily cause apparent thickening of the gastric folds, particularly in the proximal fundal region of the stomach (Fig. 2-39). These are commonly seen in association with significant portal hypertension and in patients with splenic vein thrombosis. The radiological findings usually are those of a smooth, thickened, proximal fold pattern most prominent in the fundus, but they can be seen more distally. Esophageal varices can be shown by increasing the venous distention of the varices through various techniques associated with patient positioning and respiration and usually are easily seen on CT (Fig. 2-40). These techniques tend to be less useful in gastric varices, and this is particularly the case in patients with splenic vein thrombosis.

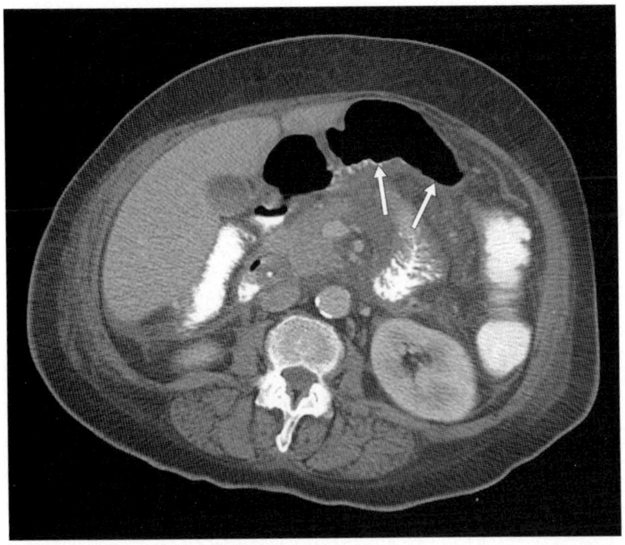

Figure 2-38 Inflammatory mass of acute pancreatic disease impressing the posterior gastric wall *(arrows)*.

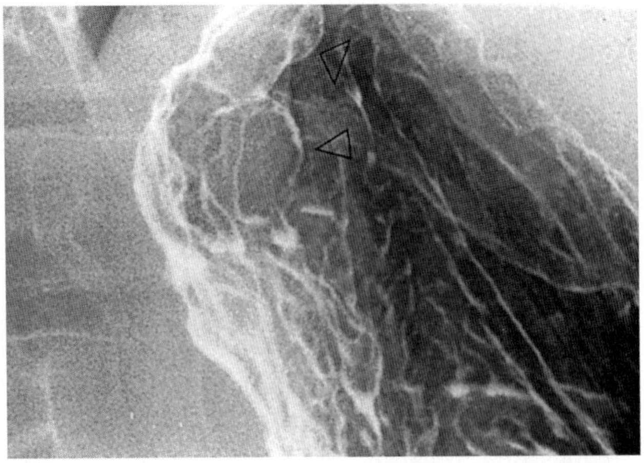

Figure 2-39 Patient with fundal gastric varices. Area of focal fold thickening and nodularity is seen. Note the smooth mucosal surface over the affected area *(arrowheads)*.

Eosinophilic Gastritis

The stomach is commonly involved in eosinophilic gastritis, a relatively rare disorder. The predilection seems to be for the gastric antrum, although the entire stomach may be involved. The disease results in eosinophilic infiltrates of the mucosal and muscular layers of the stomach. Radiological manifestations are generally those of a thickened rugal fold pattern, predominantly distally. Clinical features are nonspecific, and patients may present with early satiety, nausea, or vomiting. Involvement of the small bowel is helpful in making the diagnosis, and thickened folds are shown in the proximal small bowel wall. Isolated gastric involvement is relatively common, however. In patients with thickened gastric folds, small bowel involvement, peripheral eosinophilia, abdominal pain, history of food allergies, and no evidence of parasitic gastrointestinal infestation, the diagnosis of eosinophilic gastritis should be considered. Biopsy is crucial to the correct diagnosis.

Partial Gastrectomy

In patients with long-term gastric resection, particularly the Billroth II procedure, the presence of thickened folds

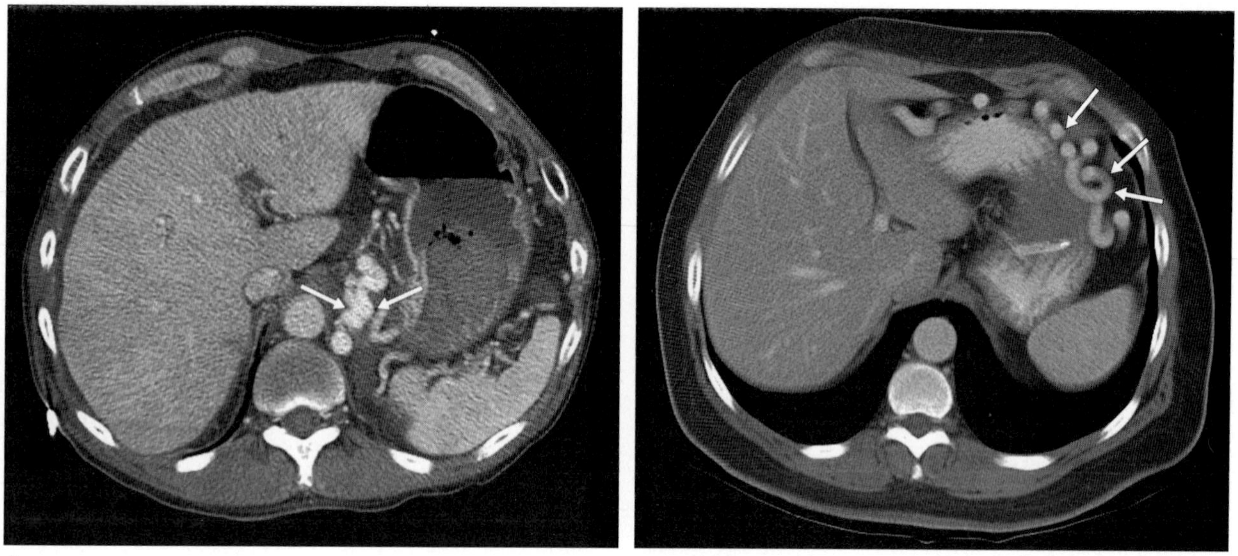
A B

Figure 2-40 **A,** Large serpentine varices *(arrows)* are seen in the gastric fundus. **B,** Coiled serpentine varices also are seen along this patient's greater curvature *(arrows)* of stomach.

within the gastric remnant is common. The exact cause is unclear. It is believed by some authors to represent the sequela of chronic bile reflux. The long-term significance also is unclear. Whether this condition predisposes these individuals to a "stump carcinoma" of the gastric remnant is uncertain.

Diffuse Thickening

Box 2-7 summarizes the causes of diffuse gastric fold thickening.

Gastritis

Virtually all forms of gastritis, including hypertrophic gastritis and phlegmonous gastritis, can diffusely involve the entire stomach. Alcoholic gastritis, although occasionally manifesting as a regional gastritis, most commonly is diffuse in its presentation and is associated with a higher incidence of positive *H. pylori* testing.

Box 2-7 The Fold Thickens: Some Causes of Diffuse Gastric Fold Thickening

- Gastritis with or without *H. pylori*
- Aspirin/NSAID-induced gastritis
- Eosinophilic gastritis
- Ménétrier's disease
- Pancreatitis
- Malignancy
- Amyloid

Pancreatitis

Occasionally, with severe involvement of the length of the pancreas, the secondary inflammatory changes involving the adjacent stomach may involve the entire length of the stomach.

Eosinophilic Gastritis

Although involvement of the stomach with eosinophilic gastritis is often limited to the antrum, all parts of the stomach may be involved.

Ménétrier's Disease

Although Ménétrier's disease is more commonly seen involving the proximal stomach, it also can involve the entire stomach, giving a diffusely thickened rugal fold pattern throughout.

Amyloidosis

Gastrointestinal involvement by amyloid is common, although involvement of the stomach seems to be rare. Diffuse infiltrative changes may be present throughout the stomach with resultant thickening of the rugal fold pattern. This thickening probably represents the most well-known presentation of gastric amyloid. Other presentations include focal changes, such as mass and ulceration. Involvement of the stomach with amyloid can be a result of primary systemic amyloidosis, secondary amyloidosis, or isolated amyloid deposition.

The secondary type of amyloidosis is associated with some chronic underlying disease that predisposes to amyloid formation and deposition in tissues. The most common antecedent diseases include rheumatoid arthritis, tuberculosis, bronchiectasis, and chronic lung disease. The site of amyloid involvement is usually the reticuloendothelial system. Primary systemic amyloid is a condition in which no underlying disease is thought to be present. The gastrointestinal system involvement with amyloid is more commonly seen with the primary systemic type. Isolated amyloid deposition, sometimes referred to as amyloid tumor, involves a single site or organ. This is probably a variant of the primary type. A fourth type of amyloidosis that should be considered and in which gastric involvement is probably extremely unusual would be amyloid formation associated with multiple myeloma.

Thickened Folds Resulting from Healed Gastric Ulcers

Occasionally, healing and scarring from a previous gastric ulcer may leave the stomach with a permanent appearance of thickened folds (Fig. 2-41); this can be very focal or involve a large portion of the stomach if the original ulcer was large. These thickened folds are not the norm, however, and most gastric ulcers heal with little or no scarring, whereas others may heal with a traction defect (owing to cicatrization) on the wall opposite the ulcer.

Diminished Gastric Folds

Normal Aging

Diminished gastric folds are a radiological dilemma. Correlation between diminished fold pattern, as seen on the UGI study and endoscopy, and histological biopsy is often poor.

In many patients, a diminished fold pattern is apparent, which primarily involves the fundus and, to a lesser degree, the body and antrum. It is often seen in older patients and, in most cases, it represents normal aging processes. Various population studies have suggested that mild to moderate atrophy and associated fold diminution are seen in patients older than age 50 years. It has been suggested that 50% of patients older than age 50 show some degree of these changes within the stomach. Histologically, this change is found to be a mild superficial and atrophic type of gastritis, with the atrophic component increasing with age. There is often accompanying intestinal metaplasia, which also seems to be age dependent. The relationship of these findings to *H. pylori* gastritis remains to be elucidated, but there is some evidence that a subset of *H. pylori* can be associated with achlorhydric states.

Diminution of fold pattern may be accompanied by prominence in the areae gastricae pattern, but these findings are controversial and not well understood. The radiologist should not presume serious disease or increased risk of malignancy on the basis of these findings. In most cases, when the stomach is otherwise normal, a simple descriptive phrase, such as "the stomach has a mild atrophic appearance with some diminution of the fold pattern," suffices. Diagnosis of atrophic gastritis should be avoided unless the stomach is totally devoid of folds.

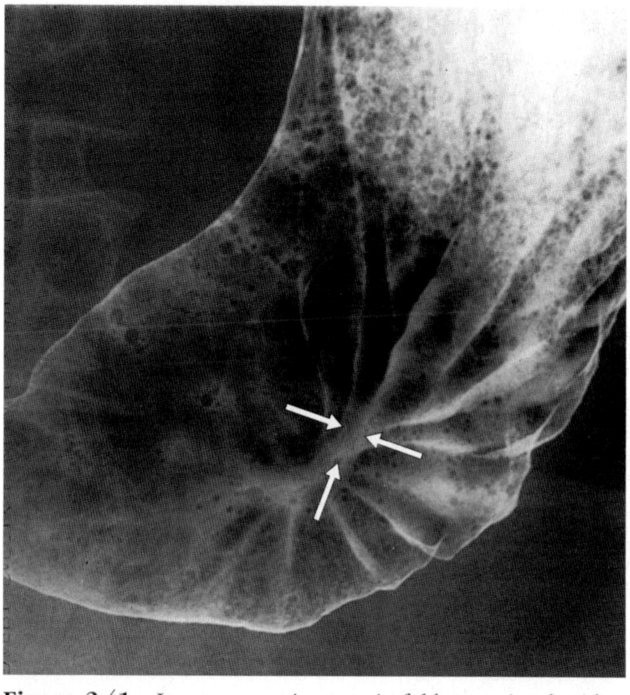

Figure 2-41 Large converging gastric folds associated with a healed gastric ulcer *(arrows)*.

Partial Gastrectomy

After partial gastrectomy, the development of gastritis is inevitable. Widened folds may be evident in most patients following gastrectomy. A diminished or absent fold pattern also may be seen in a smaller number of patients after gastrectomy. In some of these patients, no folds are discernible. These changes are more marked in the Billroth II type of anastomosis. The cause of these types of gastritis is unclear. The same bile or alkaline reflux gastritis suggested for prominent gastric folds also has been suggested as a cause for the atrophic appearance of the gastric remnant. The long-term sequela of this type of gastritis also is uncertain. The increased incidence of postgastrectomy "stump carcinoma" has been documented in the literature. It is not clear what, if any, role chronic gastritis of the gastric remnant plays in the development of carcinoma in the gastric remnant 10 to 25 years after surgery, nor is it clear if manifestations of atrophic changes in the gastric stump or prominent gastric folds in the residual stomach indicate an increased risk in these patients (Fig. 2-42).

Gastric Ulcers

Gastric ulcers, particularly chronic ulcers, tend to be associated with a diminished fold pattern throughout the

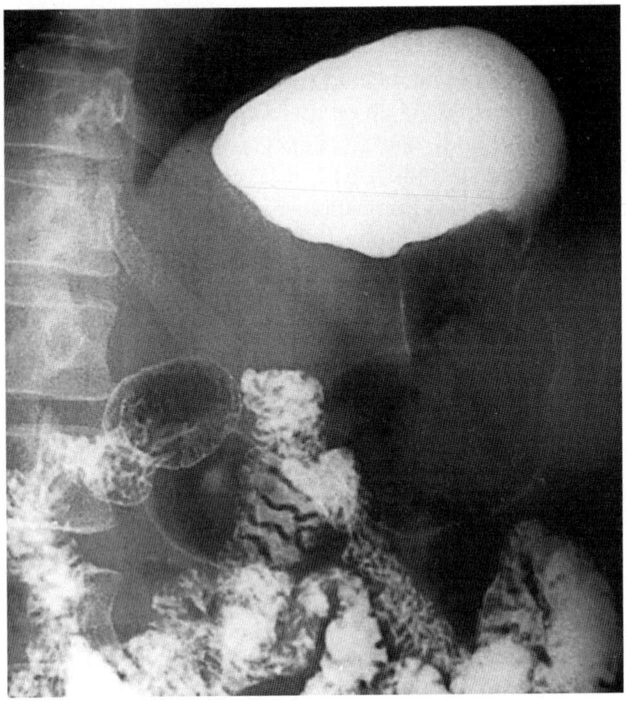

Figure 2-42 UGI study in elderly patient shows complete absence of gastric folds, giving the stomach a marked atrophic appearance.

stomach and particularly in the antrum. Histologically, atrophic superficial gastritis with intestinal metaplasia commonly accompanies the atrophic changes.

Pernicious Anemia

Addisonian pernicious anemia is a serious hematological condition that is characterized by a megaloblastic type of anemia and near-absolute achlorhydria. The Schilling test shows impaired absorption of vitamin B_{12} from the gut, which is a result of the diminished ability to secrete intrinsic factor. The stomach shows severe fundal atrophy, giving rise to the "bald fundus." The remainder of the stomach shows diminished or complete absence of a fold pattern. The stomach remains distensible and pliable at fluoroscopy. Peristaltic activity is diminished, but not absent. Histological examination shows severe mucosal atrophy, gastritis, and intestinal metaplasia. It is not unusual to see inflammatory changes within the antrum, in which case thickened folds, possibly erosions, may be encountered in a patient who otherwise presents with an absence of fold pattern throughout the remainder of the stomach.

Gastric Cancer

Cancers found in the gastric antrum and body are often associated with extensive changes of fundal atrophic gastritis and prominent intestinal metaplastic changes. This association is of questionable significance in that the intestinal metaplastic changes have been shown to be present in the aging population, and the degree and severity seem to correlate directly with age. The increased risk of gastric carcinoma in patients with the atrophic changes of the stomach secondary to pernicious anemia is well known, however. It has been estimated that such patients have three times the risk of developing gastric cancer as does the normal population. A patient with severe atrophic changes throughout the stomach and an absolute absence of gastric fold pattern presents a dilemma to the radiologist. Although the supporting evidence and the disputing evidence are controversial, such patients probably should be considered at higher risk for the development of gastric carcinoma and referred for endoscopic evaluation and sample biopsy of various portions of the stomach.

Extrinsic Masses

Many possible perigastric processes can result in an extrinsic compression defect on the stomach. The most common of these is simply an enlarged liver, particularly the left lobe. Splenomegaly also can result in a significant impression. Other processes, particularly processes arising from the pancreas, such as tumors, pseudocysts, and other forms of pancreatic cystic disease, also can result in gastric impression. These impressions are seen along the distal greater curvature of the stomach and are sometimes referred to as the "antral pad" sign on an UGI examination (Fig. 2-43). Large retroperitoneal masses, such as neurofibromatosis (Fig. 2-44), retrogastric lymph node masses, and hematomas or abscesses, can give a picture of a posterior wall impression on the stomach. Occasionally, a marked aortic aneurysm impresses the stomach, and neoplastic lesions arising from the region of the splenic flexure of the colon can result in gastric impression. Huge renal or adrenal masses also can displace the stomach.

Small Solitary Masses (<2 cm)

Gastric Polyps

Solitary gastric polyps are uncommon. Various studies have put the incidence at 0.6% to 3%. Benign spindle cell tumors are the most common type of neoplastic polyps seen in this category, with benign stromal cell tumors (leiomyomas) the most frequent lesions seen. Lipomas, hemangiomas, and neurofibromas do occur, however. These lesions tend to be small and solitary. They occasionally can grow to a large size and commonly undergo surface ulceration. Autopsy studies have suggested, however, that the incidence of multiple benign stromal cell tumors of the stomach may be higher than previously believed. A benign stromal cell tumor originates in the smooth muscle of the stomach wall and apparently can remain for a prolonged period as a small intramural

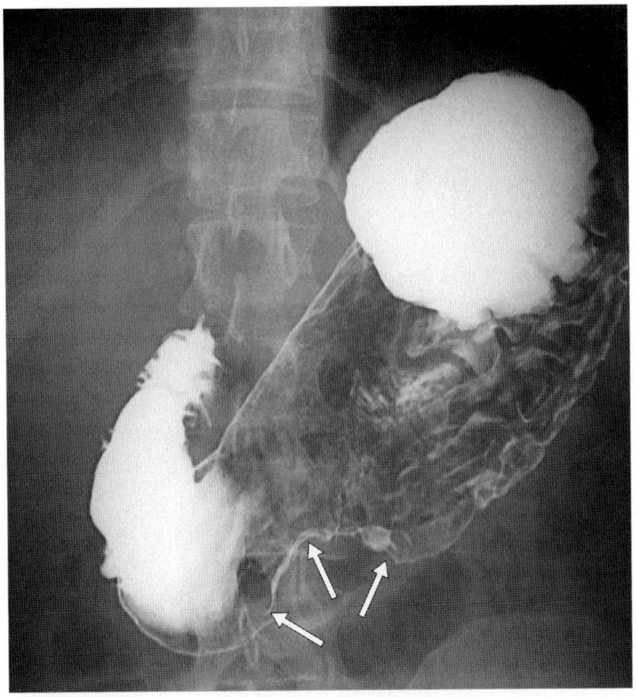

Figure 2-43 Focal impression on greater curvature of stomach secondary to pancreatic tumor, "antral pad sign" *(arrows)*.

submucosal process. If enlargement does occur, it may grow toward the gastric lumen or toward the serosal side of the bowel wall and develop as an exophytic lesion. Most benign stromal cell tumors tend to occur in the proximal part of the stomach. In general, it has been a clinical assumption that benign stromal cell tumors less than 2 cm tend to be asymptomatic, whereas larger lesions may result in symptoms.

Lipomas of the stomach are rare and generally small and asymptomatic. When they do become symptomatic, it is almost always a result of gastrointestinal bleeding. They usually occur in the distal stomach.

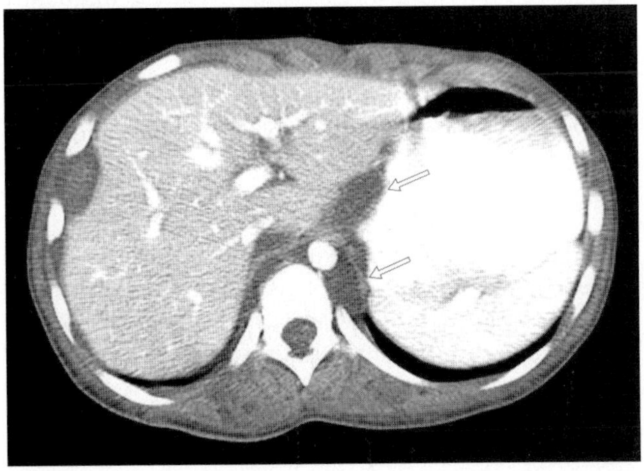

Figure 2-44 Neurofibromatosis in the retroperitoneal cavity and gastrohepatic ligament impresses the stomach wall *(arrows)*.

Glomus tumors (similar to benign stromal cell tumors in histologic appearance), although more commonly found in other sites, such as skin, can also occur in the stomach. The usual reported site is in the distal stomach, and the most common manifestation is gastrointestinal bleeding.

Ectopic Pancreas

These lesions are most commonly encountered within the antrum of the stomach, with the next most common site being the duodenum. Polypoid lesions representing ectopic pancreatic rests have been described occurring rarely in sites from the esophagus to the ileum.

The incidence varies, ranging from 1% to 14% in autopsy series. It seems to be more common than other benign polypoid conditions of the stomach, including benign stromal cell tumors.

Radiographically, these polypoid lesions are usually less than 2 cm and are generally located in the distal prepyloric antral region of the stomach. The surface of the lesion may be smooth or slightly lobulated. There may be a central depression or umbilication representing a rudimentary duct opening in approximately 50% of the cases (Fig. 2-45).

Most of these lesions are discovered incidentally in patients with nonspecific or vague gastrointestinal complaints. Occasionally, the surface of the ectopic pancreatic rests may ulcerate and bleed. Multiple gastric pancreatic rests are uncommon.

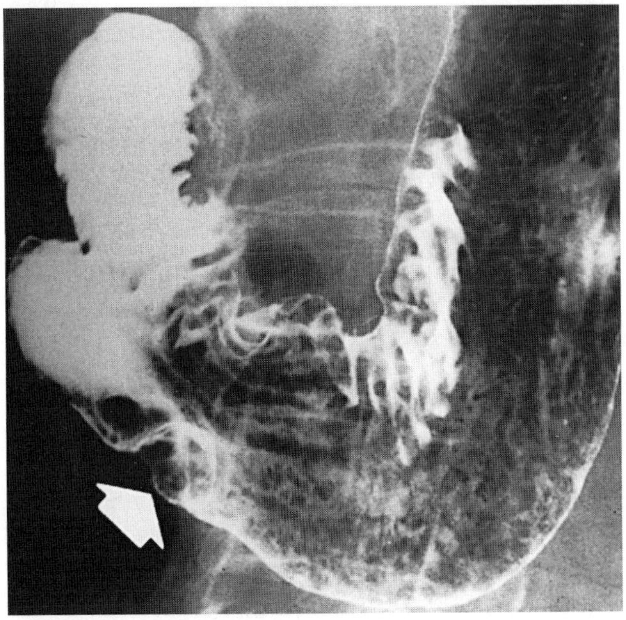

Figure 2-45 Marginal polypoid lesion is seen along the greater curvature of the antrum *(arrow)*. Endoscopic evaluation and biopsy specimen showed this to be ectopic pancreatic tissue.

Adenomas

In contrast to the colon, in which adenomatous polyp formation is common, the presence of adenomas in the stomach is unusual. Adenomatous polyps in the stomach also seem to be more predisposed to malignant degeneration. Similar to colonic adenomas, the potential for malignant degeneration increases with size. Although generally uncommon, adenomatous polyps are more common in stomachs that also harbor gastric carcinoma. The incidence has been reported to be near 60%.

Most of these lesions are sessile, although pedunculated polyps may be seen (Fig. 2-46). The most common site seems to be in the distal stomach. Tubular adenomas, which are the most common adenomas in the colon, tend to be the least common of the gastric adenomas. More frequently, the more dangerous varieties, such as villous or tubulovillous adenomas, are encountered.

Solitary polyps are more common than multiple lesions. The presence of multiple lesions should raise the possibility of one of the polyposis syndromes.

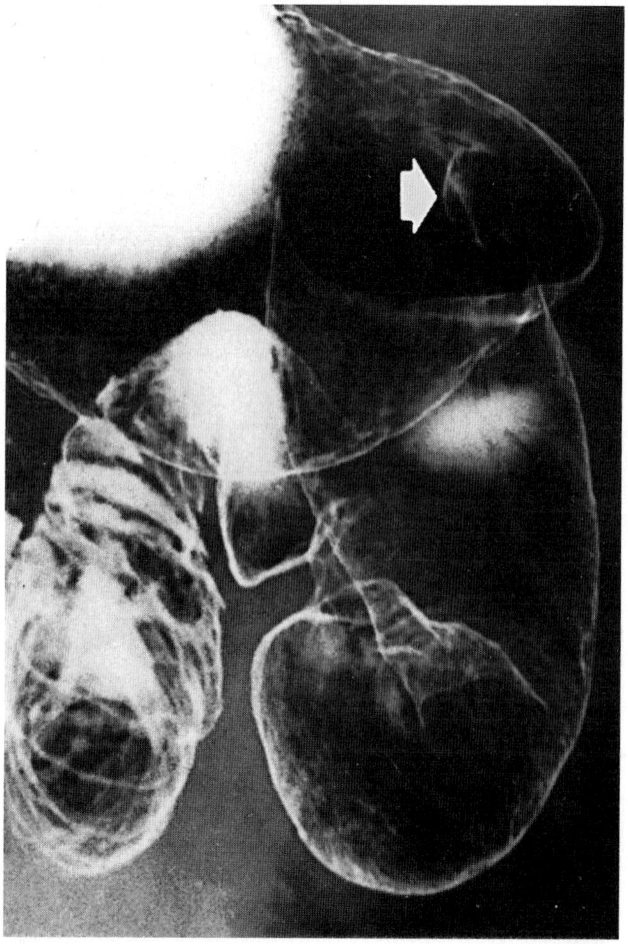

Figure 2-46 A smooth polypoid lesion *(arrow)* is seen on the anterior wall of the stomach at the junction of the body and antrum. Endoscopy showed it to be a gastric adenoma.

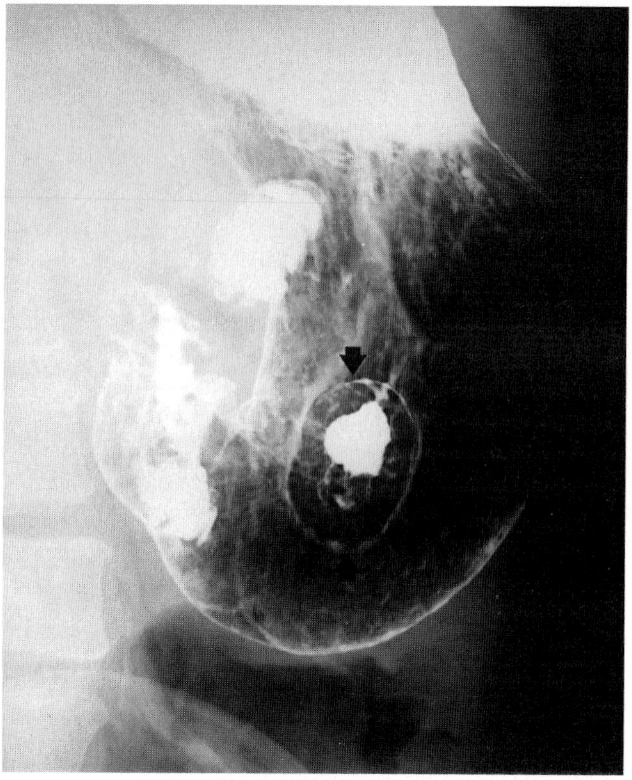

Figure 2-47 Gastric metastatic lesion. A rounded, well-defined gastric mass *(arrows)* with a central barium collection proved to be a metastatic lesion from the breast.

The radiological appearance is usually that of a mucosal lesion. It may be smooth or villous in appearance. Ulceration can occur. Most solitary adenomas are incidental findings, and most lesions are less than 2 cm.

Metastatic Lesions

Metastatic lesions to the stomach resulting in solitary, small filling defects are uncommon but do occur. Metastatic melanoma is probably the most frequently encountered lesion and occasionally can present as a single, small filling defect with typical surface ulceration and "bull's-eye" appearance. Solitary, small lesions secondary to metastatic spread of breast or lung lesions may be seen rarely with exactly the same appearance (Fig. 2-47).

Inflammatory Fibroid Polyps

Inflammatory fibroid polyps are nonadenomatous polyps characterized by an arrangement of fibrous and connective tissues infiltrated with sheets of eosinophils. These lesions also are known as eosinophilic granulomas. The lesions apparently are unrelated to eosinophilic gastroenteritis. There is no history of food allergies, and there is no peripheral eosinophilia. The lesion is usually solitary and smaller than 2 cm. It has no

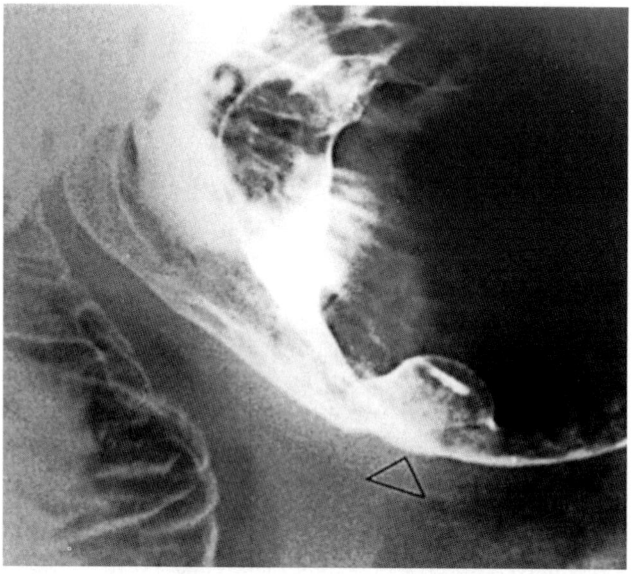

Figure 2-48 A patient with a solitary eosinophilic granuloma of the stomach *(arrowhead)* located along the greater curvature of the antrum. The lesion is smooth and mucosal in appearance. A small, linear ulceration is seen on the surface.

distinctive appearance radiologically and is seen as a smooth, sessile polypoid filling defect in the distal stomach (Fig. 2-48). Patients are usually asymptomatic, and these lesions are rarely associated with any significant symptoms. The possibility of erosions on the surface of the lesion and subsequent bleeding does exist.

Carcinoids

Carcinoids usually do not involve the stomach and are seen in this organ in less than 3% of cases. They may be seen as small, often solitary, mucosal polypoid lesions in the antrum. A more common appearance is that of a larger fungating lesion involving the antral portion of the stomach, which may be radiologically indistinguishable from an ulcerating carcinoma. Approximately 25% of gastric carcinoids have associated metastatic disease. In the stomach or duodenum, carcinoids arise from enterochromaffin-like cells. Carcinoid syndrome does not occur, however, without the presence of hepatic metastatic disease

Multiple Small Masses

Hyperplastic Polyps

Hyperplastic polyps are the most common cause of small polypoid filling defects within the stomach. They also are referred to as regenerative and sometimes inflammatory polyps and are believed to represent the sequelae of chronic inflammation. They are small and sessile and are commonly multiple in nature, although they can be solitary. They tend to be seen predominantly in the antral region (Fig. 2-49).

The hyperplastic polyp is not a neoplastic lesion. Malignant degeneration is virtually unheard of. Despite this, there is a well-documented increase in the incidence of coexisting hyperplastic polyps found in stomachs harboring gastric carcinoma.

Adenomas

The finding of multiple gastric adenomas not related to one of the polyposis syndromes is rare. Gastric polyps are reported in most polyposis syndromes. More commonly, they are seen in familial polyposis coli and Gardner's syndrome. Although these adenomatous polyps have a high malignant potential within the colon, malignant degeneration of adenomatous gastric polyps in patients with either Gardner's or familial polyposis syndrome is exceedingly rare.

Hamartomas

Hamartomatous gastric polyps develop in the stomach almost exclusively in patients with Peutz-Jeghers or Cronkhite-Canada syndromes. They are multiple, are generally small, and are seen in conjunction with the more

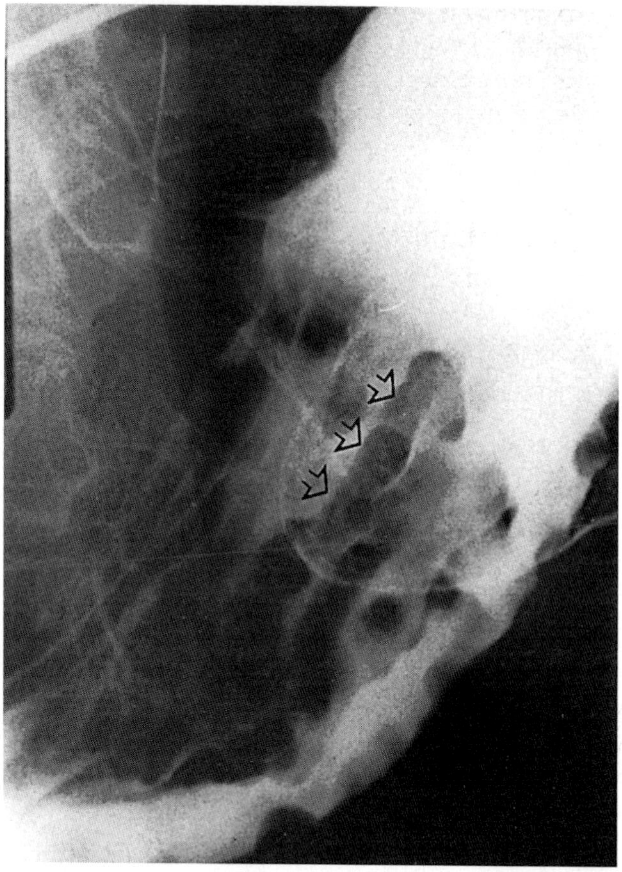

Figure 2-49 UGI study shows numerous, rounded filling defects throughout the body and antrum of the stomach *(arrows)*, which on endoscopic evaluation proved to be multiple hyperplastic polyps.

common presentation of small bowel polyps and mucocutaneous pigmentation changes. There is relatively little malignant potential related to hamartoma formation. Although a slight increase in small bowel cancer has been reported in patients with Peutz-Jeghers syndrome, there is no known increase in gastric cancer.

Multiple hamartoma syndrome (Cowden's disease) is a rare condition manifested by hamartomatous polyps within the stomach and elsewhere within the gastrointestinal tract, along with associated thyroid and breast lesions. The gastrointestinal polyps are almost always hamartomatous, although simple hyperplastic polyps have been reported.

Hemangiomas

Rarely, multiple hemangiomas are seen within the stomach, occasionally associated with typical calcification. The blue rubber bleb nevus syndrome (Bean syndrome) is rare. It is inherited as a sporadic, autosomal dominant trait in some families. It is manifested by mucosal hemangiomas, mostly reported in the stomach and associated with gastrointestinal bleeding. They are always seen as multiple, small filling defects.

Peptic Erosions

Multiple, small filling defects may be identified in patients with multiple gastric erosions. This finding relates to the edematous raised mucosa around the site of the punctate ulceration (Fig. 2-50). On single-contrast examination, these may appear as multiple, small filling defects predominantly in the distal stomach. Good-quality, double-contrast examination almost always shows the punctate ulceration present in the center of the filling defect. Often, these erosions line up on the folds of the body and antrum of the stomach.

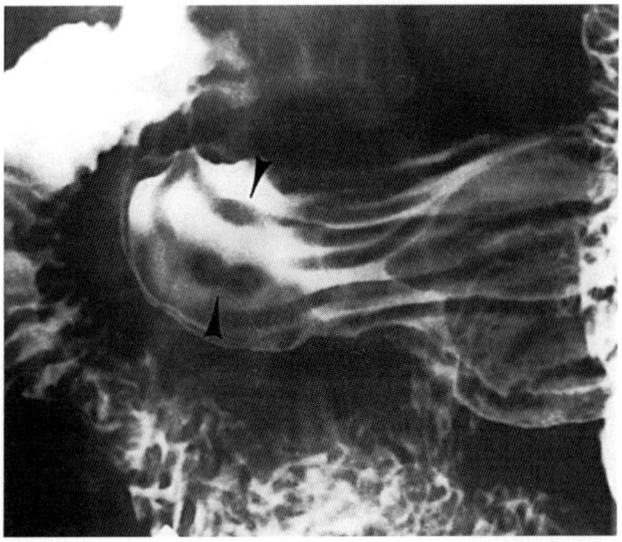

Figure 2-50 Focal swelling and beaded appearance *(arrowheads)* are shown in the distal stomach of this patient as a result of tiny superficial erosions and the associated edema surrounding each erosion.

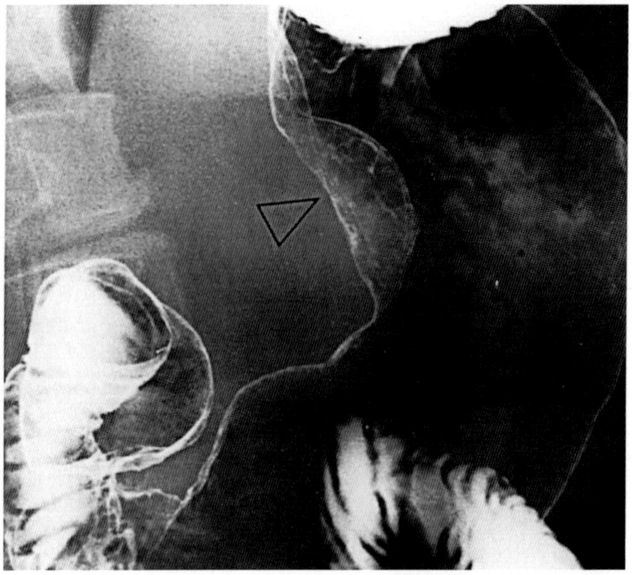

Figure 2-51 Large, smooth submucosal mass *(arrowhead)* is seen arising from the lesser curvature of the body of the stomach. This represents a large gastric stromal cell tumor (leiomyoma).

Candidiasis

With the increasing pool of immunocompromised patients in the health care system today, there is an increasing incidence of gastric candidiasis. This disease may present, as in the esophagus, with multiple, round filling defects throughout the stomach, which, if untreated, can go on to the ulcerative hemorrhagic stage commonly seen in the esophagus.

Large Solitary Masses

Adenomas

Solitary gastric adenomas greater than 2 cm are extremely uncommon but do occur and carry a high risk of malignancy. Larger adenomatous polyps within the stomach have more likelihood of being pedunculated (i.e., on a stalk).

Stromal Cell Tumors (Gastrointestinal Stromal Cell Tumors)

The most common of the stromal cell tumors of the gastrointestinal tract are those that arise from the smooth muscle of the stomach. Although multiple benign stromal cell tumors of the stomach have been reported, the solitary lesion is much more common. These lesions can be quite large, and the patients are often asymptomatic (Fig. 2-51). Occasionally, stromal cell tumors can continue to grow within the gastric wall and reach sizable proportions (Fig. 2-52). A stromal cell tumor greater than 5 cm in

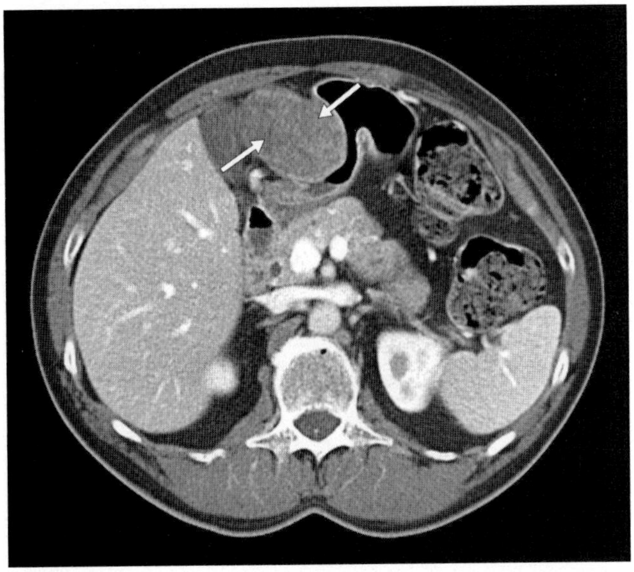

Figure 2-52 A gastric gastrointestinal stromal cell tumor is seen arising from the anterior wall of the stomach on CT *(arrows)*.

diameter is likely to be a malignant stromal cell tumor (leiomyosarcoma). These tumors often outgrow their blood supply and undergo central necrosis, often leading to large barium-filled cavities within the tumor mass. The ulcerations are usually centrally located in the tumor mass. Although stromal cell tumors seem to have a predilection for the proximal stomach, they have been described throughout the stomach. These tumors carry a relatively good prognosis, and distal metastasis is rare. Direct extension to the adjacent spleen, liver, and pancreas does occur. Lymph node spread is unusual. Symptoms are produced usually when the lesions are quite large, and patients most commonly present with bleeding. Occasionally, obstruction or perforation may be a presenting feature.

Because of the tendency for these lesions to grow in an exophytic manner, CT is helpful in identifying the limits of the tumor mass. Barium studies may show wall abnormalities, which may be evidence of extrinsic mass relating to the exophytic component of the lesion (Fig. 2-53).

Metastatic Lesions

The usual presentation of metastatic lesions is multiple polypoid or infiltrative lesions within the stomach. Occasionally, a larger, isolated metastatic lesion is encountered; this is most likely to occur in metastatic melanoma (Fig. 2-54).

Duplication Cysts

Gastric duplications are rare and may present in various sizes and configurations. A solitary filling defect within the stomach, usually along the greater curvature, is one presentation. Alternatively the cyst may communicate with the lumen and present as a large diverticulum-like barium collection along the margin of the stomach.

Polypoid Carcinomas

Approximately a quarter of gastric carcinomas present as polypoid mass lesions growing into the gastric lumen. These polypoid lesions may or may not be ulcerated on their surface (Fig. 2-55). In addition, there may be spread along the adjacent wall. It is thought that about a third of all malignant gastric carcinomas manifest

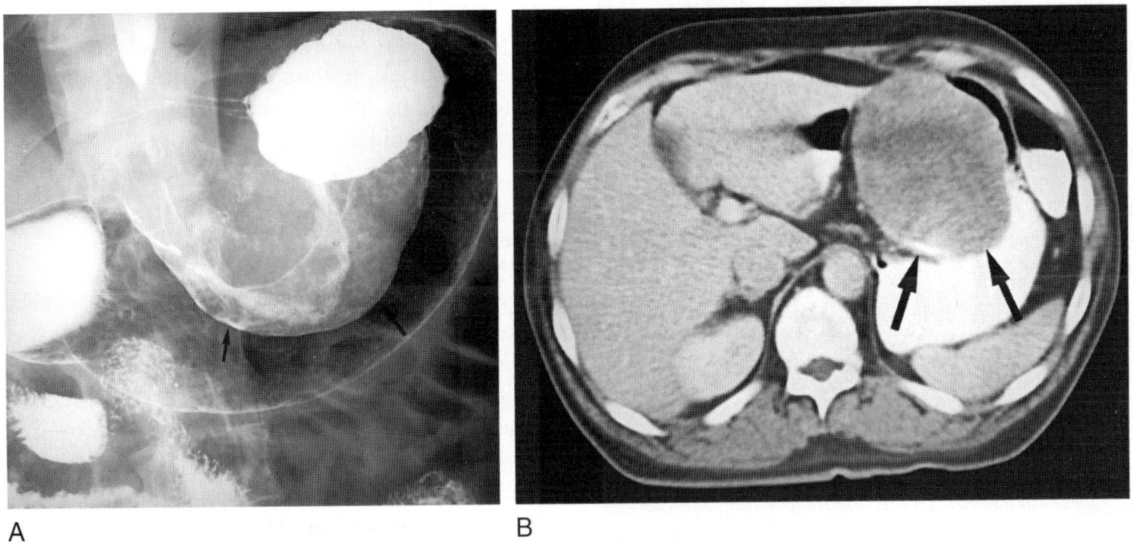

Figure 2-53 Malignant gastrointestinal stromal cell cell tumor. **A,** UGI examination shows huge gastric mass arising from lesser curve *(arrows)*. Note smooth mucosal surface over mass. **B,** Computed tomographic scan shows large soft tissue mass *(arrows)* with significant exophytic component.

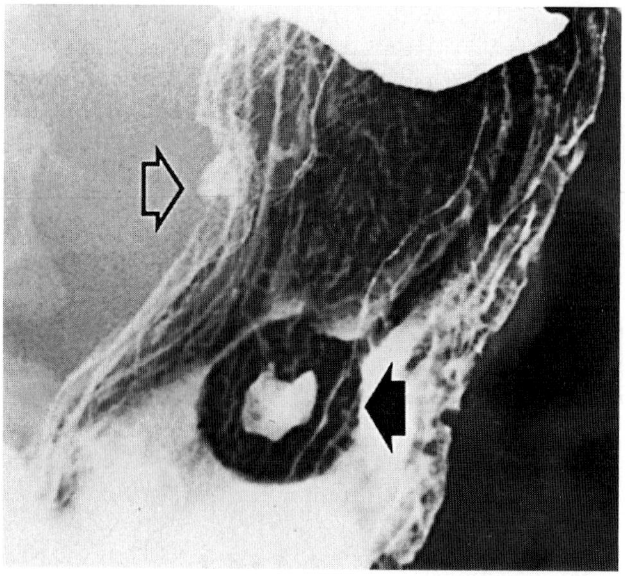

Figure 2-54 UGI study in patient with known lung cancer in which at least two bull's-eye metastatic lesions to the stomach are seen. The classic appearance of a mass with an ulcerated, barium-filled center is seen en face *(solid arrow)*, and the same type of lesion is seen profiled *(open arrow)*.

all of the characteristics of polypoid, ulcerative, and infiltrating types (Fig. 2-56).

Discrete isolated polypoid lesions tend to carry the best prognosis. The most common sites tend to be in the distal portion of the stomach, although in patients with gastric atrophy, proximal regions are more involved.

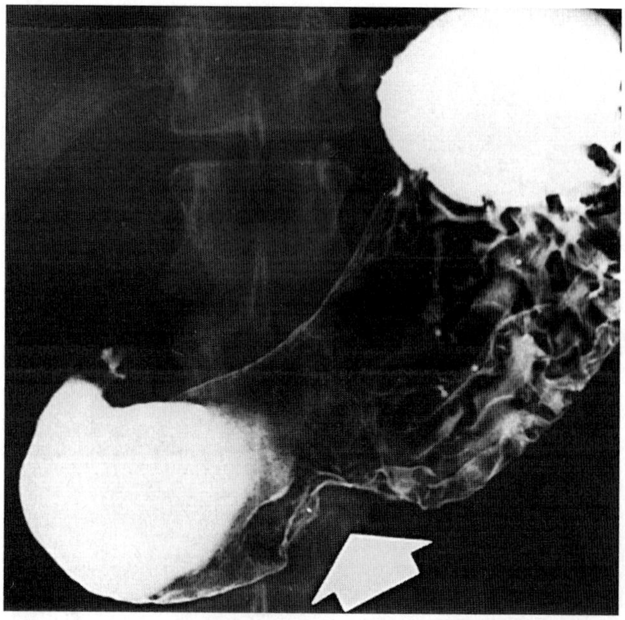

Figure 2-55 A polypoid carcinoma is seen arising from the greater curvature of the stomach at the junction of the antrum and body *(arrow)*. It is similar in appearance to the antral pad sign (see Fig. 2-43).

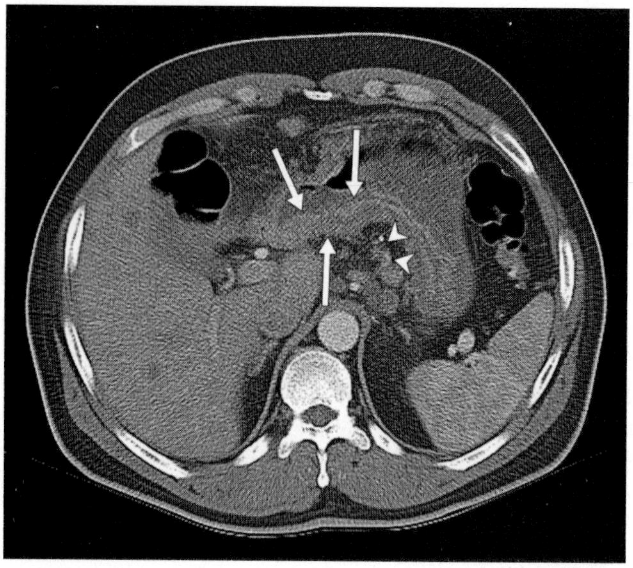

Figure 2-56 Computed tomographic scan shows infiltrating carcinoma of the stomach with thickened gastric wall *(arrows)*, extra-gastric lesions, and nodes in gastrohepatic ligament *(arrowheads)*.

Jejunal Gastric Intussusception

Of the complications associated with Billroth II partial gastrectomy, including marginal ulceration, bezoars, stump carcinoma, and chronic bile reflux gastritis, jejunal gastric intussusception is rarest. Intussusceptive changes occur within the adjacent jejunum, and retrograde progression of the intussusception results in a large filling defect within the gastric remnant. This defect has a typical radiographic appearance on barium studies of a large intragastric mass with evidence of a fold pattern within it that may or may not have the typical "coil spring" appearance. There is usually a significant degree of obstruction to the distal flow of barium.

Gastric Bezoars

Small, asymptomatic bezoars can be seen as a filling defect within the stomach. These are usually less than 2 cm and mobile.

Multiple Large Masses

Metastatic Disease

As already suggested, metastatic disease to the stomach can be eclectic in appearance. Multiple, large nodular lesions can be seen in metastatic melanoma. Occasionally, metastatic lesions arising from breast and lung lesions may present in such a fashion. Often, these types of metastatic lesions are sharply circumscribed and have the typical bull's-eye or "target lesion" appearance when associated with central ulceration. The lesions, particularly melanoma, may remain silent for some time and increase in size. Bleeding usually is the first manifestation of gastric involvement.

Benign Stromal Cell Tumors (Leiomyomas)

Stromal cell tumors (gastrointestinal stromal cell tumors) occasionally can occur in the stomach as multiple, large submucosal masses. These lesions can grow large, and the patient can be entirely asymptomatic. The usual presentation is bleeding associated with ulceration on the surface of one of the stromal cell tumors.

Neurogenic Tumors

Neurofibromas occur as isolated tumors of the stomach. They can be multiple, however, and in a patient with generalized neurofibromatosis, there may be involvement of the stomach with multiple neurofibromas. Apart from the possibility of ulceration and bleeding, they are generally asymptomatic.

Kaposi's Sarcoma

Kaposi's sarcoma is a vascular endothelial tumor that was described approximately 100 years ago. There has been significant resurgence in the incidence of Kaposi's sarcoma with the advent of the acquired immunodeficiency syndrome (AIDS) epidemic. Involvement of the gastrointestinal tract is common, and the gastrointestinal tract is probably the most frequent site of involvement after the skin. It is estimated that 40% to 50% of patients with Kaposi's sarcoma lesions of the skin have gastrointestinal involvement. Nearly any level of the gastrointestinal tract may be involved, from the pharynx to the rectum, although most lesions are in the upper tract. The gastrointestinal lesions are almost always seen in homosexual men. Gastric involvement can be either diffuse or in the form of large discrete nodules (Fig. 2-57). The nodules may or may not have central ulceration. CT is helpful in defining the extent of wall involvement and the presence or absence of perigastric disease. The lesions themselves are generally asymptomatic, although they can bleed.

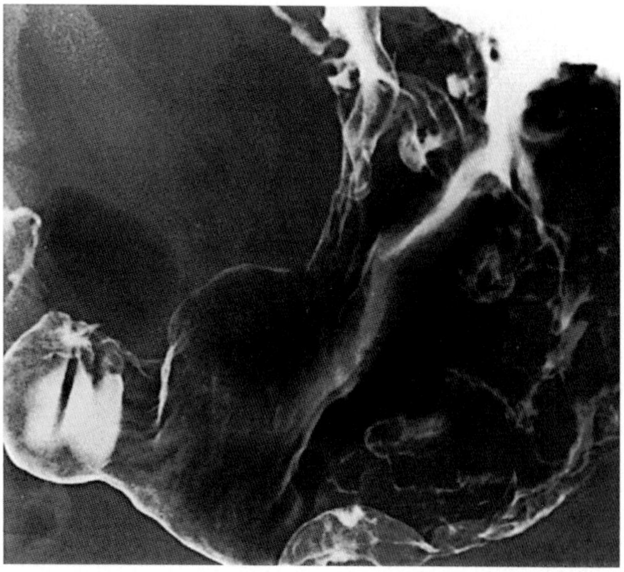

Figure 2-57 Patient with Kaposi's sarcoma of the stomach. Numerous rounded, ulcerated masses of the stomach are seen.

Lymphoma

Primary lymphoma of the stomach is much less common than adenocarcinoma and accounts for less than 5% of malignant lesions of the stomach. As with gastric adenocarcinoma, patients may present with nonspecific complaints of abdominal pain, nausea, vomiting, and weight loss. The radiological manifestations of lymphoma can be quite variable. Ulcerating, infiltrating lesions and multiple polypoid filling defects within the stomach are common (Fig. 2-58). Lymphoma can imitate numerous conditions, and radiological differentiation can be difficult. When faced with multiple large nodules in the stomach, factors that favor the possibility of lymphoma include relative preservation of the pliability of the stomach, associated fold thickening, and extension of the lesion into the duodenum (Fig. 2-59).

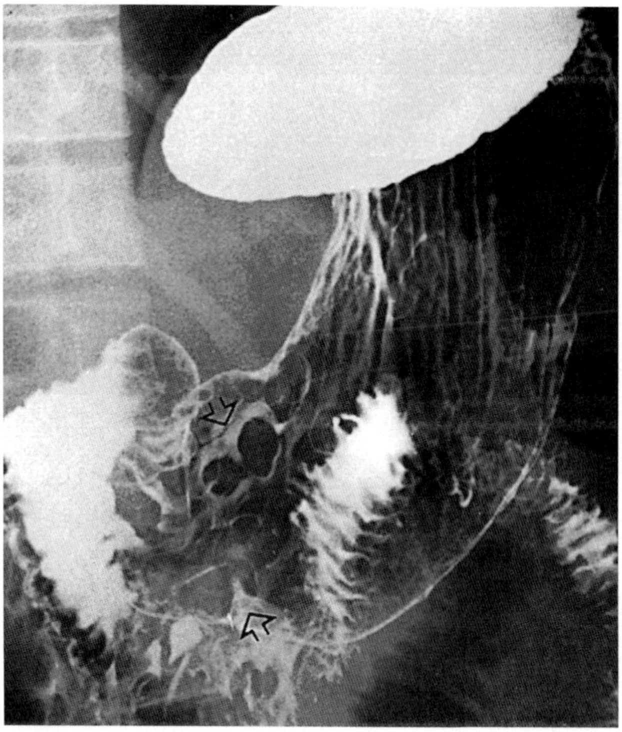

Figure 2-58 Lymphoma of the stomach presenting as multiple polypoid lesions in the antrum *(arrows)*.

Infiltrating Masses

Adenocarcinoma

The incidence of gastric cancer has decreased strikingly during the past 4 decades, and it continues to decrease. In Asia, particularly in Japan, however, gastric cancer is

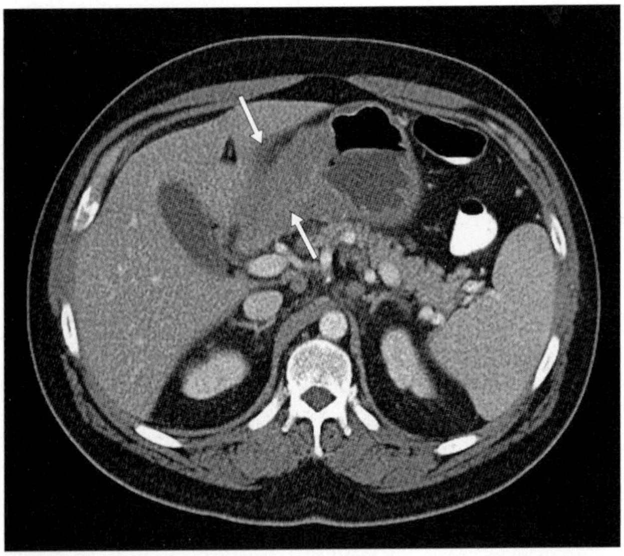

Figure 2-59 Computed tomographic scan shows gastric lymphoma of the distal stomach *(arrows)* with marked wall thickening, but no evidence of obstruction.

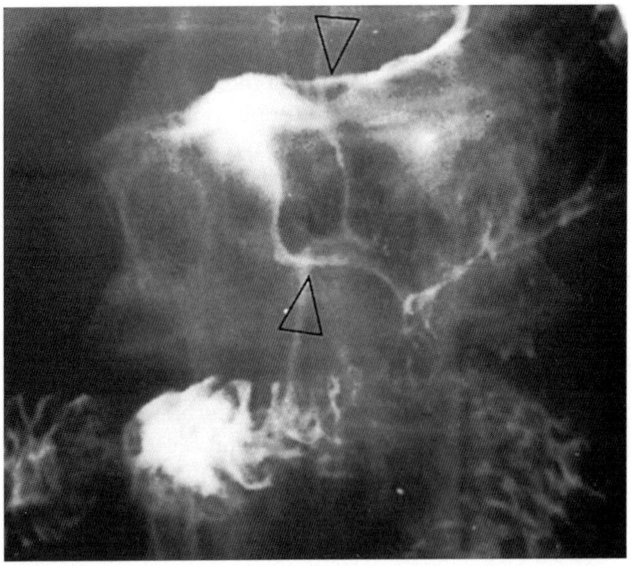

Figure 2-60 Patient with lymphomatous infiltration of the distal stomach giving a narrow, tubular appearance without obstruction *(arrowheads)*.

a common carcinoma and a cause of mortality. There may be some slight decline in the rate in Japan, possibly associated with intensive screening programs. In the United States, the median age of diagnosis is about 72 years, slightly younger in women, with mortality being approximately 2:1 male to female. There is an identifiable group of younger patients in which the male-to-female ratio is about 1:1, there is a family history of malignancy, and there is also a preponderance of type A blood among the patients.

Historically, adenocarcinoma, which manifests as a diffuse infiltrative process within the stomach, is described as a scirrhous type of lesion and is the most common cause of the linitis plastica configuration of the stomach seen on UGI studies. The diffuse infiltrative process results in desmoplastic changes in the wall of the stomach, rendering the stomach tubular, narrow, and rigid (see Fig. 2-16).

Lymphoma

Primary gastric lymphoma may have a multiplicity of presentations in the stomach. A marked increase in the fold pattern and infiltrative changes is the most common presentation (Fig. 2-60); this can be accompanied by ulceration. The stomach may be involved in part or in whole. Evaluation of radiographs may present difficulty in distinguishing between lymphoma and carcinoma. Fluoroscopic examination can be helpful in many cases of lymphoma because of the relative pliability of the stomach despite the apparent extent of disease. In many cases, degrees of peristalsis also are retained. These findings relate to the overall lack of fibrosis and desmoplastic reaction associated with lymphoma but commonly seen with adenocarcinoma. The exception would be a Hodgkin's-type lymphoma.

Pseudolymphoma

Although pseudolymphoma or lymphoreticular hyperplasia of the stomach is a benign condition, it is virtually impossible to distinguish this benign process from malignant disease of the stomach, such as lymphoma or carcinoma. The spectrum of radiological problems presented by this disease includes gastric masses with associated ulceration and infiltrative disease of the stomach, commonly with associated ulceration. The etiological origins of this process, also occasionally referred to as "lymphofollicular gastritis," are unclear. It is believed by some to represent an unusual late stage of peptic ulceration of the stomach, whereas others have suggested that it is the least aggressive of the spectrum of lymphoma types. Focal lymphoreticular hyperplastic changes have been reported elsewhere in the bowel, often associated with ulcers. Microscopic examination of this lesion presents some difficulty to the pathologist who is attempting to differentiate it from lymphoma. This is particularly the case on a frozen section.

Metastatic Lesions

As previously discussed, metastatic lesions, particularly in the breast and lung, can present as focal and diffuse infiltrative changes in the stomach. A local contiguous spread, such as from adjacent pancreatic malignancy, rarely may give a similar appearance.

Leukemic Infiltration

All types of leukemia may involve the gastrointestinal tract. Autopsy studies suggest that virtually all patients have some degree of gastrointestinal involvement. In the stomach, this generally is an infiltrative, diffuse process resulting in thickened irregular folds and is virtually indistinguishable from adenocarcinoma. There may be associated ulcerations and bleeding.

Gastric Erosions and Ulcers

A gastric erosion is a superficial mucosal defect, which, in contrast to a gastric ulcer, does not penetrate into the submucosa. These are virtually impossible to see on single-contrast examinations and can be detected relatively frequently using a high-quality, double-contrast technique. An integral part of the double-contrast technique consists of washing barium over the portions of the stomach most likely to harbor erosions and obtaining a barium pool sufficiently thin to show the erosions.

These erosions may be seen in any portion of the stomach, but are most common within the antrum (Fig. 2-61). The distribution can be asymmetrical. There is a tendency for erosions to line up on folds. A small lucent halo around an erosion is commonly shown and has been referred to as a complete erosion. This halo represents a circular area of edema around the erosive defect. Erosions lacking this edematous halo have been referred to as incomplete erosions and are often difficult to show even on high-quality, double-contrast studies. Often, these are short, linear erosions (Fig. 2-62).

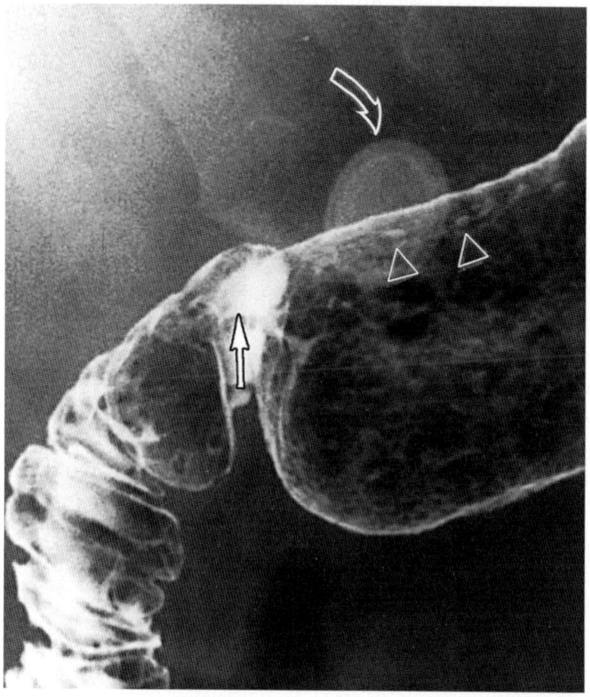

Figure 2-61 Patient with chronic peptic disease and numerous tiny erosions *(arrowheads)* and a 1.5-cm pyloric channel ulcer *(arrow)* and a laminated gallstone *(curved arrow)*.

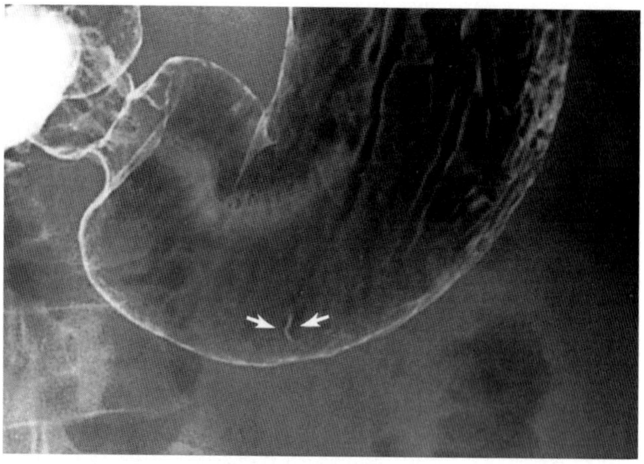

Figure 2-62 Air-contrast UGI examination shows short, superficial linear ulcer along the greater curvature of the stomach *(arrows)*.

There is considerable controversy regarding gastric erosions and their cause and clinical course. High-quality, double-contrast evaluations of the stomach show that these lesions are much more common than was previously thought.

Under normal circumstances, the gastric mucosa is protected from the acidic environment of the stomach by a surface layer of mucus in which secreted bicarbonate results in a pH gradient near neutral at the cellular level. In addition, prostaglandins within the gastric mucosa seem to play an important part in maintaining and supporting the epithelium in the presence of potentially harmful acid.

Gastric mucosal erosive changes may be acute or chronic. Erosive changes seem to be most common in patients with peptic disease and hyperacidity. It may be a manifestation of *H. pylori*-induced peptic ulcer disease in many patients. There is also a higher incidence of gastric erosions associated with excessive ingestion of alcohol or salicylates. Other medications, including indomethacin, reserpine, corticosteroids, ibuprofen, and potassium chloride, also have been implicated. Gastric erosive changes are a common cause of UGI bleeding, and hemorrhagic erosive gastritis is thought to be responsible for 10% to 20% of upper tract bleeding.

Other causes that may result in gastric mucosal erosions include Crohn's disease and viral gastritis, such as cytomegalovirus or herpesvirus. Such lesions also have been described in Behçet's syndrome. There is also reason to suspect that a significant proportion of erosive gastritis, particularly of the chronic nature, may be idiopathic, distinctively different from that induced by peptic ulcer disease, aspirin, alcohol, other medications, or *H. pylori* gastritis.

A different manifestation of multiple superficial gastric erosions is related to patients who are undergoing acute, severe physiological or emotional stress. This stress has been described as a relatively common occurrence in patients with extensive burns, in which the superficial ulcers have been referred to as "Curling's ulcers." These ulcers are identical to gastric superficial ulcers that have been described as a complication in patients with intracranial disease, severe head trauma, or after craniotomy. These stress-type ulcers (Cushing's ulcer) are almost always superficial, virtually never perforate, and in many patients are painless, with an incidence of gastrointestinal bleeding of 10% to 20%.

Malignant versus Benign Gastric Ulceration

The widespread use of high-quality, double-contrast technique in evaluation of the stomach has improved the ability of the radiologist to detect and classify ulcers as benign versus malignant. Various distinguishing features of gastric ulceration have been suggested to classify gastric ulcers successfully as benign versus malignant. The features listed in Table 2-1 can be helpful in making this differentiation. Some of the items are more useful than others, but taken together, they can give the radiologist direction as to how to classify gastric ulcerations.

There are three radiological classifications of gastric ulcers—benign, malignant, and indeterminate. In general, it has been found that when ulcers contain well-defined radiological features of benignity, they are almost always benign, and ulcerations that blatantly display the features of malignancy are almost always malignant. There is, however, a large category in which there may be benign and malignant features. In such instances, the disposition to assign the ulcer to one category or another is unclear, and such ulcers are categorized as indeterminate in nature. In patients with radiologically malignant or indeterminate gastric ulcers, follow-up gastroscopy and biopsy are always indicated. In patients in whom benign radiological features are overwhelming, automatic gastroscopy and biopsy are probably poor uses of medical resources, personnel, and health care dollars.

- *Location.* About 90% of all benign gastric ulcers are located in the antrum, and 75% of these are on the lesser curvature. Although most malignant ulcers occur in the antrum, various studies suggest that they occur here with less frequency than do benign ulcers, and malignant ulcers can be seen anywhere in the stomach. In particular, ulcers seen on the greater curvature or in parts of the stomach other than the antrum should be viewed with greater degrees of suspicion.
- *Convergence of folds.* In virtually all benign ulcers, gastric folds can be identified up to the edge of the ulcer crater (Fig. 2-63). It is extremely common for the rugal pattern to stop short of the crater margin of a malignant ulcer. This differentiation is one of the most important radiological differences between the types of ulcers.
- *Fold shape.* In benign ulcers, the adjacent fold pattern can be normal, or it may show the uniform or beaded widening secondary to edema and swelling. As previously stated, however, these folds proceed to the edge of the ulcer crater. The malignant ulcer may show a variety of abnormal fold patterns in the adjacent mucosal surface; this can include amputated, fused, or clubbed folds, all of which are

Table 2-1 Malignant versus Benign Ulceration: Radiological Distinguishing Features

Feature	Benign	Malignant
Location	Mostly antrum, 75% lesser curvature	Most lesions in antrum, but can occur anywhere
Convergence of folds	To edge of crater	Stop short of crater edge
Fold shape	Normal or uniformly swollen (edematous)	Amputated, fused, or clubbed folds that may fail to reach crater edge
Projections beyond expected confines of gastric wall	Yes	No
Position of ulcer mound or mass	Round or linear	Irregular
Ulcer collar	Yes, well-defined	May be present, but shaggy and irregular
Multiplicity	Increased frequency 10%-30%	Less frequent
Associated duodenal ulcer disease	Increased association 50%-60%	Less frequent
Carman's sign and Kirklin complex	No	Yes
Crescent sign	Yes	No
Response to therapy	Reduction of size in 4-6 weeks	No reduction in size; ulcer may enlarge

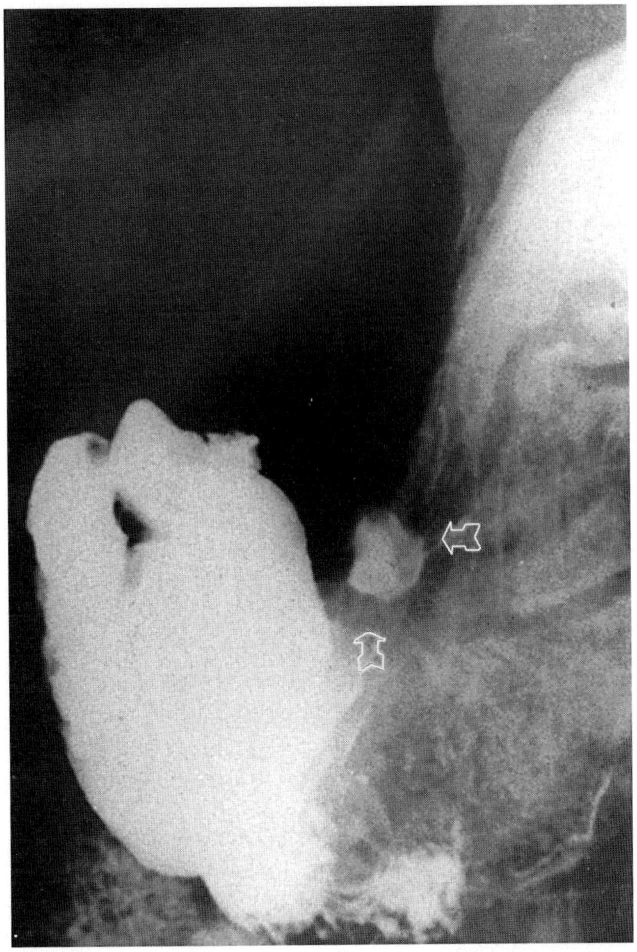

Figure 2-63 A large benign ulcer is seen along the lesser curvature of the body of the stomach. Note the gastric folds coming up to the edge of the ulcer crater *(arrows)*.

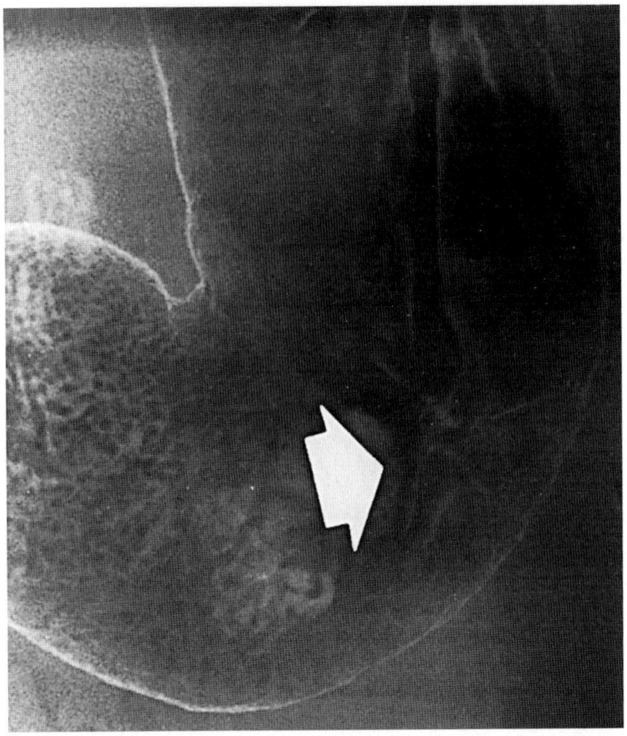

Figure 2-64 A shallow gastric ulcer *(arrow)* is seen with associated adjacent clubbed and amputated folds indicative of malignant lesion.

abnormal and often fail to reach the crater edge (Fig. 2-64). Fold configuration represents an important differentiating factor.

- *Projections beyond expected confines of gastric wall.* This has been an acceptable and reliable sign of differentiation for decades. Benign ulcers tend to excavate into the normal mucosal wall, giving a distinct impression of projecting beyond the adjacent mucosal boundaries. A malignant ulcer representing ulceration in a mass quite frequently gives the impression of ulceration that does not extend beyond the adjacent mucosal confines of the stomach. Some care should be taken with the interpretation of this sign, however. A chronic gastric ulcer in which some degree of alternating healing and exacerbation has occurred can give a configuration identical to that of a malignant ulcer as a result of fibrosis, cicatrization, and contraction of the adjacent gastric wall.
- *Position of the ulcer on the mound or mass.* Benign ulcers excite inflammatory and edematous changes in the adjacent tissues in a concentric distribution around the ulcer crater (Fig. 2-65). The appearance is that of a centrally located ulcer on a raised mass or mound of edematous tissue. Conversely, the point of ulceration that occurs on a malignant tumor is not predictable and is often eccentric.

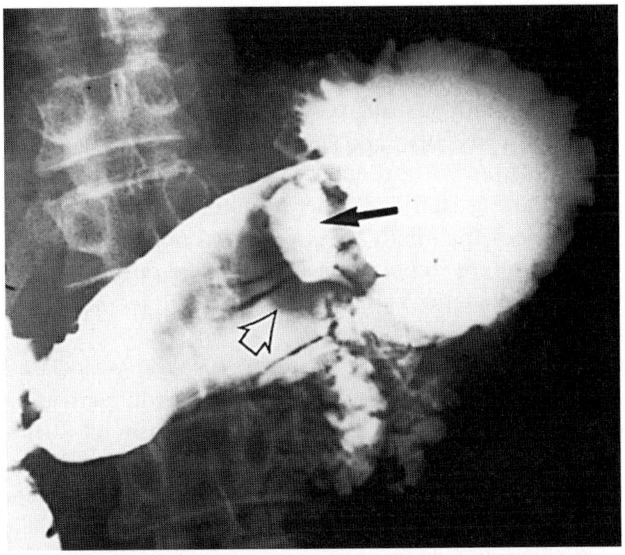

Figure 2-65 A large, benign gastric ulcer with barium-filled ulcer crater *(solid arrow)* and an edematous ulcer collar *(open arrow)* are seen.

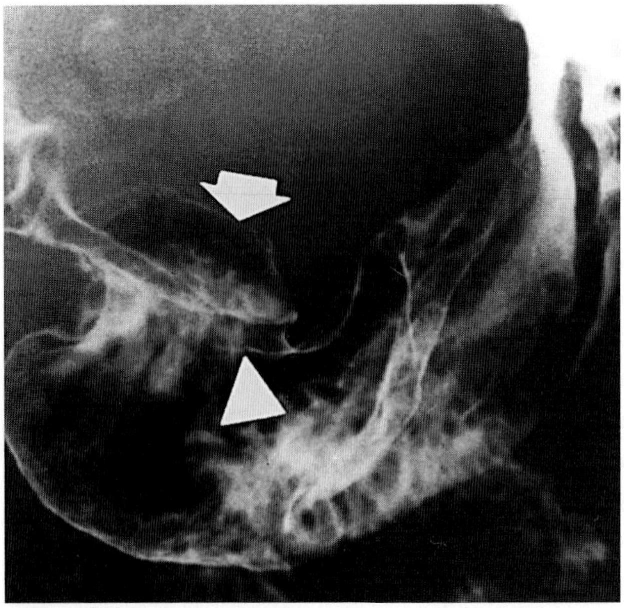

Figure 2-66 A huge gastric ulcer is seen along the lesser curvature of the stomach *(arrow)*. A well-defined ulcer collar *(arrowhead)* is seen at the margin of the ulcer.

- *Ulcer shape.* Benign ulcers are generally round. Distinct linear ulcers almost always are benign. Malignant ulcers occasionally can be round and well defined, but more often are found to be irregular with poor definition of the margins.
- *Ulcer collar.* A uniform ulcer collar around a centrally located ulcer is a good sign for benignity (Fig. 2-66). Undermining of the adjacent soft tissue and subsequent edematous changes result in the appearance of an ulcer collar. When the edematous changes are restricted to the overhanging mucosa around the crater margin, the configuration in profile may be that of a thin, well-demarcated lucent ulcer collar, known as a "Hampton line." Ulcer collars may be present on malignant ulcers, but they are generally thick, irregular, and shaggy in appearance.
- *Multiplicity.* Although this cannot be considered a strong sign for either benignity or malignancy, it does apparently have some statistical significance. Literature reports have suggested an increased potential for benignity when multiple ulcers are present (Fig. 2-67).
- *Associated duodenal ulcer disease.* Associated duodenal ulcer disease is a statistically differentiating point that must be correlated with all other distinguishing features. The increased association between benign gastric ulcers and duodenal ulcers has been reported with considerable variance.
- *Carman's meniscus sign and Kirklin complex.* First described by Carman in the late 1920s, Carman's sign (Box 2-8) is thought to be diagnostic of a particular type of ulcerated neoplasm. The ulcer is almost always located on the saddle portion of the stomach on the lesser curvature of the antrum and body. The malignant lesion lacks significant mass effect. The type of ulceration is usually large and flat, with raised edges. In single-contrast, barium-filled examination of the stomach with compression of this saddle region, the heaped-up edges of the ulcer approximate and entrap barium within the flat ulcer bed, giving a meniscoid configuration to the trapped barium within the ulcer, in which the inner margin is concave toward the lumen (Fig. 2-68). Where the heaped-up margins of the ulcer approximate and meet and entrap barium, as a result of compression, the lucent margin that surrounds the concavity of the ulcer represents the approximated heaped-up ulcer edges. This is called the "Kirklin complex." Because of the special

Box 2-8 Recipe for Carman's Meniscus Sign: Necessary Ingredients

Flat tumor with heaped-up edges
Located on saddle area of lesser curve of antrum of stomach
Seen in single-contrast examination or single-contrast phase of biphasic examination
Seen only with compression

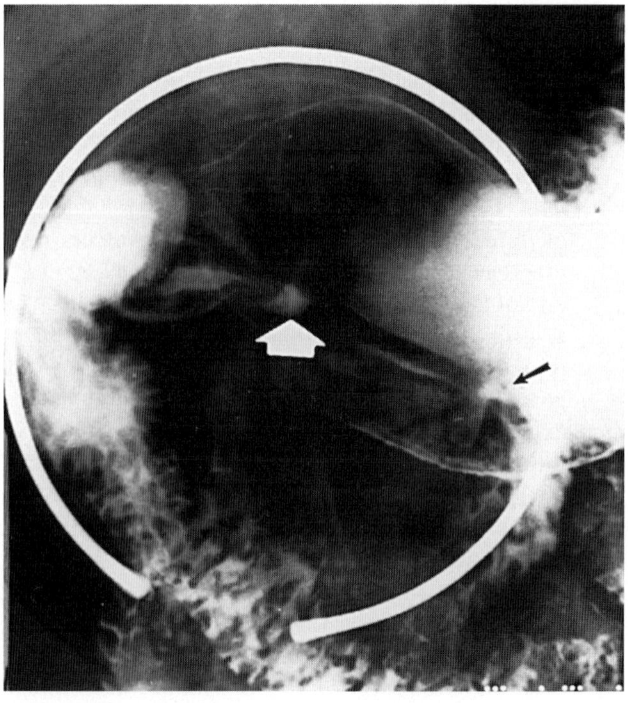

Figure 2-67 Multiple, small gastric ulcers are shown *(arrows)*.

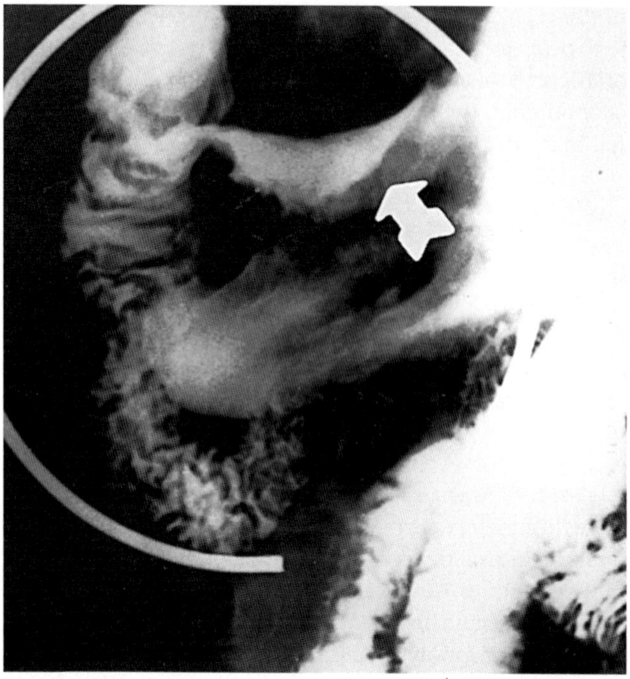

Figure 2-68 Large ulcer along the lesser curvature of the antrum of the stomach, under compression, shows concavity of the ulcer crater *(arrow)* along its luminal side. This is Carman's meniscus sign of malignancy.

circumstances regarding the nature of the mass, configuration and location of the ulcer, and the need for the barium-filled stomach and compression views, this sign rarely is identified on double-contrast views of the stomach.

- *Crescent sign.* Benign ulcers occurring along the greater curvature of the antrum or body and in which significant mucosal undermining has occurred may show the configuration of a crescent-shaped ulceration with its concavity directed away from the gastric lumen.
- *Response to therapy.* With adequate treatment, almost all benign gastric ulcers undergo a reduction of size in a 4- to 6-week period. Expected deformity changes associated with scarring and cicatrization also can be identified. Alternatively, there is no change in malignant ulcers, or they increase in size. This differentiating factor is significant, although it has been noted that on rare occasions, a malignant ulcer may undergo some decrease in size with peptic ulcer treatment.

Miscellaneous Findings

Diverticula

Fundal Diverticula

The most common of diverticula encountered in the stomach arise from the cardiofundal region, usually seen on the posterior wall of the stomach (Fig. 2-69). It is a true diverticulum, containing all the layers of the stomach, and can range in size from 1 to 10 cm. These are considered to be congenital and, for the most part, of no clinical significance. Reports of bleeding from gastric diverticula exist in the literature, citing incidences of 14%. This incidence is probably considerably higher, however, than the experience of most endoscopists and gastrointestinal radiologists. Additionally, if a diverticulum becomes sufficiently large, impaired emptying and stasis may result, although this is also a rare complication.

Antral Diverticula

Antral diverticula are unusual intramural projections of mucosa in the gastric wall. They are almost always located along the greater curvature of the antrum of the stomach. There has been an association with ectopic pancreatic tissue reported in approximately 10% to 15% of cases (Fig. 2-70).

Radiologically, the partial diverticulum on the greater curvature of the antrum has a "collar-button" appearance and is often misdiagnosed as a benign gastric ulcer. The persistent appearance, lack of inflammatory changes around the partial diverticulum, and lack of tenderness when compressing this region should help the radiologist avoid this mistake (Fig. 2-71).

Postoperative Stomach

The most common types of gastric surgeries are the partial gastrectomy and gastrojejunostomy (Billroth II), antrectomy and gastroduodenostomy (Billroth I), diverting gastrojejunostomy, and gastric partitions for morbid obesity. Radiographic abnormalities seen in complications of gastric resection include the following.

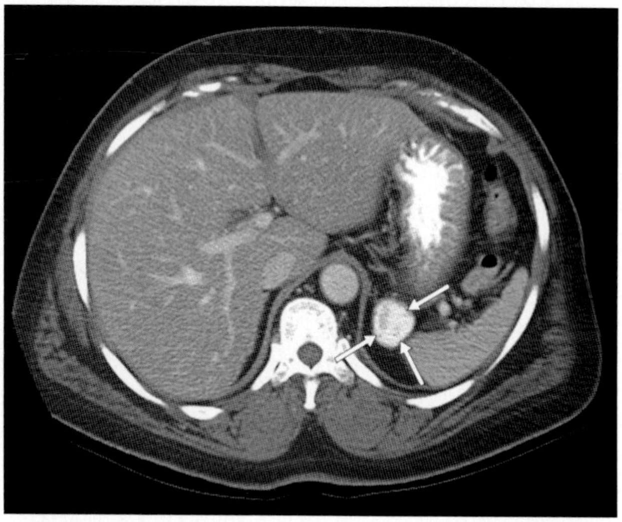

Figure 2-69 Computed tomographic scan shows a rounded collection of contrast material *(arrows)* arising from the posterior gastric fundus; this represents a fundal diverticulum.

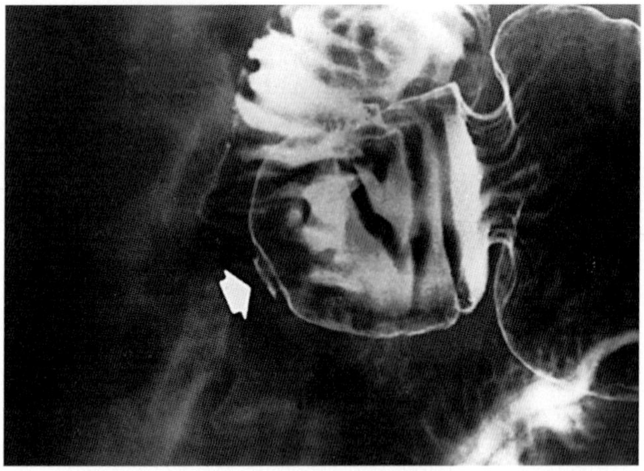

Figure 2-70 On UGI examination, a small, shallow protrusion along the greater curvature of the stomach *(arrow)* was diagnosed to be a shallow gastric ulcer. Note the absence of inflammatory changes around the area. Endoscopy showed no evidence of inflammation or ulceration and a small antral diverticulum.

Pseudomass

Pseudomass can be seen after a Billroth I or Billroth II procedure, although it is more common in the latter. It represents the plication deformity that results when the divided end of the stomach is oversewn to restrict the size of the stoma (Fig. 2-72). The radiological problem presented in this situation is that of a masslike filling defect seen at or near the anastomotic site. It is generally more prominent on immediate postoperative examinations secondary to the edematous changes that persist in the region. On subsequent examinations, it may seem less prominent and over time may appear static in its configuration and size. Without a baseline postoperative examination, the deformity can easily simulate neoplastic recurrence.

Postoperative Gastric Bezoars

As previously discussed, bezoar is a common complication of gastric surgery (see Fig. 2-9). The bezoars encountered in this setting are almost always phytobezoars and can be asymptomatic. If the bezoar becomes sufficiently large, obstruction of the stoma, distention of the gastric remnant, and irritation and erosion of the mucosa can occur.

Gastric Stump Carcinoma

Although controversy continues regarding the incidence and occurrence of carcinoma in the gastric remnant, the postoperative stomach is at higher risk for carcinoma than the nonoperated stomach. These lesions are most commonly seen in patients 10 years after partial gastrectomy and, as previously discussed, may be due to chronic gastritis secondary to bile reflux (Fig. 2-73).

Chronic Gastric Remnant Gastritis

One of the more common postoperative complications seen in the stomach is chronic gastritis. It is hypothesized that the lack of pyloric protection results in chronic reflux of bile and pancreatic secretions stimulating inflammatory changes in the gastric remnant. The common radiological appearance is of enlarged

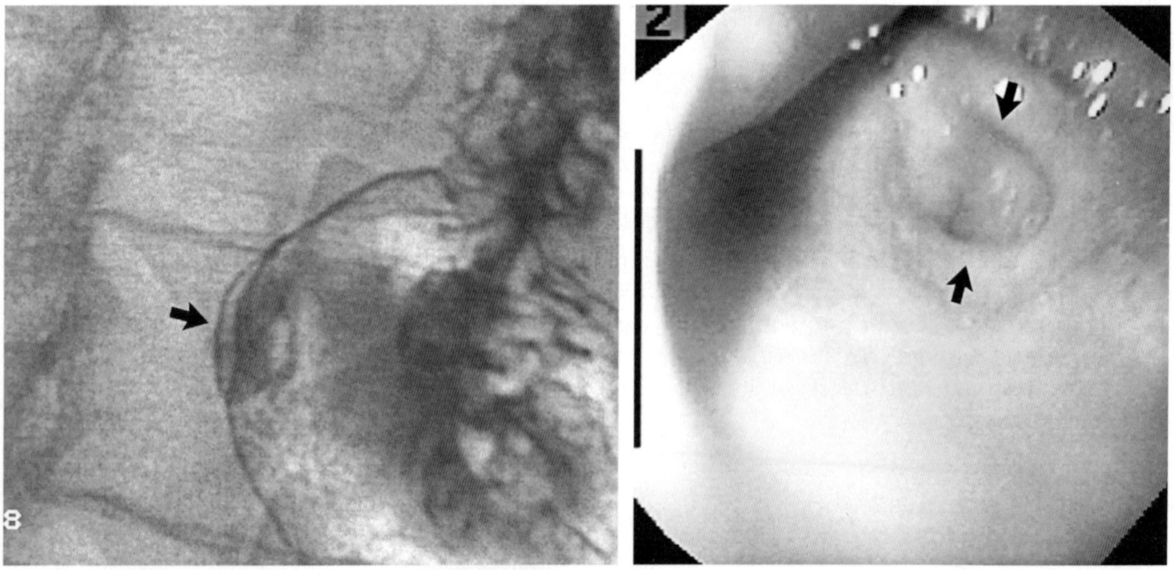

A B

Figure 2-71 Antral diverticulum. **A,** Digital image of distal stomach shows a shallow excavation in antrum *(arrow)*. Note lack of edematous changes in the area. **B,** Endoscopic image of area shows the margins of the antral diverticulum *(arrows)*. Note normal mucosa in and around the diverticulum.

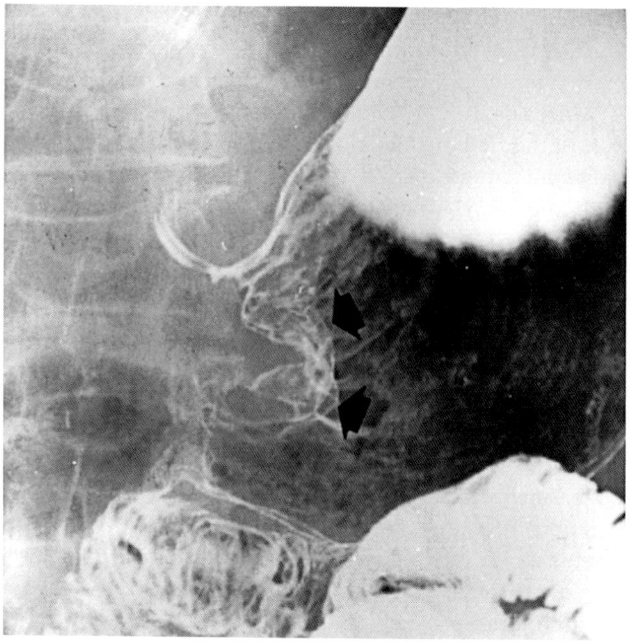

Figure 2-72 This patient has had a Billroth II gastric resection. UGI examination shows a large mass along the margin of the gastric stump *(arrows)*. Ominous as this appears, it represents only a prominent plication defect.

gastric rugae, although erosions and even ulcers have been associated with chronic gastritis.

Stomal Ulceration

Recurrent ulceration after partial gastrectomy for peptic ulcer disease commonly appears on the jejunal side of the gastrojejunostomy and is known as a stomal or marginal ulcer (Fig. 2-74). When these ulcers are sufficiently large, they are difficult to miss. Smaller marginal ulcers are readily missed on UGI studies, however, particularly on single-contrast examinations. The presence of recurrent ulcers on the anastomotic margin is probably unrelated to chronic small bowel reflux and more likely suggests the possibility of inadequate gastric resection, the possible existence of an antral remnant inadvertently left behind, or even the presence of a pancreatic islet cell Zollinger-Ellison–type tumor. Additionally, some have suggested that an excessively long afferent loop may predispose to marginal ulcers.

Chronic Gastroesophageal Reflux

Patients with partial gastric resections experience an increased incidence of gastroesophageal reflux. Any patient undergoing any surgery involving mobilization of the stomach may experience increased reflux and subsequent reflux esophagitis.

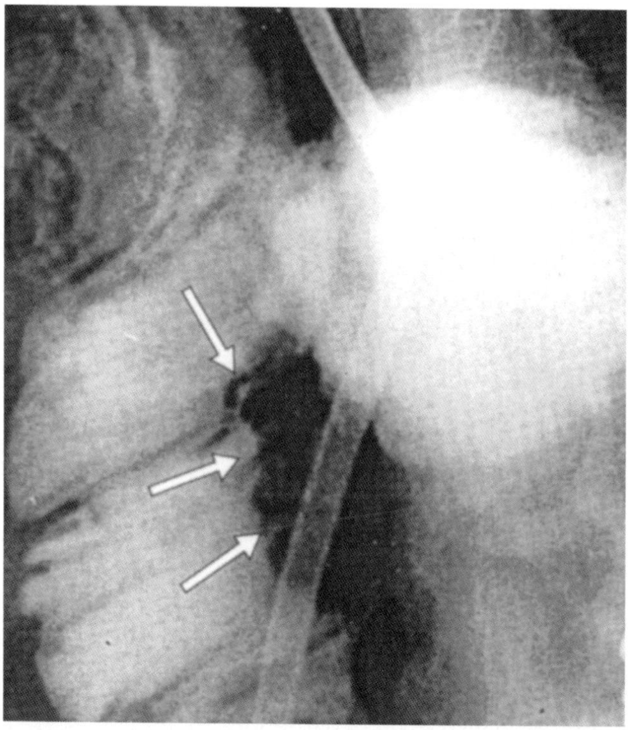

Figure 2-73 UGI study in a patient with previous gastrectomy. The anastomosis is open. There is nodularity *(arrows)* along the margin of the efferent loop, which proved to be a recurrent adenocarcinoma.

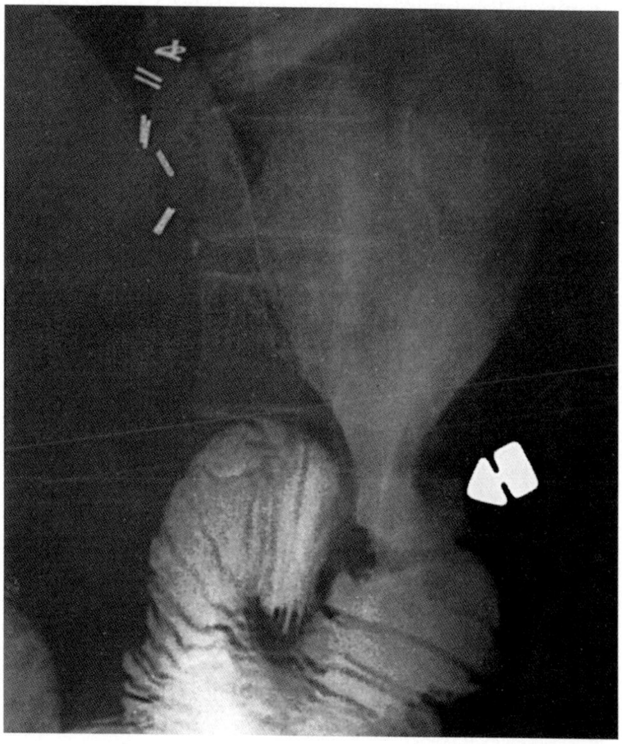

Figure 2-74 Patient with previous gastrectomy and Billroth II resection presented with recurrent pain. UGI study shows large stomal ulcer *(arrow)*.

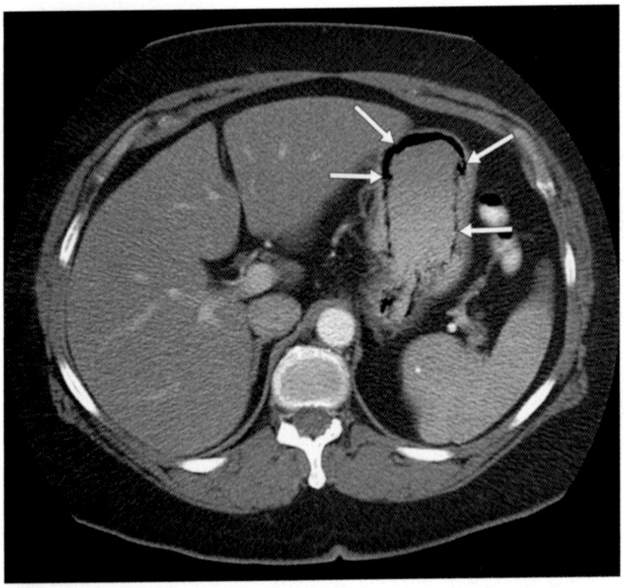

Figure 2-75 Computed tomographic scan shows air in gastric wall *(arrows)* after instrumentation.

Jejunal Gastric Intussusception

Jejunal gastric intussusception is infrequent, but when it does occur, it can be seen as an acute or chronic recurrent process. The acute intussusception is often a surgical emergency with compromise of the blood supply in the intussuscepted small bowel loops. These patients present with severe abdominal pain, nausea and vomiting, and evidence of UGI obstruction. Patients with the chronic recurring type may have no more symptoms than occasional vague upper abdominal discomfort. The intussusception may decompress spontaneously after several minutes.

A large intraremnant filling defect often suggestive of intussusception in its configuration and barium pattern is seen. In the chronic transient variety, the patient may have vague upper abdominal symptoms, and unless the intussusception is occurring at the time of examination, the diagnosis probably will not be considered.

Gastric Wall Emphysema

Gastric intramural pneumatosis is an unusual finding. The most common cause relates to the ingestion of corrosive acidic material with subsequent necrosis of the mucosa. In addition, it can be seen in the phlegmonous type of gastritis, in which the offending bacterial agent is a gas-producing organism. Air in the gastric wall also has been associated with gastric ulcers and with instrumentation of the stomach, for example, endoscopy and placement of tubes (Fig. 2-75).

DUODENUM

The evaluation of the duodenum is normally included as part of the UGI examination. It should include air-contrast views and compression views, particularly of the duodenal bulb region. Hypotonic duodenography also has been helpful in evaluating this region. The desired result is usually achieved with 0.1 to 0.5 mg of intravenous glucagon (Fig. 2-76). Although the use of glucagon has diminished significantly with the increased number of immunocompromised patients being seen over the last 2 decades, the quality of the study done without the use of parenteral glucagon can be at least as good if the radiologist is patient and committed to high-quality work. Occasionally, the duodenum can be located in a posterior position directly behind the gastric antrum. Under such circumstances, profiling the duodenal bulb, particularly for air-contrast views, can be difficult. In the left lateral position, the air-filled bulb may be overlapped by portions of the antrum. Angulation of the x-ray tube during fluoroscopy, if this facility is available, may be helpful in separating the duodenal bulb from the antrum. When angulation is not available, a few simple maneuvers may be undertaken. The first is an attempt to evaluate the duodenum in the left oblique position while the patient is upright. The weight of the barium within the stomach may pull the gastric antrum sufficiently downward to

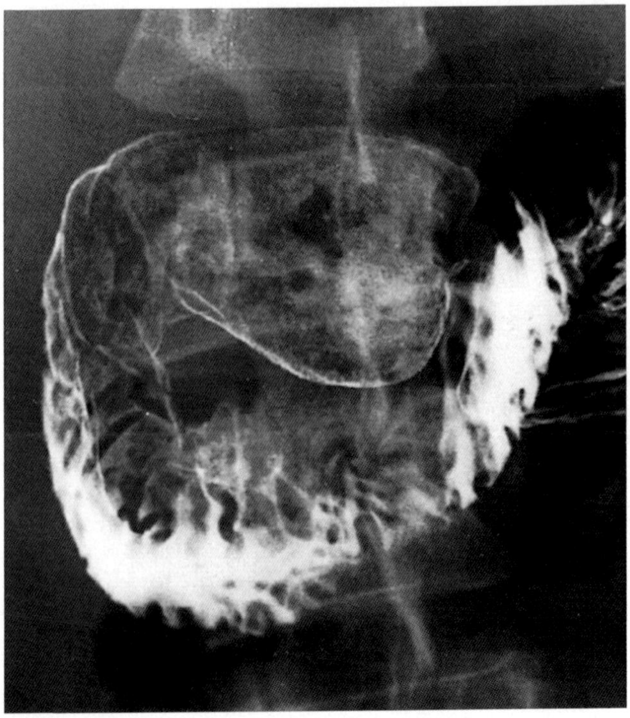

Figure 2-76 Air-contrast view of normal duodenal bulb using 0.1 mg intravenous glucagon.

allow visualization of the duodenal bulb, which tends to be fixed. Alternatively, with the patient recumbent and in the left lateral position, a bolster (inflated balloon or pillow) is placed in the patient's epigastrium, and the patient is asked to roll downward toward the bolster and the table (left anterior oblique position). This maneuver often displaces the stomach away from the duodenum, permitting an unobstructed profile view of the air-filled duodenum and pyloric channel (Fig. 2-77).

Most of the radiological problems associated with the duodenum also are common to the remainder of the small bowel. For this reason, discussion of these entities in this section is limited; more detail can be found in Chapter 3.

Dilated (Nonobstructed) Lumen

Neuromuscular abnormalities account for most of the findings of a dilated flaccid duodenum during UGI examination. They include scleroderma, idiopathic intestinal pseudoobstruction, and diabetes mellitus. Patients taking anticholinergic atropine-like medication may exhibit similar findings (Fig. 2-78).

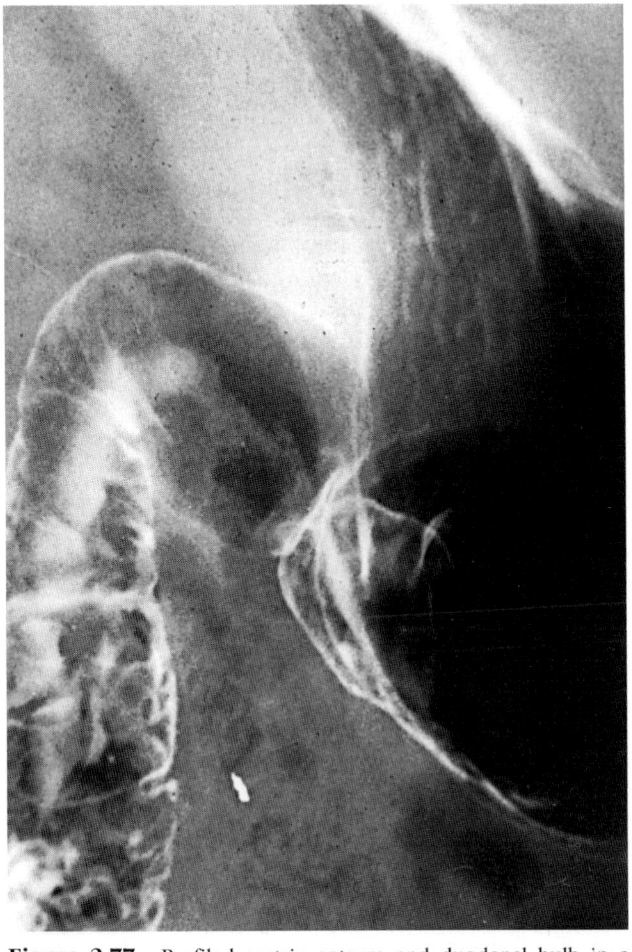

Figure 2-77 Profiled gastric antrum and duodenal bulb in a posteriorly located duodenum.

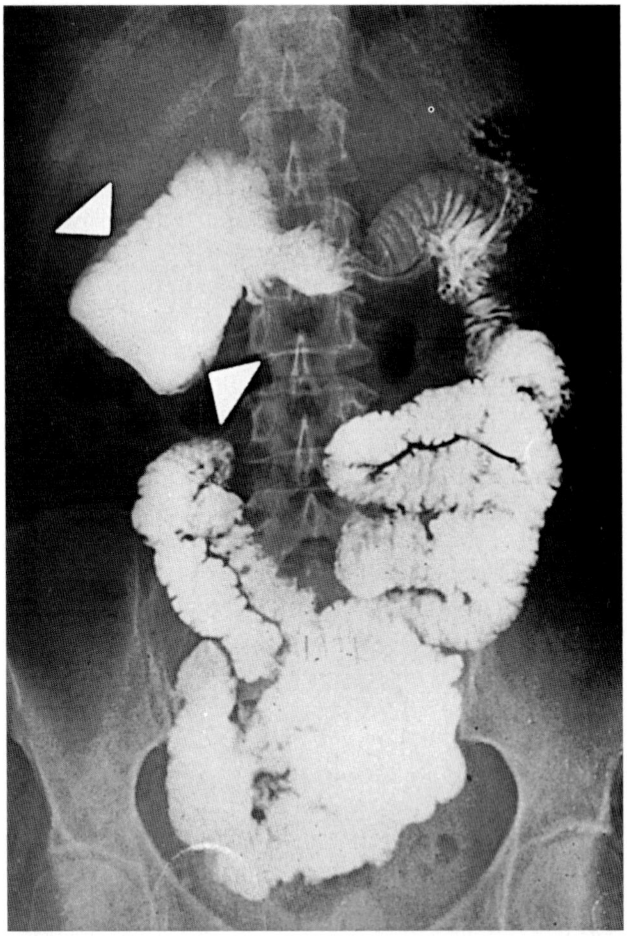

Figure 2-78 Megaduodenum *(arrowheads)* in a patient with scleroderma.

In patients with nontropical sprue, dilatation of the small bowel is a common finding and may be seen within the duodenum as well. Most of the other findings associated with sprue tend to be confined to the more distal small bowel.

Occasionally, a dilated nonobstructed duodenal sweep may be seen in patients with severe acute illnesses, trauma, or burns. In these patients, distention of the stomach and occasionally the duodenum may be encountered. Intraabdominal processes, which result in an adynamic ileus, also can involve the duodenum, causing dilatation. Although the esophagus is the main gastrointestinal site of involvement in patients with Chagas' disease, the intramural plexus of the duodenum can also be damaged by the trypanosomes, resulting in diminished peristalsis and dilatation. Dilated duodenum has been described in eating disorders, such as anorexia nervosa or postpartum cachexia.

Narrowed Lumen

More than 90% of peptic ulcer disease involving the duodenum affects the duodenal bulb. It can occur as an acute episode, recurrent disease, or chronic disease. In recurrent and chronic disease, duodenal bulb deformity is common, and a small, contracted, narrow duodenal bulb often is seen in patients with chronic peptic ulcer disease. This deformity occasionally can result in obstruction and a dilated stomach.

Approximately 10% of duodenal ulcers are postbulbar in location. They are radiologically difficult to see. Often the radiological findings are thickened, irregular folds, with an area of focal narrowing. Crohn's disease or tuberculosis involving the duodenum, although relatively uncommon, can produce an identical appearance (Fig. 2-79). Inflammatory changes affecting adjacent pancreas or, less commonly, the gallbladder, also can result in postbulbar stricture. Malignancy arising from the pancreatic head also can invade any portion of the duodenal sweep, resulting in strictured narrowing (Fig. 2-80); this most commonly occurs in the descending and proximal transverse portion of the duodenum.

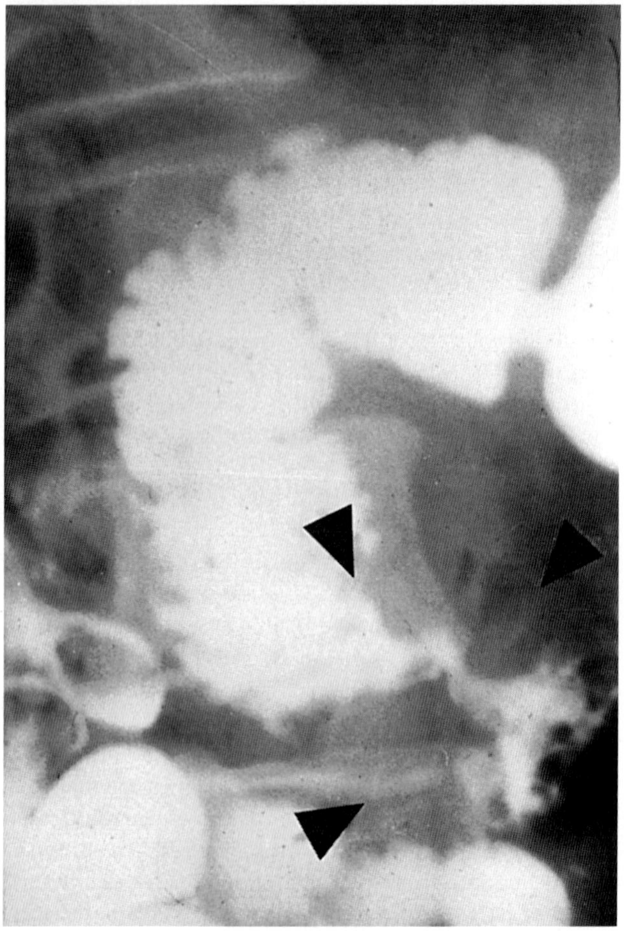

Figure 2-79 Crohn's disease involving the duodenal sweep with resultant stricture *(arrowheads)*.

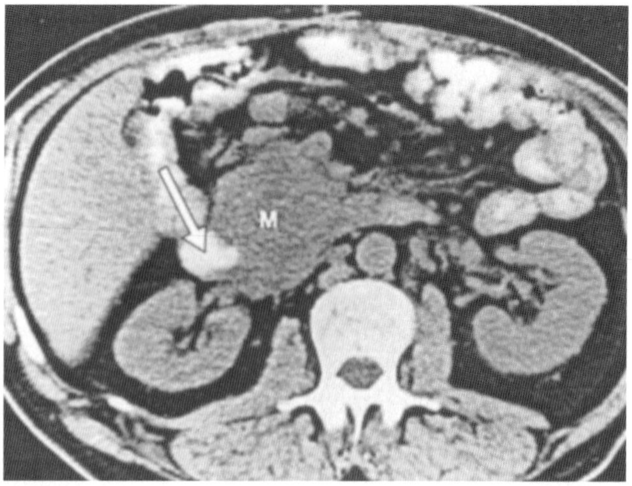

Figure 2-80 CT through the pancreas shows a large mass *(M)* invading the adjacent contrast-filled duodenal sweep *(arrow)*.

Annular pancreas is an unusual condition involving the descending duodenum. It represents an embryological abnormality of pancreatic development in which the ventral bud of the pancreas encircles the duodenum. This abnormality produces circumferential indentation of the descending duodenum by the surrounding pancreatic tissue. It is often diagnosed in infancy or childhood, although many of these patients are not identified until adolescence or adulthood. Occasionally, periduodenal fibrosis of the duodenal wall can develop at the site of the long-standing stricture resulting from the annular pancreatic tissue. For this reason, surgical relief of the annular extrinsic compression may not always be curative, and occasionally a gastroenterostomy bypass may be indicated.

The intraluminal diverticulum of the duodenum, or "wind sock deformity," is a thin, intraluminal web or membrane (Fig. 2-81). The wind sock configuration occurs as a result of the web being stretched and billowed into the distal lumen by the prolonged and constant effect of peristaltic activity. Bleeding into the duodenal wall, as a result of trauma or other causes such as Henoch-Schönlein purpura, hemophilia, or anticoagulation therapy, can present as a discrete intramural mass or diffuse infiltrative changes with thickened fold pattern, or a combination, with associated narrowing.

The superior mesenteric artery syndrome is a condition in which duodenal obstruction occurs as a result of narrowing of the angle between the aorta and the superior mesenteric artery at the point at which the duodenum passes between them. This condition is most commonly seen in burn patients, patients in body casts, or patients who have experienced acute severe illness with substantial weight loss. It is thought that the loss

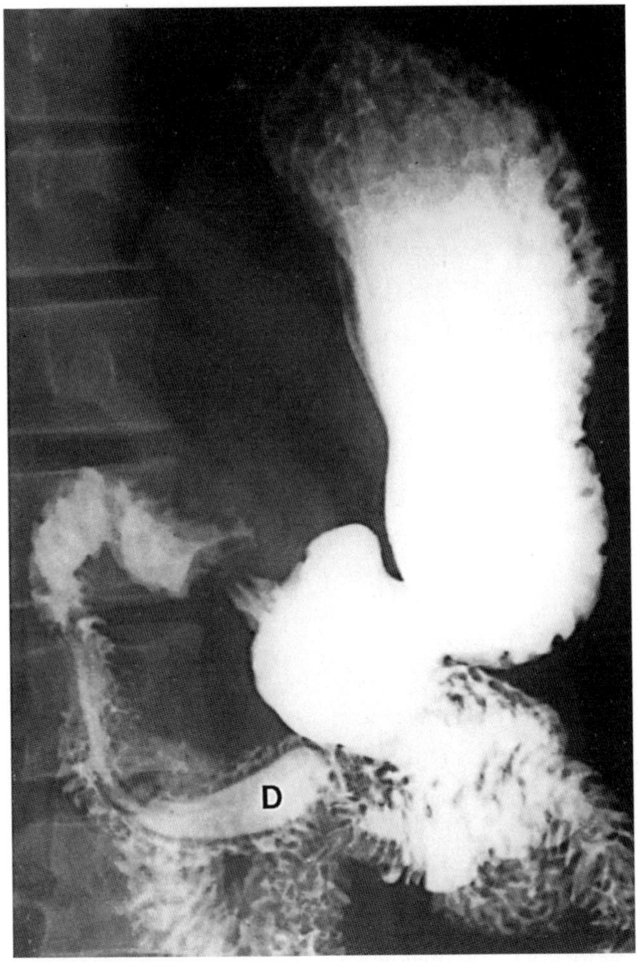

Figure 2-81 UGI study demonstrates intraluminal diverticulum or wind sock configuration *(D)*.

of retroperitoneal fat results in a narrowing of the angle between the vessels. Another condition that can result in duodenal narrowing and potential obstruction is midgut volvulus, seen in patients with incomplete rotation of the midgut. The volvulus can occur as a result of fibrous bands overlying the proximal portion of the duodenum, around which the midgut can rotate (Ladd's bands) and twist. Volvulus also can occur as a result of rotation of the midgut around a markedly abbreviated small bowel mesentery that may occur as a result of incomplete rotation.

Aortoduodenal fistulas are usually complications of prosthetic aortic Dacron grafts. They originally were described as complications of aortic abdominal aneurysms. The distal portion of the duodenum, in contact with the graft or aneurysm, breaks down as a result of focal pressure or erosion of the aorta dissecting into the duodenal wall. The condition is potentially fatal. Contrast examination of the distal duodenum can show several possible findings, including mass effect, luminal narrowing, ulceration, and even tracking of contrast material along the outside of the graft. Complete obstruction of the intestinal lumen in the neonate (duodenal atresia) results from failure of cannulization of the duodenum during early intrauterine life. The incidence is higher in infants with Down syndrome; often these patients present within several hours of birth with the classic "double-bubble" sign, representing an air-filled and distended stomach and duodenal bulb. Another congenital cause of duodenal narrowing is duodenal duplication. Although this condition is rare, it can result in a large periduodenal mass impressing and narrowing the duodenum. The duplicated segment also may be continuous with the main lumen.

Adenocarcinoma of the duodenum, although rare, occurs most commonly in the distal half of the duodenum and in most instances has the typical apple-core configuration (Fig. 2-82). Metastasis to the duodenum also is uncommon but can occur as an encircling obstructing mass, often in the distal portion of the duodenal sweep (Fig. 2-83).

Thickened Folds

The most common causes of thickened duodenal folds, particularly in the more proximal duodenum, are peptic ulcer disease and pancreatitis. The changes are a result of edema from direct inflammatory changes involving the duodenum and indirect changes involving the pancreatic head.

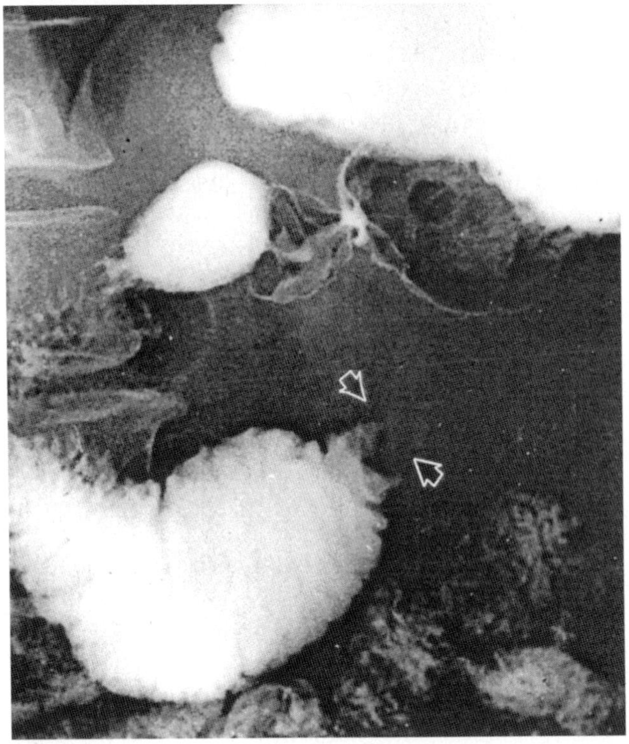

Figure 2-82 Primary adenocarcinoma of the duodenum with annular narrowing and obstruction *(arrows)*.

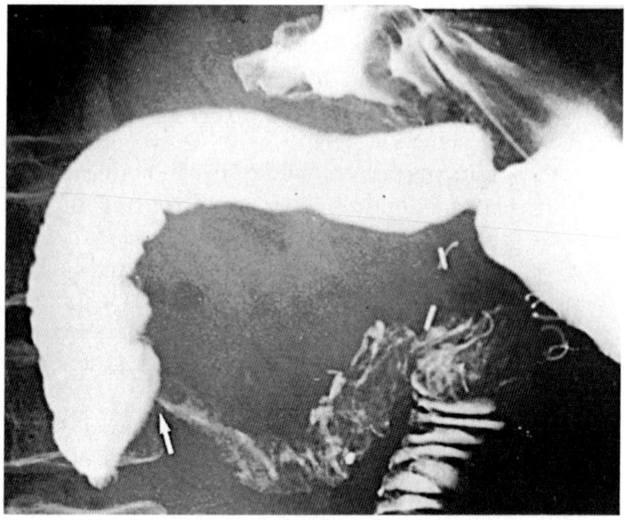

Figure 2-83 Metastatic disease involving the duodenal sweep *(arrow)*, eccentrically narrowing the lumen.

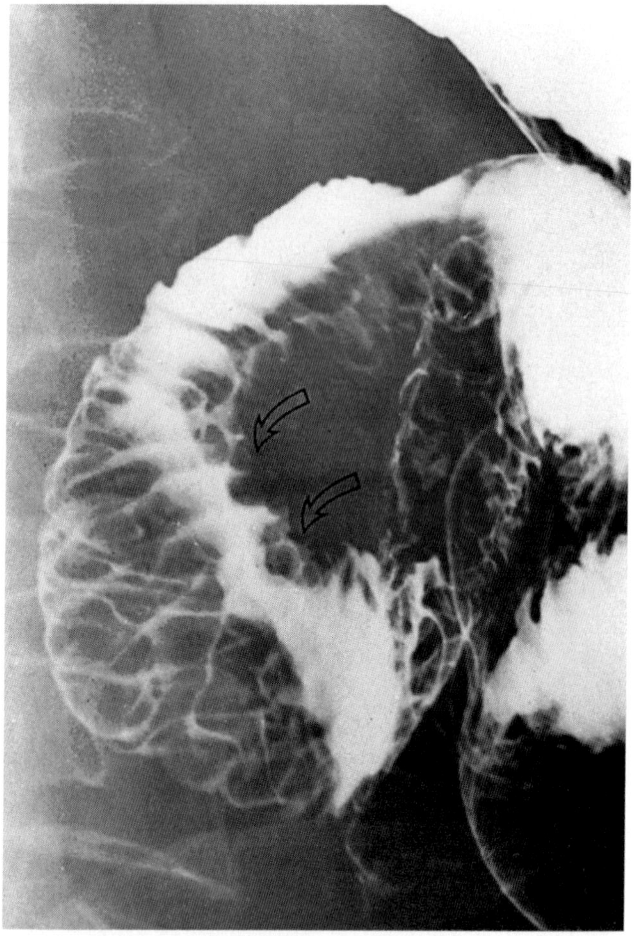

Figure 2-84 UGI study in a patient with acute severe pancreatitis resulting in marked thickening of duodenal folds and the reverse figure 3 configuration on the inner margin *(arrows)*.

In acute pancreatitis, the changes may be limited to the medial inner curve of the duodenal sweep. There may be thickening and tethering of folds that can result in the "reverse figure 3" sign (also seen with pancreatic carcinoma) described on the UGI examination (Figs. 2-84 and 2-85).

Patients with Zollinger-Ellison syndrome always have fold prominence within the duodenum as a result of the marked amount of gastric acid secretion stimulated by pancreatic gastrinoma. A few patients with this uncommon disease have the offending gastrinoma located within the duodenum. Crohn's disease of the duodenum is most commonly seen as thickened folds (Fig. 2-86).

Parasitic infection in the small bowel commonly involves the duodenum and results in thick, irregular folds. *Ascaris lumbricoides* commonly involves the distal small bowel. *Strongyloides stercoralis* and intestinal hookworm, *Ancylostoma duodenale,* have a marked preference for the proximal small bowel, particularly the duodenum. *Giardia lamblia* is a relatively common protozoan parasite that involves the duodenum and jejunum, with resultant fold thickening and irregularity (Fig. 2-87). Hypersecretion and hypermotility also may be seen in patients with giardiasis. Additionally, the presence of lymphoid hyperplasia has been observed in some patients with giardiasis.

Fold thickening also can be observed in patients with eosinophilic gastroenteritis. These patients often present with abdominal pain, nausea, vomiting, and eosinophilia on their peripheral blood smear. Fold thickening usually involves the gastric antrum and duodenum. Whipple's disease involves the proximal small bowel with thickened and irregular folds in the duodenum and proximal jejunum.

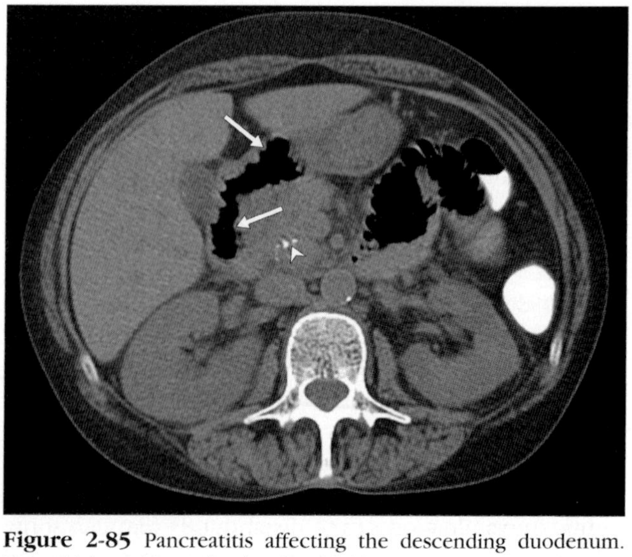

Figure 2-85 Pancreatitis affecting the descending duodenum. Note thickened irregular duodenal folds *(arrows)* and calcification in the head of pancreas *(arrowhead)*.

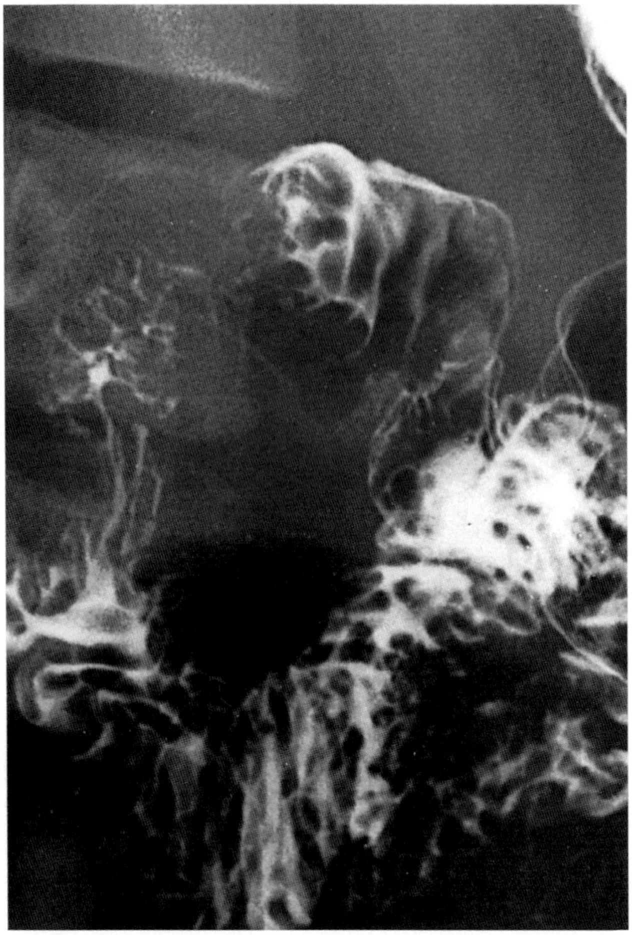

Figure 2-86 Thickening of folds in the duodenal bulb and postbulbar region secondary to Crohn's disease.

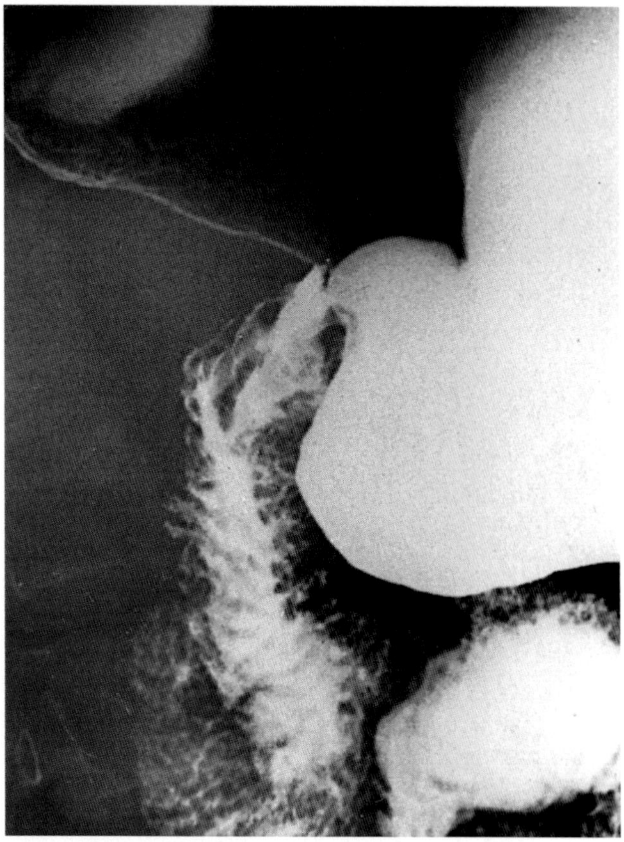

Figure 2-87 Thickened, irregular folds with fine nodularity are seen in a patient with giardiasis.

Occasionally, patients with portal hypertension and esophageal varices also may manifest varicoid formation within the proximal duodenum; this is seen as thickened and smooth serpiginous folds. Frequently, the presence of duodenal varices is an indication of portal vein occlusion. Duodenal intramural bleeding also may manifest as thickened regular folds with the classic "stack of coins" appearance.

Lymphomas may have multiple physical manifestations within the small bowel, among which is diffuse fold thickening. Its presence in the duodenum is rare and, when present, is similar to lymphomas elsewhere in the gut; it almost never obstructs. Patients in chronic renal failure or on long-term dialysis commonly show thickened folds within the duodenum. There is also an increased incidence of peptic ulcer disease in such patients, although the persistent thickened folds probably are not peptic in origin. Uniform thickening of folds within the duodenum, jejunum, and ileum can occur in primary and secondary amyloidosis.

Filling Defects

Flexural Pseudopolyp

One of the most common and troublesome of duodenal filling defects is the flexural pseudopolyp (Fig. 2-88). This phenomenon is usually seen in thin patients with a sharp, acute angle between the apex of the duodenal bulb and the descending duodenum. Because of the acuteness of the angle, mucosa can pile up on the medial inner aspect of the duodenum at the level of the apex of the bulb; this results in a filling defect that can easily be diagnosed as a nonexistent polypoid mass. Demonstration of this mass in a thin individual with a sharp bulbar duodenal angle should alert the radiologist to the possibility of a flexural pseudotumor. This condition can be confirmed by evaluating the area in question with the patient in different positions, particularly supine positions that may open the bulbar duodenal angle and change the configuration of the filling defect.

Pancreatic Rests

Pancreatic rests or ectopic pancreatic tissue within the duodenum can result in a well-defined filling defect (Fig. 2-89). These are not neoplastic lesions and are of embryonic origin. They are smooth, can be round or

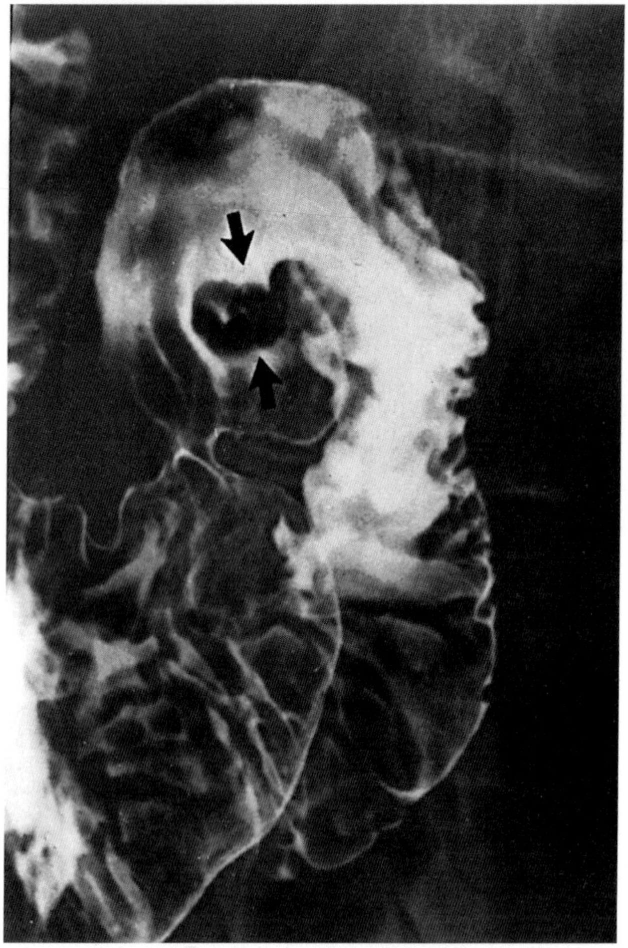

Figure 2-88 Polypoid filling defect in the duodenal bulb *(arrows)* proved to be a flexural pseudotumor. No polyps were identified at endoscopy.

lobulated, and usually measure 1 to 2 cm in diameter. They more commonly present as solitary filling defects in the duodenal bulb or second portion of the duodenum. They also can be seen in the gastric antrum. A characteristic radiological finding is the central collection of barium (dimple) that may be confused with a small ulcer on the surface of a neoplastic polypoid lesion.

Mesenchymal Tumors (Gastrointestinal Stromal Cell Tumors)

Mesenchymal benign tumors, such as stromal cell tumors (leiomyomas) and lipomas, are the most common benign lesions of the duodenum. They are usually solitary and submucosal in origin and have a smooth surface. These can ulcerate on the surface, although this is uncommon in the duodenum. The duodenal variety is usually smaller than the tumors seen elsewhere in the bowel. Neurofibroma and hemangioma also can occur within the duodenum but are rare.

Adenoma

Duodenal adenomas are uncommon. When present, they are seen radiologically as mucosal polypoid lesions usually no more than 1 cm in diameter. The exception is the villous adenoma, which when symptomatic is commonly 2 to 3 cm (Fig. 2-90). Patients may present with either gastrointestinal bleeding or symptoms related to intussusception. These lesions have a high potential for malignant degeneration.

Carcinoid/APUDoma

Similarly, carcinoid tumors arising from argentaffin cells within the mucosa can be seen in the duodenum and particularly in the peripapillary region of the second

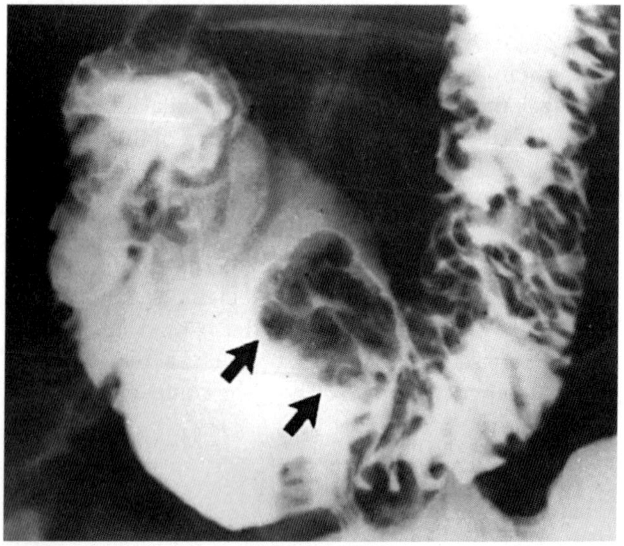

Figure 2-89 A lobulated filling defect *(arrows)* is seen in the duodenal bulb with a small, central barium collection (dimple) representing a pancreatic rest.

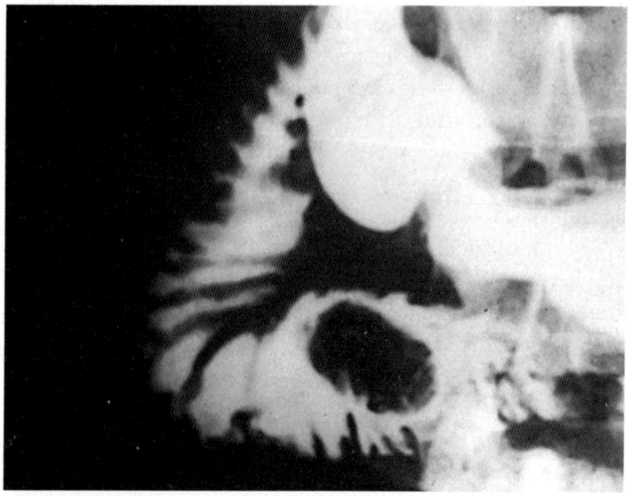

Figure 2-90 A well-defined, lobulated filling defect in the transverse portion of the duodenum representing a villous adenoma is seen.

portion of the duodenum. The radiological appearance varies and may involve discrete smooth polyps or irregular infiltrating processes. A variant of this, the APUDoma, can arise from amine precursor uptake and decarboxylation (APUD) cells. These tumors are histologically similar to ileal carcinoid tumors and are frequently associated with multiple endocrine neoplasia syndromes. Various polypoid syndromes also may have polyps within the duodenum, including familial polyposis, Peutz-Jeghers syndrome, Cronkhite-Canada syndrome, and Cowden's disease.

Brunner's Gland Hyperplasia and Brunner's Gland Adenoma

Multiple filling defects in the duodenal bulb are also a presentation of Brunner's gland hyperplasia (Fig. 2-91). This process also can extend into the second portion of the duodenum. The cause of this condition is unclear. Normal function of Brunner's glands, which produce alkaline secretion to protect the sensitive duodenal

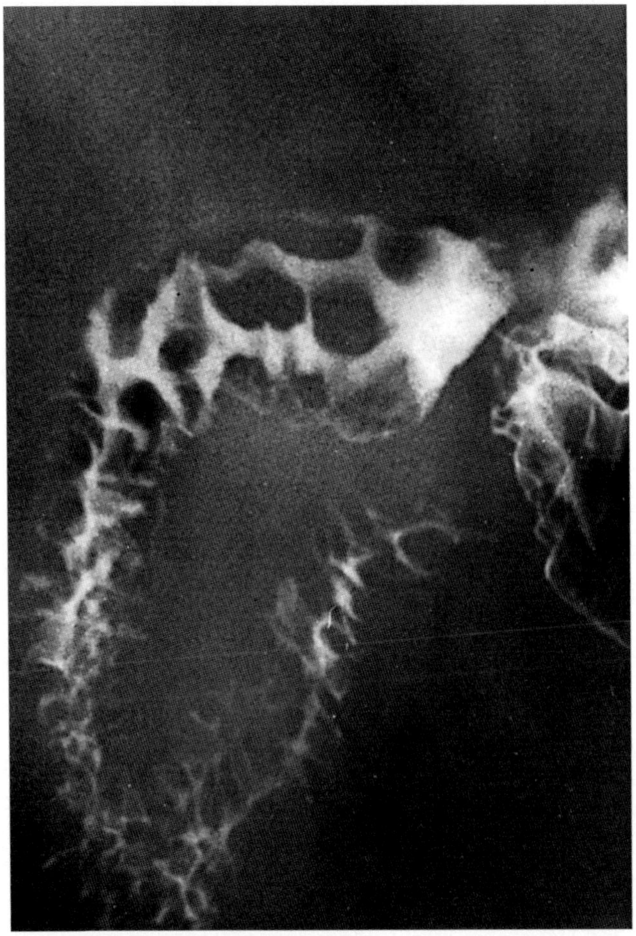

Figure 2-91 Multiple, large, rounded nodular filling defects in the duodenal bulb and postbulbar region representing Brunner's gland hyperplasia are seen.

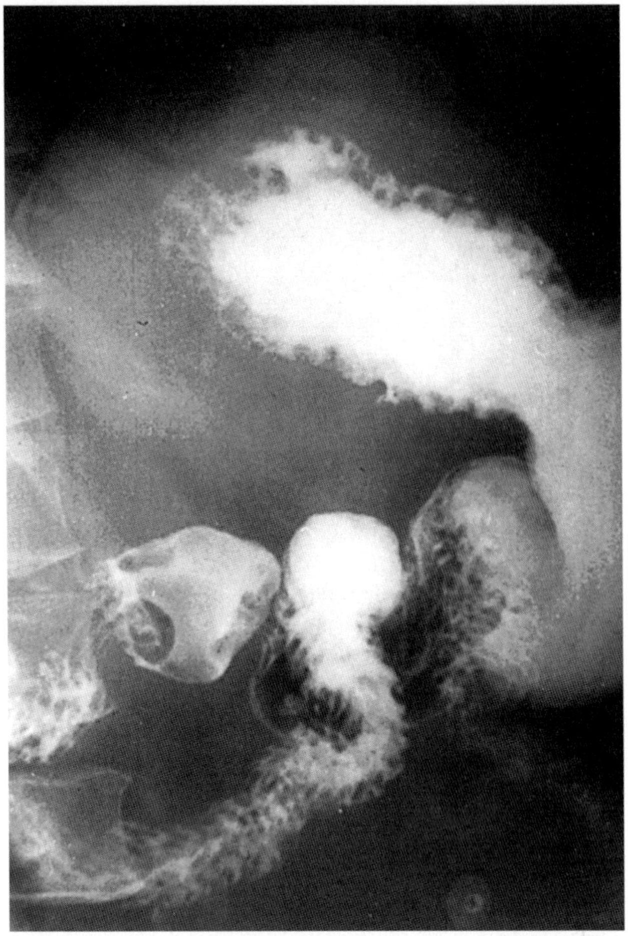

Figure 2-92 A solitary filling defect near the apex of the duodenal bulb suggests the possibility of a flexural pseudotumor. This was found to be a Brunner's gland adenoma.

mucosa from damaging effects of gastric acid, does not seem to be impaired. A variation of this is Brunner's gland adenoma or hamartoma, which is a rare lesion caused by focal overgrowth of the tissue elements of Brunner's glands in the proximal duodenum (Fig. 2-92). They are usually seen as smooth polypoid masses, often about 1 cm in size.

Lymphoid Hyperplasia

Benign lymphoid hyperplasia of the duodenum with multiple small filling defects may be a normal finding in children, although in adults the condition has been associated with hypogammaglobulinemia and the concomitant presence of giardiasis.

Choledochocele

Occasionally, a round, smooth defect arising in the region of the papilla is seen and is a result of choledochocele formation. This is a variation of the choledochal cyst (Fig. 2-93).

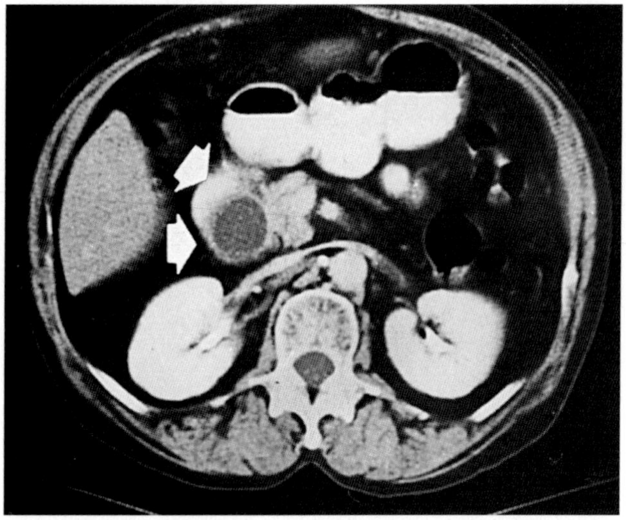

Figure 2-93 Computed tomographic scan shows large cystic dilatation in the common bile duct representing a choledochal cyst *(arrows)* impressing the duodenum.

Kaposi's Sarcoma

Kaposi's sarcoma is a relatively common lesion seen in AIDS patients. The major sites of involvement include the stomach and small bowel, although lesions may be visible within the duodenum. The appearance is that of multiple polypoid lesions, frequently ulcerated on the surface. Hematogenous metastatic disease, particularly breast or melanoma, may have a similar appearance.

Papillitis

Abnormalities of the papilla of Vater also may manifest as a duodenal filling defect. Most commonly, this is papillitis, resulting from inflammation and an enlargement of the major papilla, usually resulting from traumatic stone passage or peripapillary fibrotic changes.

Heterotopic Gastric Mucosa

An uncommon cause of multiple plaquelike filling defects in the duodenal bulb is heterotopic gastric mucosa (Fig. 2-94). These filling defects can vary in size and configuration and form a mosaic pattern usually in the base of the duodenal bulb; they can easily be missed on single-contrast examination. The exact clinical significance of this condition is unclear. There seems to be no malignant potential.

Extrinsic Processes

Pancreatic Disease

The most common extrinsic process involving the duodenal sweep is a result of pancreatic disease in the head of the pancreas. This disease can be inflammatory, with diffuse enlargement of the pancreas or pseudocyst formation. Also, benign or malignant pancreatic neoplasms can impress the duodenum.

Kidney and Adrenal Gland Diseases

Disease processes arising from the right kidney or adrenal gland, if sufficiently large, can impress the outer aspect of the descending portion of the duodenal sweep (Fig. 2-95).

Enlarged Common Bile Duct, Gallbladder, and Liver

Abnormalities arising in the liver and biliary system can also occasionally result in extrinsic impression of the duodenum. This includes an enlarged gallbladder, whether it be from obstructive causes or passive dilatation. An enlarged common bile duct occasionally can impress the duodenal sweep at the level of the apex of the bulb (Fig. 2-96).

Other Causes

Large choledochal cysts also can result in a significant duodenal impression. Retroperitoneal lymph node masses in the peripancreatic region also can lead to an extrinsic impression on the duodenal sweep (Fig. 2-97).

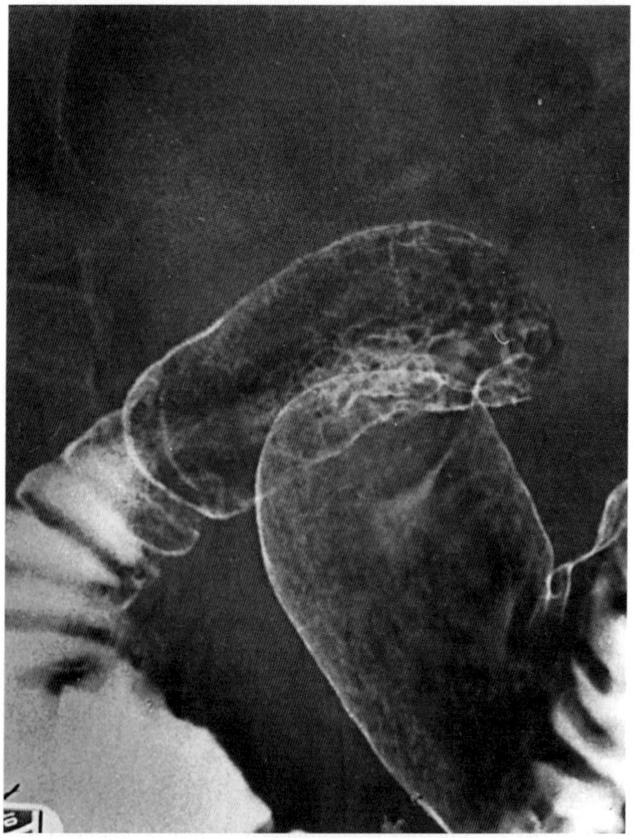

Figure 2-94 Multiple, irregular, plaquelike filling defects at the base of the duodenal bulb represent heterotopic gastric mucosa.

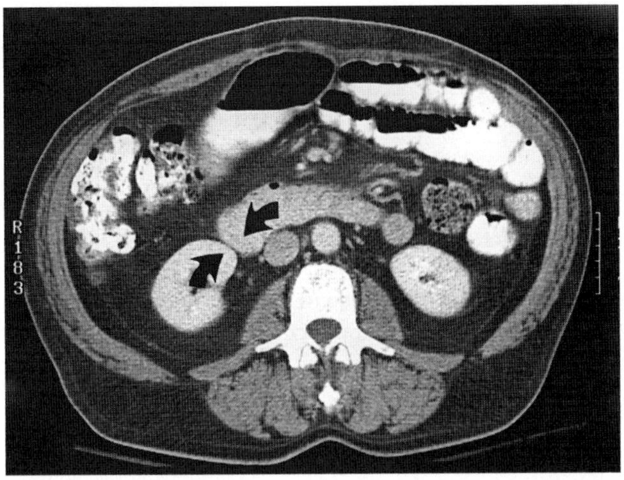

Figure 2-95 Relationship of the right kidney and the proximal duodenal sweep. Computed tomographic section through this region shows intimate relationship between contrast-filled duodenum and anterior-medial aspect of the kidney *(curved arrows)*.

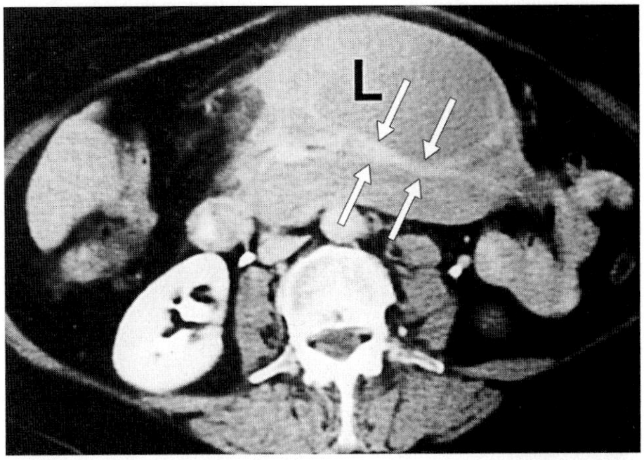

Figure 2-97 Computed tomographic scan shows large, retroperitoneal lymph node mass *(L)* sandwiching and compressing the retroperitoneal portion of the duodenal sweep *(arrows)*.

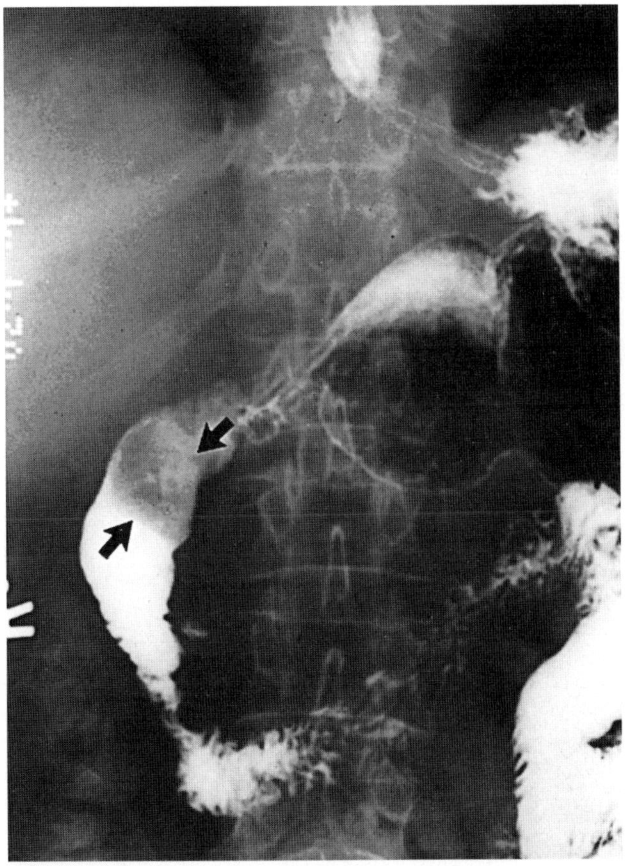

Figure 2-96 Obstruction of the biliary system and extrinsic impression of the postbulbar duodenum *(arrows)* by a dilated common bile duct.

Duodenal Ulceration

Peptic Ulcer Disease

Duodenal peptic ulcer disease is a common entity and accounts for a sizable portion of health care costs expended on gastrointestinal diseases. The relationship between *H. pylori* and peptic ulcer disease was discussed earlier. It is estimated that 10% to 15% of North American men have had duodenal ulcer disease at some time in their lives. The incidence is less for women. The disease is a direct effect of the corrosive effect of gastric acid on the duodenal mucosa and the breakdown of normal protective antacid mechanisms within the duodenal bulb. Various risk factors also are thought to play an important role in the possible etiological origins of the disease. These include *H. pylori,* alcohol, and certain types of drugs, such as aspirin and other NSAIDs that also have a direct corrosive effect.

The presence of duodenal ulcer disease is probably not an isolated phenomenon and is simply a manifestation of one facet of the spectrum of peptic ulcer disease involving the distal esophagus, gastric antrum, and duodenal bulb. Careful evaluation of the stomach of patients with duodenal ulcer disease almost always reveals gastritis. The incidence of peptic esophagitis in these patients also is increased.

Radiological diagnosis traditionally has been based on a persistent barium collection seen within the duodenal bulb (Fig. 2-98). However, the advent of widespread use of endoscopy resulted in numerous assertions that the radiological evaluation of the duodenum for peptic ulcer disease was quite insensitive. The ability of the radiologist to show duodenal ulceration can be significantly improved if the examination of the duodenal bulb includes good air-contrast views and single-contrast views with compression (Fig. 2-99). Occasionally, a good portion,

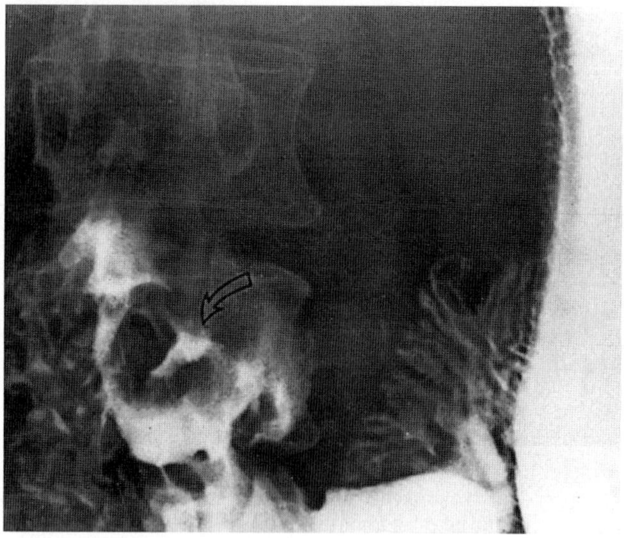

Figure 2-98 Typical appearance of duodenal bulb ulcer is seen, with central ulcer crater *(curved arrow)* and surrounding edema.

if not all, of the duodenal bulb may be ulcerated, resulting in a "giant duodenal ulcer" (Fig. 2-100). These ulcers may assume the triangular configuration of the duodenal bulb and, as a result, be missed during UGI study, which adds credence to the old saw that "the only things radiologists miss are the very small or the very large." Certain factors should alert the radiologist to the possibility of a giant duodenal ulcer (Box 2-9). These include the unusual persistence of barium within the duodenal bulb, little or no discernible fold pattern within the bulb, and postbulbar narrowing or spasm (Fig. 2-101). Postbulbar duodenal ulceration can be difficult to detect radiologically (Box 2-10).

Other Causes

Duodenal ulcerations or erosions may be seen in a variety of other conditions, including Zollinger-Ellison syndrome, Crohn's disease of the duodenum, tuberculosis of the small bowel, and ulceration resulting from viral diseases.

Duodenal Diverticulosis

Duodenal diverticula are seen on approximately 5% of routine UGI studies. They represent serosal and mucosal herniations through the muscular wall and are not true diverticula (Fig. 2-102). They usually occur in the second portion of the duodenum along the inner margin of the duodenal C-loop within 1 to 2 cm of the major papilla. Duodenal diverticula are usually only incidental findings. Complications such as hemorrhage, infection, and enterolith formation have been reported. Occasionally, the papilla of Vater may empty directly into a duodenal diverticulum, resulting in the potential of difficult cannulation and possible perforation during endoscopic retrograde cholangiopancreatography.

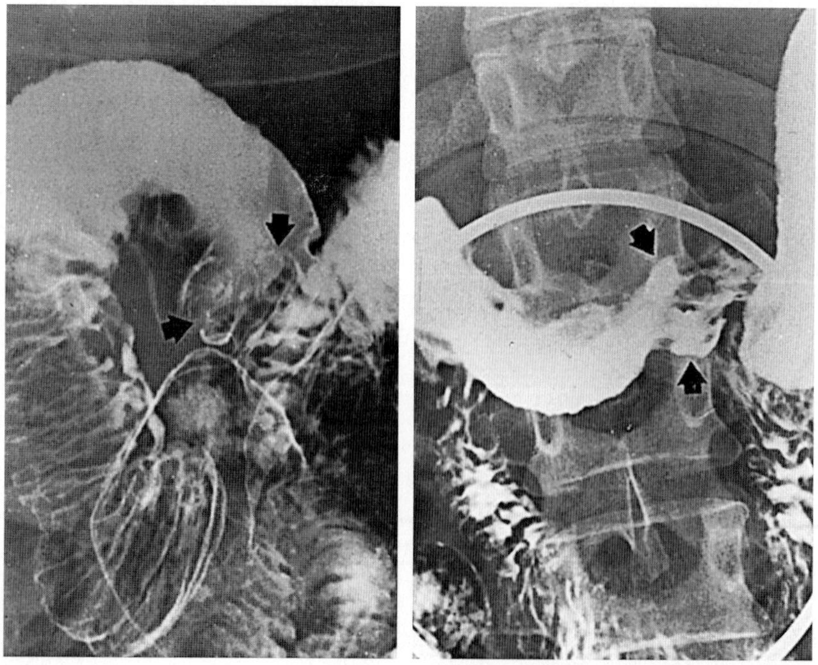

A B

Figure 2-99 **A,** Air-contrast views suggest possibility of ulcer craters in the form of "ring shadows" *(arrows)*. **B,** Single-contrast compression views of the same area show two well-defined ulcer craters *(arrows)*.

Box 2-9 Subtle Giant: Giant Duodenal Ulcer: Radiological Signs

Little, if any, fold pattern in duodenal bulb
No change in configuration of bulb
Always with postbulbar narrowing
Barium retained, especially on delayed images

Duodenal Positional Abnormalities

Midgut Malrotation

Midgut malrotation is a result of incomplete rotation of the midgut during intrauterine life. Although this condition can predispose to midgut volvulus in children, it is more often seen as degrees of incomplete rotation and often as an incidental finding. The location of the ligament of Treitz (marking the duodenal-jejunal junction) is key to making this diagnosis. The ligament is located inferiorly and medially to its expected position. In cases of complete malrotation, it is located to the right of the spine. The position of the cecum varies, but in complete malrotation it is located largely in the left abdomen.

Displacement of C-Loop by Extrinsic Mass

Any large mass in the upper abdomen can displace the C-loop of the duodenum. The most common are masses arising from the pancreas, stomach, kidney, or adrenals.

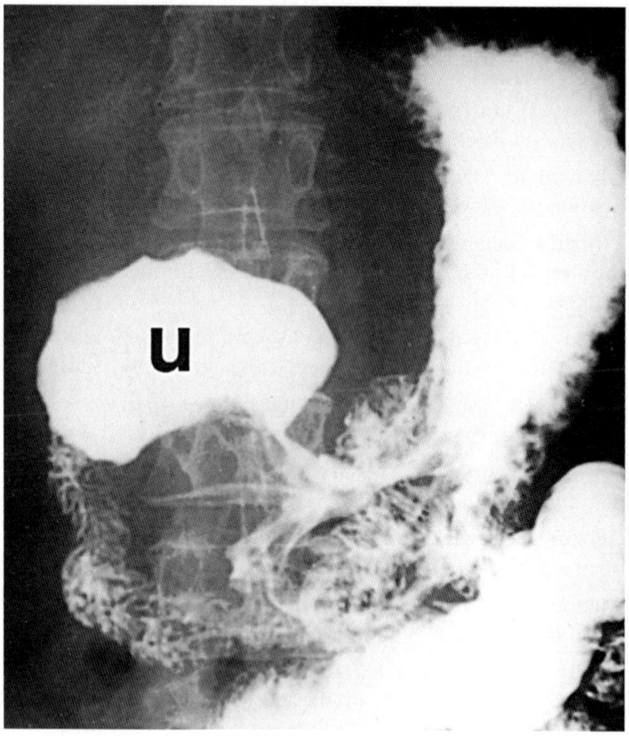

Figure 2-100 A giant duodenal ulcer *(u)* is shown.

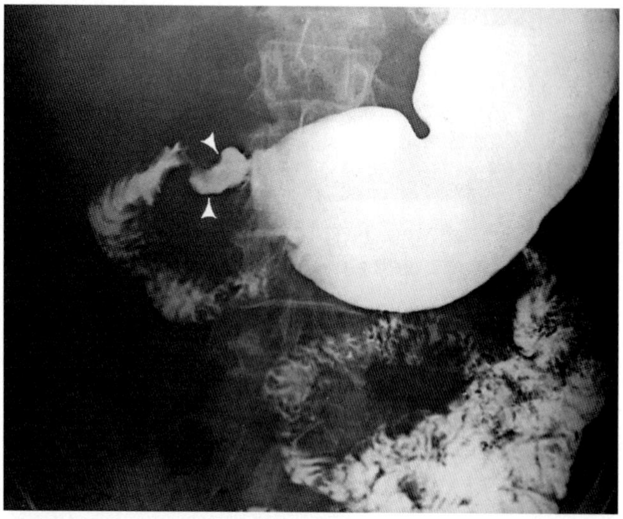

Figure 2-101 A large, triangular barium collection *(arrowheads)* looks like a deformed duodenal bulb. Note (1) absence of folds in "duodenal bulb," (2) postbulbar narrowing, and (3) persistence of barium in "bulb" on delayed films. These three signs are suggestive of a giant duodenal ulcer, which this proved to be.

Paraduodenal Hernias

Paraduodenal hernias occur when there is incomplete fixation of the posterior peritoneum and potential spaces develop. Bowel loops can be sequestered in these potential spaces. If the paraduodenal hernia is on the right, the ligament of Treitz and the entire C-loop may be displaced. Left-sided paraduodenal hernias are two to three times more common. These conditions may be associated with vague upper abdominal symptoms or can be found as an incidental finding on an UGI study (Fig. 2-103).

Intrathoracic Stomachs

Displacement and distortion of the duodenal sweep also can be seen in patients with exceedingly large hiatal hernias, in which most of the stomach is intrathoracic in position. The ligament of Treitz may be pulled medially.

Box 2-10 Postbulbar Ulcers: A Hard-to-Track Animal That Leaves Tracks

Persistent postbulbar narrowing/spasm
Postbulbar fold thickening
Rarely results in obstruction
Actual ulcer crater may be difficult to see on UGI studies

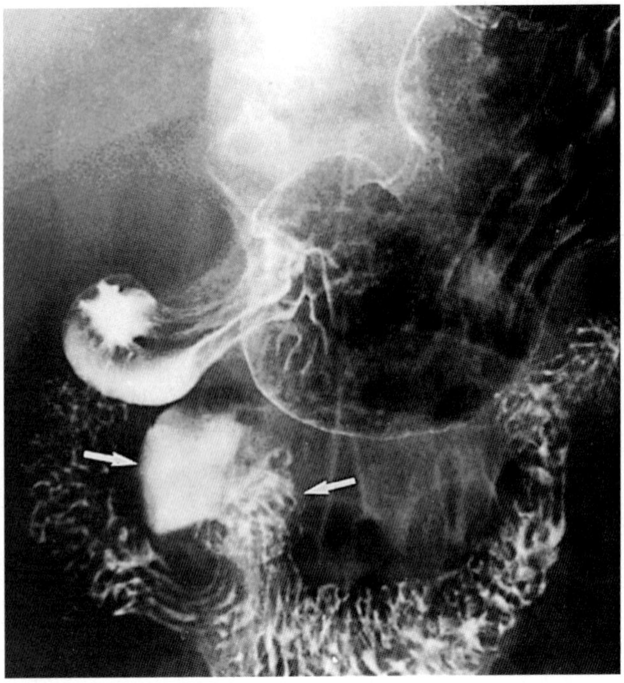

Figure 2-102 Duodenal diverticulum *(arrows)* arising from the medial aspect of the transverse duodenum.

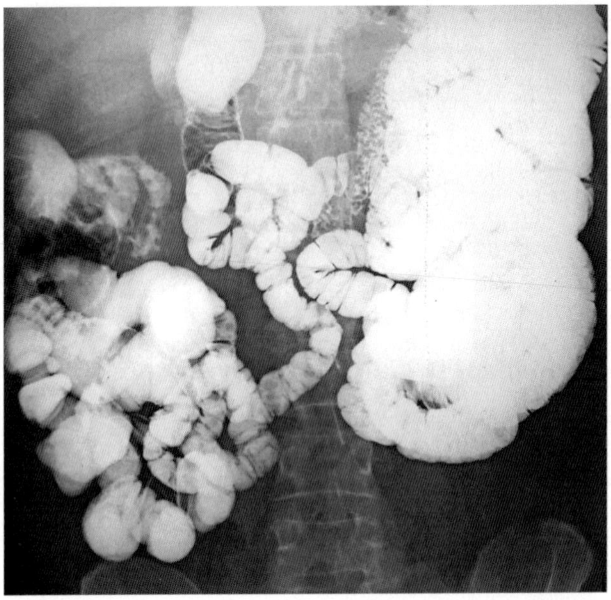

Figure 2-103 Left paraduodenal hernia in patient with vague upper abdominal complaints. UGI study and small bowel follow-through disclosed sequestration of small bowel loops in the left upper quadrant. Only a few loops of ileum are seen before cecum is reached.

Lesser Sac Hernias

Lesser sac hernias are uncommon and result when loops of bowel pass through the foramen of Winslow (epiploic foramen) and become sequestered in the lesser sac behind the stomach.

SUGGESTED READINGS

Abbara S, Kalan MMH, Lewicki AM: Intrathoracic stomach revisited. AJR 181:403-414, 2003.

Asrani AV: The antral pad sign. Radiology 229:421-422, 2003.

Balfe DM, Koehler RE, Karstaedt N, et al: Computed tomography of gastric neoplasms. Radiology 140:431-436, 1981.

Balthazar EJ, Rosenberg H, Davidian MM: Scirrhous carcinoma of the pyloric channel and distal antrum. AJR Am J Roentgenol 134:669-673, 1980.

Blaser MJ: Gastric *Campylobacter*-like organisms, gastritis, and peptic ulcer disease. Gastroenterology 93:371-383, 1987.

Blaser MJ: In a world of black and white, *Helicobacter pylori* is gray (editorial). Ann Intern Med 130:695-697, 1999.

Camblos JF: Acute volvulus of the stomach. Am Surg 35:505-509, 1969.

Choi SH, Sheehan FR, Pickren JW: Metastatic involvement of the stomach by breast cancer. Cancer 17:791-797, 1964.

Chuang VP, Wallace S, Stroehlein JR, et al: Hepatic artery infusion chemotherapy: gastroduodenal complications. AJR Am J Roentgenol 137:347-350, 1981.

Clements JL, Jinkins JR, Torres WE, et al: Antral mucosal diaphragms in adults. AJR Am J Roentgenol 113:1105-1111, 1979.

Correa P, Haenswel W, Cuello C, et al: A model for gastric cancer epidemiology. Lancet 2:58-59, 1975.

Delikaris P, Golematis B, Missitziz J, et al: Smooth muscle neoplasms of the stomach. South Med J 76:440-442, 1983.

Dooley CP, Cohen H: The clinical significance of *Campylobacter pylori*. Ann Intern Med 108:70-79, 1988.

Edelman MJ, March TL: Eosinophilic gastroenteritis. AJR Am J Roentgenol 91:773-778, 1964.

Farman J, Faegenburg D, Dallemand S, et al: Crohn's disease of the stomach: the "ram's horn" sign. AJR Am J Roentgenol 123: 242-251, 1975.

Feczko PJ, Halpert RD, Ackerman LV: Gastric polyps: radiological evaluation and clinical significance. Radiology 155:581-584, 1985.

Feliciano DV, Van Heerden JA: Pyloric antral mucosal webs. Mayo Clin Proc 52:650-653, 1977.

Felson B, Berkmen YM, Anastacio MH: Gastric mucosal diaphragm. Radiology 92:513-517, 1969.

Gerson DE, Lewicki AM: Intrathoracic stomach: when does it obstruct? Radiology 119:257-264, 1976.

Goldberg HI: Radiographic evaluation of peptic ulcer disease. J Clin Gastroenterol 3(suppl 2):57-65, 1981.

Goldstein HM, Cohen LE, Hagen R, et al: Gastric bezoars: a frequent complication in the postoperative ulcer patient. Radiology 107:341-344, 1973.

Goldstein SS, Lewis JH, Rothstein R: Intestinal obstruction due to bezoars. Am J Gastroenterol 79:313-318, 1984.

Gonzalez G, Kennedy T: Crohn's disease of the stomach. Radiology 113:27-29, 1974.

Goodwin CS, Armstrong JA, Marshall BJ: *Campylobacter pyloridis,* gastritis and peptic ulceration. J Clin Pathol 39:353-365, 1986.

Hyson EA, Burrell M, Toffler R: Drug-induced gastrointestinal disease. Gastrointest Radiol 2:183-212, 1977.

Ishikura H, Sato F, Naka H, et al: Inflammatory fibroid polyp of the stomach. Acta Pathol Jpn 36:327-335, 1986.

Ivey KJ: Drugs, gastritis, and peptic ulcer. J Clin Gastroenterol 3(suppl 2):29-34, 1981.

Jacobs DS: Primary gastric lymphoma and pseudolymphoma. Am J Clin Pathol 40:379-394, 1963.

Joffe N: Some unusual roentgenologic findings associated with marked gastric dilatation. AJR Am J Roentgenol 119:291-299, 1973.

Jolobe OM, Montgomery RD: Changing clinical pattern of gastric ulcer: are anti-inflammatory drugs involved? Digestion 29: 164-170, 1984.

Katelaris PH, Seow F, Lin BPC, et al: *Helicobacter pylori* infection and gastritis with atrophy of serum gastrin and gastric acid secretion in healthy men. Gut 34:1032-1037, 1993.

Kilman WJ, Berk RN: The spectrum of radiological features of aberrant pancreatic rests involving the stomach. Radiology 123:291-296, 1977.

Kim HC, Lee JM, Kim SH, et al: Primary gastrointestinal stromal tumors in the omentum and mesentery: CT findings and pathologic correlations. AJR Am J Roentgenol 182:1463-1467, 2004.

Kim TS, Shijo H, Kokawa, et al: Risk factors for hemorrhage from gastric varices. Hepatology 25:307-312, 1997.

Koyama T, Veda H, Togashi K, et al: Radiologic manifestations of sarcoidosis in various organs. Radiographics 24:87-104.

Laufer I, Hamilton J, Mullens JE: Demonstration of superficial gastric erosions by double contrast radiography. Gastroenterology 68:387-391, 1975.

Llaneza PP, Salt WB: Gastric volvulus: more common than previously thought? Postgrad Med 80:279-288, 1986.

Loo FD, Palmer DW, Soergel KH, et al: Gastric emptying in patients with diabetes mellitus. Gastroenterology 86:485-494, 1984.

Lucas CE, Sugawa C, Riddle J, et al: Natural history and surgical dilemma of "stress" gastric bleeding. Arch Surg 102:266-273, 1971.

Marks IN, Bank S, Werbeloff L, et al: The natural history of corrosive gastritis: report of five cases. Am J Dig Dis 6:509-524, 1963.

Martel W, Abell MR, Allan TNK: Lymphoreticular hyperplasia of the stomach (pseudolymphoma). AJR Am J Roentgenol 127: 261-265, 1976.

Menuck L: Plain film findings of gastric volvulus herniating into the chest. AJR Am J Roentgenol 126:1169-1174, 1976.

Menuck LS, Amberg JR: Metastatic disease involving the stomach. Am J Dig Dis 20:903-913, 1975.

Muhletaler CA, Gerlock AJ, Desoto L, et al: Gastroduodenal lesions of ingested acids: radiographic findings. AJR Am J Roentgenol 135:1247-1252, 1980.

Neimark S, Rogers AI: Gastric polyps: a review. Am J Gastroenterol 77:585-587, 1982.

Op den Orth JO, Dekker WL: Gastric adenomas. Radiology 141: 289-293, 1981.

Ott DJ, Chen YM, Gelfand DW, et al: Radiographic accuracy in gastric ulcer: comparison of single-contrast and multiphasic examination. AJR Am J Roentgenol 147:697-700, 1986.

Overholt BF, Jeffries GH: Hypertrophic hypersecreting protein-losing gastropathy. Gastroenterology 58:80-87, 1970.

Patterson CP, Combs MJ, Marshall BJ: *Helicobacter pylori* and peptic ulcer disease: evolution to revolution to resolution. AJR Am J Roentgenol 168:1415-1420, 1997.

Pillari G, Weinreb J, Vernace F, et al: CT of gastric masses: image patterns and a note on potential pitfalls. Gastrointest Radiol 8:11-17, 1983.

Pruitt BA, Goodwin CW: Stress ulcer disease in the burned patient. World J Surg 5:209-222, 1981.

Raotma H, Angervall L, Dahl I, et al: Clinical and morphological studies of giant hypertrophic gastritis (Ménétrier's disease). Acta Med Scand 195:247-252, 1974.

Read NW: Functional dyspepsia: a case of indecision, Gastroenterology 116:761-762, 1999.

Scatarige JC, Fishman EK, Jones B, et al: Gastric leiomyosarcoma: CT observations. J Comput Assist Tomogr 9:320-327, 1985.

Schuman BM, Waldbaum JR, Hiltz SW, et al: Carcinoma of the gastric remnant in the U.S. population. Gastrointest Endosc 30:71-73, 1984.

Sohn JS, Levine MS, Furth EE, et al: *Helicobacter pylori* gastritis: radiographic findings. Radiology 195:763-767, 1995.

Spechler SJ: Adenocarcinoma of the gastroesophageal junction. Clin Perspect Gastroenterol 2:95-97, 1999.

Thoeni RF, Gedgaudas RK: Ectopic pancreas: usual and unusual features. Gastrointest Radiol 5:37-42, 1980.

Thompson G, Somers S, Stevenson GW: Benign gastric ulcer: a reliable radiologic diagnosis? AJR Am J Roentgenol 141: 331-333, 1983.

Wallace RG, Howard WB: Acute superior mesenteric artery syndrome in the severely burned patient. Radiology 94:307-310, 1970.

CHAPTER 3

Small Bowel

EXAMINATION TECHNIQUES

The mesenteric small bowel extends from the ligament of Treitz to the ileocecal valve (almost 20 ft) and consists of the jejunum and ileum, which are entirely intraperitoneal and are attached posteriorly to a mesentery. Plain films of the abdomen are often the first radiological examination obtained in evaluating suspected small bowel disease, particularly obstruction or adynamic ileus. The role of x-rays is confined mainly to emergency and postoperative patients. The standard supine film (kidneys, ureters, and bladder) can be supplemented with upright or lateral decubitus films to detect air-fluid levels or free intraperitoneal air.

A wide variety of fluoroscopic procedures using barium are available for studying the mesenteric small bowel. Nonintubation methods include the small bowel follow-through (SBFT) examination (often performed in conjunction with an upper gastrointestinal series) and the dedicated small bowel study (in which only the small bowel is examined) (Fig. 3-1). Both methods use an approximately 40% weight/volume barium suspension. A dedicated small bowel study should include intermittent fluoroscopy with palpation and spot filming of suspect areas, along with routine overhead films.

If the suspected area of pathology is the stomach or duodenum, SBFT is often included as an attempt to "cover all the bases." SBFT is, at best, a good survey examination of the small bowel, however, and its sensitivity leaves much to be desired. If the suspected pathology is in the small bowel (i.e., Crohn's disease of the ileum), a dedicated small bowel study should be undertaken. This examination differs from SBFT in that there is no mixture of differing densities of barium and no carbon dioxide gas to break up the barium column. A good dedicated small bowel study done properly is an excellent examination. The radiologist should endeavor to keep the stomach full of barium during the course of the examination (to try to ensure continuous filling of the small bowel with no breakup of the column). Instead of a schedule of overhead films being obtained, the dedicated small bowel study is radiologist intensive and requires the radiologist periodically, under fluoroscopy, to press out the small bowel so that all bowel from the ligament of Treitz to the ileocecal valve can be visualized and examined. Thin patients, especially when the bony pelvis prohibits bowel compression, can be problematic. The number of thin patients seems to be decreasing, however. Using compression, the fluoroscopist should ensure the bowel is soft and pliable, the fold pattern should be assessed, and the loops should be examined for filling defects.

Intubation methods (small bowel enema or enteroclysis) are performed by injecting barium directly through a tube (12F to 14F) placed fluoroscopically into the

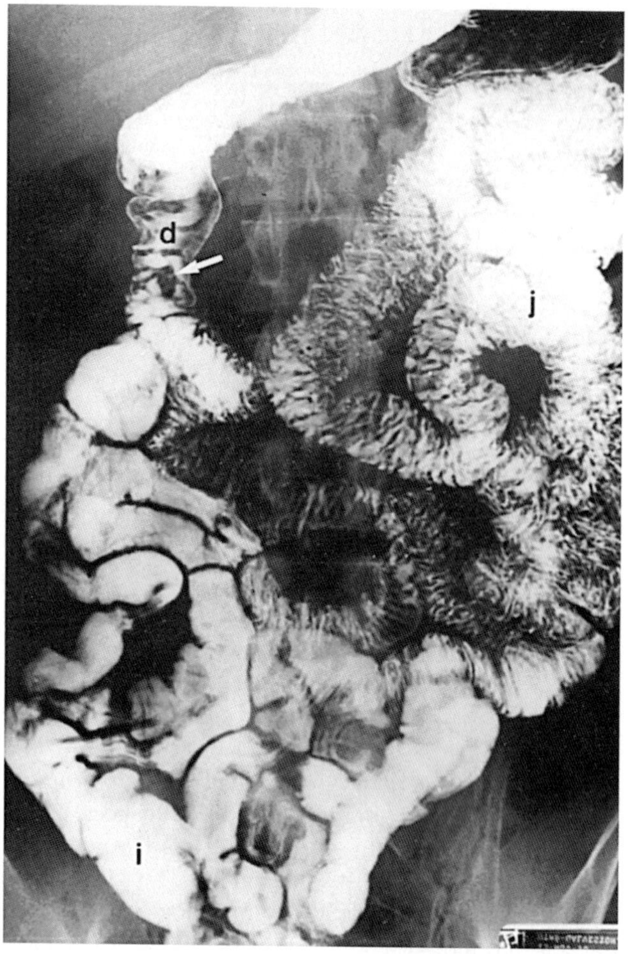

Figure 3-1 Normal SBFT examination shows fold patterns of duodenum *(d)*, jejunum *(j)*, and ileum *(i)*. An ovoid filling defect in the mid-descending duodenum *(arrow)* represents the normal ampulla seen en face.

jejunum. These procedures include single-contrast techniques (using barium alone) and double-contrast techniques (using air or methylcellulose in addition to barium) (Fig. 3-2). This method employs a denser barium, typically 50% to 80% weight/volume, depending on the method used. Careful graded compression under fluoroscopy is imperative in nonintubation and intubation examinations to unfold and separate overlapping small bowel loops. Drawbacks to the intubation methods include higher radiation dose because of increased fluoroscopy, discomfort to the patient (some patients require mild sedation), and complications related to the intubation or reflux of contrast material with aspiration. This method also has an increased yield, however, in detecting subtle mucosal pathology or mass lesions.

A peroral pneumocolon is an infrequent examination sometimes used to improve visualization of the distal small bowel. This procedure is performed during SBFT examination or small bowel meal. When barium has reached

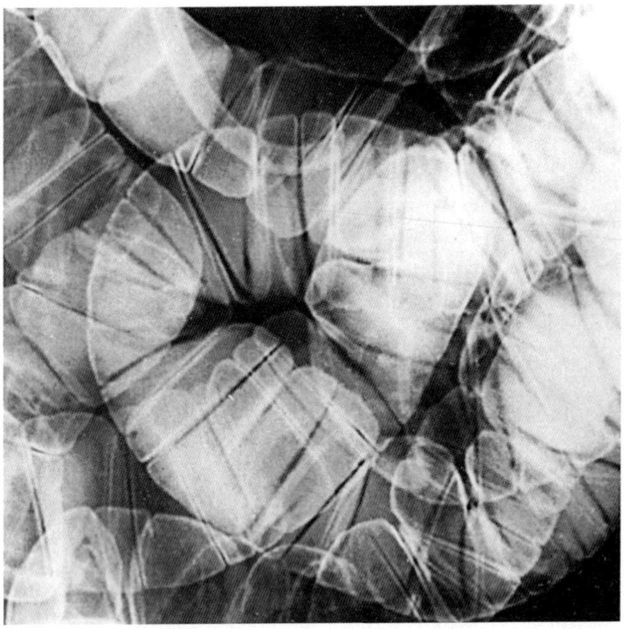

Figure 3-2 Spot film from a double-contrast enteroclysis examination shows jejunal fold pattern.

the terminal ileum or cecum, air is insufflated into the rectum. Intravenous glucagon usually is given to promote reflux of air from the colon through the ileocecal valve. This reflux distends the distal small bowel lumen and creates a double-contrast appearance. The distal small bowel also can be examined by retrograde injection of barium, either through a preexisting ileostomy or through the colon with reflux across the ileocecal valve. The tendency for reflux of barium to occur across the ileocecal valve seems to be higher in single-contrast examinations.

Water-soluble contrast material generally is used to confirm the position of jejunostomy tubes (or other percutaneously placed small bowel catheters). In the case of perforation, barium injected into the peritoneal cavity through an incorrectly positioned tube may cause peritonitis. Water-soluble contrast material is not useful, however, for routine evaluation of the small bowel because the hyperosmolar contrast material draws fluid into the bowel lumen, causing progressive dilution of the contrast material and rendering the study nondiagnostic. In cases of suspected small bowel obstruction, hyperosmolar water-soluble contrast material is contraindicated because it causes worsening of the luminal distention.

Multidetector computed tomography (CT) is useful for studying many forms of small bowel disease (Fig. 3-3). Its excellent evaluation of the bowel wall and extrinsic processes is complementary to conventional contrast studies, which are better for showing motility and mucosal abnormalities. The rapid scanning times now widely available with CT, particularly multidetector CT, lessen image degradation by peristalsis of bowel loops. Adequate bowel opacification is essential for optimal display of small bowel abnormalities on CT. Four 8-oz cups of dilute barium or dilute water-soluble contrast material are administered before scanning.

Ultrasonography may detect distended fluid-filled loops of small bowel in cases of obstruction and a thickened bowel wall resulting from inflammatory or neoplastic disease. The usefulness of ultrasonography is limited, however, because of deflection of sound waves and degradation of the image by air within the small bowel lumen. Because ultrasonography is often one of the first modalities used in evaluating patients with acute abdominal complaints, however, it may detect unsuspected small bowel pathology before other studies.

The most commonly used nuclear imaging technique pertaining to the small bowel is Meckel's scan (for detecting ectopic gastric mucosa in Meckel's diverticula), which

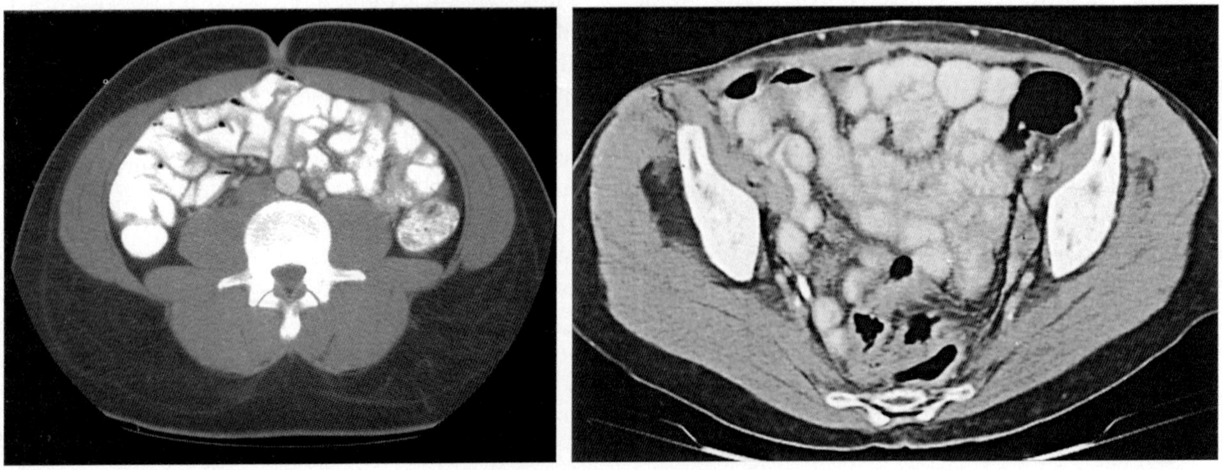

A B

Figure 3-3 **A,** Example of normal small bowel in the upper abdomen with contrast agent on CT study. **B,** CT lower in the abdomen shows normal opacified ileal loops.

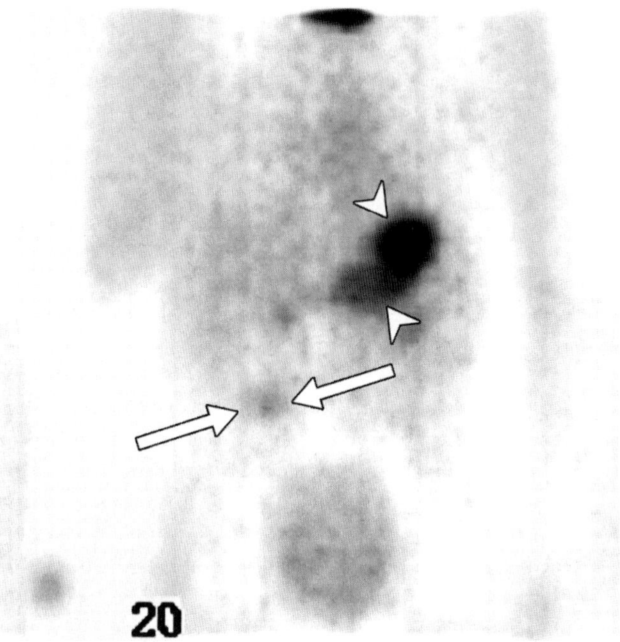

Figure 3-4 Technetium-99m pertechnetate nuclear scan shows uptake in a focal area in the right lower quadrant *(arrows)*, which turned out to be a bleeding Meckel's diverticulum. Also note normal excretion of radionuclide from parietal cells in stomach *(arrowheads)*.

uses technetium-99m pertechnetate, which is excreted by gastric mucosa (Fig. 3-4). Another frequent use of nuclear studies is a gastrointestinal bleeding scan, using radioactive sulfur colloid or labeled red blood cells (Fig. 3-5). Occasionally, radionuclides that detect inflammatory

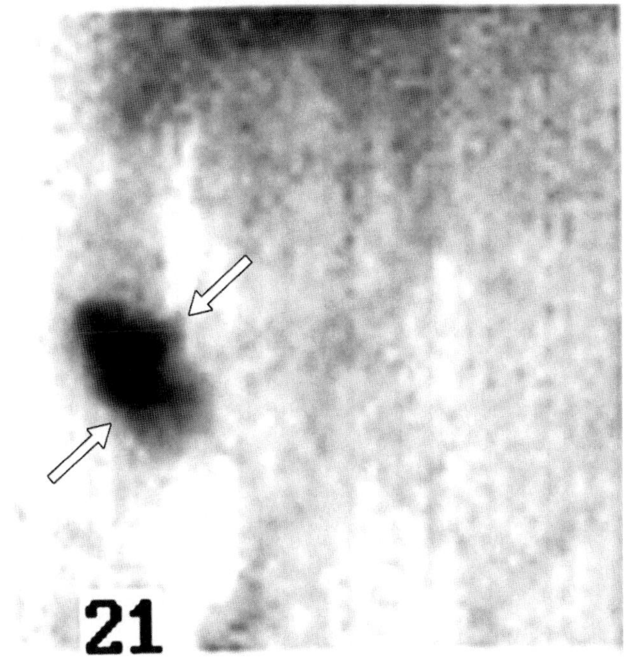

Figure 3-5 Labeled red blood cell scan shows focal uptake in the cecum *(arrows)* in an anemic patient. This turned out to be an adenocarcinoma.

conditions are used in evaluating the small bowels of patients with Crohn's disease and other inflammatory conditions.

Angiography is used primarily for showing and treating vascular thrombosis and hemorrhage involving the small bowel, in acute and chronic states. Angiography is unique in that treatment of these small bowel conditions can be performed in selected circumstances. As the technology of multidetector CT improves, however, the evaluation of the vascular system using CT arteriography is quickly gaining adherents, with the potential of major and even smaller vascular structures, whether mesenteric or cardiac, being shown in multiplanar images and three-dimensional reconstruction (Fig. 3-6).

Various drugs have an effect on small bowel motility, and these can be employed sometimes to assist in small bowel evaluation. Metoclopramide has a dual effect on the intestinal tract. First, it aids in increasing gastric emptying, helping deliver barium to the small bowel faster. Second, it increases small bowel peristalsis. It can be given intravenously for immediate effect or given orally, which usually requires 30 minutes for action. It is primarily used during intubation examination of the small bowel.

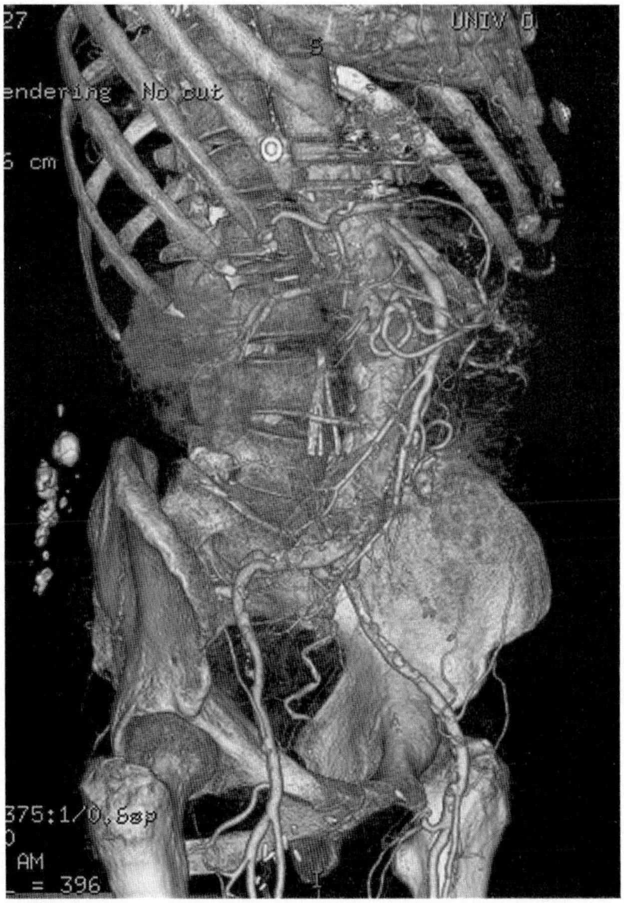

Figure 3-6 Sixteen-track multidetector CT with three-dimensional reconstruction shows the visceral arterial system nicely.

A variety of drugs decrease small bowel motility. The most commonly used is glucagon. Doses smaller than 1 mg can have a profound hypotonic effect on the small intestine and can last 15 to 30 minutes. Glucagon must be given intramuscularly or intravenously. Anticholinergics, such as morphine compounds, atropine, and diphenoxylate, also affect small bowel transit.

RADIOLOGICAL EVALUATION

As noted earlier, the radiologist has a variety of modalities available to evaluate for possible small bowel disease. It is beyond the scope of this book to indicate which methods are most efficacious for evaluating a particular small bowel condition, whether suspected or real. Currently, there is some controversy concerning these different methods, and each has its own proponents. In choosing what study to perform, other factors enter into the decision, particularly what equipment may be available (multidetector CT) and the particular skill or comfort level of the radiologist with a technique. Perhaps the most important factor is the clinician managing the patient. Often clinicians have a particular approach to a clinical situation with which they feel comfortable, and radiologists must communicate with clinicians regarding what they believe is the best modality to use.

Regardless of the imaging methods, several features of the small bowel are consistent with all examination types and are referred to frequently throughout this chapter.

- *Diameter.* The maximum normal diameter of the small bowel is about 3 cm. With intubation methods, this diameter is frequently exceeded, and differences in bowel diameter, rather than the actual size, become more important for evaluation.
- *Fold thickness.* The folds of the small bowel (valvulae conniventes) are typically 1.5 to 2 mm in size. When the size of the folds begins to reach or exceed 3 mm over a segment of bowel and is fairly consistent during the study, it should be considered abnormal.
- *Bowel wall thickness.* The distance between two loops of bowel is the width of two bowel walls. Because each bowel wall is usually less than 1.5 mm in diameter, the distance between bowel loops should not exceed 3 mm. This distance must be measured at adjacent loops of bowel that are adequately distended.
- *Differential air-fluid levels.* Differential levels are evaluated on upright abdominal radiographs and indicate the difference in air-fluid levels in a single loop of bowel. When this difference exceeds 1 cm, the likelihood of a mechanical obstruction increases.

Box 3-1 Rule of 3s: Abnormal Small Bowel Measurements

Small bowel diameter—≥3 cm
Small bowel folds—≥3 mm
Small bowel wall thickness—≥3 mm
Difference between air-fluid levels in a single loop of bowel—≥1 cm (usually indicates mechanical obstruction rather than adynamic ileus)

- *Secretions.* Typically in a fasted patient, there is no discernible fluid in the small bowel. If excess fluid is encountered, seen as dilution of the barium column, this should be considered abnormal.
- *Transit time.* There is a great variation in transit time and many dependent factors. Normally, one might expect barium to reach the cecum in 1 to 3 hours. It can be only 30 minutes, however. Transit time may be quite prolonged in the presence of obstruction further down the bowel, a generalized ileus, certain types of medications, and chronic constipation. Generally, if the right colon is collapsed and empty, it results in increased contractions in the small bowel and a faster transit time.
- *Rule of 3s.* One rule of thumb to use in evaluating the small bowel is the rule of 3s. In reviewing the above-listed criteria, it is apparent that most small bowel measurements are considered abnormal when they reach 3 or greater (Box 3-1).

Radiologists frequently use an algorithmic approach in evaluating an organ in which a multitude of diseases may occur, such as the small bowel. Figure 3-7 shows one such algorithm. Many diseases do not lend themselves to simple classification, however. Also, some diseases, such

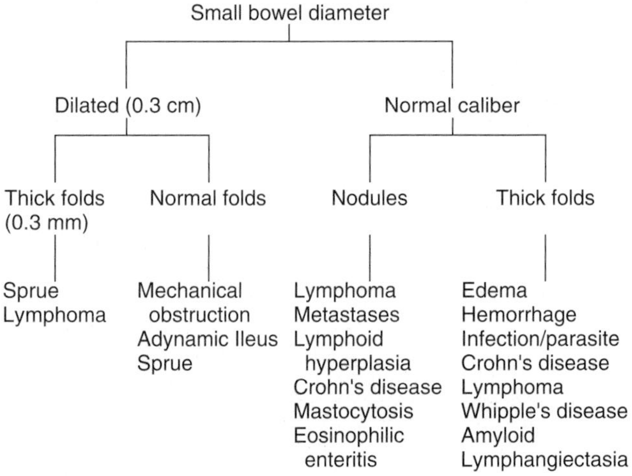

Figure 3-7 Basic algorithm for small bowel disease. Many diseases have a variable appearance.

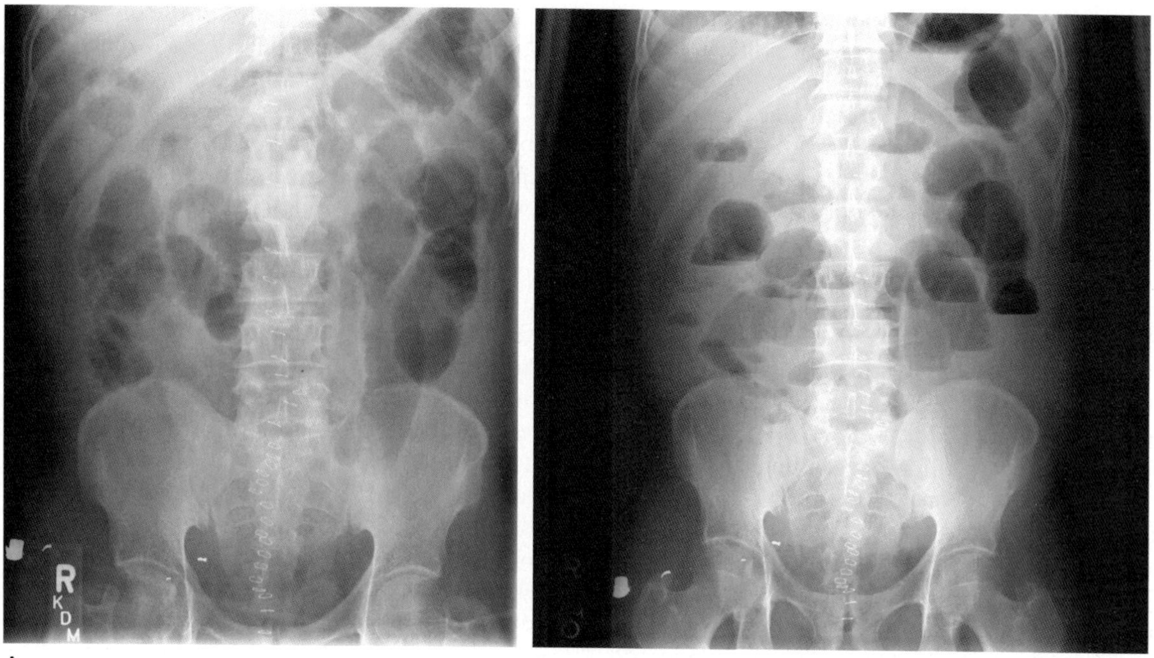

A B

Figure 3-8 **A,** Supine plain film of the abdomen shows numerous dilated loops of small bowel in a patient with small bowel obstruction secondary to adhesions. **B,** Upright film shows differential air-fluid levels indicating mechanical small bowel obstruction.

as lymphoma or Crohn's disease, can present with a variety of appearances. The algorithmic approach is nevertheless helpful in sorting through the various disease entities that affect the small bowel and allowing one to make some intelligent guesses regarding diagnosis.

DILATED SMALL BOWEL

Mechanical Obstruction Resulting in Distention

Adhesions

Dilatation of the small bowel occurs in a wide variety of conditions, some associated with mechanical obstruction and others in which no obstructing lesion is present. The most common obstructing lesion causing distention of the mesenteric small bowel is an adhesion or band, usually resulting from previous abdominal surgery. Supine plain films typically show distended air-filled loops of small bowel, identified by the linear folds traversing the circumference of the bowel lumen (valvulae conniventes or plicae circulares). Distended loops may lay in a tiered or stepladder pattern, and variable amounts of air are present in the colon, depending on the level, grade, and duration of the obstruction. Distended small bowel loops containing mostly fluid (with little or no air) usually appear as a gasless abdomen on supine films.

On erect or lateral decubitus films, the small amounts of air rise within the dilated, fluid-filled loops to form a series of bubbles or short air-fluid levels ("string of pearls"). When more air is present, air-fluid levels are longer and often appear at different heights within the same bowel loop (differential levels) (Fig. 3-8). Significant (>1 cm) differential air-fluid levels almost always indicate mechanical obstruction. Occasionally, minor degrees of differential air-fluid levels may be seen early in a small bowel ileus (Fig. 3-9).

To understand the concept of differential air-fluid levels, it is helpful if one considers what is happening in the small

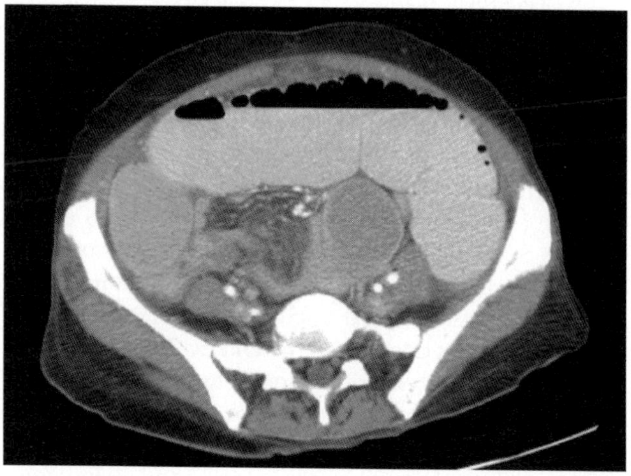

Figure 3-9 Axial computed tomographic scan through lower abdomen shows dilated small bowel in a patient with small bowel obstruction.

bowel during these pathologies. In the case of mechanical obstruction, there is initially increased amplitude and frequency in the contractions of the small bowel in an attempt to force the bowel content through the narrowed or obstructed area. These contractions result in the classic sounds heard when one applies a stethoscope to the abdomen of a patient with bowel obstruction—high-pitched rushes of fluid moving back and forth as the bowel contracts. The fluid tends to move in both directions when the bowel is working hard to overcome an obstruction. As a result, water is distributed unevenly, and when the patient is put in the upright position, this uneven distribution of fluid gives the classic differential air-fluid level with fluid levels at differing heights *within the same loop of bowel*. One can identify differential air-fluid levels only if the levels are within the same loop of bowel. Otherwise, differing levels can be seen in the bowel of patients with an ileus. Early in an ileus, one may see a small differential air-fluid level in the same bowel. Seeing differential air-fluid levels in an ileus is not the usual case, however. As the bowel wall contractions become more hypotonic and eventually cease, there is little movement of fluid, and water (always seeking its own level) is seen as nondifferential air-fluid levels when the patient is raised into the upright position. In a high-grade prolonged small bowel obstruction, the muscular contractions of the small bowel eventually weaken and cease altogether, after which there may be no differential air-fluid levels. In such cases, diagnosis can be difficult, and the radiologist must pay careful attention to the distal bowel. If the small bowel is distended and fluid-filled, while the colon is collapsed or of normal caliber, this is presumptive evidence of small bowel obstruction. Regardless, the evaluation of the distal bowel is an important part of every evaluation of potential small bowel pathology, either on routine anteroposterior images or multidetector CT.

Differential or nondifferential air-fluid levels apply only to the small bowel. The colon should be considered as one continuous loop of tethered bowel, and whether it is affected with the hypotonicity of an ileus or an obsructing process, there often are differing fluid levels. As a result, this sign is meaningless in the colon.

The use of water-soluble contrast material versus barium in the face of mechanical obstruction continues to be a problem sometimes. A good rule of thumb is this: If there is any evidence of obstruction, use barium. The reasoning here is not complicated. When water-soluble contrast material encounters dilated fluid-filled loops of bowel, it dilutes into the enteric fluid and quickly disappears. It may contribute to the further distention of the bowel by its hypertonic nature, drawing additional fluid across the mucosa into the lumen. Barium may become dilute, but never disappears, and being inert it does not draw fluid across the mucosal barrier. Additionally, the use of barium may allow the radiologist to determine the site or level of the obstruction and the degree of obstruction and in some instances may determine even the nature of the obstructing process. The use of water-soluble contrast material for any small bowel obstructive process beyond the first several feet of jejunum is probably a waste of time. Also, most obstructions secondary to adhesions are seen distally.

Most small bowel obstructions resulting from an adhesion spontaneously resolve with nasogastric suction and decompression. Continued or worsening symptoms may lead to barium studies, however, to delineate the level, cause, and severity of the obstruction. In an incomplete small bowel obstruction, a transition zone can be detected between the dilated loops proximal to the obstruction and the normal-caliber loops distal to it. An adhesion appears as a well-defined linear impression crossing the bowel lumen at the site of obstruction or as the center of a star-shaped collection of bowel loops all pointing at the same spot (Fig. 3-10). That spot, or the center of the star, is the adhesion. Entrapment of a loop of bowel by one or more adhesions may result in a closed-loop obstruction.

A single-contrast enema (either barium or water-soluble contrast material) is used by some radiologists to evaluate for small bowel obstruction and to rule out the possibility of a colonic obstruction. It is necessary to rule out colonic obstruction, and this is done easily via this method. To comment on small bowel obstruction, however, it is necessary to reflux contrast material through the ileocecal valve. Refluxed contrast material into a collapsed or normal-caliber terminal ileum in the face of proximal

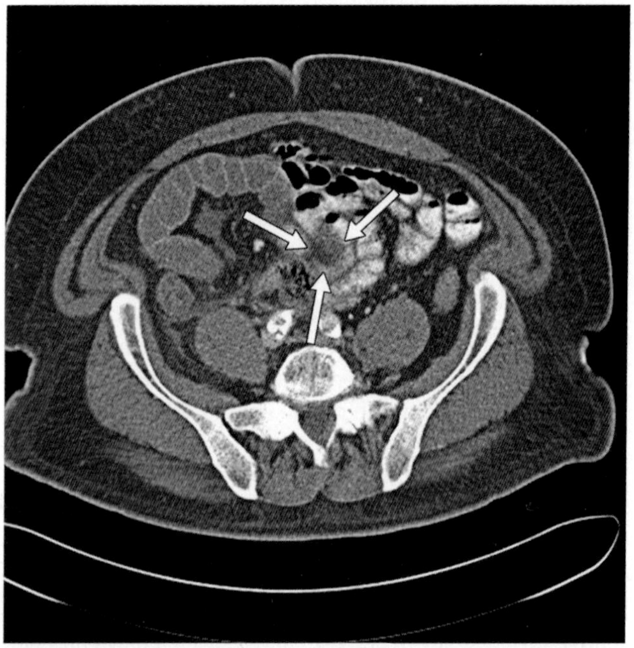

Figure 3-10 Transition between dilated small bowel and normal-caliber small bowel owing to adhesions *(arrows)* is seen.

small bowel dilatation is presumptive evidence of small bowel obstruction.

Multidetector CT is becoming more useful for evaluating suspected small bowel obstruction. In addition to possibly determining the site of obstruction, CT can provide information about intramural and extraintestinal disease, which may indicate the cause of obstruction.

Hernias

External and internal hernias containing small bowel may be associated with obstruction and proximal distention and, similar to adhesive bands, sometimes cause closed-loop obstruction. Inguinal hernias are common and may contain a variable length of ileum. Paraumbilical hernias, incisional hernias involving the anterior or lateral abdominal wall, and spigelian hernias (caused by weakness at the lateral aspects of the rectus abdominis muscles) all may contain loops of small bowel. Other unusual external hernias include femoral, obturator, sciatic, peristomal, and lumbar types.

Internal hernias usually represent defects in the mesentery or peritoneum through which bowel has passed to become sequestered and in some cases entrapped and narrowed. The peritoneal defects may be congenital, posttraumatic, or postsurgical. If the patient is not frankly obstructed, the symptoms can be nonspecific and diagnosis challenging. These hernias include left and right paraduodenal (about 55%), pericecal (10% to 15%), foramen of Winslow (6% to 10%), transmesenteric (8% to 10%), intersigmoid (4% to 8%), and perivesicular (1% to 3%) herniation (Fig. 3-11).

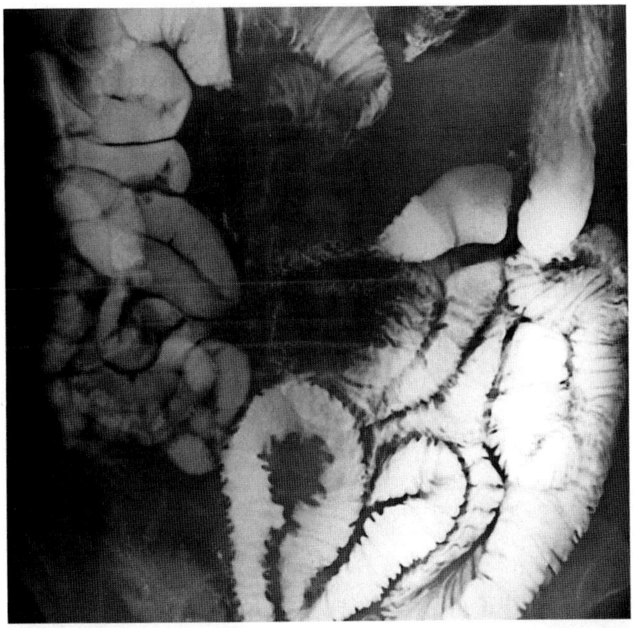

Figure 3-11 Note small bowel loops in the right upper quadrant with displacement of the duodenum. This patient has a paraduodenal hernia.

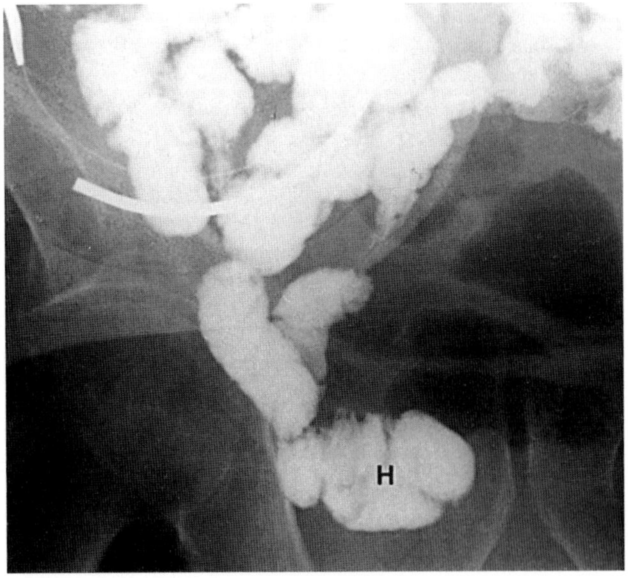

Figure 3-12 A loop of distal ileum *(H)* overlying the right pubic bone lies in an inguinal hernia.

On contrast studies, hernias containing small bowel may be indicated by abnormal location or clustering of loops (Fig. 3-12). Smooth extrinsic compression on the loops as they enter and exit the hernia also is a useful finding on contrast studies. Supplementary examination in the lateral position is usually necessary to detect herniation through the anterior abdominal wall because this is easily obscured on frontal films. CT is often useful in displaying the abnormal location of herniated loops of bowel and may define other hernia contents, including colon and omentum (Fig. 3-13).

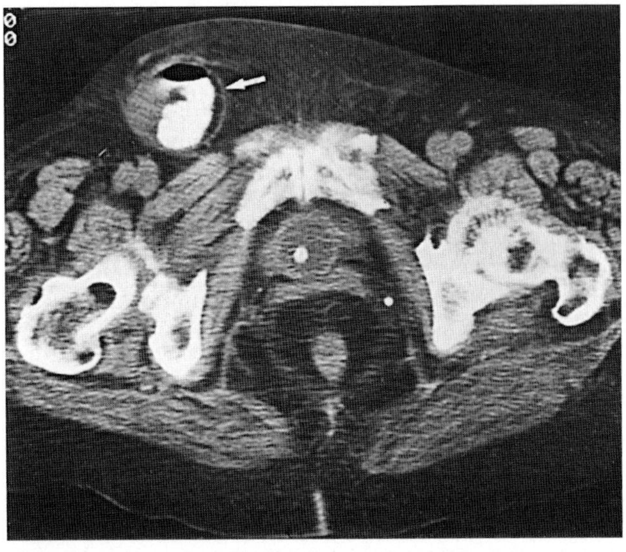

Figure 3-13 Computed tomographic scan shows an opacified loop of bowel in a right inguinal hernia *(arrow)*.

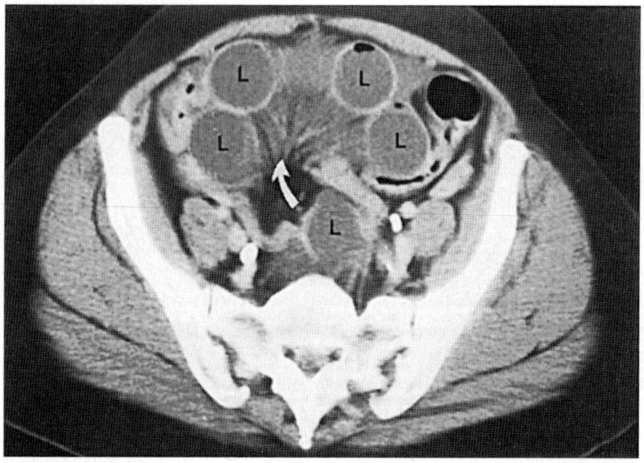

Figure 3-14 CT shows fluid-filled small bowel loops *(L)* around edematous mesentery *(curved arrow)*. (From Goodman P, Raval B: CT diagnosis of acquired small bowel volvulus. Am Surg 56:628, 1990.)

Volvulus

Small bowel volvulus occurs when a loop of bowel twists around its mesenteric axis. Primary volvulus is seen mostly in children as a result of intestinal malrotation, whereas secondary volvulus occurs in adults and is associated with preexisting factors, including adhesions, internal hernias, and tumors. Torsion of a bowel loop causes constriction of its mesenteric vascular supply and often results in ischemia or infarction if not treated promptly. Plain films and barium studies are frequently nonspecific, but CT is useful in showing dilated loops of small bowel radially distributed around the twisted edematous mesentery (Fig. 3-14).

Intussusception

Intussusception represents invagination or telescoping of a bowel loop to form an inner loop (intussusceptum) enclosed within an outer loop (intussuscipiens). The inner loop and its associated mesentery may become edematous and cause a small bowel obstruction. In adults, a tumor or other mass acting as a nidus or lead point usually causes small bowel intussusception, and symptoms are often sporadic. On barium examination, small bowel intussusception typically has a coil-spring appearance, denoting barium trapped between the inner and outer loops of bowel (Fig. 3-15). CT shows the inner loop and its mesentery surrounded by the outer loop and may identify the lead mass (Figs. 3-16 and 3-17).

Neoplasms

Various intrinsic primary and metastatic neoplasms can occlude the small bowel lumen (Figs. 3-18 and 3-19).

Nonneoplastic Strictures

Intrinsic inflammatory, infectious, and ischemic processes can lead to stricture formation with distention of proximal small bowel loops. Postoperative anastomotic strictures also may cause proximal obstruction.

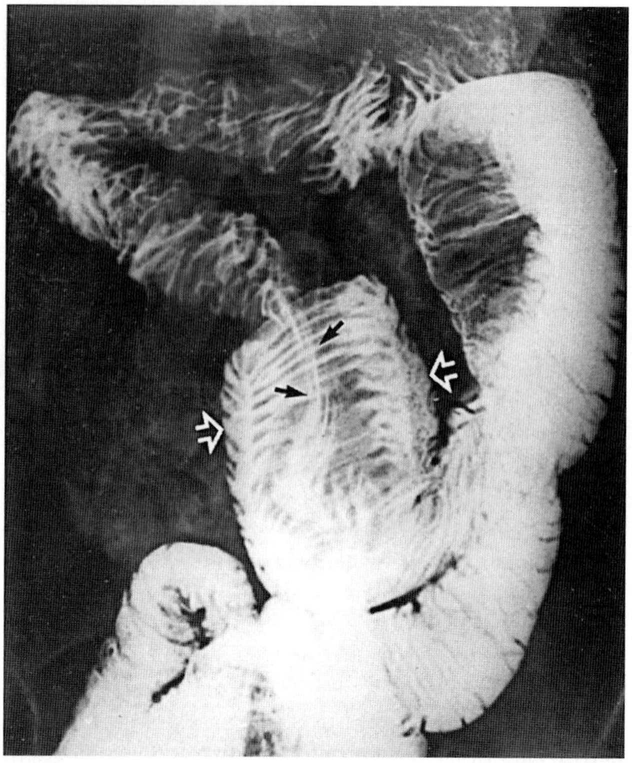

Figure 3-15 Small bowel intussusception shows intussusceptum *(arrows)* and intussuscipiens *(open arrows)*.

Intraluminal Masses

Intraluminal masses may cause small bowel obstruction by occluding the lumen. These masses most commonly lodge at the ileocecal valve and include impacted foreign bodies and gallstones (gallstone ileus).

In meconium ileus equivalent, inspissated fecal material obstructs the distal ileum in children or adults with cystic fibrosis. This complication may be prevented by routine ingestion of pancreatic enzyme supplements.

Extrinsic Masses

Extrinsic inflammatory and neoplastic masses can compress and obstruct adjacent small bowel loops. This obstruction is less important in the mesenteric small bowel than in the duodenum, which is fixed and in close proximity to many organs, including the pancreas, right kidney, gallbladder, biliary tract, and liver.

Colonic Lesions

Colonic lesions, particularly carcinoma of the ascending colon or the region of the ileocecal valve, may result in distended fluid-filled loops of small bowel with little or no air in the colon. These loops mimic a distal small bowel obstruction on conventional abdominal images, but are easily evaluated with a barium enema.

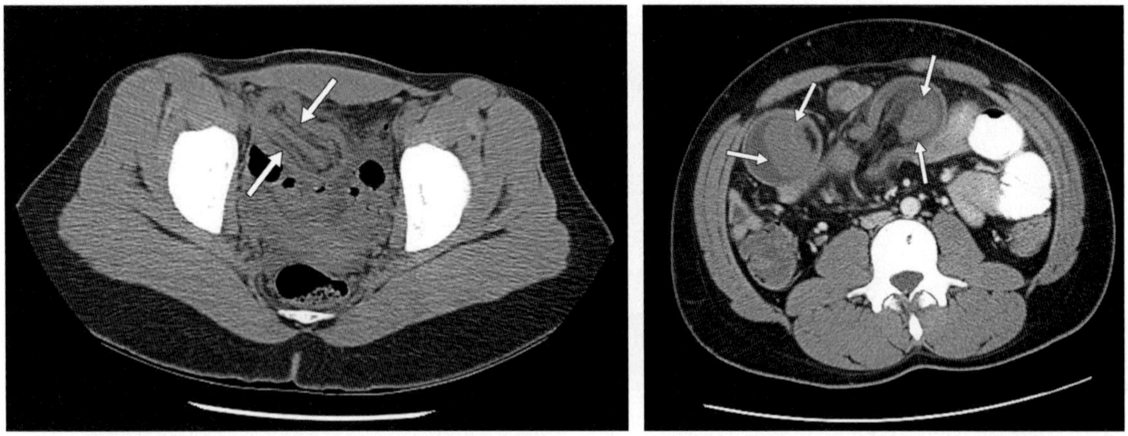

A B

Figure 3-16 **A** and **B,** Two examples of small bowel intussusception in which invaginated small bowel (intussusceptium) is shown (*arrows*).

Appendicitis

Acute appendicitis typically has one of four plain film presentations, the most common being a normal abdominal series. In some instances, there are findings of a focal ileus in the right lower quadrant. An even less frequent finding is a radiopaque appendolith. Additionally, acute appendicitis may present with an appearance of a distal small bowel obstruction on plain film images of the abdomen. This appearance probably is caused by the inflammatory process in and around the appendix being adjacent to the distal ileum, resulting in an intense high-grade focal spasm in the distal ileum. If the appendix is perforated, the process may be a combination of true obstruction and spasm secondary to abscess and inflammation. The clinical history and physical findings are usually more definitive, however, than this unusual presentation on plain film. Multidetector CT is the most effective imaging method to make the diagnosis of appendicitis in any scenario.

Distention without Obstruction (Adynamic Ileus)

Sprue

Small bowel distention also can occur in the absence of a mechanical obstruction. Nontropical sprue (celiac disease) is a mostly reversible condition caused by malabsorption of dietary gluten found in wheat and bread. Refractory cases of nontropical sprue exist. The association of wheat and celiac disease in children was first noted in the Netherlands at the conclusion of World War II. Because of the scarcity of wheat in the Netherlands during the war, other grains were substituted in the making of bread. Dutch physicians noted the improvement of the

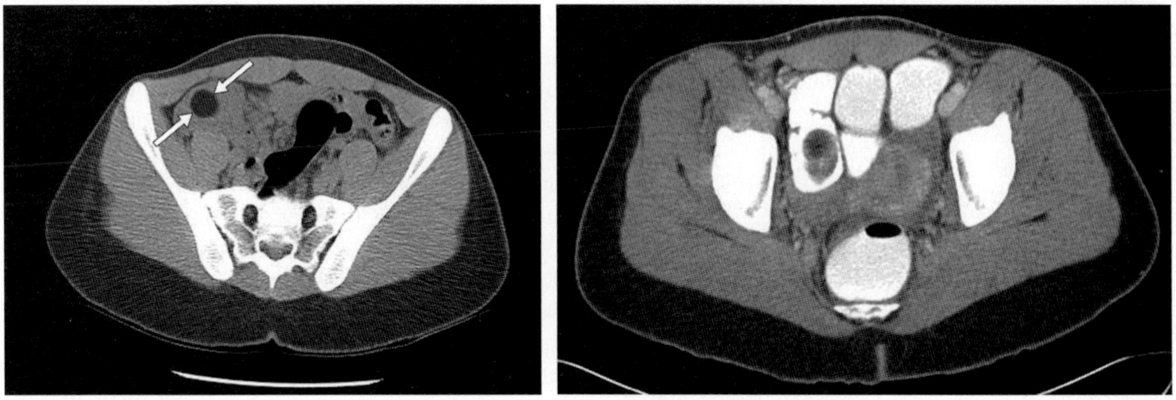

A B

Figure 3-17 **A,** A young patient has an intussusception-like clinical presentation. Rounded, fatty density *(arrows)* is the lead point of a small bowel intussusception on noncontrast CT. **B,** Same patient with opacification of the small bowel shows the lead point of the intussusception as a lipoma.

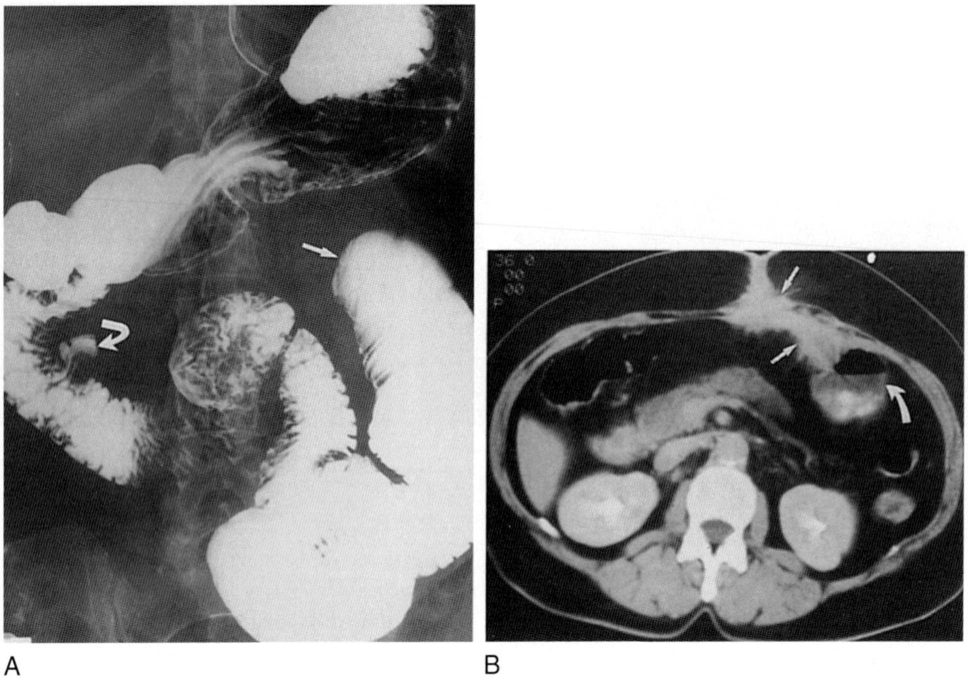

Figure 3-18 **A,** Complete jejunal obstruction *(arrow)* with proximal dilatation. A duodenal diverticulum is also noted *(curved arrow)*. **B,** CT shows an irregular soft tissue mass *(arrows)* in the anterior abdominal wall adjacent to a distended bowel loop *(curved arrow)*. This represents metastatic colon carcinoma.

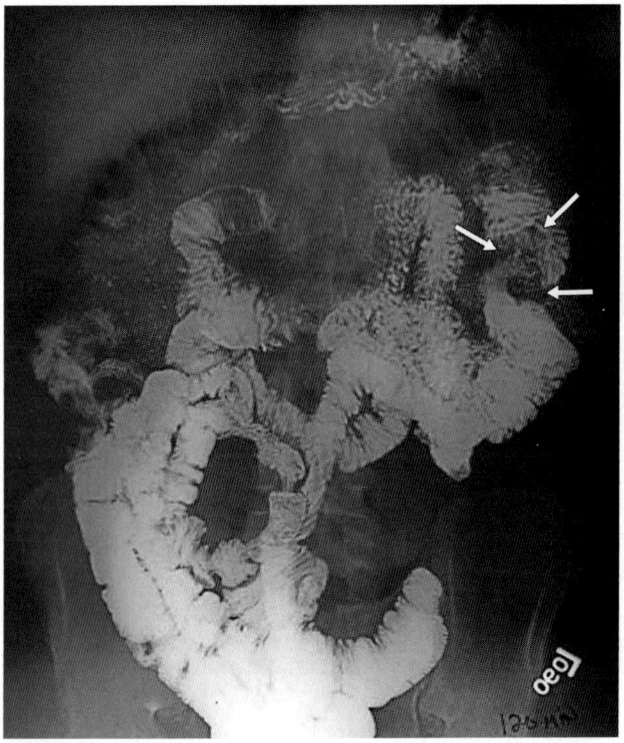

Figure 3-19 Subtle findings of fold irregularity and mucosal destruction *(arrows)* in the jejunum in an anemic patient with no obstruction.

celiac patients during this time and, in particular, took note of the return of symptoms at the conclusion of the war, when wheat became readily available again. Most patients with immunological evidence of gluten enteropathy are either minimally symptomatic or asymptomatic. As a result, prevalence of the disease is usually a reflection of patients sick enough to seek medical attention; in North America, that is about 1:3000. The clinical presentation includes diarrhea, steatorrhea, flatulence, and weight loss.

Of patients who are symptomatic enough to command medical attention, the disease typically produces dilatation of proximal small bowel loops secondary to hypersecretion of fluid within the bowel; this is manifested as dilution of the barium column. Flocculation, segmentation, and a moulage (featureless or castlike) appearance of the barium column previously were considered classic features of sprue, but are less often shown with the improved barium suspensions now widely available. An increase in separation of jejunal folds suggests the bowel atrophy of sprue and is best shown with enteroclysis technique, but also commonly can be seen on SBFT examination. Sprue is associated with an increased incidence of small bowel intussusception, which occurs without a lead mass and is typically transitory and asymptomatic (Fig. 3-20). Other complications of sprue include small bowel ulcerations or strictures (ulcerative enteritis) and a slight increased

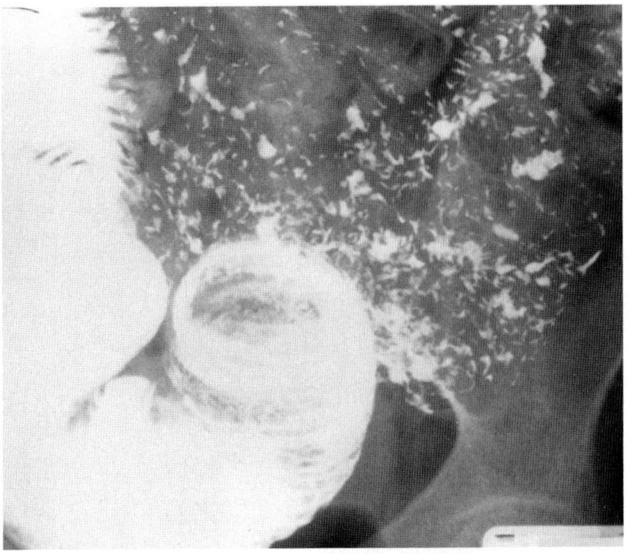

Figure 3-20 Classic coil-spring appearance in distal small bowel in a patient with sprue. Intussusceptions in sprue are usually transient.

risk (3% to 5%) for lymphoma and adenocarcinoma of the proximal small bowel. These patients also have a slightly increased risk for small bowel lymphoma and adenoma (Box 3-2).

Tropical sprue occurs in certain tropical locations and radiographically appears similar to nontropical sprue. In contrast to nontropical sprue, the tropical form is much more complicated and thought by some authors to be associated with vitamin B_{12} and folic acid deficiencies and megaloblastic anemia; others assert these conditions are not a cause, but a reflection of malabsorption in patients with chronic bowel infection or enteric parasitic infestation. Tropical sprue may respond to folic acid or antibiotic therapy, but not to a gluten-free diet.

Lactose Intolerance and Other Hypersecretory States

Lactose intolerance is a common cause of malabsorption in adults that results from acquired deficiency of the enzyme lactase in the small bowel. After a lactose-containing meal, hypersecretion of fluid into the small bowel causes luminal distention and symptoms of bloating and cramps. Lactose intolerance is easily treated by either eliminating dairy products from the diet or supplementing the diet with commercially available lactase enzymes. Other hypersecretory states, including Zollinger-Ellison syndrome and cryptosporidial enteritis, likewise may cause small bowel distention as a result of increased fluid content.

Box 3-2 Complications of Celiac Disease (Nontropical Sprue)

Malabsorption
Intussusception
Ulceration and strictures
Lymphoma
Adenocarcinoma
Carcinoma (squamous) of the esophagus
Hyposplenism
Cavitating lymph node syndrome

Neuromuscular and Motility Abnormalities

Various neuromuscular and motility abnormalities can affect the small bowel and lead to luminal distention. The best known of these is scleroderma (progressive systemic sclerosis), in which smooth muscle atrophies and is replaced by fibrous tissue (Fig. 3-21). In the mesenteric small bowel, smooth asymmetric sacculations (pseudodiverticula) are sometimes seen. Crowding of folds ("hidebound bowel") is a characteristic finding of scleroderma involving the small bowel. Traumatic spinal cord injuries also can result in bowel dilatation, often on a chronic basis.

Chagas' disease, a parasitic infection common in Brazil, can cause distention of the duodenum and mesenteric small bowel by destroying the neural plexus. Associated abnormalities are often seen in the esophagus, colon, and heart.

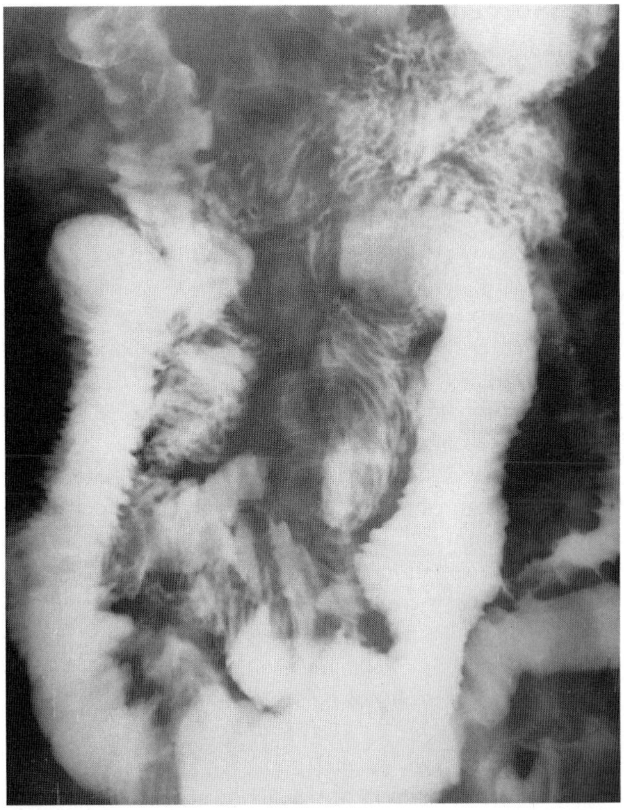

Figure 3-21 Diffuse mild dilatation of the small bowel as seen in scleroderma.

Peritonitis or Severe Abdominal Pain

Peritonitis, severe abdominal pain, and recent abdominal surgery are important causes of adynamic ileus, a condition characterized by decreased peristalsis of the bowel. Supine abdominal films reveal distention of small bowel, colon, or both, and upright films typically show air-fluid levels to be at equal heights within the same bowel loop (nondifferential air-fluid levels). Localized abdominal pain caused by conditions such as appendicitis, cholecystitis, or pancreatitis may be associated with focal bowel dilatation and focal air-fluid levels (sentinel loops).

Other Causes

Other causes of adynamic ileus include drugs (anticholinergics, morphine), metabolic disorders resulting in electrolyte imbalance, and previous vagotomy. Idiopathic pseudoobstruction is a chronic form of adynamic ileus of unknown origin. Ischemia resulting from thromboembolic disease, vasculitis, or low-flow states may decrease small bowel motility and increase distention. Associated fold thickening caused by intramural edema or hemorrhage also may be present.

NARROWED SMALL BOWEL

Narrowing Resulting from Intrinsic Abnormality

Narrowing of the small bowel lumen can result from numerous intrinsic and extrinsic processes.

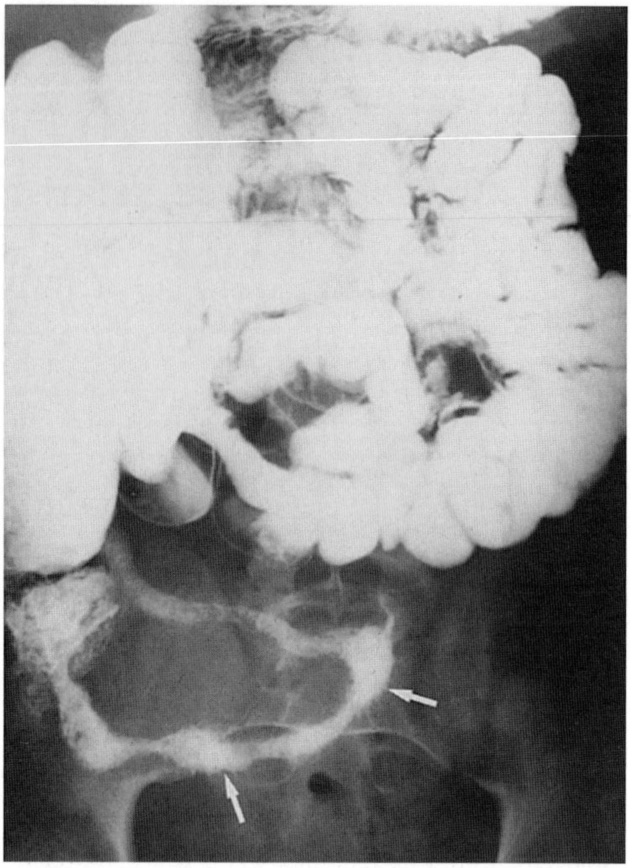

Figure 3-22 Narrowing and mucosal irregularity of the distal ileum *(arrows)* is associated with separation of bowel loops in a patient with Crohn's disease.

Crohn's disease

Crohn's disease (regional enteritis) usually is confined to the distal ileum and the colon, but may involve any portion of the small bowel. Until the time Koch (1882) identified the tuberculosis bacillus as the cause of terminal ileal disease in some patients and its absence in others, regional enteritis was thought to be a bowel manifestation of tuberculosis. Although a granulomatous transmural inflammatory process, no organisms have been isolated, and its cause continues to be elusive.

Early in the disease, spasm and edema associated with ulcerations can cause luminal narrowing, and later in the disease, continued inflammation and fibrosis often lead to stricture formation (Figs. 3-22 and 3-23). Skip lesions consisting of narrowed segments of small bowel separated by normal or dilated segments are sometimes noted. These can produce bizarre radiographic findings, although clinically the patient may not be symptomatic.

Neoplasms

Primary neoplasms of the small bowel, including adenocarcinoma, lymphoma, leiomyosarcoma, and carcinoid tumor, can cause focal narrowing of the lumen (Fig. 3-24). Primary tumors do this by infiltration of the bowel wall, which is more typically seen with carcinoma. Lymphomas and sarcomas may narrow or dilate the lumen. Carcinoid tumors narrow the lumen by their associated desmoplastic response, producing fibrosis and kinking. Metastatic spread to the small bowel through contiguous, peritoneal, or hematogenous routes also can lead to one or more areas of narrowing (Fig. 3-25).

Zollinger-Ellison Syndrome

Involvement of the distal duodenum and proximal jejunum is uncommon in peptic ulcer disease, but sometimes occurs in severe ulcer diathesis, as seen in Zollinger-Ellison syndrome, because of the increased acidity in the proximal small bowel.

Ischemia and Radiation

Small bowel ischemia can cause luminal narrowing secondary to spasm, intramural edema (Fig. 3-26) or hemorrhage, or stricture formation. Similar findings are sometimes seen after radiation and are caused by endarteritis and subsequent small bowel ischemia (Fig. 3-27).

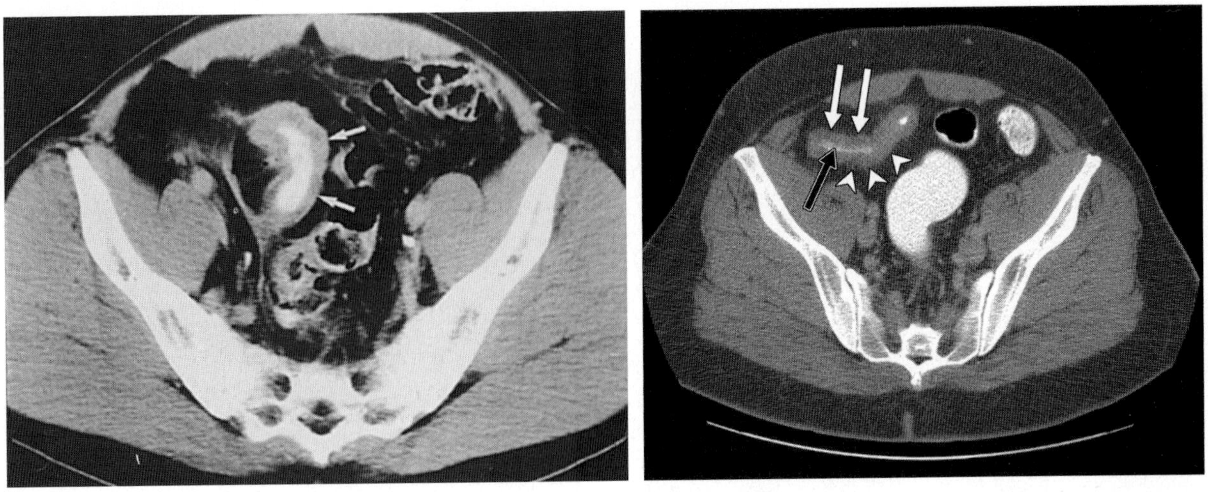
A
B

Figure 3-23 **A,** CT shows thickened wall *(arrows)* of distal ileum in a patient with Crohn's disease. **B,** Changes of Crohn's disease in the terminal ileum include thickened wall *(white arrows)*, narrowed lumen *(black arrow)*, and linear stranding into the peri-ileal fat *(arrowheads)*.

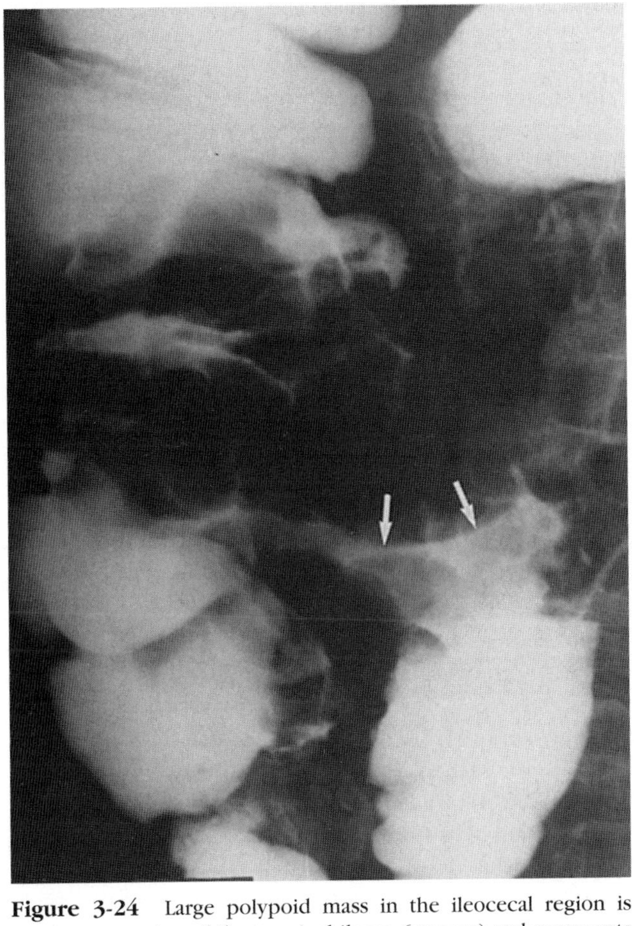

Figure 3-24 Large polypoid mass in the ileocecal region is causing narrowing of the terminal ileum *(arrows)* and represents non-Hodgkin's lymphoma.

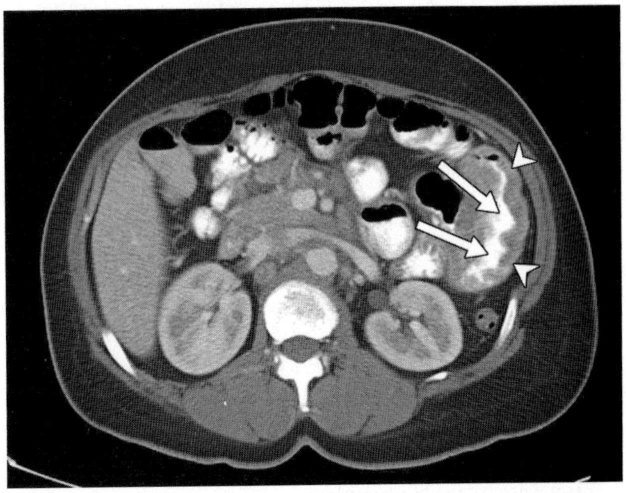

Figure 3-25 Metastatic disease from lung infiltrating jejunum is seen, with wall thickening *(arrowheads)* and narrowed lumen *(arrows)*.

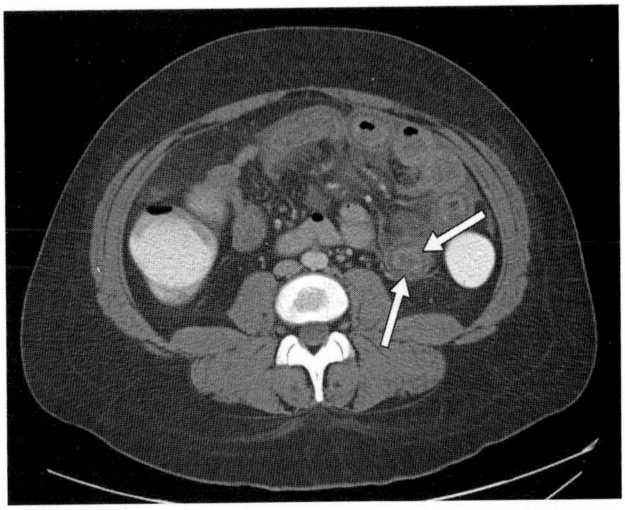

Figure 3-26 This patient has small bowel edema of the wall with "target sign" *(arrows)*.

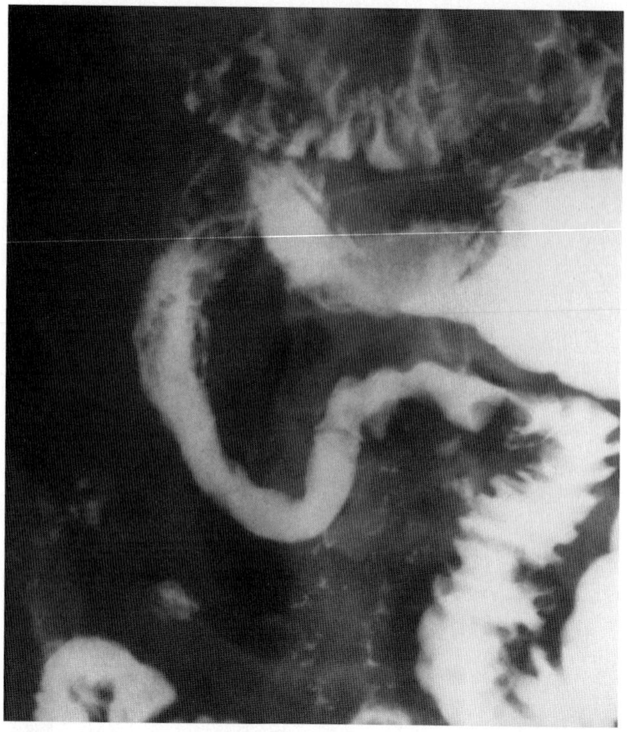

Figure 3-27 Narrowed, featureless segment of small bowel is a sequela of ischemia.

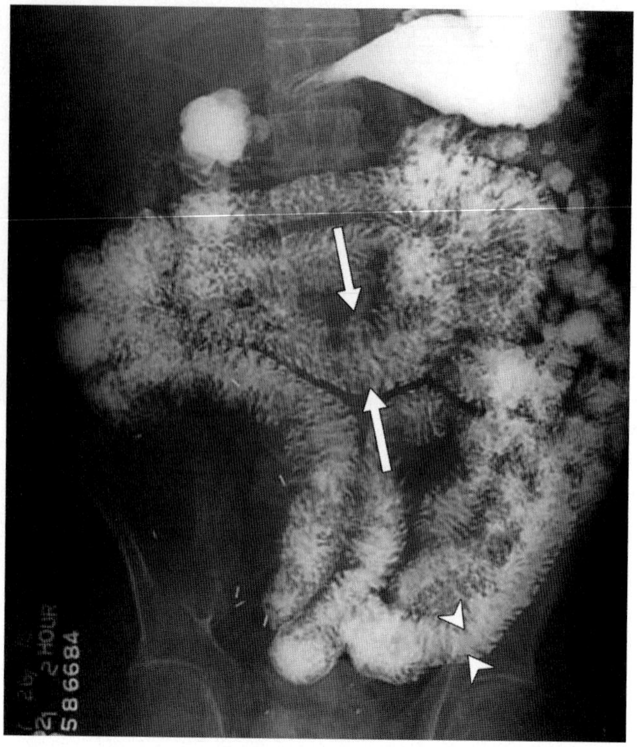

Figure 3-28 SBFT examination shows thickened folds *(arrows)* and areas of diminished luminal caliber *(arrowheads)*.

Drug-Induced Narrowing

Various drugs have been associated with small bowel narrowing because of their local toxic effects. These include potassium chloride tablets and floxuridine and other related chemotherapeutic agents.

Postoperative Narrowing

Narrowing at surgical anastomoses usually is related to edema in the immediate postoperative period and fibrosis with stricture formation later on.

Volvulus and Intussusception

In small bowel volvulus, narrowing results from torsion of a loop of bowel, whereas in intussusception, edema of the intussuscepted loop and its mesentery causes narrowing.

Infection

Several infectious agents can cause small bowel narrowing. The protozoan *Giardia lamblia* may cause narrowing secondary to thickening of folds in the duodenum and proximal jejunum. The roundworm *Strongyloides stercoralis* (Fig. 3-28) causes similar findings and may cause tubular narrowing of the bowel lumen resulting from spasm or stricture formation (Table 3-1).

Tuberculosis of the small bowel caused by *Mycobacterium tuberculosis* may result from drinking unpasteurized milk or swallowing infected sputum. The ileocecal region is most often involved, with narrowing sometimes causing marked distortion of this area. As previously mentioned, small bowel intestinal tuberculosis may be difficult to distinguish from Crohn's disease. Other infections in which fold thickening and luminal narrowing are usually localized to the distal ileum include *Campylobacter fetus jejuni, Yersinia enterocolitica,* and *Salmonella typhi* (typhoid fever). *Anisakis,* a small roundworm transmitted by eating raw fish, has been reported to cause narrowing of the jejunum or ileum secondary to spasm and ulceration.

Cytomegalovirus (CMV) enteritis occurs with increased frequency in immunocompromised patients, especially patients with acquired immunodeficiency syndrome (AIDS). CMV enteritis can cause diffuse small bowel narrowing, ulcerations, and effacement of folds. Associated esophagitis, gastritis, or colitis also may be present in patients with disseminated CMV infection.

Graft-versus-Host Disease

Graft-versus-host disease is a potential complication of bone marrow transplantation in immunocompromised patients and represents rejection of the patient's own tissues by the donor bone marrow lymphocytes. Diffuse narrowing of the small bowel with effacement of folds has been compared with the appearance of ribbon or toothpaste, hence the "ribbon sign."

Table 3-1 Infectious and Parasitic Diseases of the Small Bowel

	Genus/Species or Expanded Name	Origin	Area of Involvement
Bacteria			
Yersinia	*Yersinia enterocolitica*	Water	Terminal ileum
Tuberculosis	*Mycobacterium tuberculosis*	Milk, pulmonary	Distal small bowel
	Mycobacterium avium-intracellulare	Soil	Entire small bowel
Dysentery	*Salmonella typhi*	Water, food	Distal small bowel
	Shigella dysenteriae	Water, food	Distal small bowel
Helicobacter	*Helicobacter fetus jejuni*	Ingested	Distal small bowel
Virus			
Herpes	Herpes simplex	Person	Distal small bowel
CMV	Cytomegalovirus	Person	Entire small bowel
HIV	Human immunodeficiency virus	Person	Entire small bowel
Fungus			
Blastomycosis	*Paracoccidioides brasiliensis*	Soil	Distal small bowel
Histoplasma	*Histoplasma capsulatum*	Pulmonary	Entire small bowel
Candida	*Candida albicans*	Ingested	Entire small bowel
Protozoan			
Cryptosporidiosis	*Cryptosporidium enteritis*	Water	Proximal small bowel
	Isospora belli	Water	Proximal small bowel
Giardiasis	*Giardia lamblia*	Water	Proximal small bowel
Amebiasis	*Entamoeba histolytica*	Water	Proximal small bowel

Narrowing Resulting from Extrinsic Abnormality

Adhesions

Extrinsic narrowing of the small bowel is usually related to an adhesion and probably ranks as the primary cause of small bowel obstruction. The adhesion usually results from prior surgery or inflammatory conditions of the abdomen, with fibrous bands of tissue developing in the peritoneal cavity as a result (Fig. 3-29). Adhesions are rarely detected by any of the imaging methods, and their presence is inferred from the clinical history and lack of other findings on radiographic studies.

Hernias

Hernias are a frequent cause of small bowel obstruction. The hernia itself does not produce the problem. Instead, the size of the opening into the hernia has a significant effect on any bowel loops passing through it. The smaller the opening, the more likely that loops of bowel entering it will be affected. The bowel lumen, and possibly vascular supply, becomes more easily compromised by a small opening, resulting in obstruction.

Serosal Metastases and Other Extrinsic Masses

Various extrinsic masses can compress and narrow the small bowel lumen. The most common of these are serosal metastases. The primary tumor usually arises within the abdomen, most commonly ovarian or gastric cancer. Extraabdominal tumors, such as breast or lung, can produce intraperitoneal deposits of tumor, causing multifocal areas of narrowing. Whenever multiple areas of obstruction are encountered, metastatic tumor should be a primary consideration. Other abdominal masses, such as cysts and mesenchymal tumors, also can produce narrowing of the small bowel by extrinsic compression (Fig. 3-30).

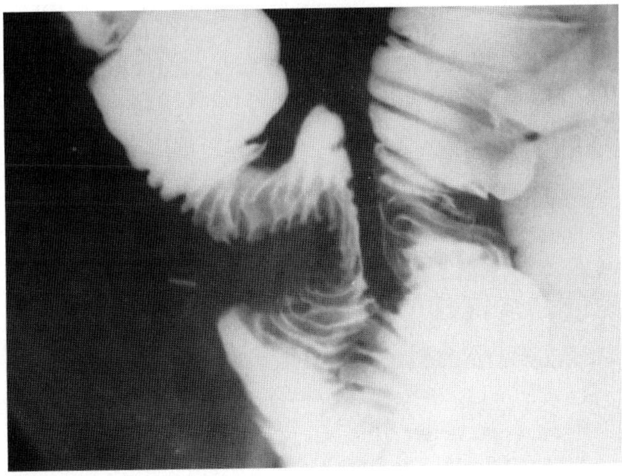

Figure 3-29 The distal small bowel is narrowed and kinked owing to adhesions.

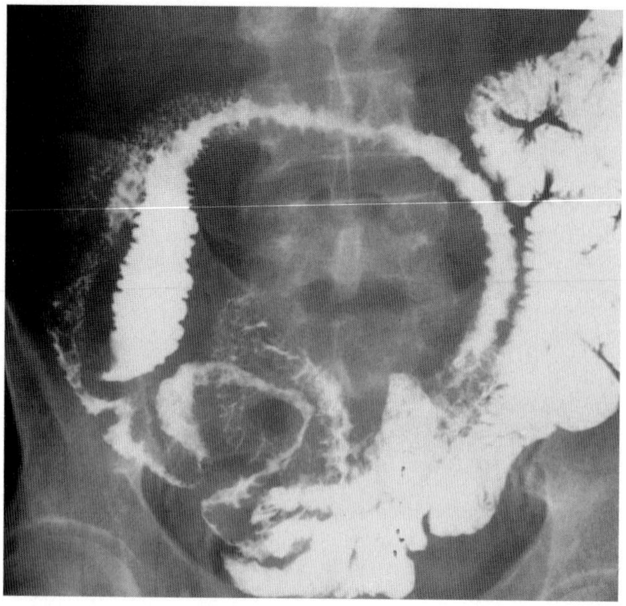

Figure 3-30 Extensive narrowing of distal small bowel is secondary to extensive mesenteric involvement by lymphoma.

NARROWED TERMINAL ILEUM

The category of a narrowed terminal ileum deserves a separate discussion because it is one of the more common abnormalities encountered during small bowel examinations.

Crohn's Disease

In most practices, Crohn's disease is the most common cause of terminal ileal narrowing. This narrowing can be due to either active disease with ulceration or chronic disease with fibrosis. The classic term "string sign," originally applied to Crohn's disease, refers to a narrowed terminal ileum with displacement of the adjacent bowel loops (Box 3-3). The encroachment of hardened mesenteric fat on the chronically inflamed bowel ("fingers of fat") (Fig. 3-31) may contribute to some degree to narrowing, but overall it is a secondary cause.

Box 3-3 Complications of Crohn's Disease

Strictures and obstruction
Fistulas and sinus tracts
Perforation and abscesses
Malignancy (adenocarcinoma, rarely lymphoma)

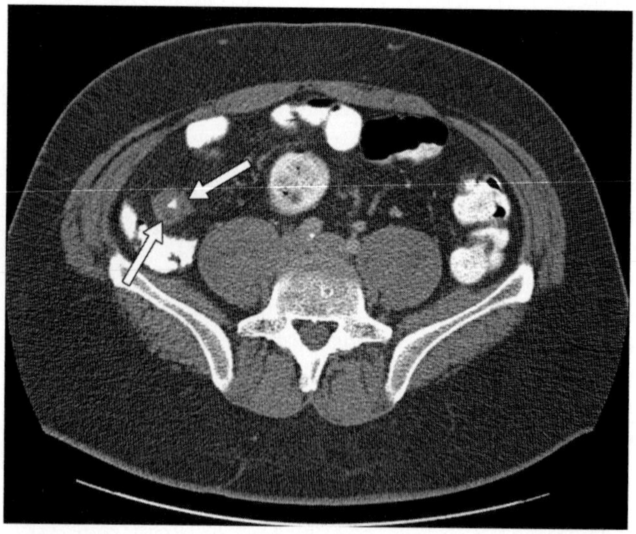

Figure 3-31 Thickened irregular terminal ileum with low-density areas of fat *(arrows)* on outer surface of bowel wall is seen.

"Backwash ileitis" (Fig. 3-32) from ulcerative colitis never produces narrowing of the terminal ileum, even after healing. The appearance is that of a mildly dilated terminal ileum with atrophy of the folds. Mild inflammatory changes have been reported.

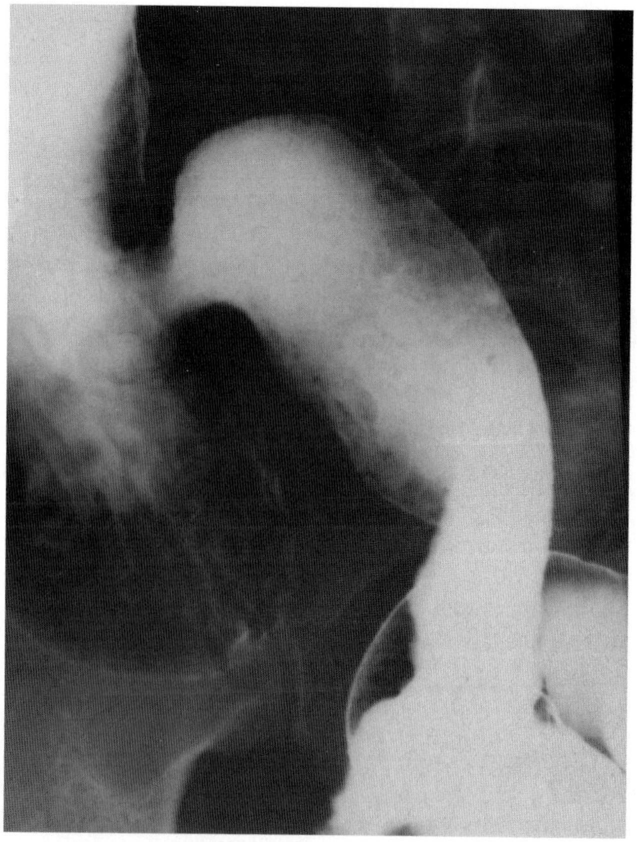

Figure 3-32 "Backwash ileitis" in a patient with ulcerative colitis shows dilatation and atrophy of the terminal ileum.

Infection

The next most common cause for narrowing of the terminal ileum is usually some type of infectious process. Tuberculosis can produce changes in the terminal ileum that are identical to Crohn's disease (Fig. 3-33), but in the presence of acid-fast bacterium. Tuberculosis is usually encountered in large cities in which there is a large immigrant population or in persons who travel overseas. In the last 2 decades, there has been an upsurge of gastrointestinal tuberculosis as a result of the AIDS epidemic. A patient with gastrointestinal tuberculosis almost always had some degree of pulmonary tuberculosis until recent times. Today, most patients with gastrointestinal tuberculosis have normal chest x-rays.

Another infectious process that also frequently appears is *Yersinia enterocolitica,* a gram-negative rod more commonly seen in Europe than in North America. The infection tends to be more common in children and is self-limiting. This bacterial infection sporadically can infect the terminal ileum and can produce a radiological picture similar to Crohn's disease (although fistulous tracts are not seen in *Yersinia*). The infection produces inflammatory changes in the terminal ileum that usually resolve over a few weeks or months. Many other infections of the bowel can involve the terminal ileum and produce inflammatory changes with narrowing. These often involve the rest of the small bowel, however, and typically are not isolated to the terminal ileum.

Neoplasms

Lymphoma is more frequent in the distal small bowel and is the most common neoplastic process to involve the terminal ileum. It can infiltrate through the bowel wall, producing narrowing and irregularity or nodularity of the folds (Fig. 3-34), although it seldom obstructs (Fig. 3-35). Carcinoid also occurs in that region. The narrowing it produces is related to the desmoplastic changes that occur in the adjacent mesentery. The ileum is also a common area for metastases, particularly from serosal spread of intraabdominal tumors (Fig. 3-36); this is related to the flow of ascitic fluid in the abdomen. Ovarian and upper abdominal tumors have been known to produce marked narrowing of the terminal ileum. Tumors of the cecum or ileocecal valve can extend in a retrograde fashion to involve the terminal ileum. Rarely, primary carcinoma of the small bowel could occur in the region.

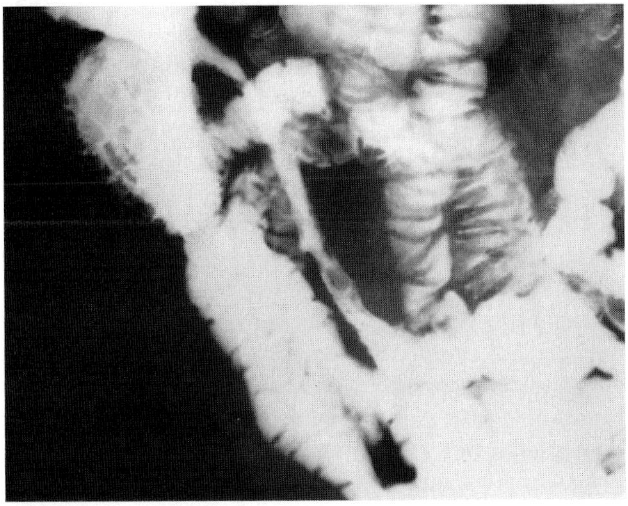

Figure 3-33 Narrowed and ulcerated terminal ileum and cecum. Although this is due to tuberculosis, the changes are identical to those seen in Crohn's disease.

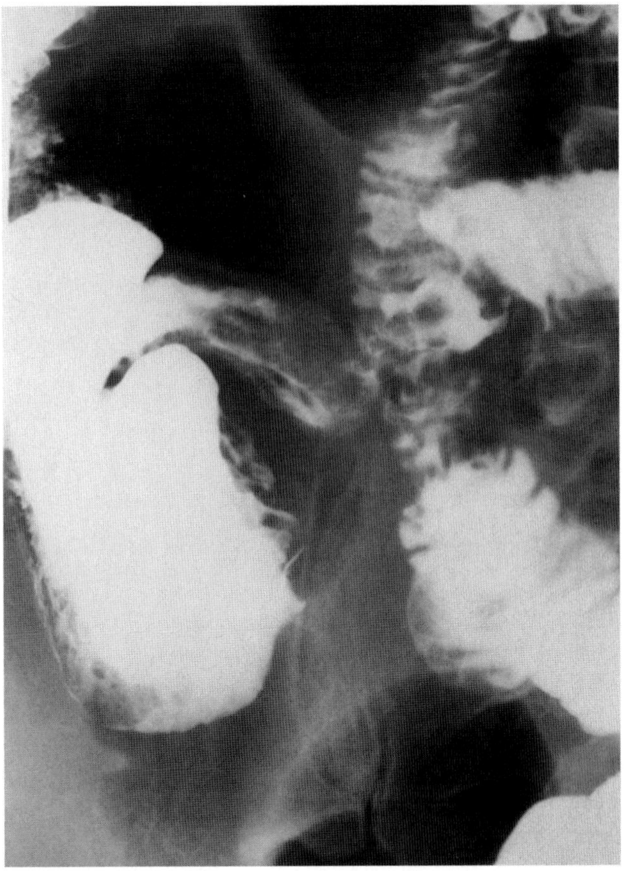

Figure 3-34 A short segment of narrowing of the terminal ileum results from lymphoma.

Extrinsic Masses

The pelvis and right lower quadrant are frequent sites for abscesses or intraabdominal masses or tumors. Because the terminal ileum is on a relatively short mesentery, it is not as free to move as the rest of the intestines, and the terminal ileum may become secondarily involved by these adjacent processes. When the terminal ileum abuts an abscess, such as can be

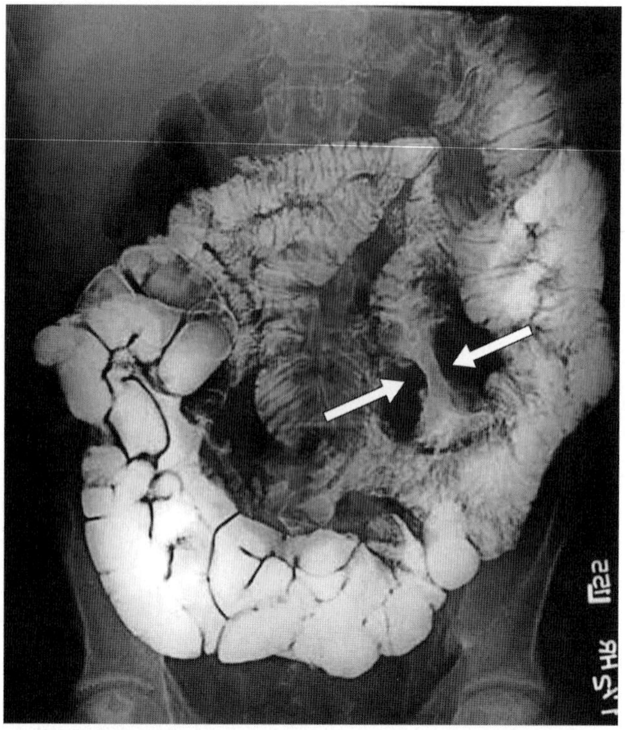

Figure 3-35 Large lymphoma involving the jejunum without evidence of obstruction. Note example of bowel replacement with tumor *(arrows)* and aneurysmal dilatation.

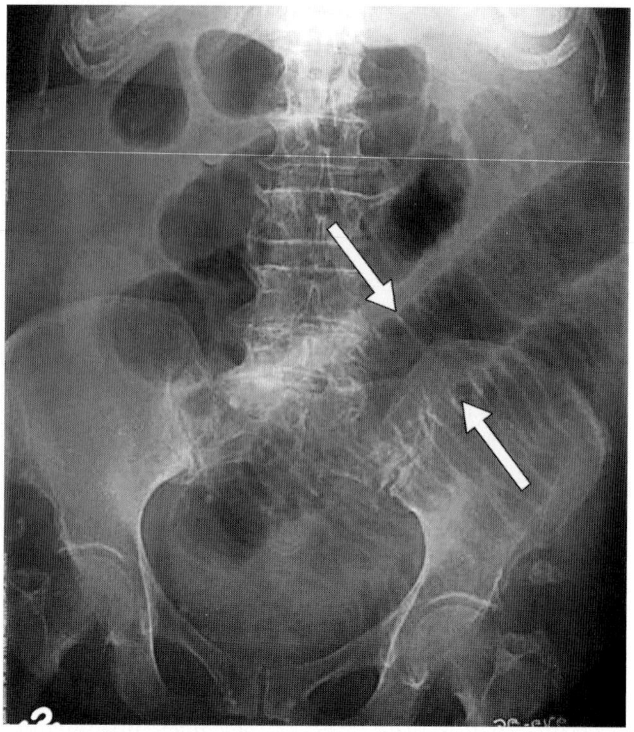

Figure 3-37 Patient with periappendiceal abscess resulting in narrowing and occlusion of the terminal ileum has the appearance of a small bowel obstruction *(arrows)*.

encountered with a periappendiceal abscess, the terminal ileum narrows and becomes spastic (Fig. 3-37). These changes may mimic Crohn's disease or other inflammatory processes. Terminal ileal narrowing also can be seen in mesenteric panniculitis and pseudomyxoma peritonei.

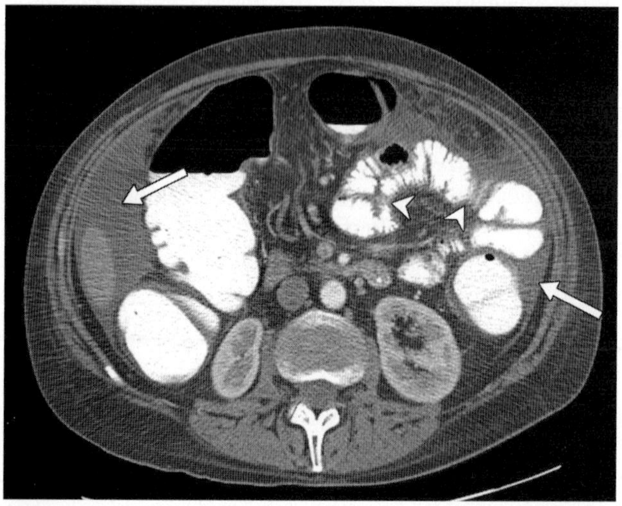

Figure 3-36 Axial computed tomographic scan shows malignant ascites *(arrows)* and attachment of peritoneal metastatic disease to small bowel *(arrowheads)*.

THICKENED FOLDS

Fold thickening is characteristic of a variety of abnormalities affecting the small bowel. In some conditions, folds appear uniformly or regularly thickened, whereas in other conditions, thickening is nodular or irregular. Fold thickening also can be focal or diffuse, depending on the underlying disease or the extent or severity of the disease. These features provide a pattern-based approach to the differential diagnosis of thickened small bowel folds.

Uniformly Thickened Folds

Intramural Hemorrhage

Uniformly thickened small bowel folds are typical of intramural hemorrhage. In these conditions, blood or transudate infiltrates into the submucosal layer of the bowel wall. As the folds become thicker, the space between adjacent folds becomes shorter, with the overall appearance likened to a stack of coins (Fig. 3-38). Small bowel hemorrhage is caused by various insults, including hemophilia, mesenteric ischemia or infarction, vasculitis, coagulopathy, anticoagulant medications, and trauma. Unusual disease entities, such as Henoch-Schönlein purpura and idiopathic thrombocytopenic purpura, also can have this appearance (Fig. 3-39). The changes typically

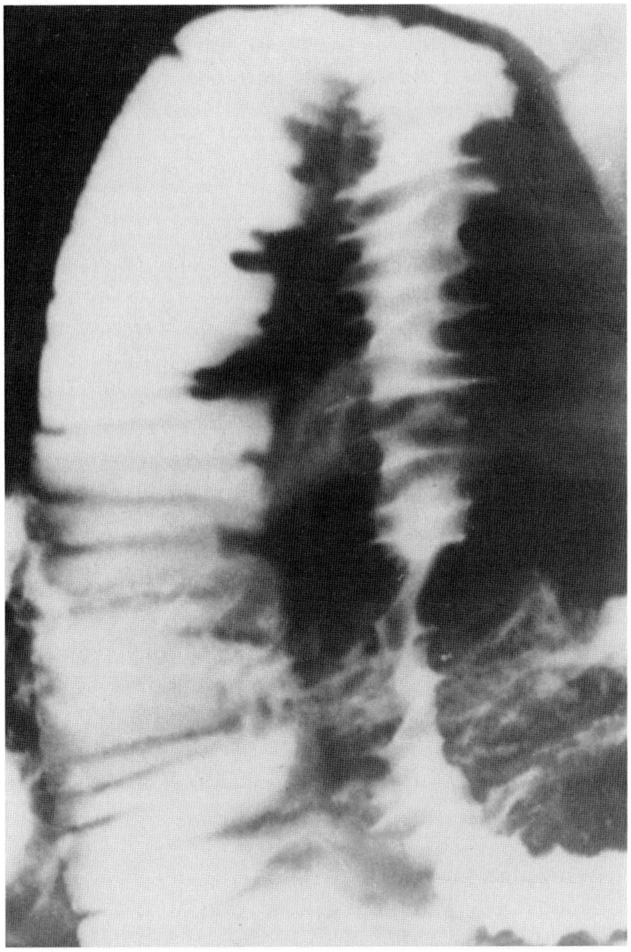

Figure 3-38 Thickened folds and luminal narrowing represent segmental small bowel hemorrhage caused by oral contraceptive drug.

involve a short segment of bowel and rarely involve the entire bowel. This segmental involvement along with the appropriate clinical history helps differentiate it from edema.

Edema

Edema of the small bowel may complicate mesenteric ischemia or infarction, congestive heart failure, and hypoproteinemia (resulting from hepatic, renal, or gastrointestinal disease). Edema probably is seen most frequently in patients with end-stage liver disease because of a combination of hypoproteinemia and portal venous congestion (Fig. 3-40). Angioneurotic edema is an unusual cause of small bowel edema. In this disease, an autosomal dominant genetic defect in the complement inactivation system can trigger episodes of transudation of fluid rapidly into extravascular spaces, resulting in small bowel edema, hives, and life-threatening laryngeal edema. Between attacks of angioneurotic edema, patients are asymptomatic and the small bowel folds appear normal.

Lymphangiectasia represents dilatation of intestinal lymphatic channels, resulting in inadequate lymph drainage. It is seen most commonly distally in the small bowel and is seen mostly as uniform fold thickening. In some cases, it may have a slightly more irregular fold appearance and appear radiologically similar to Whipple's disease, which, by comparison, tends to occur more proximally in the small bowel. There also can be an associated hypoproteinemia. The disease may be congenital or acquired and typically shows diffuse thickening of small bowel folds (Fig. 3-41). Other causes of small bowel edema that are associated with nonuniform or nodular fold thickening are discussed later in this section.

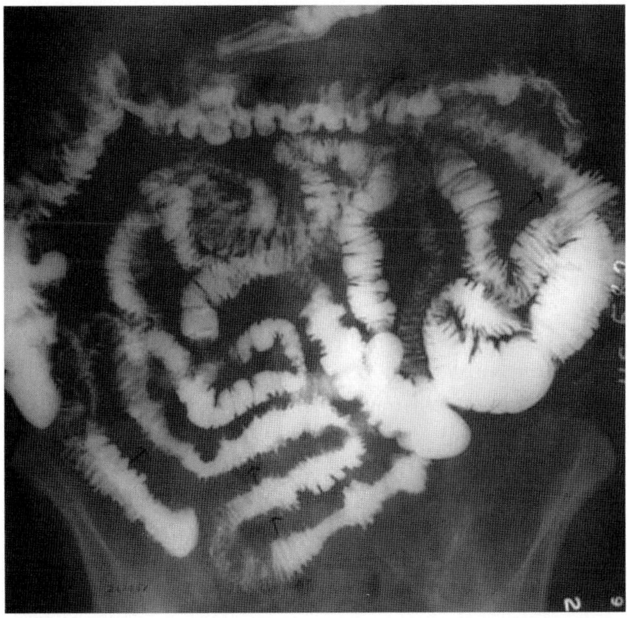

Figure 3-39 A 51-year-old woman with Henoch-Schönlein purpura and bleeding into the wall of most of her ileum is seen.

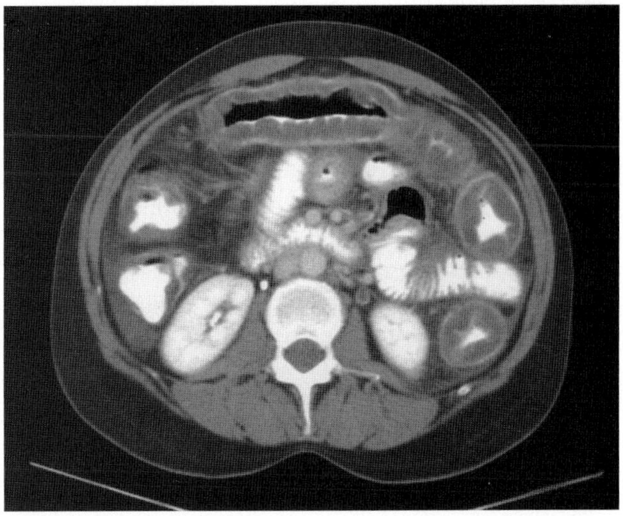

Figure 3-40 Widespread edema of the small bowel and colon is seen.

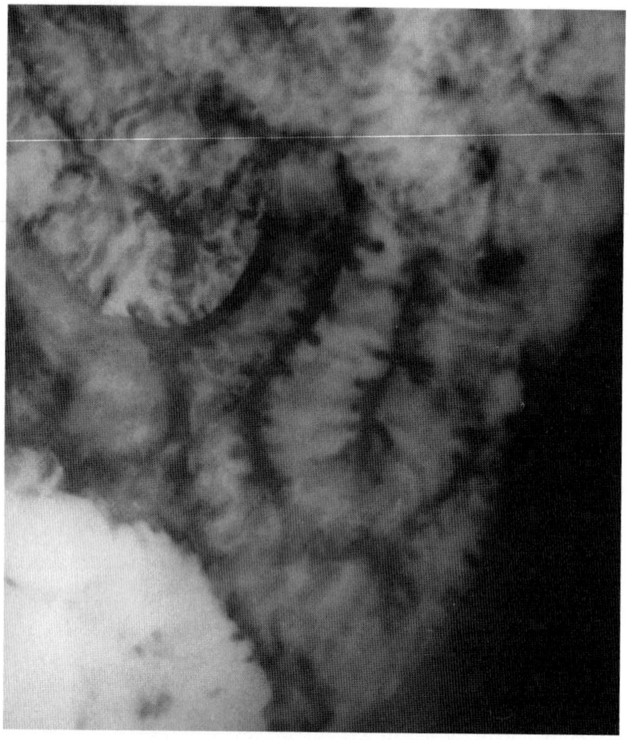

Figure 3-41 Diffuse small bowel fold thickening is represented, as seen in lymphangiectasia.

Radiation

Radiation to the abdomen or pelvis can lead to endarteritis in small bowel loops within the radiation port. Similar to other forms of ischemia, radiation enteritis causes uniform thickening of small bowel folds.

Eosinophilic Enteritis

Eosinophilic enteritis is characterized by excessive eosinophilic infiltration of the gastrointestinal tract and degranulation of these cells. The granular protein content of these cells has been shown to cause tissue damage. The exact cause of infiltration and degranulation is unknown. Food allergies, parasitic infiltration, and defects in the gut epithelium that invite eosinophilic congregation have been postulated. This disease most often affects the stomach or small bowel and may be transmural or confined to the mucosa, muscularis, or serosa. With primary mucosal involvement of the small bowel, folds often appear thickened. The thickening may be uniform or nodular, focal or diffuse. Associated fold thickening or luminal narrowing of the gastric antrum and proximal duodenum also may occur. Peripheral eosinophilia and a history of allergy may suggest the diagnosis of eosinophilic enteritis, and are present in about 80% of cases.

Radiological findings are nonspecific, and there may or may not be gastric involvement. Thickened folds are seen throughout small bowel (and possibly the stomach). The bowel may be mildly dilated, and some nodularity of the fold pattern may be present. Jejunealization of the ileum has been reported associated with this disease. CT may show thickened bowel wall and possibly some free intraperitoneal fluid resulting from "seepage" from the serosal surface.

Abetalipoproteinemia

Abetalipoproteinemia is a rare genetic disease, probably autosomal recessive, in which abnormal lipid metabolism leads to fat malabsorption, cerebellar degeneration, and acanthocytosis (pointed red blood cells). Deposits of fat in epithelial cells of the duodenum and jejunum produce uniform or nodular thickening of folds with relative sparing of the ileum. Similar findings have been noted in small bowel xanthomatosis, an extremely rare condition in which lipid-laden macrophages infiltrate the bowel wall.

Nodular or Irregularly Thickened Folds (Focal and Diffuse)

In contrast to the straight thickened folds typical of intramural hemorrhage, nodular or irregular fold thickening is featured in numerous diseases affecting the small bowel. In some, involvement is primarily focal or segmental, whereas in others, the small bowel is diffusely abnormal.

Whipple's Disease

Since 2000, Whipple's disease, previously thought to be a chronic systemic disease of unknown origin, has been the target of numerous microbiological and immunological studies. Considerable suspicion has fallen on the bacterium *Tropheryma whippelii*. Besides protein loss, diarrhea, and malabsorption, seen in the small bowel involvement, the disease also manifests systemically as joint pain and swelling, fever, skin pigmentation abnormalities, and dementia. In the proximal small bowel, Whipple's disease causes nodular thickened folds in the duodenum and proximal jejunum (Fig. 3-42). Macrophages containing abundant periodic acid–Schiff–positive material are found throughout the lamina propria layer of the bowel wall, and characteristic rod-shaped, gram-positive bacilli (*T. whippelii*) have been identified within these cells. Whipple's disease occurs mostly in middle-aged men; presenting symptoms include diarrhea, arthralgias, fever, and adenopathy. The pleura, pericardium, and central nervous system also may be involved. Long-term treatment with antibiotics is often curative (Box 3-4).

Infection

Numerous organisms can affect the small bowel and many cause nodular fold thickening, including bacteria, viruses, protozoa, worms, and fungi (see Table 3-1). Overall, the changes they produce in the small bowel are similar, and it is typically impossible to distinguish the

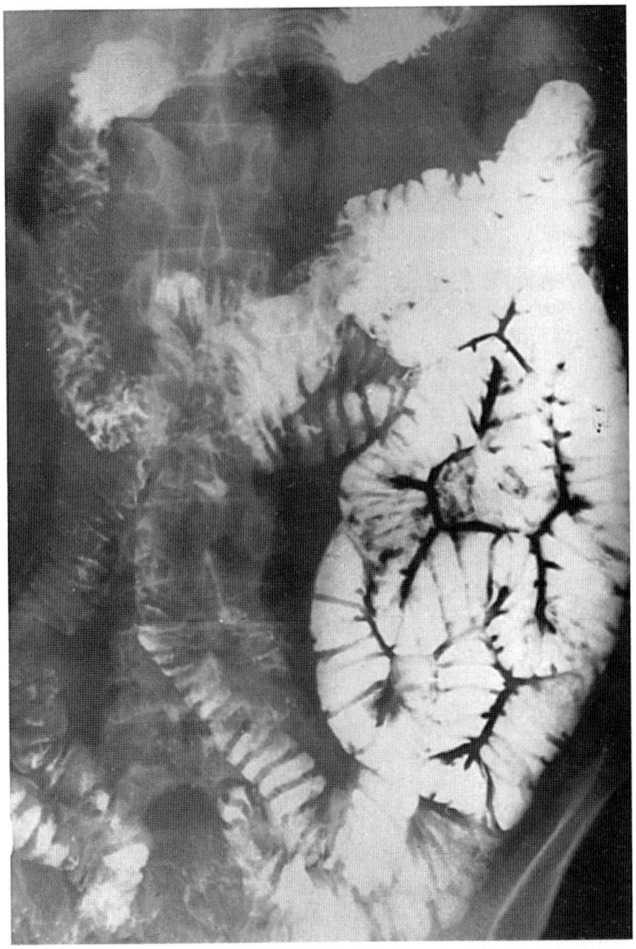

Figure 3-42 Diffuse small bowel fold thickening represents Whipple's disease.

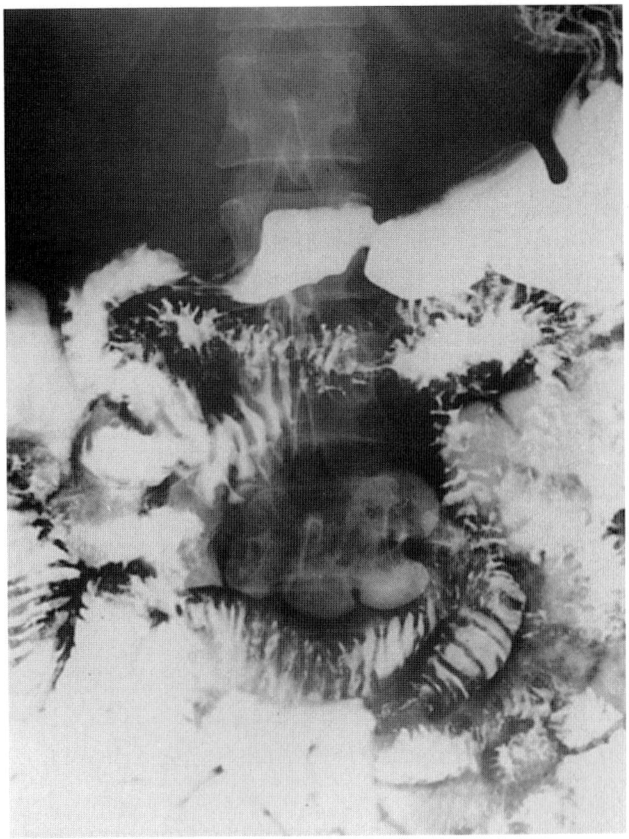

Figure 3-43 Diffuse, irregular small bowel fold thickening in a patient with giardiasis is seen.

different organisms by their radiographic appearance except for a select few. Sometimes the distribution of the abnormalities can help in narrowing the possibilities. The parasites *Strongyloides* and *Giardia* usually are localized to the duodenum and proximal jejunum (Fig. 3-43). A similar appearance has been described in hookworm infestation (ancylostomiasis). Focal involvement of the distal ileum suggests tuberculosis, typhoid fever, and *Yersinia* or *Campylobacter* enteritis.

In AIDS, otherwise unusual types of small bowel infections occur frequently, with most causing focal or diffuse thickening and nodularity of folds. Etiologies include CMV, *Mycobacterium avium-intracellulare, Cryptosporidium,* and *Isospora belli* (Figs. 3-44 and 3-45, Box 3-5).

Thickened folds in eosinophilic enteritis and abetalipoproteinemia can appear straight or nodular. Involvement in eosinophilic enteritis may be focal or diffuse, whereas in abetalipoproteinemia, the ileum is usually spared.

Box 3-4 Whipple's Disease

- Occurs predominantly in middle-aged men
- Clinical symptoms include diarrhea, arthralgias, fevers, and neurologic symptoms
- Glycoprotein-laden macrophages in bowel wall (periodic acid–Schiff stain positive)
- *Tropheryma whippelii* bacilli also evident in bowel wall and thought to be causative agent
- Also may affect heart valves, central nervous system, and joint capsules
- Potentially fatal, but responds dramatically to antibiotics

Crohn's Disease

Crohn's disease of the small bowel may show coarsely thickened folds. This represents edema or inflammation. Although it is typically in the terminal ileum, other portions of the bowel may be involved, even with sparing of the terminal ileum. Associated findings include ulcerations, eccentric involvement, and skip lesions.

Lymphoma

Nodular thickened folds are one of many manifestations of small bowel lymphoma. The infiltration of malignant

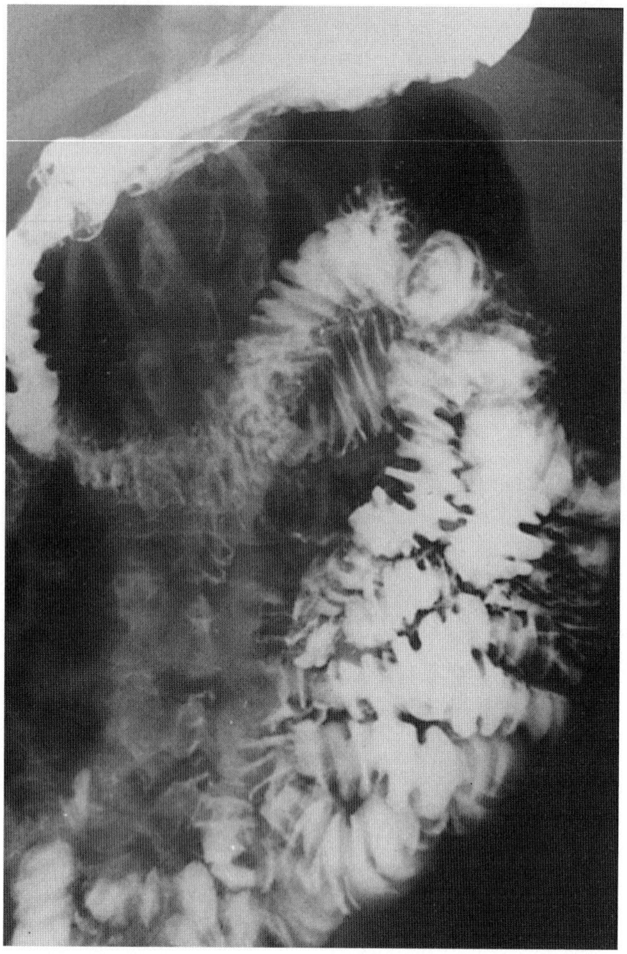

Figure 3-44 This represents diffuse small bowel fold thickening caused by *M. avium-intracellulare* in a patient with AIDS.

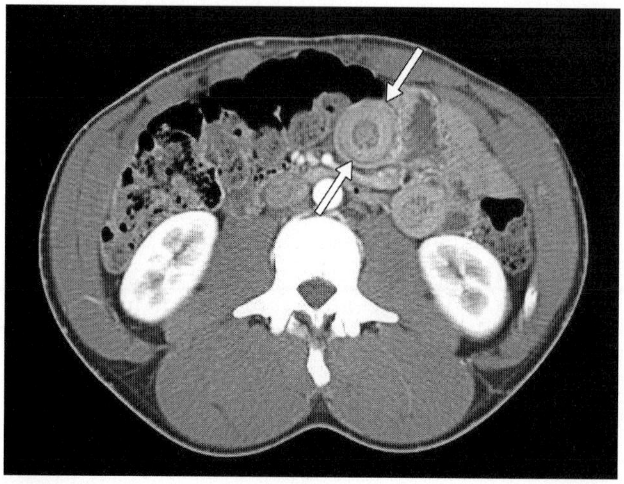

Figure 3-45 Patient with AIDS and involvement of the small bowel. Note thickened wall *(arrows)*.

Box 3-5 Manifestations of AIDS in the Small Bowel

Thickened folds—usually a manifestation of infection, occasionally Kaposi's sarcoma
Masses—malignancy, either lymphoma or Kaposi's sarcoma
Bull's-eye lesions—metastatic Kaposi's sarcoma
Adenopathy—neoplastic, either lymphoma or Kaposi's sarcoma
Infectious—*M. avium-intracellulare*

lymphocytes into the mucosal and submucosal layers of the bowel wall may be focal or diffuse.

Mastocytosis

Mastocytosis is an uncommon disease characterized by the proliferation of histamine-secreting mast cells. Although often localized to the skin (urticaria pigmentosa), the disease also may involve lymph nodes, liver, spleen, and bone (osteoblastic lesions). Gastrointestinal tract involvement produces fold thickening and nodularity throughout the small bowel and occasionally in the distal stomach. Episodes of flushing, pruritus, headache, and diarrhea may occur after the release of histamine from the mast cells (Fig. 3-46). The classic presentation of mastocytosis for the radiologist is that of images of SBFT with thickened, irregular small bowel folds and white, sclerotic bones in the background.

Eosinophilic Enteritis and Graft-versus-Host Disease

Eosinophilic enteritis and graft-versus-host disease can cause a similar alteration of the small bowel fold pattern. These changes are typically more diffuse.

Amyloidosis

Amyloidosis is a systemic disease in which extracellular deposits of amyloid occur throughout the body, including the gastrointestinal tract. Small bowel folds may appear diffusely thickened and nodular. This disease most often occurs in patients with underlying multiple myeloma or chronic inflammatory conditions, but sometimes may be primary in nature.

Edema

Small bowel edema, although typically causing uniform fold thickening, is sometimes associated with coarsened or nodular thickened folds. In Zollinger-Ellison syndrome, the markedly elevated levels of gastric acid result in severe inflammation and edema of the proximal duodenum and may cause similar findings in the distal duodenum and proximal jejunum. Nodular thickened folds also are seen

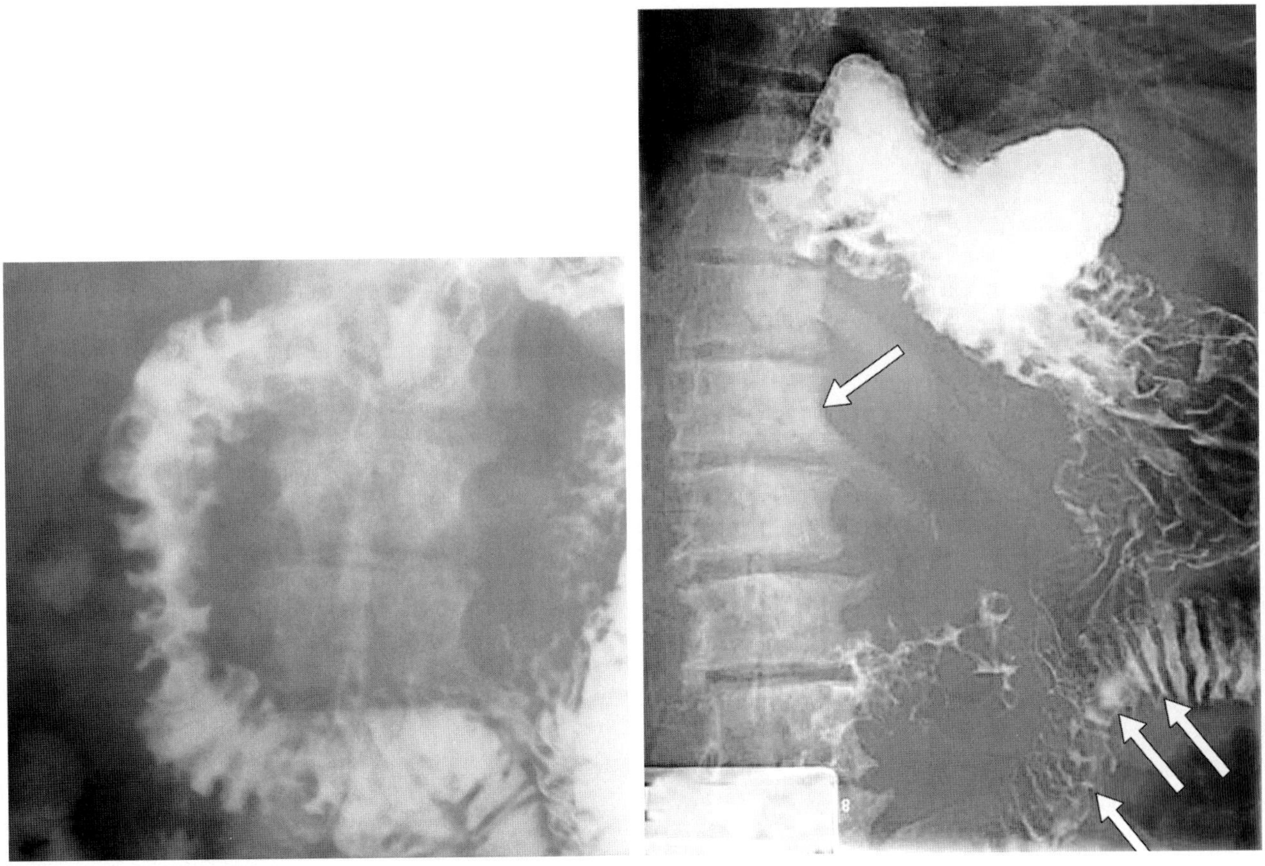

A B

Figure 3-46 **A,** Nodular, asymmetrical fold thickening of the duodenum from mastocytosis is seen. **B,** Note sclerotic bones *(arrows)*.

in edematous small bowel adjacent to an inflammatory mass; this can involve the jejunum (pancreatitis) or ileum (appendicitis, tuboovarian abscess).

Waldenström's Macroglobulinemia

Waldenström's macroglobulinemia, a rare disease caused by proliferation of IgM-producing plasma cells, may involve the small bowel. Diffuse fold thickening and tiny mucosal nodules result.

DIMINISHED OR EFFACED FOLDS

Loss of the normal small bowel fold pattern results in a tubular appearance that may be focal or diffuse. This appearance is not always the result of actual loss of the folds, but in some conditions the folds become so thickened that no barium can penetrate between the valvulae, and the folds no longer become discernible. This condition is often associated with thickening and rigidity of the bowel wall. It may be preceded by focal or diffuse fold thickening and can be considered at the end of the spectrum of small bowel fold thickening. Complete absence of any folds is often termed a "moulage" pattern.

Infection

Several infectious agents can cause effacement of small bowel folds and narrowing of the lumen. In CMV enteritis and cryptosporidiosis, small bowel involvement is typically diffuse, whereas in strongyloidiasis, disease is localized to the duodenum and proximal jejunum (Fig. 3-47).

Graft-versus-Host Disease

In graft-versus-host disease, donor lymphocytes from a bone marrow transplant attack host tissues. The gastrointestinal tract is usually affected, and a tubular appearance of the small bowel is frequently noted (Fig. 3-48) secondary to infiltration and edema of the bowel wall. This condition is a good example of when the apparent loss of fold pattern is actually due to severe fold thickening, not allowing any barium to pass in between the folds (ribbon sign).

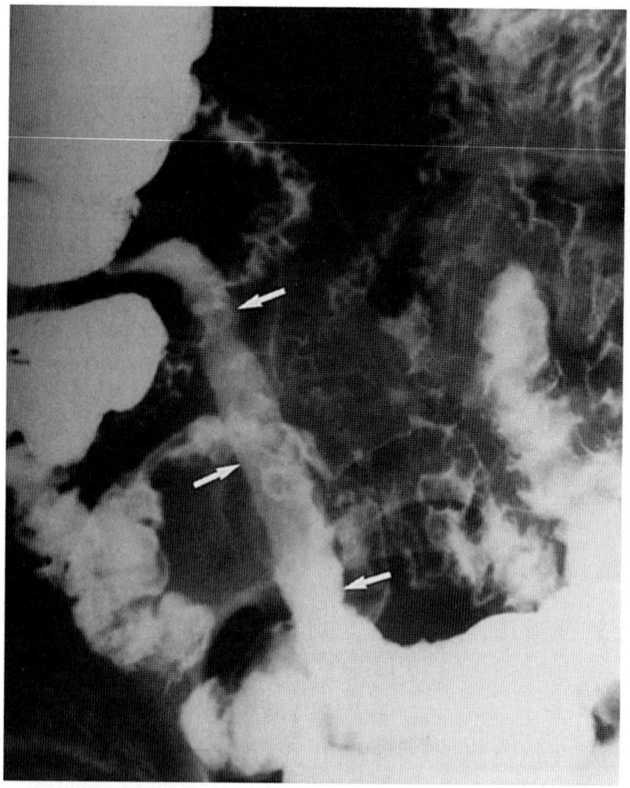

Figure 3-47 Tubular distal ileum *(arrows)* resulting from CMV enteritis in a patient with AIDS is seen.

Sprue

Sprue (celiac disease) is associated with a decrease in the number of folds per inch in the duodenum and proximal jejunum. Occasionally, folds may be absent, resulting in a tubular-shaped lumen. In contrast to most other causes of diminished small bowel folds, however, sprue may produce luminal dilatation rather than narrowing.

Crohn's Disease

In Crohn's disease, small bowel loops may appear featureless and narrowed secondary to edema or fibrosis. The length of bowel involved varies, but the condition is often seen in long-standing disease (Fig. 3-49).

Scleroderma

Scleroderma results in fibrotic changes in the bowel wall. Usually the fold pattern is more prominent because of the combination of fibrosis and crowding of the valvulae (hidebound small bowel). In severe end-stage disease, the small bowel loops become featureless with a diminished fold pattern.

Other Causes

Small bowel ischemia or infarction sometimes causes effacement of the fold pattern. Dilatation or narrowing of the lumen and scalloping of the bowel wall (thumbprinting) also may be noted. Similar findings in radiation enteritis reflect the underlying endarteritis and subsequent ischemia.

Toxic chemicals, introduced either by direct ingestion (potassium chloride tablets) or by vascular infusion (floxuridine and related chemotherapeutic agents), can reduce or eliminate small bowel folds. A tubular-appearing small bowel may result from infiltration of the bowel wall. This appearance has been described in amyloidosis, lymphoma, and other infiltrative diseases.

Featureless dilatation of the terminal ileum (backwash ileitis) sometimes occurs in patients with chronic ulcerative pancolitis. A similar finding can result from long-term cathartic abuse (cathartic colon). In both conditions, the ileocecal valve is patulous (see Fig. 3-32).

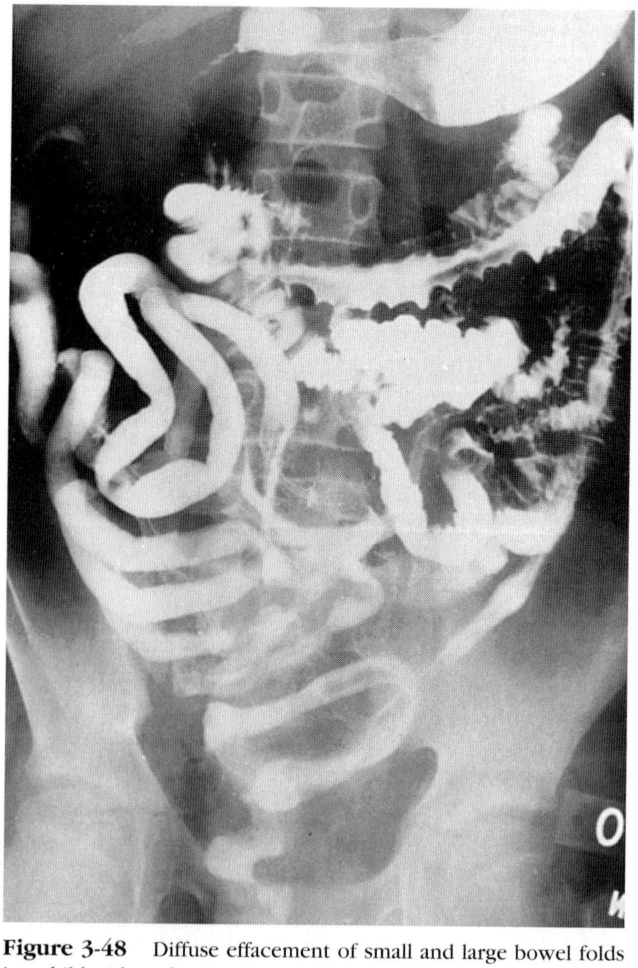

Figure 3-48 Diffuse effacement of small and large bowel folds in a child with graft-versus-host disease. Note ribbon-like appearance of small bowel.

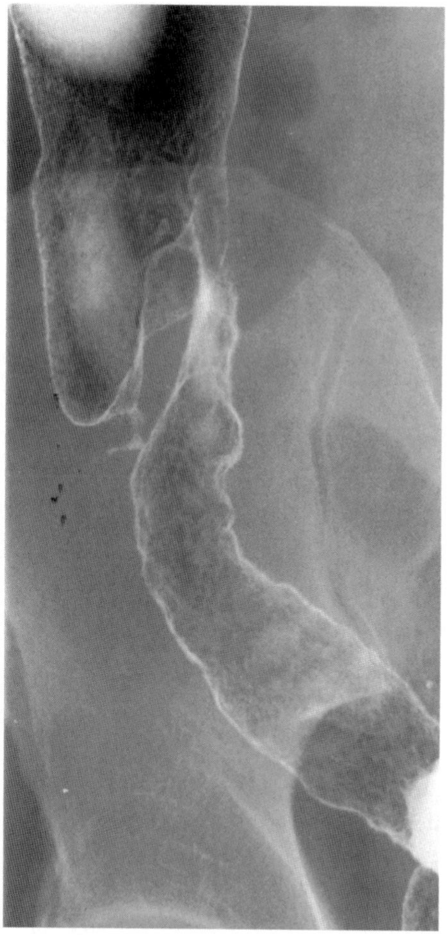

Figure 3-49 Featureless terminal ileum and cecum from long-standing ulcerative colitis is seen.

TINY NODULES

Discrete tiny nodules in the small bowel are sometimes associated with thickened folds. This pattern is seen in Whipple's disease, mastocytosis, Waldenström's macroglobulinemia, and small bowel infection (*Yersinia* enteritis, *M. avium-intracellulare,* disseminated histoplasmosis).

Tiny nodules also can be seen in the absence of fold thickening. In nodular lymphoid follicular pattern, prominent lymphoid follicles in the small bowel wall appear as tiny, round, uniform nodules (Fig. 3-50). This condition is often termed *lymphoid hyperplasia,* but it is not really pathologic, and it is not always associated with a disease. This condition is a normal finding in children and young adults, especially in the terminal ileum, where lymphoid tissue is most abundant. It is encountered as a normal finding in older adults with no underlying disease. The small bowel folds appear normal in these patients. Fold thickening is often present in older patients with diffuse nodular lymphoid hyperplasia associated with immunoglobulin deficiency or giardiasis of the small bowel.

SOLITARY MURAL MASSES

Malignant Tumors

Adenocarcinoma

Adenocarcinoma, although the most common primary malignant neoplasm of the duodenum, occurs with decreasing frequency from the proximal jejunum to distal ileum. It arises in the mucosal layer and typically infiltrates the bowel wall to cause a short annular narrowing with mucosal destruction, circumferential wall thickening, and overhanging margins (Fig. 3-51). If encountered in its early stages, small bowel adenocarcinoma appears as a polypoid intraluminal mass. Clinical symptoms associated with adenocarcinoma include obstruction, bleeding, and abdominal pain. Because it often does not produce early symptoms, obstruction is the most frequent presentation. An increased incidence of adenocarcinoma has been noted in the duodenum and proximal jejunum (Fig. 3-52) in patients with celiac disease and in the ileum in patients with Crohn's disease (Table 3-2).

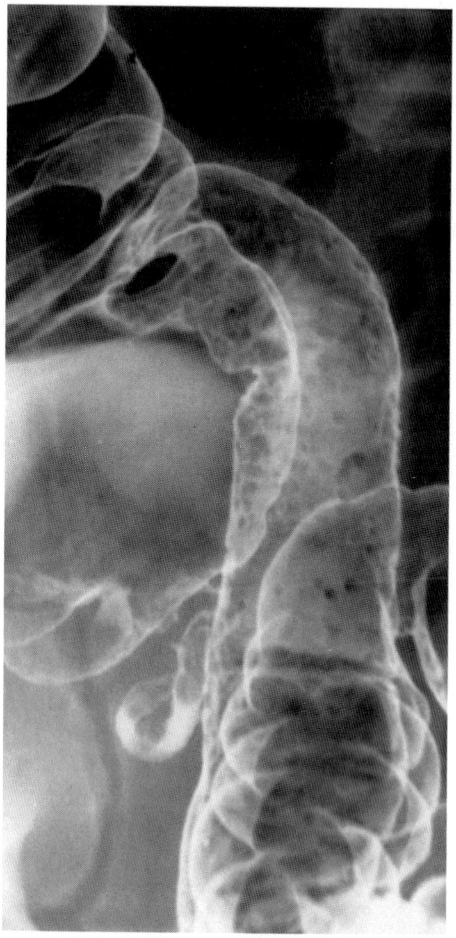

Figure 3-50 Multiple small, uniform nodules in the terminal ileum of a 17-year-old patient represent nodular lymphoid hyperplasia.

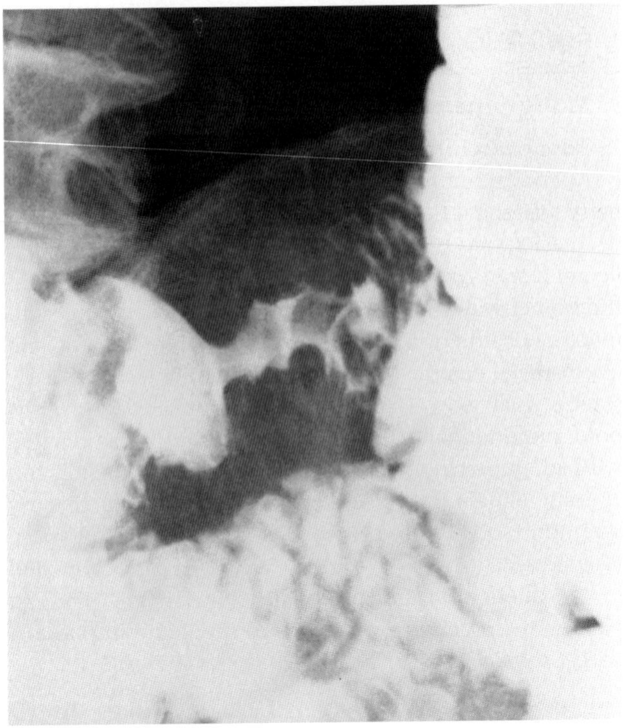

Figure 3-51 Annular lesion of small bowel from primary adenocarcinoma is seen.

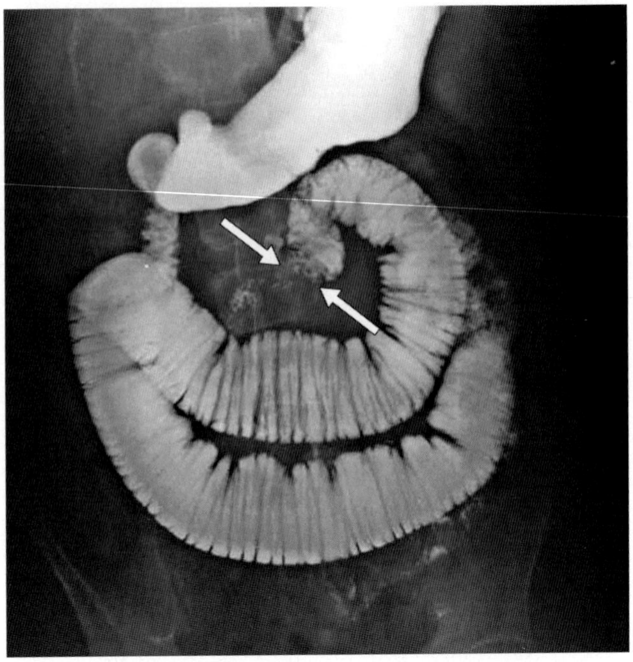

Figure 3-52 Obstructing adenocarcinoma *(arrows)* is seen in the proximal jejunum.

Gastrointestinal Stromal Cell Tumors

Leiomyosarcoma of the small bowel arises in the muscular or submucosal layer and grows either away from the lumen (exoenteric) or toward it (endoenteric) (see Table 3-2). Malignant stromal cell tumors (leiomyosarcomas) are more common in the jejunum and ileum than in the duodenum and account for approximately 9% of primary malignant neoplasms of the small bowel (Fig. 3-53).

Exoenteric lesions often produce few symptoms until they have attained a large size and have outgrown their blood supply. Central necrosis and cavitation of the tumor lead to ulceration and hemorrhage into the adjacent bowel lumen. Contrast studies may show either extrinsic compression of bowel loops by the large intramural mass or an irregular collection of barium within the necrotic portion of the tumor itself. CT is useful in showing the enhancing peripheral component and the necrotic or gas-containing central component of the lesion.

Table 3-2 Neoplasms of the Small Bowel

Type	Location	Characteristics
Malignant		
Adenocarcinoma	Usually jejunum	Mass or annular lesion
Lymphoma	Usually ileum, but can occur anywhere	Variable appearance from solitary to multiple nodules, strictures or dilatation, mesenteric masses
Carcinoid	Usually ileum	Nodule or mass, bowel kinking and mass effect; variable malignancy; can be multiple
Leiomyosarcoma	Anywhere	Mass, often extending extraluminally
Metastases	Anywhere	Single or multiple intraluminal polyps, mural masses, intussusception, ulceration
Benign		
Leiomyoma	Usually jejunum	Solitary mass; variable ulceration
Adenoma	Usually ileum	Solitary intraluminal polyp; may intussuscept
Lipoma	Usually ileum	Same as adenoma
Neurofibroma	Usually ileum	Luminal or submucosal polyp
Hemangioma	Anywhere	Sessile polyps, phleboliths

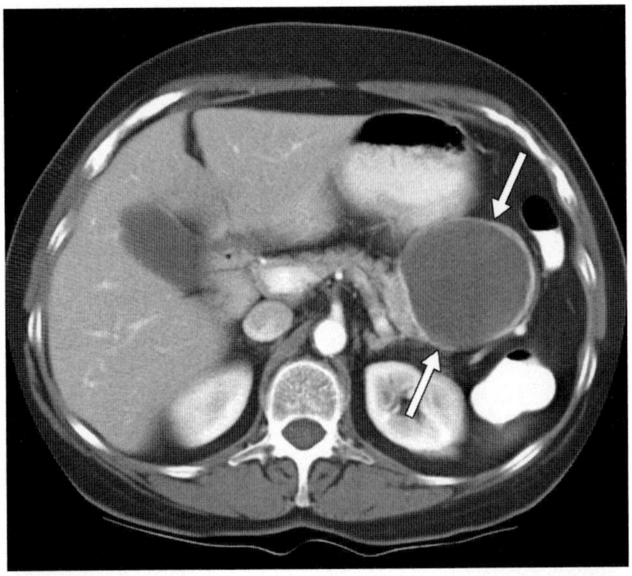

Figure 3-53 Large stromal cell tumor of the jejunum *(arrows)*. Note the exophytic growth of this large lesion.

The endoenteric form of small bowel leiomyosarcoma usually appears as a compressible intraluminal mass. This mass may cause bleeding, intussusception, or obstruction. Malignant stromal cell tumors may be difficult to distinguish from benign tumors radiographically and histologically. Metastases usually occur through hematogenous spread to the liver or lungs.

Lymphoma

Lymphoma affects the small bowel more often than any other portion of the gastrointestinal tract; this usually represents secondary involvement by non-Hodgkin's lymphoma and occurs with greatest frequency in the distal ileum because of the predominance of lymphoid tissue there (Box 3-6). Small bowel lymphoma has a variety of radiographic appearances, including fold thickening or effacement, luminal narrowing, aneurysmal dilatation, diffuse nodularity, and extrinsic compression by mesenteric masses (Fig. 3-54). Solitary or multiple focal mural masses also can be seen. With continued enlargement, these masses may become exoenteric, undergoing excavation and ulceration (aneurysmal dilatation), or endoenteric, producing an intraluminal polypoid mass with the potential for intussusception. The presence of a large gastrointestinal mass involving and destroying the small bowel without evidence of obstruction should be considered a sign of non-Hodgkin's lymphoma (Fig. 3-55).

Box 3-6 Lymphoma

- Non-Hodgkin's lymphoma (Hodgkin's type rare)
- More common in distal small bowel (ileum)
- Variable appearance—mass or polyp
- Multiple polyps (polyposis)
- Infiltrative (aneurysmal dilatation)
- Endo- or exoenteric
- Mesenteric (adenopathy)
- Predisposing conditions—sprue, immunosuppression (AIDS, transplant recipients)

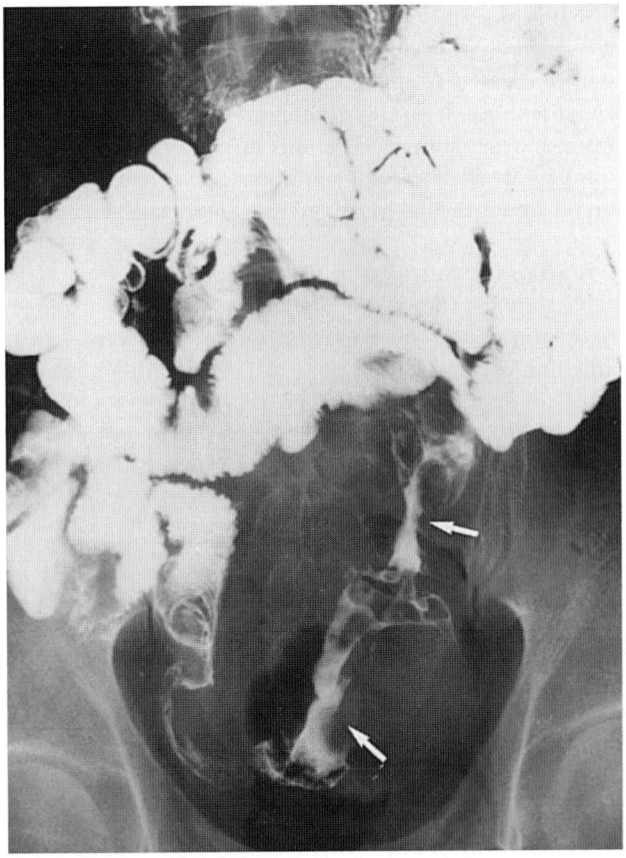

Figure 3-54 Distorted, irregular ileal loop *(arrows)* represents non-Hodgkin's lymphoma.

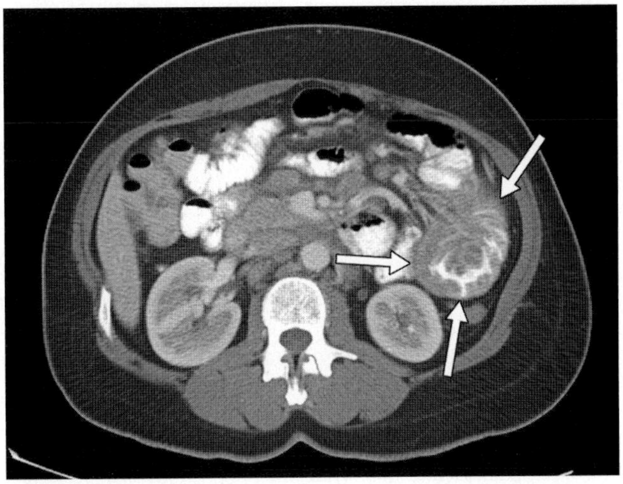

Figure 3-55 This is non-Hodgkin's lymphoma affecting the small bowel *(arrows)* without evidence of obstruction.

Non-Hodgkin's lymphoma of the small bowel is a recognized complication of celiac disease. It also occurs with increased frequency in patients with immunodeficiency as a result of AIDS or immunosuppression resulting from antirejection medications after organ transplantation. In Mediterranean lymphoma, diffuse small bowel involvement results in severe intestinal malabsorption.

Carcinoid Tumor

Carcinoid tumor is the most common primary neoplasm of the small bowel (Box 3-7). It arises from argentaffin cells in the crypts of Lieberkühn and occurs most commonly in the distal ileum. Carcinoid tumors less than 1 cm in diameter usually cause no symptoms and rarely metastasize. A carcinoid tumor may be noted incidentally on contrast studies as a smooth, round submucosal mass.

As the tumor enlarges, it may extend into the overlying mucosa and lead to ulceration or intussusception. Outward extension into the muscular and serosal layers may induce a local desmoplastic reaction consisting of angulation, tethering, and "kinking" of the bowel and partial obstruction (Fig. 3-56). This reaction represents the local effects of serotonin, which is produced by the tumor from the dietary amino acid tryptophan. Carcinoid tumors measuring 1 to 2 cm in diameter metastasize in about 50% of cases, and tumors larger than 2 cm metastasize in about 90% of cases. Regional metastases are usually located in the mesentery or lymph nodes and are commonly larger than the primary tumor. On CT, these lesions may show a stellate appearance or dystrophic calcifications.

Box 3-7 Carcinoid Tumor

Amine precursor uptake and decarboxylation tumor, may be found anywhere in gastrointestinal or genitourinary tract or bronchi
Location—appendix most common, then small bowel (typically ileum)
All potentially malignant, >2 cm most likely to metastasize
Hormonally active—secrete serotonin
Serotonin is converted in liver and lungs to 5-HIAA, which is elevated in urine
May provoke a desmoplastic reaction in small bowel
Usually asymptomatic
Carcinoid syndrome—occurs with liver metastases (95%)
Intestinal hypermotility—diarrhea and cramping
Vasomotor—flushing
Bronchoconstriction—wheezing
Endocardial fibrosis—right-sided heart valves

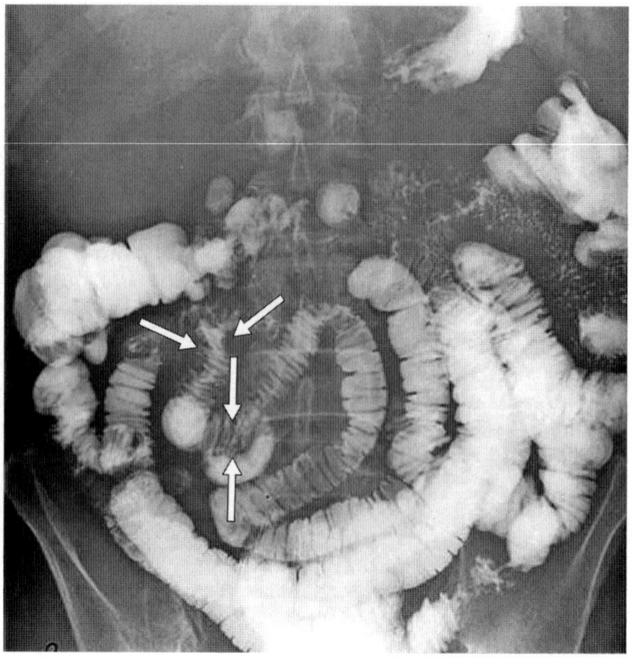

Figure 3-56 Areas of tethering, nodularity, and fold separation *(arrows)* are seen in this patient with carcinoid syndrome.

Metastasis

Liver metastases from carcinoid tumor are usually hypervascular and are the usual cause of carcinoid syndrome, characterized by episodic cutaneous flushing, wheezing, and diarrhea. The liver normally degrades serotonin into 5-hydroxyindoleacetic acid (5-HIAA) and prevents it from entering the systemic circulation. In the presence of liver metastases, however, serotonin may pass through the right heart into the lungs, producing carcinoid syndrome and damaging the right heart valves before being broken down in the lungs to 5-HIAA. Bone metastases from carcinoid tumor are typically osteoblastic.

Metastatic disease to the small bowel occurs through hematogenous, peritoneal, contiguous, or lymphatic spread and can cause a variety of radiographic findings. Although metastases are often multiple, solitary lesions are sometimes shown.

Benign Tumors

Mesenchymal tumors

Benign tumors arising in mesenchymal tissues of the small bowel wall include leiomyoma, lipoma, neurofibroma, and hemangioma, in order of descending frequency. The most common of these is leiomyoma, a hypervascular, nonencapsulated smooth muscle tumor (Fig. 3-57). Leiomyoma, similar to its malignant counterpart leiomyosarcoma, can undergo endoenteric or exoenteric growth with resultant complications of intussusception or tumor necrosis and ulceration.

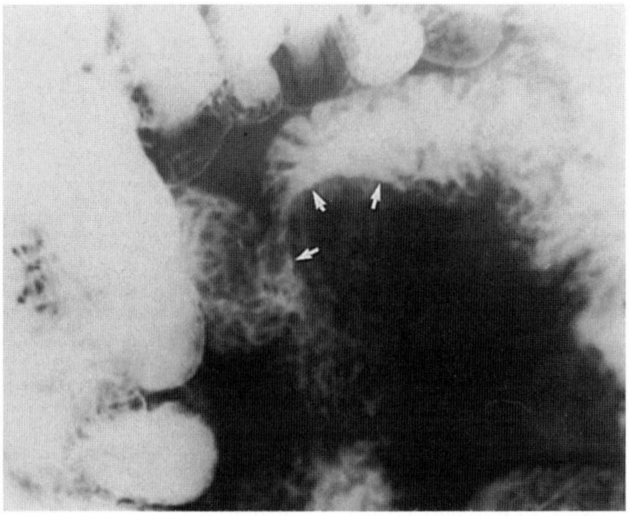

Figure 3-57 Submucosal mass *(arrows)* represents a jejunal leiomyoma.

Lipoma, an encapsulated fatty tumor, is characterized fluoroscopically by its softness and compressibility during palpation. Continued stretching of the tumor by bowel peristalsis may form a pedunculated intraluminal mass that can ulcerate or act as a lead point for intussusception (Fig. 3-58).

Neurofibroma and other neural tumors are unusual solitary mural masses in the small bowel. Occasionally, they may be multiple in nature, particularly if the patient has neurofibromatosis (Fig. 3-59).

Hemangioma represents a focal proliferation of vascular channels. Although phleboliths are uncommonly shown, their presence in association with a submucosal mass indicates a hemangioma.

Adenoma

Adenomas, benign mucosal tumors arising in glandular epithelium, may appear sessile or pedunculated. They are the second most common small bowel tumor encountered, after benign leiomyoma. They may develop anywhere in the small bowel, but are more common in the ileum.

Carcinoid Tumor and Inflammatory Fibroid Polyp

Carcinoid tumor of the small bowel has variable malignant potential. Inflammatory fibroid polyp (eosinophilic granuloma) is composed primarily of connective tissue and appears as a smooth submucosal mass in the small bowel, stomach, or colon. Although eosinophilic infiltration of the mass is characteristic, the focal nature of the mass and the absence of associated peripheral eosinophilia differentiate it from eosinophilic gastroenteritis. Complications of inflammatory fibroid polyp include ulceration and intussusception.

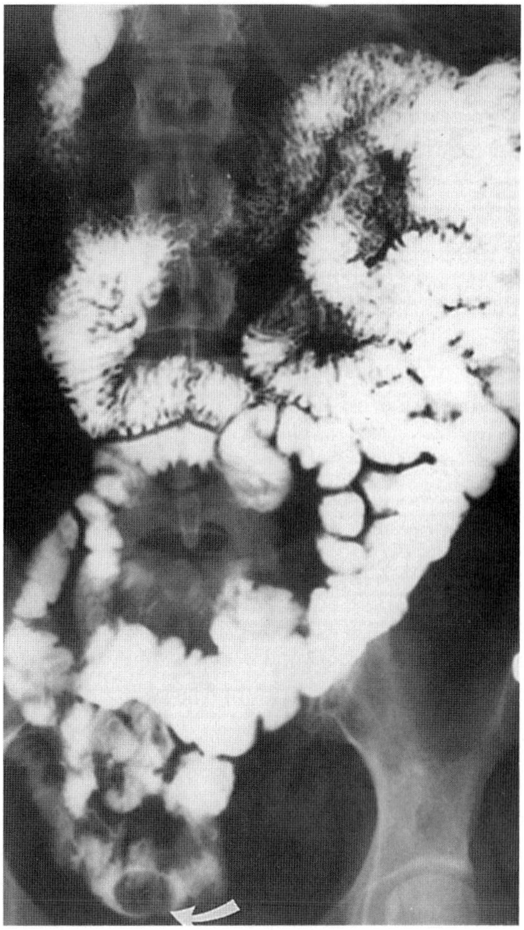

Figure 3-58 Ovoid mass *(curved arrow)* in the distal ileum represents a lipoma.

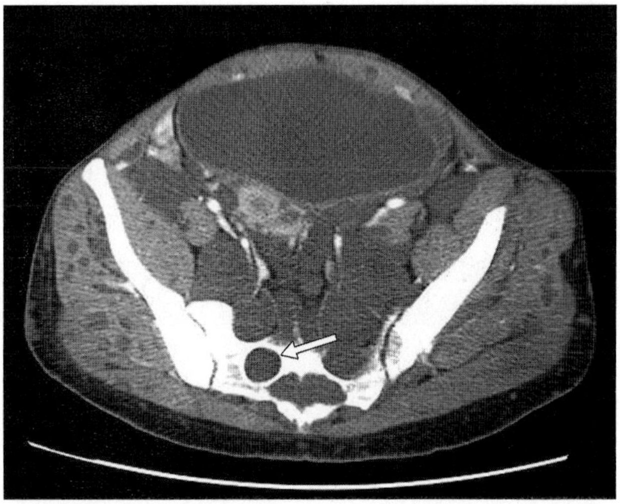

Figure 3-59 A patient with neurofibromatosis with severe involvement of the bowel. Note the widened neuroforamen in the sacrum *(arrow)*.

Other Masses

Endometrioma

Endometrioma of the small bowel represents a focal deposit of ectopic endometrial tissue on the serosal surface of the distal ileum in women. The cause of endometriosis is uncertain; proposed theories include reflux of endometrial tissue through the fallopian tubes, hematogenous or lymphatic spread, and metaplasia of coelomic epithelium. The sigmoid colon is most commonly affected, and small bowel involvement is uncommon and may appear as a focal mass with associated serosal tethering resulting from repeated episodes of intramural hemorrhage and subsequent fibrosis.

Duplication Cyst

Duplication cyst is an embryologic abnormality that can occur anywhere in the small bowel. These cysts are tubular or round and may communicate with the adjacent bowel lumen. Although often discovered in childhood, duplication cysts occasionally are recognized incidentally in adults as a smooth intramural mass seen on contrast examination.

Hematoma

In contrast to duodenal hematoma, focal hematoma of the mesenteric small bowel rarely causes a focal masslike appearance, possibly because of the tamponading effect of the circumferential serosal layer there.

Inverted Meckel's Diverticulum

An inverted Meckel's diverticulum also can appear as a smooth, round or oval mass on contrast studies. With inverted Meckel's diverticulum, the possibility of an intussusception increases.

MULTIPLE MURAL MASSES

Many of the lesions that can occur as solitary mural masses also can occur as multiple mural masses. These lesions were described in greater detail in the previous section (Table 3-3).

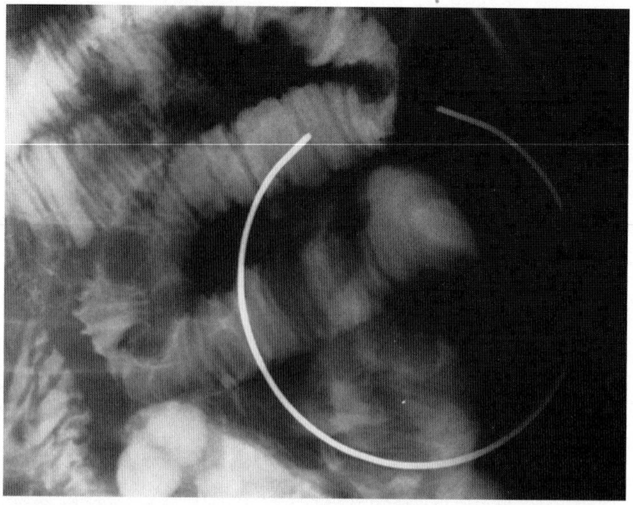

Figure 3-60 Multiple small bowel nodules from metastatic lung carcinoma.

Malignant Tumors

Metastasis

Metastasis to the small bowel can occur through peritoneal, hematogenous, lymphatic, or contiguous spread. Lesions are often multiple and may show variability in size secondary to repeated episodes of seeding (Fig. 3-60). Hematogenous dissemination can affect any segment of the small bowel. This dissemination occurs most frequently in malignant melanoma and less often in breast or lung carcinoma. Metastatic melanoma typically produces submucosal nodules that may contain a central ulceration (target lesions). With further growth, these lesions may become primarily exoenteric (with subsequent necrosis and ulceration) or endoenteric (with subsequent intussusception). Small bowel metastases from breast carcinoma rarely result in focal scirrhous-type narrowing similar to that seen more commonly in the stomach.

Peritoneal spread through ascitic fluid leads to seeding of tumor on the serosal surface of the small bowel. Peritoneal fluid accumulates in the mesenteric reflections of the small bowel, especially at the ileocecal

Table 3-3 Polyposis Syndromes Affecting the Small Bowel

Title	Type	Other Features
Peutz-Jeghers syndrome	Hamartomas	Polyps throughout gastrointestinal tract; mucocutaneous pigmentation
Cronkhite-Canada syndrome	Hamartomas	Alopecia, nail dystrophy, protein malabsorption
Juvenile polyposis	Hamartomas	Colon polyps
Neurofibromatosis	Neurofibromas	Cutaneous fibromas and café au lait spots
Gardner's syndrome	Adenomas	Colonic polyps, osteomas, desmoid tumors
Familial polyposis	Adenomas	Typically colon tumors. Rarely small bowel tumors, but without Gardner's stigmata

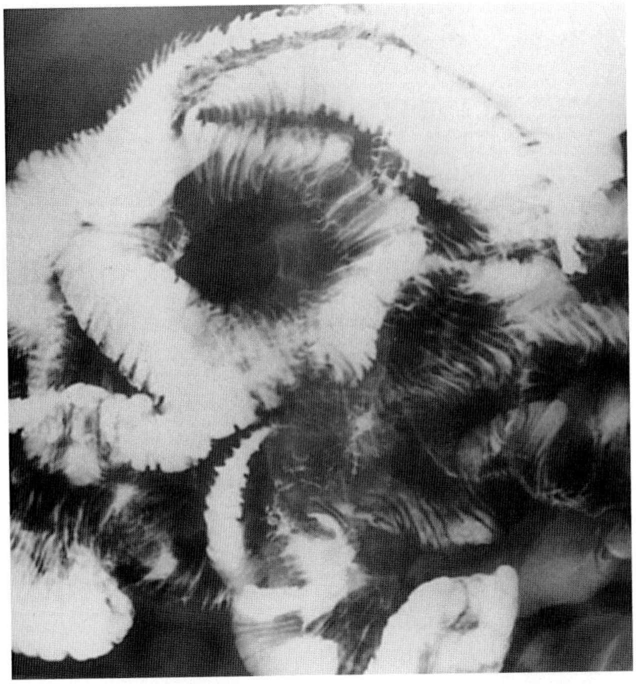

Figure 3-61 There is diffuse distortion and angulation of small bowel loops caused by peritoneal spread of colon carcinoma.

region because of its relatively dependent position. Serosal metastases most often occur secondary to gastrointestinal or gynecological malignancies, particularly ovarian carcinoma. In addition to the nodular masses representing serosal tumor implants, associated fibrous reaction may cause tethering of folds and angulation of bowel loops (Fig. 3-61). CT shows associated findings of peritoneal tumor spread, including ascites, peritoneal implants, and mesenteric infiltration (omental cakes).

Direct or contiguous spread of tumor may involve the mesenteric small bowel, as seen in invasion of the distal ileum by pelvic or cecal tumors. Lymphatic spread has been reported to involve the distal ileum after ileocolic anastomosis for colon carcinoma.

Kaposi's Sarcoma

Kaposi's sarcoma is a vascular tumor of the skin that also can affect visceral organs, including the gastrointestinal and respiratory tracts. Although previously a rare disease, Kaposi's sarcoma is a common neoplasm in AIDS, particularly in homosexual men with AIDS, although the incidence seems to have declined since the early 1990s. Submucosal nodules of Kaposi's sarcoma in the small bowel often resemble hematogenous metastases. Similar to metastatic malignant melanoma, Kaposi's sarcoma nodules may contain a central ulceration and at times act as a lead point for small bowel intussusception.

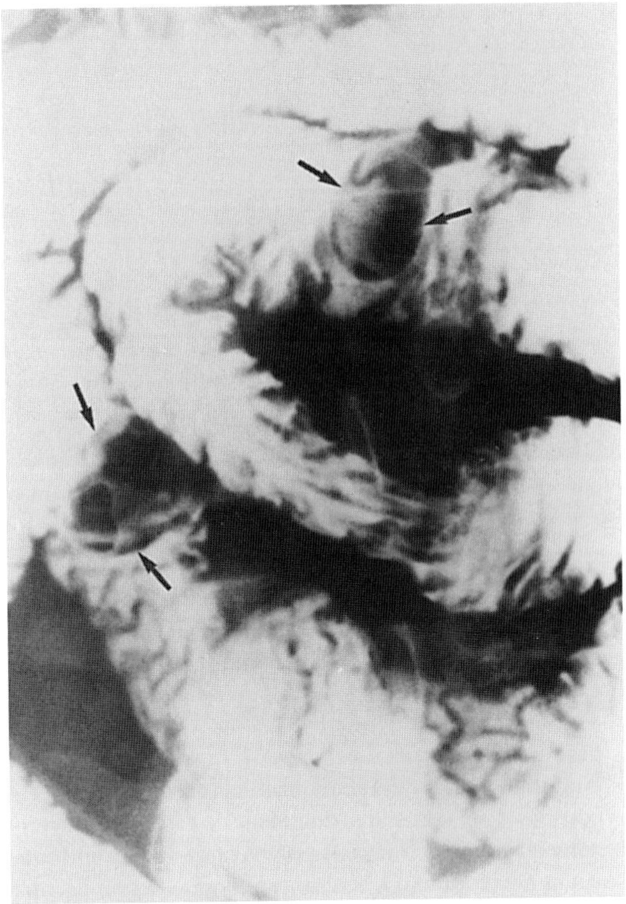

Figure 3-62 Submucosal masses *(arrows)* represent non-Hodgkin's lymphoma in a patient with AIDS.

Lymphoma

Non-Hodgkin's lymphoma of the small bowel can produce multiple, discrete mural masses or diffuse nodularity. Non-Hodgkin's lymphoma most often involves the ileum as a result of the normal abundance of lymphoid tissue there (Fig. 3-62).

Carcinoid Tumor

Carcinoid tumors of the small bowel are multiple in approximately one third of cases (Fig. 3-63).

Benign Tumors

Hamartoma

Multiple hamartomas of the small bowel occur in several polyposis syndromes, including Peutz-Jeghers, Cronkhite-Canada, juvenile polyposis, and Cowden's syndromes. Peutz-Jeghers syndrome is an autosomal-dominant disease characterized by mucocutaneous pigmentation and multiple small bowel polyps that may cause transient intussusception (Fig. 3-64). Cronkhite-Canada syndrome consists of multiple gastrointestinal polyps, ectodermal abnormalities, and intestinal malabsorption.

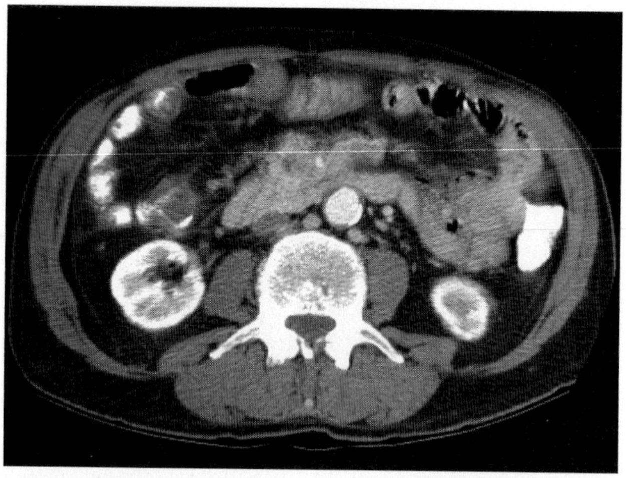

Figure 3-63 CT in a patient with carcinoid tumor in the small bowel mesentery.

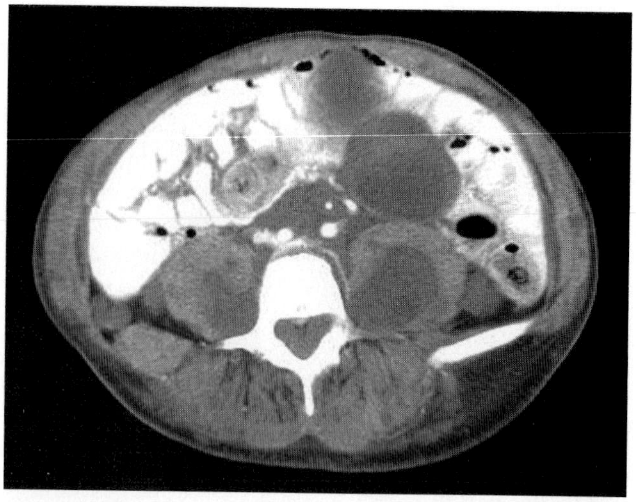

Figure 3-65 Axial computed tomographic scan shows multiple neurofibromas involving retroperitoneum and root of small bowel.

Gastrointestinal juvenile polyposis may involve any portion of the gastrointestinal tract. In Cowden's syndrome, gastrointestinal polyps are associated with tumors of the breast, thyroid, and skin.

Adenoma

Multiple small bowel adenomas can occur in Gardner's syndrome. This autosomal-dominant disease is characterized by diffuse adenomatous polyps of the colon and subsequent development of colon carcinoma. Extraintestinal tumors, including osteomas of the facial bones, sebaceous cysts, and desmoid tumors of the mesentery, also occur. The polyps that occur in the small bowel can be adenomatous and have a malignant potential, in contrast to the other polyposis symptoms described, which have no malignant potential. Patients with Gardner's syndrome have an increased incidence of ampullary carcinoma.

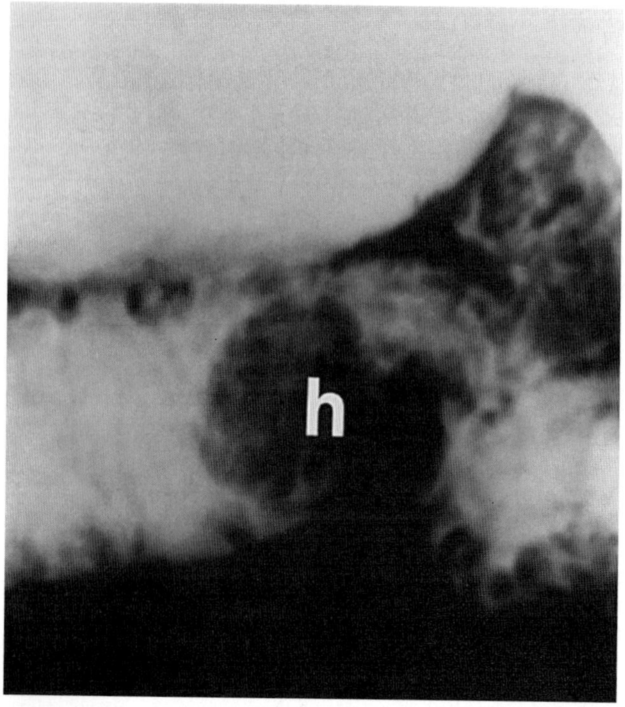

Figure 3-64 Polypoid mass *(h)* in the jejunum represents a hamartoma in a patient with Peutz-Jeghers disease.

Mesenchymal Tumor

Benign mesenchymal tumors of the small bowel, although usually solitary, may be multiple; this is especially true in neurofibromatosis, a genetic disease in which neural tumors can involve the skin, visceral organs, or central nervous system. Multiple neurofibromas of the small bowel in neurofibromatosis typically occur along the antimesenteric border (Fig. 3-65). Small bowel lipomatosis is a rare condition characterized by multiple lipomas of the small bowel. Carcinoid tumors exhibit variable malignant potential and are multiple in approximately one third of cases.

Other Masses

Postinflammatory Polyps

Postinflammatory polyps of the small bowel are similar to polyps seen in the colon in the healing stages of inflammatory bowel disease. In the small bowel, these are typically well-defined round polyps of varying size and most often involve the terminal ileum. They may be secondary to Crohn's disease or, very rarely, ulcerative pancolitis with backwash ileitis. The small branching (filiform) polyps are far less commonly seen in the small bowel.

Pneumatosis Cystoides Intestinalis

Pneumatosis cystoides intestinalis is a disorder of variable origin in which multiple subserosal cystic collections of gas indent the lumen of the small bowel or colon. The most interesting theory is "Macklin's pathway." In 1938, Macklin described the route of air leaking from microalveolar ruptures in the lung along the bronchovascular interstitial route to the mediastinum, from whence it traveled north and south. Small amounts of air traveling upward were unnoticed and eventually reabsorbed in the soft tissues of the neck, whereas air traveling down the mediastinum through the hiatus of the diaphragm collected in the retroperitoneum. From there, the air trickled along the mesenteric folds and eventually came to rest as small subserosal cysts in the lowest of the mesenteric compartments, the sigmoid mesentery. There, a universally abrupt termination of the cystic type of pneumatosis at the peritoneal reflection off the bladder is seen (representing the rectosigmoid border). Any air detected in the wall of the rectum cannot be benign pneumatosis. The typical radiolucent appearance of these apparent "mural masses" on plain films or CT is characteristic of this benign form of intestinal pneumatosis. Pneumatosis involving the small bowel more often presents as intramural streaking and may have more ominous significance, such as ischemic or necrotic changes, peptic ulceration, or instrumentation. Small to large amounts of intramural air can be seen postoperatively on plain film radiographs if the bowel has been resected.

Varices

Varices of the mesenteric small bowel are unusual, but can produce smooth submucosal masses similar to those seen in esophageal or gastric varices.

OTHER INTRALUMINAL ABNORMALITIES

Intraluminal masses in the small bowel include worms, bezoars, tubes, ingested foreign bodies, and calculi. Other lesions, such as pedunculated tumors and inverted diverticula, may simulate intraluminal masses.

Worms

The most common worm encountered in the small bowel is *Ascaris lumbricoides*. This roundworm is seen frequently, especially in tropical areas. On contrast studies, ascaris worms appear as long tubular intraluminal filling defects. A thin white line sometimes shown to bisect the length of the worm represents ingested barium in the worm's own gastrointestinal tract (Fig. 3-66). Ascaris worms can be solitary or multiple and when especially numerous may cause a small bowel obstruction.

Tapeworms also can produce linear intraluminal filling defects on contrast examinations. These flatworms are usually much longer than ascaris worms and never show a thin white line bisecting their length because they do not have a continuous gastrointestinal tract (Table 3-4).

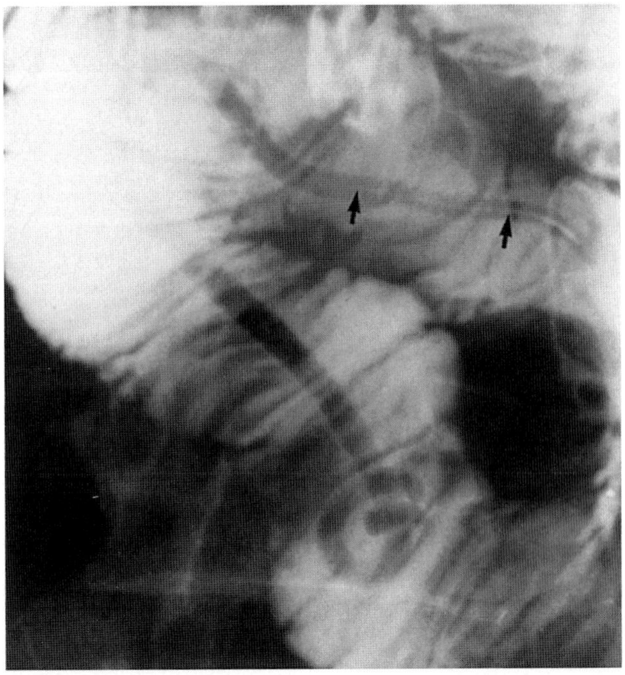

Figure 3-66 Tubular intraluminal filling defect in the jejunum represents an ascaris worm. The thin white line bisecting part of the length of the worm *(arrows)* indicates barium in the worm's gastrointestinal tract. (From Goodman P: Diagnostic radiology case number 16. Intern Med 12:46, 1991.)

Bezoars

Bezoars are uncommon in the small bowel. Phytobezoars (concretions of vegetable matter) usually result from ingestion of a large amount of high-fiber foods, such as citrus fruit. An increased incidence of small bowel phytobezoars also has been reported in patients with previous gastric outlet surgery and recent ingestion of persimmons. Phytobezoars can cause an obstruction anywhere in the jejunum or ileum and may resemble a villous tumor on contrast studies as a result of barium filling numerous interstices.

Other Foreign Bodies

Ingested foreign bodies sometimes become obstructed at the ileocecal valve because of physiological narrowing there. Prune pits have a characteristic biconvex shape. Radiopaque objects, such as coins, keys, and screws, are sometimes seen in the small bowel of psychiatric patients and are easily identified on abdominal plain films (Fig. 3-67). Ingested packets of heroin, cocaine, and other illegal drugs may appear on abdominal plain films as round or oval opacities, sometimes surrounded by a thin crescent of air ("double condom" sign). These drug packets may

Table 3-4 Intestinal Worms in the Small Bowel

Type	Genus/Species	Origin	Area of Involvement
Hookworm	*Necator americanus*	Soil	Proximal small bowel
	Ancylostoma duodenale	Soil	Proximal small bowel
Tapeworm	*Taenia saginata*	Beef	Entire small bowel
	Taenia solium	Pork	Entire small bowel
	Diphyllobothrium latum	Fish	Entire small bowel
Roundworm	*Ascaris lumbricoides*	Water	Entire small bowel
Strongyloidiasis	*Strongyloides stercoralis*	Water	Entire small bowel
Anisakiasis	*Anisakis* species	Raw fish	Entire small bowel

cause mechanical bowel obstruction or drug intoxication when leakage or rupture of a packet occurs.

Various iatrogenically placed feeding or drainage catheters may become dislodged and pass into the small bowel, where they appear as tubular filling defects. These include surgical or endoscopic gastrostomy and jejunostomy tubes. Balloon-tip catheters may show the inflated balloon and the tubular portion of the catheter (Fig. 3-68). The Garren-Edwards gastric bubble, an intragastric balloon previously used to treat morbid obesity, also has been reported to deflate spontaneously and migrate into the small bowel, where it can cause obstruction.

Gallstone Ileus

Erosion of a gallstone into the duodenum can lead to gallstone ileus, a mechanical obstruction caused by impaction of the gallstone in the small bowel, usually at the ileocecal valve. The ectopic gallstone is visible on plain films in approximately 25% of cases. On contrast studies, it may appear as a round or oval filling defect in the distal small bowel. Associated findings include distal small bowel obstruction and air in the biliary tree, seen in about 50% of cases (caused by reflux of air through the biliary-enteric fistula). A similar case has been reported in which a renal

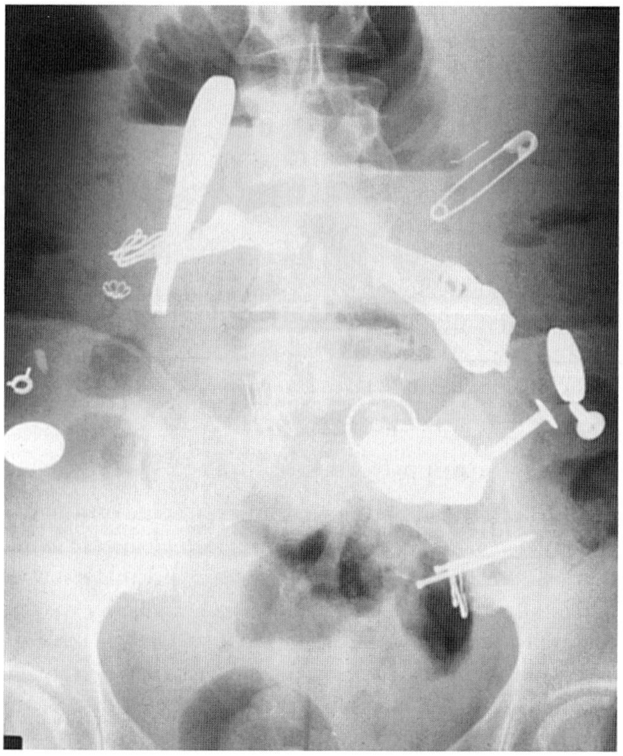

Figure 3-67 Small bowel obstruction is seen in a psychiatric patient who has ingested multiple metallic objects.

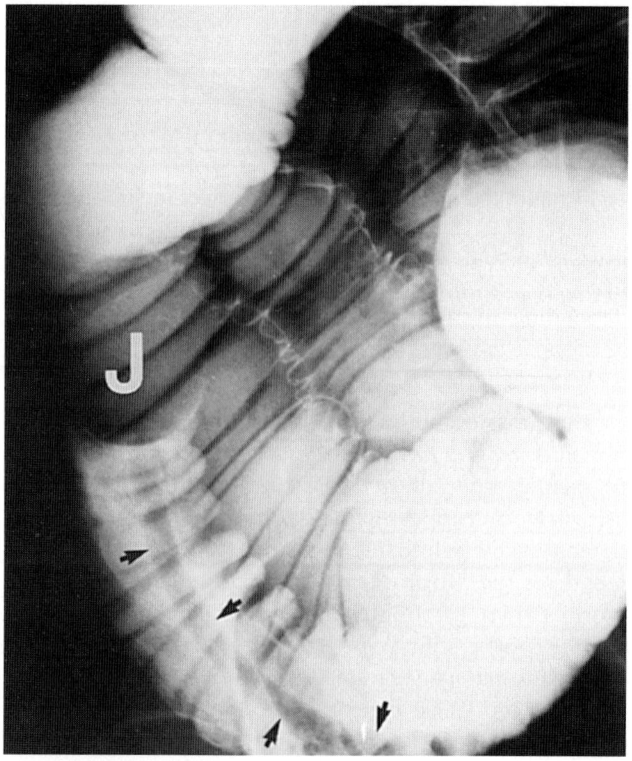

Figure 3-68 Small bowel obstruction is caused by migration of a jejunostomy tube *(arrows)* and impaction of the balloon tip *(J)*.

staghorn calculus eroded into the duodenum and subsequently became impacted at the ileocecal valve.

Air Bubbles and Stool

Air bubbles anywhere in the small bowel, and fecal debris refluxed across the ileocecal valve into the distal ileum also appear as intraluminal filling defects. Rarely, in patients with gastrointestinal bleeding or after surgical procedures, a blood clot may be seen within the lumen. Characteristically, they conform to the dimensions of the bowel.

Inverted Diverticulum

Any diverticulum may invert and appear almost entirely intraluminal. Classically, this entity is seen in the duodenum, but is also rarely encountered in the rest of the small bowel, particularly with inverted Meckel's diverticula.

EXTRINSIC PROCESSES

Adhesions

Extrinsic compression of small bowel loops may result from postsurgical adhesive bands. Although these adhesions are extremely common, they are not usually shown by imaging methods. Their presence may be suspected, however, when tethering or "pointing" of bowel loops (several loops of relatively fixed bowel all pointing to one spot in the abdomen) occurs.

Organomegaly and Adenopathy

Focal or diffuse enlargement of abdominal or pelvic organs and distention of other hollow viscera may compress or displace adjacent small bowel. These extrinsic masses cause a spectrum of radiographic appearances depending on their size, location, and relationship to the peritoneal cavity (Fig. 3-69). Although the mass effect typically is smooth, an extrinsic inflammatory or neoplastic mass may evoke serosal tethering or fold thickening. Marked adenopathy caused by inflammatory, infectious, or neoplastic disease can cause similar findings.

Metastatic Disease

As discussed previously, peritoneal metastases can occur from abdominal (gastric, ovarian, and pancreatic) and extraabdominal (breast, lung, and melanoma) tumors. Metastases are probably the most common cause of multiple extrinsic masses affecting the small bowel (Fig. 3-70).

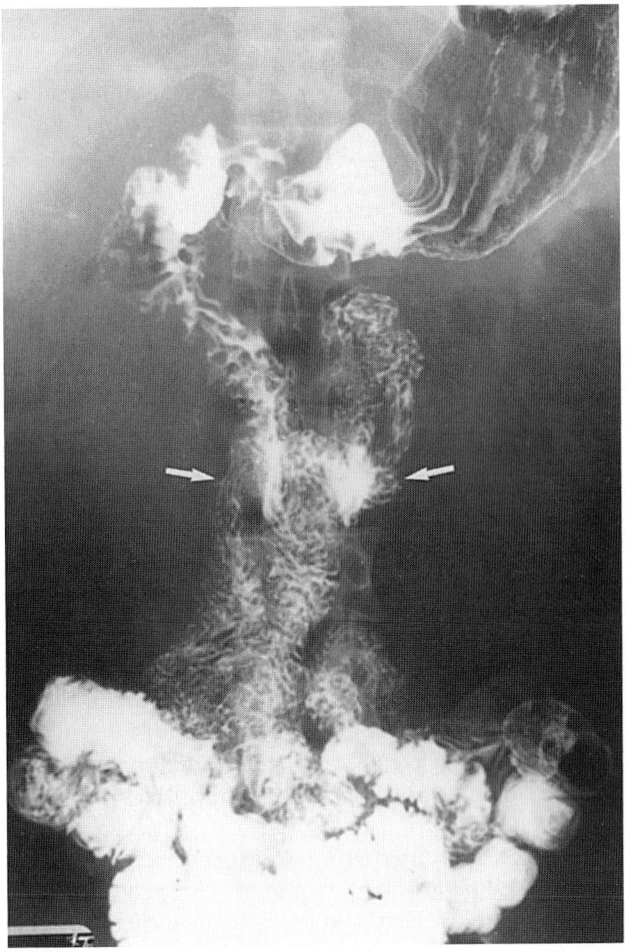

Figure 3-69 Medial displacement of mid–small bowel loops *(arrows)* results from bilateral huge polycystic kidneys.

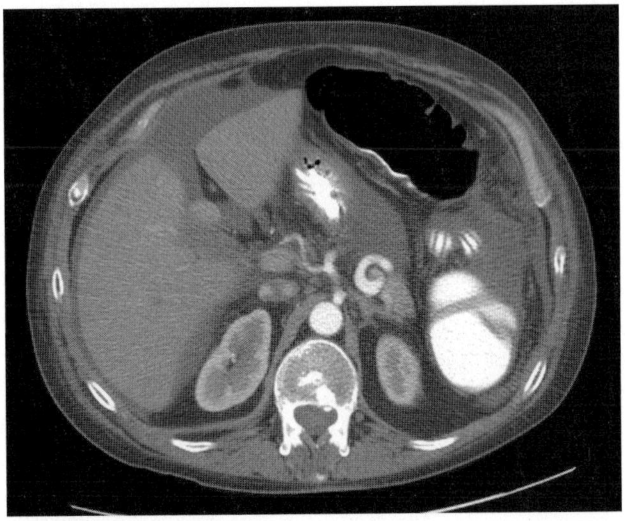

Figure 3-70 Widespread metastatic disease involving the peritoneum from colonic primary tumor is seen.

Aortic Aneurysm

An abdominal aortic aneurysm causing extrinsic compression of small bowel may be recognized by curvilinear calcifications outlining the aneurysm or by a pulsatile appearance on fluoroscopy.

Other Masses

Mesenteric masses (cysts, tumors, and abscesses) typically cause focal displacement of bowel loops. Mesenteric extension of malignant stromal cell tumor (leiomyosarcomas) or other exoenteric masses arising from the bowel wall also can compress or displace adjacent bowel (Fig. 3-71). Diffuse inflammation or infiltration of the mesentery may produce separation of bowel loops throughout the abdomen and pelvis. Focal peritoneal abscesses can produce localized mass effect and inflammation of nearby small bowel.

When a mucinous adenocarcinoma of the abdomen ruptures, it seeds the lower abdomen with tumor implants. These implants can continue to produce mucin, which usually fills the lower abdominal cavity with a mixture of gelatinous fluid and tumor cells. This mixture can result in numerous extrinsic impressions or displacement of the bowel (Fig. 3-72).

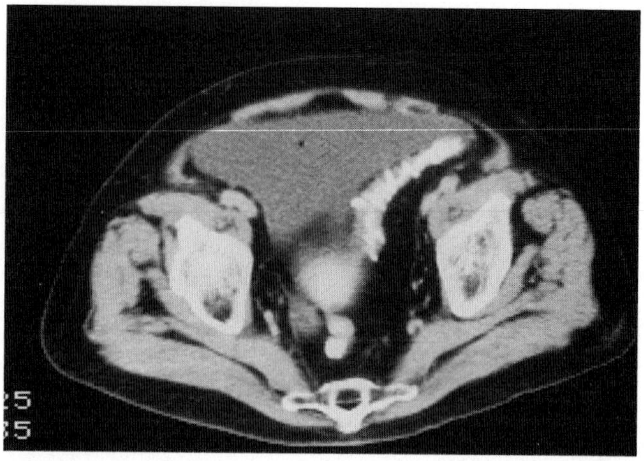

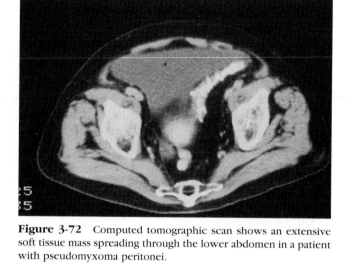

Figure 3-72 Computed tomographic scan shows an extensive soft tissue mass spreading through the lower abdomen in a patient with pseudomyxoma peritonei.

Retractile mesenteritis or sclerosing mesenteritis (two of its several names) is a rare disease that produces fatty and fibrotic thickening of portions of the mesentery. This thickening consists of a combination of inflammation, fibrosis, and fatty infiltration. When inflammation is the predominant pathologic feature of this process, it is often termed *mesenteric panniculitis*. These processes usually involve the distal small bowel mesentery, but sometimes can affect the sigmoid mesentery. The cause is obscure. Some cases have been associated with drugs (ergotamine and methysergide). Complications include ureteral or vascular obstruction. Desmoid tumors are fibrous mesenchymal tumors involving the mesentery and peritoneal cavity (Fig. 3-73). These are seen in Gardner's polyposis syndrome.

Ascites

In the presence of diffuse ascites, supine films show small bowel loops floating together in the central portion of the abdomen. Sometimes the ascites may be loculated and appear as localized masses. Ascites is seen occasionally in patients on peritoneal dialysis for renal failure.

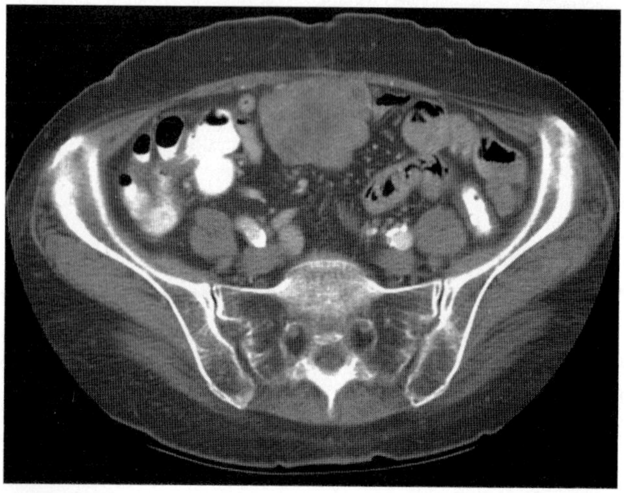

Figure 3-71 Computed tomographic scan shows gastrointestinal stromal tumors in small bowel mesentery, displacing bowel loops.

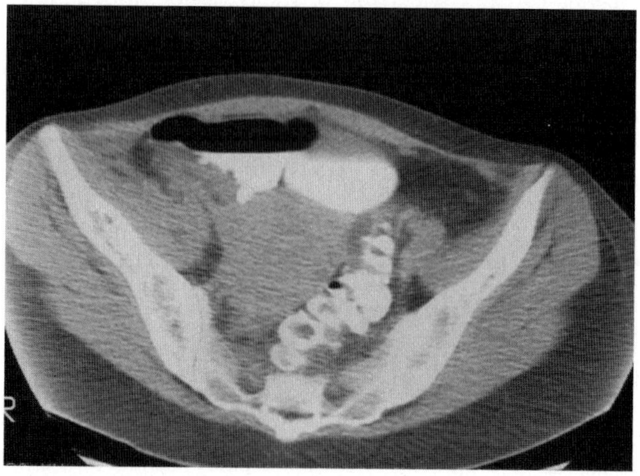

Figure 3-73 Abdominal masses (desmoids) can be seen in Gardner's syndrome.

Fatty Mesenteric Infiltration

Obese patients sometimes may have pronounced fatty changes in their mesentery, which result in separation and displacement of small bowel loops. In these patients, the mesenteric fat is diffuse in nature. Pelvic lipomatosis produces more focal fatty or fibrotic changes in the pelvic region. Although it usually involves the rectum, lipomatosis can produce displacement or compression of small bowel loops in the pelvis. More localized fatty infiltration can be seen in patients with Crohn's disease or isolated lipodystrophy of the mesentery.

ULCERATIONS

Nonneoplastic

Zollinger-Ellison Syndrome

Marked gastric hyperacidity as seen in Zollinger-Ellison syndrome can produce an ulcer diathesis affecting the proximal duodenum and less commonly the distal duodenum and proximal jejunum. Marginal ulcerations may complicate subtotal gastrectomy with gastrojejunal anastomosis. These ulcers occur most often in patients with underlying severe peptic ulcer disease and are usually located in the efferent loop just distal to the anastomotic site.

Crohn's Disease

Ulcerations as a result of Crohn's disease can affect any portion of the small bowel and have a variety of radiographic appearances. Aphthoid ulcers are small, round, and uniform and consist of a central ulceration surrounded by a radiolucent rim of edema (Fig. 3-74).

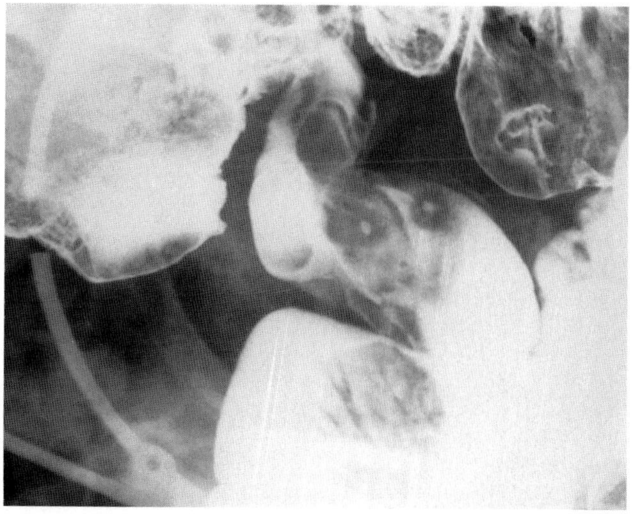

Figure 3-74 Two distinct aphthous ulcers of the terminal ileum are seen in this patient with Crohn's disease.

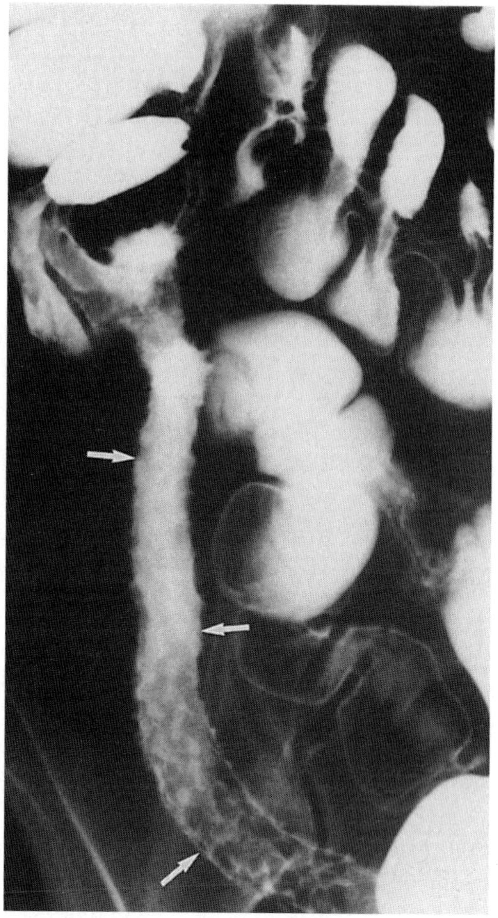

Figure 3-75 Diffuse ulceration of the neoterminal ileum *(arrows)* represents recurrent Crohn's disease.

Deeper transverse and longitudinal ulcerations may combine to form a "cobblestone" pattern, in which residual islands of preserved mucosa are separated by the crisscrossing transmural ulcers (Figs. 3-75 and 3-76).

Infection

Small bowel infections also may cause ulceration. Gastrointestinal tuberculosis most often involves the ileocecal area, where it can cause ulcers and appear radiographically similar to Crohn's disease. CMV enteritis in AIDS may result in ileal ulceration and subsequent perforation. Ileal ulcerations also are seen in enteritis caused by *Salmonella* (typhoid fever), *Yersinia,* and *Campylobacter*. Parasitic infection by *Strongyloides* and *Anisakis* roundworms also may cause ulcers in the small bowel.

Behçet's disease

Behçet's disease (the "silk route disease" because of its Mediterranean origins) is a rare systemic vasculitis in which ulcerations occur in the mouth, genitalia, eyes, and gastrointestinal tract. Ileal ulcerations in this disease may

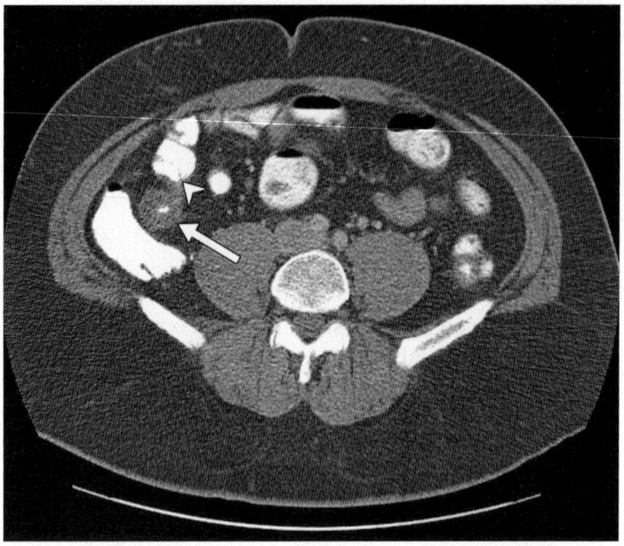

Figure 3-76 Thickened distal ileum *(arrow)* and fistulous tract to adjacent bowel *(arrowhead)* are seen in a patient with Crohn's disease.

appear either aphthoid or linear. Behçet's disease mimics the radiographic appearance of Crohn's disease.

Other Causes

Ulcerative ileojejunitis is an uncommon condition, either idiopathic or secondary to sprue, in which ulcerations in the small bowel may lead to fibrosis and focal stricture formation. Small bowel ulcerations also can result from mucosal irritation by ingested enteric-coated potassium chloride tablets.

Neoplastic

Benign Mesenchymal Tumors

In addition to the many inflammatory causes of small bowel ulceration, various neoplastic masses in the small bowel can ulcerate. Benign mesenchymal tumors, including leiomyomas and lipomas, sometimes bleed because of ulceration of the overlying mucosa (Fig. 3-77). Bleeding is one of the most frequent presenting symptoms because these tumors often remain asymptomatic.

Metastases

Ulcerating metastases to the small bowel most often result from hematogenous spread of malignant melanoma and less commonly breast or lung carcinoma. These masses vary in size and number and may radiographically resemble bull's-eye targets because of the central location of the ulcers.

Kaposi's Sarcoma

Kaposi's sarcoma can produce similar ulcerated masses in the duodenum and less commonly in the mesenteric small bowel.

Malignant Mesenchymal Tumors

Leiomyosarcomas and other less common primary malignant mesenchymal tumors of the small bowel may undergo extensive necrosis and subsequent ulceration. Contrast studies and CT show contrast material filling the large, irregular excavated portion of the mass.

Lymphoma, Adenocarcinoma, and Carcinoid Tumor

Lymphoma, adenocarcinoma, and hematogenous metastases may cause a similar appearance because of infiltration of the bowel wall and resultant ulceration. Carcinoid tumors, which show variable malignant potential, may rarely cause similar findings, but ulceration is not a major feature.

FISTULAS AND SINUS TRACTS

Small bowel sinus tracts and fistulas may result from extension of preexisting small bowel ulcerations. Fistulas are connections between two mucosal-lined organs, such as between two loops of bowel or between the bowel

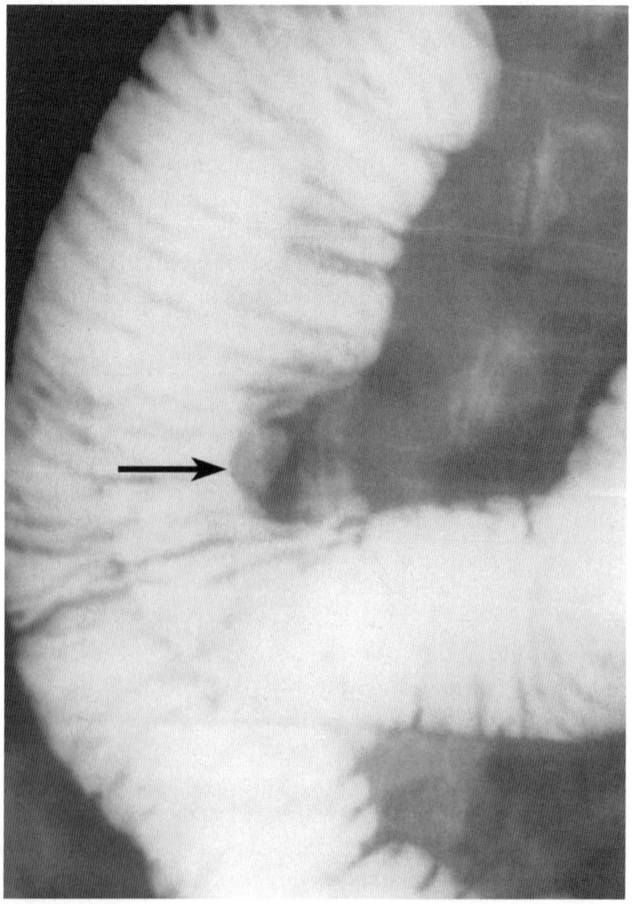

Figure 3-77 Polyp with central ulceration *(arrow)* was a surgically proven leiomyoma.

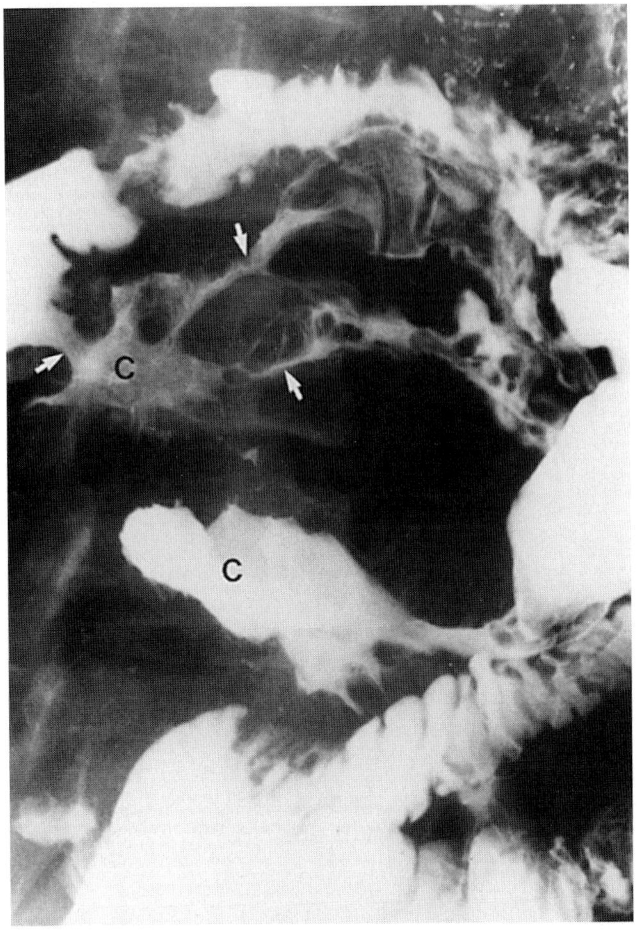

Figure 3-78 Multiple enteric fistulas *(arrows)* and irregular barium collections *(C)* are seen in a patient with Crohn's disease.

and skin. Sinus tracts are confined areas of perforation that end blindly, often in inflammatory tissue, and do not connect to other organs.

Sinus tracts and fistulas are common features of severe Crohn's disease and may form between small bowel and adjacent colon, urinary bladder, abdominal wall, or other loops of small bowel (Fig. 3-78; see Fig. 3-76). Similar findings can be seen in intestinal tuberculosis; the two entities cannot be distinguished by their radiographic features. Small bowel fistulas sometimes occur as a late complication of radiation therapy to the abdomen or pelvis. Fistulas forming from radiation therapy are the sequelae of multiple processes, including ischemia and necrosis of bowel loops and matting of bowel loops from fibrosis and adhesions.

Postoperative sinus tracts and fistulas (enterocutaneous and enteroenteric) may result from a variety of factors. Often they are simply the result of a breakdown or interruption at an enteric anastomosis. Sometimes they result from ischemia and necrosis of a portion of bowel whose blood supply may have been compromised at surgery.

Involvement of the small bowel by extrinsic processes can lead to the formation of sinus tracts or fistulas. Inflammatory masses of the gallbladder, pancreas, kidney, colon, or pelvic organs may become adherent to an adjacent loop of small bowel and erode into it.

Various neoplastic masses can form fistulous connections involving the small bowel. Primary tumors of the small bowel may invade adjacent bowel loops or other viscera, most commonly occurring with lymphoma. More typically seen are tumors from the colon or stomach with direct extension into the small bowel secondarily producing fistulas. Serosal metastases also may be a source of fistulas involving the small bowel, but fistulas are rarely due to hematogenous metastases.

DIVERTICULA

Jejunal and Ileal Diverticula

Jejunal and ileal diverticula are less common than duodenal diverticula. They occur along the mesenteric aspect of the bowel wall, where penetrating blood vessels have produced focal defects in the muscular layer. Jejunal diverticula may be multiple and usually are large (Fig. 3-79). The main clinical concern is that they may develop bacterial overgrowth from stasis of bowel contents, leading to malabsorption and anemia. Ileal diverticula, although often multiple, are usually small and located in the terminal portion of the ileum (Fig. 3-80). Diverticulitis, enterolith formation, hemorrhage, and perforation are rare complications of jejunal and ileal diverticula. When ileal

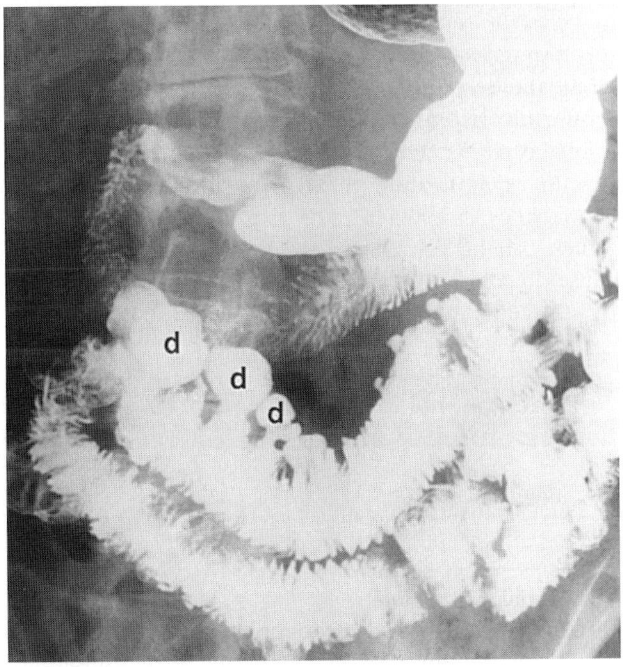

Figure 3-79 Multiple jejunal diverticula *(d)* are seen.

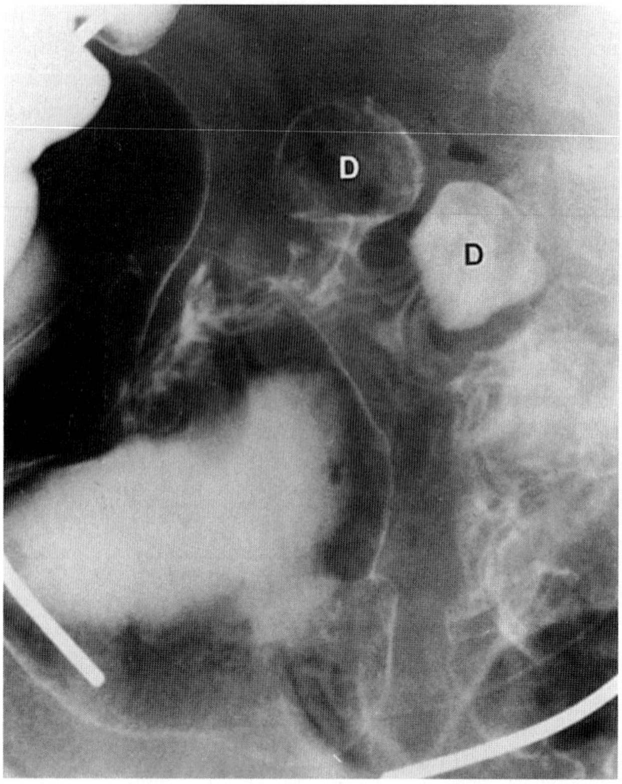

Figure 3-80 Diverticula *(D)* of the terminal ileum are seen.

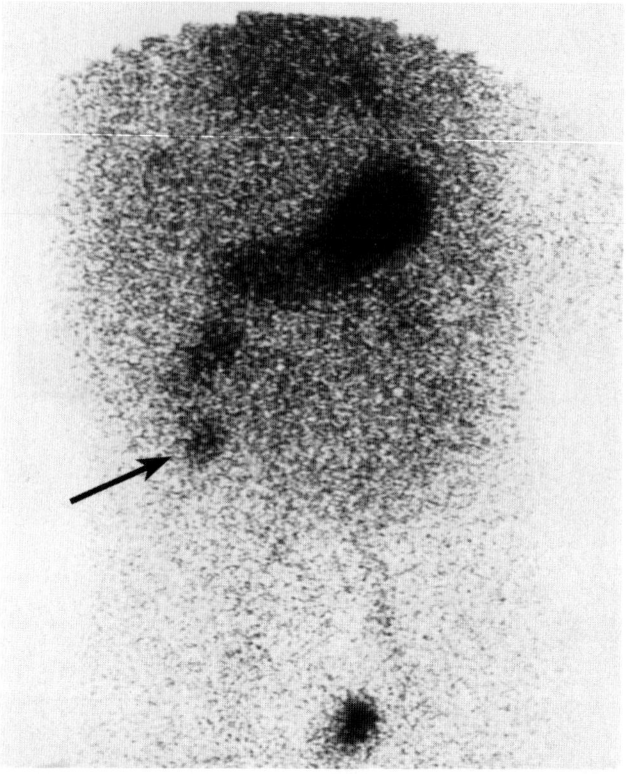

Figure 3-81 Meckel's diverticulum is detected by increased uptake of the radiotracer by the ectopic gastric mucosa *(arrow)*.

diverticula become inflamed, the condition can mimic appendicitis.

Meckel's Diverticulum

Meckel's diverticulum is a congenital abnormality seen in 3% of the population (Box 3-8). Partial persistence of the omphalomesenteric duct results in a diverticulum along the antimesenteric aspect of the ileum, usually within 100 cm of the ileocecal valve. Meckel's diverticulum contains all layers of the bowel wall. Typically, they remain asymptomatic throughout life. Less than half of Meckel's diverticula have gastric mucosa, however, which can be functional and produce acid. This acid causes ulceration in mucosa of the diverticulum or in the adjacent ileum, resulting in gastrointestinal bleeding.

Box 3-8 Meckel's Diverticulum

- Occurs in 3% of the population
- True diverticulum has all layers of bowel wall
- Most are asymptomatic
- Ectopic gastric mucosa in 20% to 30%—detectable by technetium-99m pertechnetate
- Clinical problems—bleeding, perforation, intussusception, enteroliths

This ectopic gastric mucosa accounts for its positive uptake on a technetium-99m pertechnetate scan (Fig. 3-81). Occasionally, it may first present during adulthood, usually secondary to obstruction because the diverticulum may invaginate and be the lead point for intussusception. Diverticulitis, enterolith formation, perforation, and neoplastic transformation are less commonly seen manifestations of Meckel's diverticulum.

Careful fluoroscopy using graded compression is often necessary to show a Meckel's diverticulum on SBFT examination because otherwise it is obscured by overlapping bowel loops (Fig. 3-82). Enteroclysis has proved useful for revealing Meckel's diverticula and showing the characteristic triradiate fold pattern at the junction of the diverticulum and the adjacent segment of ileum. A Meckel's scan using radioactive technetium-99m pertechnetate is sensitive for detecting diverticula that contain ectopic gastric mucosa.

Pseudodiverticula

Various abnormalities in the mesenteric small bowel may mimic diverticula. Any process that produces asymmetrical inflammation or fibrosis or both can result in asymmetrical sacculations or pseudodiverticula (Fig. 3-83). Classically, Crohn's disease can be an asymmetrical inflammatory process that may produce asymmetrical fibrosis

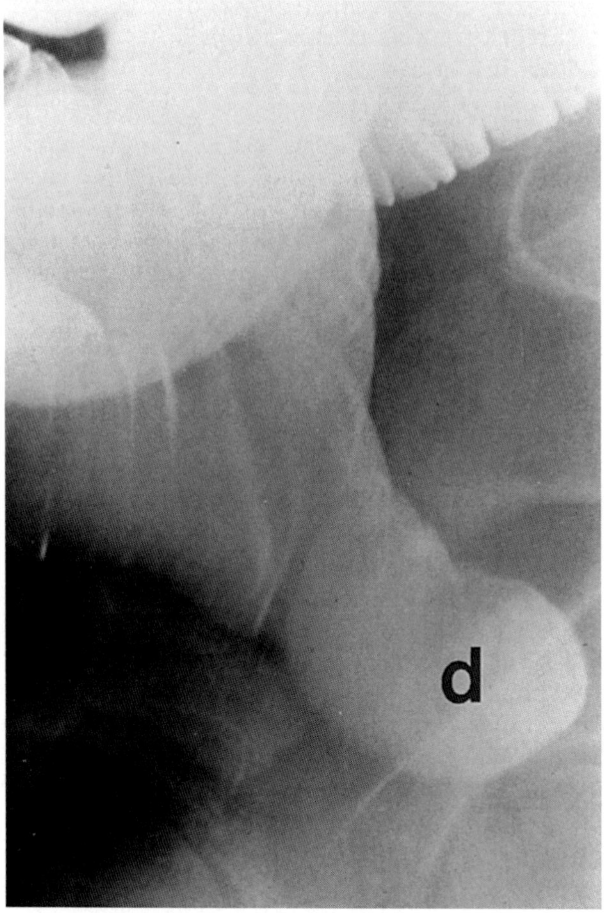

Figure 3-82 Meckel's diverticulum *(d)* extends from the distal ileum.

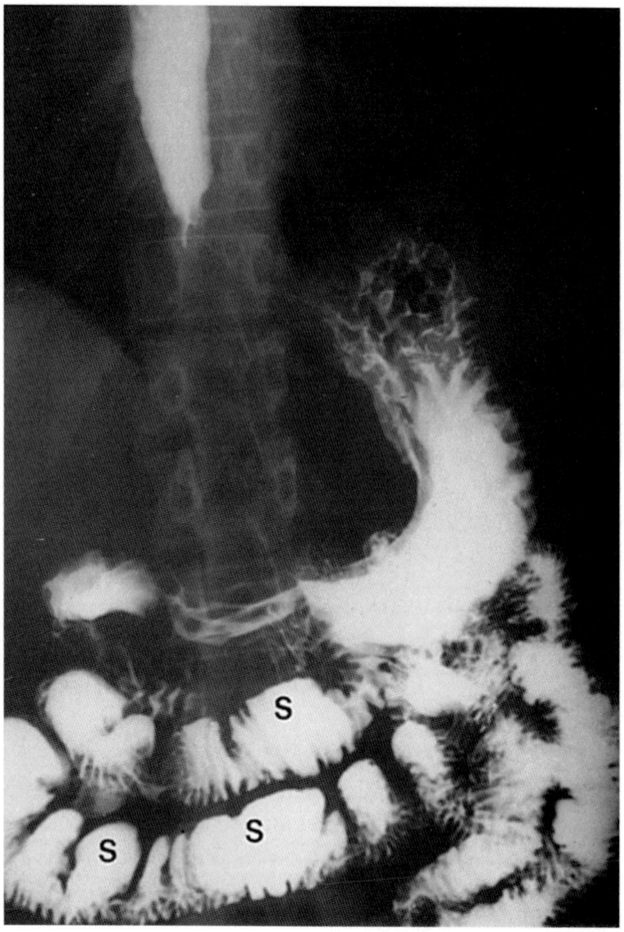

Figure 3-83 Multiple eccentric sacculations *(S)* in the jejunum in a patient with scleroderma. Note the retained barium in the distal esophagus.

of the bowel wall with subsequent pseudosacculations (Fig. 3-84). The fibrosis that is seen in scleroderma also may produce unusual sacculations of the bowel wall. Surgically created blind loops and communicating congenital duplications of the small bowel also can resemble diverticula.

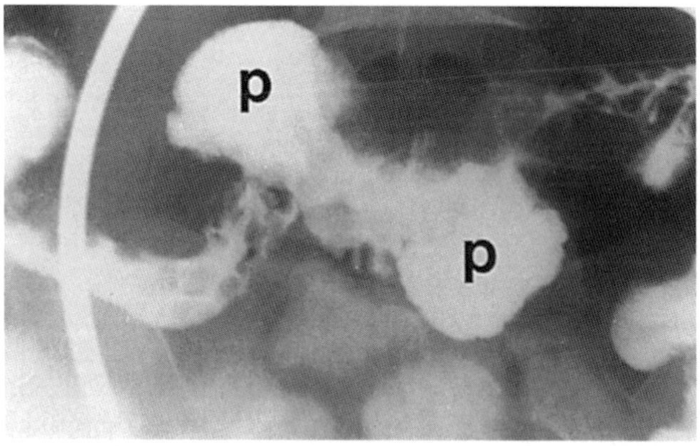

Figure 3-84 Pseudosacculations *(p)* in the small bowel are seen in a patient with Crohn's disease.

In lymphoma, focal aneurysmal dilatation of the lumen, either fusiform or asymmetrical, may result from destruction of the autonomic neural plexus by tumor infiltration. Focal saccular dilatation of the ileum also may be seen in ileal dysgenesis, a rare condition of uncertain origin.

PNEUMATOSIS INTESTINALIS

Idiopathic Causes

Pneumatosis intestinalis indicates air in the bowel wall. This condition is idiopathic in approximately 15% of cases and secondary to various underlying diseases in the remaining 85%. Patients with idiopathic pneumatosis are asymptomatic, and the air collections are usually cystic and subserosal in appearance. In secondary pneumatosis, the air collections are linear and intramural, and the patients may have signs or symptoms of gastrointestinal or pulmonary disease (Fig. 3-85) relating to ischemia or necrosis. Even this form of pneumatosis can be benign, resulting from recent bowel surgery, bowel ulceration, or recent instrumentation.

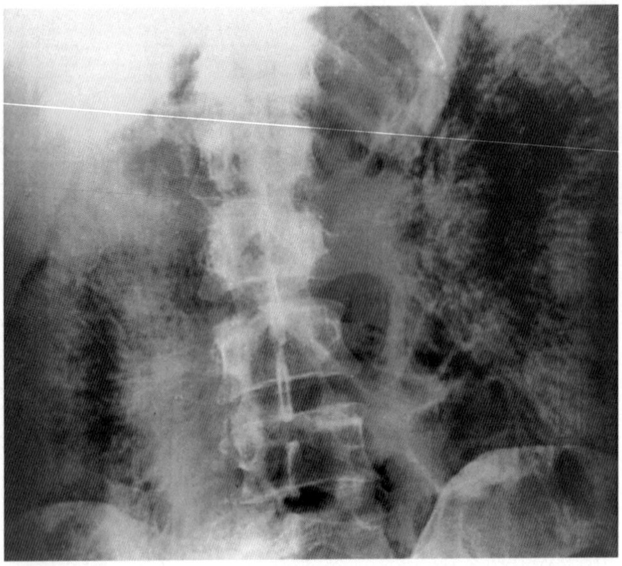

Figure 3-85 Diffuse linear collections of air in the small bowel wall represent pneumatosis intestinalis.

Ischemia and Infarction

Small bowel ischemia or infarction can cause mucosal necrosis and extension of luminal air into the bowel wall (Fig. 3-86). Air in the mesenteric and portal veins or pneumoperitoneum may follow, with a high incidence of morbidity and mortality.

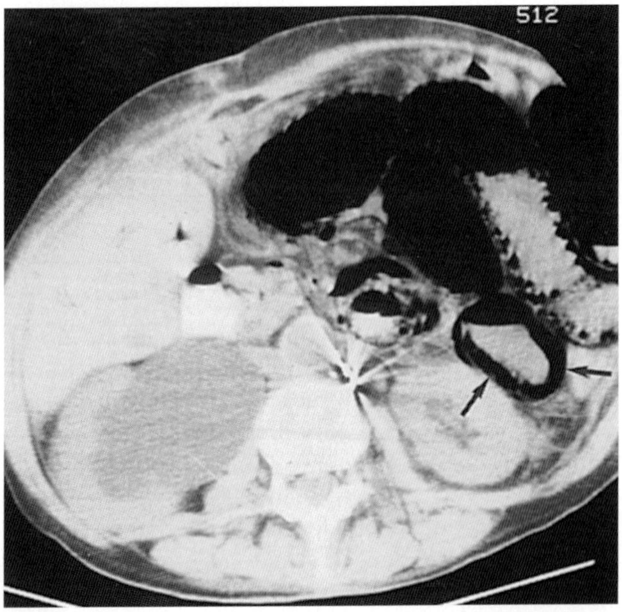

Figure 3-86 Computed tomographic scan shows extensive intramural air *(arrows)* surrounding intraluminal fluid in a patient with small bowel infarction.

Infection and Inflammation (Noninfectious)

Infectious and noninfectious enteritis also may cause pneumatosis because of luminal air passing into the bowel wall through mucosal ulcerations. Other factors, including luminal distention proximal to strictures and infection of the bowel wall by gas-forming organisms, also may play a role in the development of pneumatosis in these cases.

Other Causes

Pneumatosis has been reported after focal perforation of a small bowel diverticulum and iatrogenic trauma caused by indwelling catheters or previous enteric anastomoses. Scleroderma, celiac disease, and other related conditions are rarely complicated by pneumatosis of the small bowel. Obstructive pulmonary disease can produce pneumatosis secondary to alveolar rupture and subsequent passage of air along interstitial pathways to the mediastinum and, through defects in the diaphragm, to the retroperitoneum, mesentery, and bowel wall. Pneumatosis also has been reported in patients receiving steroids, but may be related to the patients' underlying disease rather than to the steroids themselves.

POSTOPERATIVE SMALL BOWEL

Resection

Segmental resection of small bowel with end-to-end anastomosis is a commonly performed procedure in cases of small bowel infarction, perforation, or stenosis. The most frequent complication of this procedure is development of adhesions. In Crohn's disease, segmental small bowel resection is usually avoided whenever possible because of the high incidence of recurrent disease or fistulas at the margins of resection.

Anastomoses

Various enteric anastomoses to the stomach, colon, biliary tree, and pancreas have been described. In Billroth II subtotal gastrectomy, afferent and efferent loops of small bowel are anastomosed to the greater curvature of the gastric remnant. The afferent loop has a closed end and consists of the duodenum and a variable length of proximal jejunum. Current surgical construction of the anastomosis favors emptying of the stomach into the efferent loop, avoiding distention of the afferent loop (afferent loop syndrome). A Roux-en-Y anastomosis can be performed simultaneously, connecting the afferent loop to the efferent loop beyond the gastrojejunostomy site. This procedure prevents bile in the duodenum from refluxing into the gastric remnant, where it may cause severe bile reflux gastritis.

Several complications involving the small bowel may occur after the Billroth II procedure. Marginal ulcerations representing peptic ulceration of the jejunal mucosa typically involve the efferent loop just distal to the gastrojejunal anastomosis. In afferent loop syndrome, continued distention of the afferent loop may lead to bacterial overgrowth. Gastrojejunal and jejunogastric intussusception are unusual complications resulting from antegrade or retrograde intussusception at the anastomotic site.

In cases of gastric outlet obstruction, gastrojejunostomy can be used to bypass narrowing of the distal stomach, pylorus, or duodenum. Gastrojejunostomy also is performed in gastric bypass procedures for morbid obesity. Staples form a small gastric pouch that is anastomosed side-to-side with a loop of proximal jejunum. Important complications of this procedure include anastomotic leakage and obstruction.

Intestinal Bypass

Many intestinal bypass procedures previously used for treating morbid obesity have been abandoned because of the high incidence of complications (Fig. 3-87). Because of the decreased length of functioning small bowel, malabsorption occurred with subsequent development of gallstones, renal oxalate stones, and liver disease. Bacterial overgrowth also occurred in the lengthy bypassed segment (blind-loop syndrome).

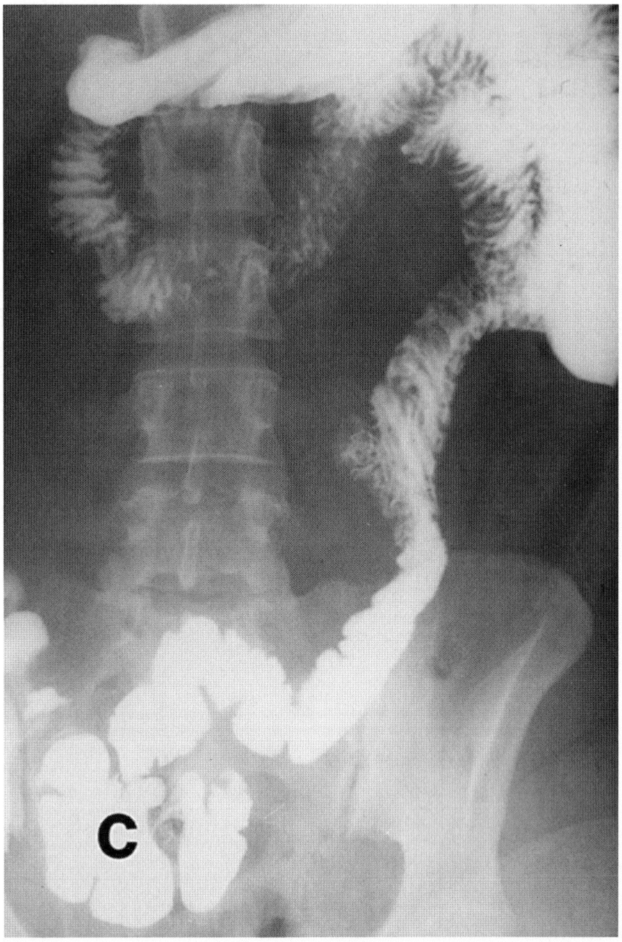

Figure 3-87 Shortened small bowel secondary to intestinal bypass surgery for obesity. The cecum *(C)* is filled early in the examination.

Stomas and Reservoirs

Various ileostomy procedures have been developed for patients with total colectomy. The conventional ileostomy consists of a loop of ileum that is brought to the skin surface and empties into a bag. Kock's continent ileostomy represents a surgically created internal ileal pouch just beneath the abdominal wall. A segment of ileum acts as a valve in Kock's continent ileostomy, and the patient empties the pouch by intubating it at regular intervals.

Ileoanal reservoir represents anastomosis of the ileum to the distal rectum after resection of rectal mucosa. After the ileum is folded on itself in the shape of a J or S, the ileal pouch is created, and ileoanal anastomosis is performed.

INTUSSUSCEPTION

Intussusception is the invagination of one bowel loop into another, with the resulting intestinal peristalsis producing increasing movement of the proximal segment (intussusceptum) into the distal segment (Box 3-9). Intussusception can result in obstruction, ischemia, and sometimes perforation. Typically, an intraluminal lesion, such as a polyp, serves as a nidus or lead point, which gets carried by the peristaltic action into the distal segment. A lead point is not necessary, however, for intussusception to occur. Radiographically, an intussusception has a coiled-spring appearance as the contrast material outlines the intussusceptum (see Fig. 3-15). With cross-sectional imaging techniques, the multiple layers of bowel within each other produce a bull's-eye target appearance.

Box 3-9 Causes of Small Bowel Intussusception

- Tumors, primary or metastatic
- Idiopathic (typically in children)
- Celiac disease (sprue)
- Meckel's diverticulum
- Intestinal tubes
- Cystic fibrosis

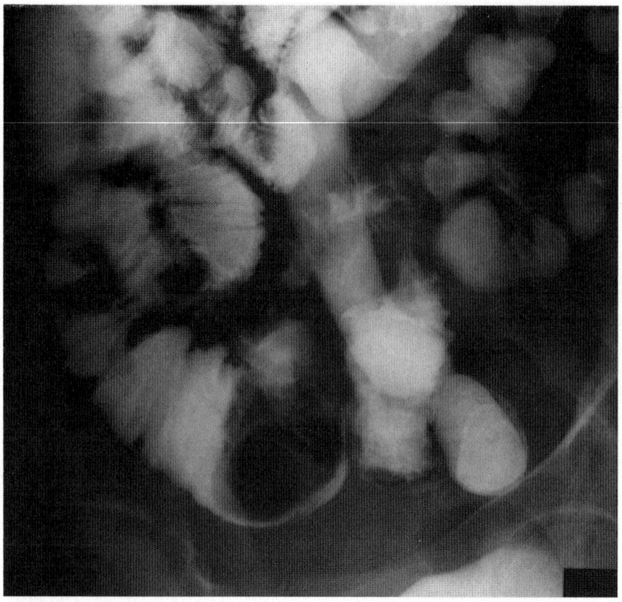

Figure 3-88 This large intussusception was produced by a polyp in a patient with Peutz-Jeghers syndrome.

Neoplastic

Neoplasms are the most frequent cause of intussusception in adults. Usually, they are benign tumors such as a lipoma or adenoma that serve as lead points for the intussusceptums (Fig. 3-88). These benign tumors often are pedunculated, which aids in the development of intussusception. Malignant tumors, such as carcinoma or lymphoma, rarely intussuscept because they infiltrate through the bowel wall and not into the lumen. Malignant sarcomas have the potential for intussuscepting, however. Also, metastases that develop intraluminal polypoid lesions have been known to produce intussusception rarely; these include melanoma, breast, and lung.

Nonneoplastic

Approximately a quarter of intussusceptions have no known cause. Intussusceptions that occur in infants and children typically have no known cause. Patients present with abdominal pain and bleeding. These intussusceptions sometimes can be reduced by a fluoroscopically guided enema, depending on the duration of the intussusception and the clinical state of the patient.

Sprue is another cause of benign intussusception, although the exact reason why it develops in these patients is uncertain. Intussusception in sprue is usually intermittent or transient in nature and rarely requires any intervention (see Fig. 3-20).

With the increasing use of intestinal tubes, particularly for hyperalimentation, the incidence of intussusception related to tubes is becoming more frequent. Some tubes have a balloon or bag at their end, which serves as a lead point, dragging not only the tube, but also a segment of bowel along with it into the distal bowel. Usually removal of the tube solves the problem.

Rarely, diverticula (particularly Meckel's diverticula) may invert and be a lead point for an intussusception. Also, ectopic tissue, foreign bodies, and adhesions may serve as a site for intussusception.

POSITIONAL ABNORMALITIES

The intestines develop outside the abdominal cavity and with time return within the abdomen. As they do this, they rotate 270 degrees counterclockwise with the superior mesenteric artery acting as the central axis point. The final location is with the jejunum in the left upper quadrant and the cecum and ileum in the right lower quadrant. If this rotation is stopped before completion, any sort of positional variation can occur.

Rotational Abnormalities

Nonrotation is when there is no rotation of the intestines as they return to the abdomen. The ligament of Treitz is not present, the jejunum and ileum are on the right side of the abdomen, and the colon is on the left (Fig. 3-89). Malrotation refers to any degree of rotational abnormality between nonrotation and normal. Often, patients are

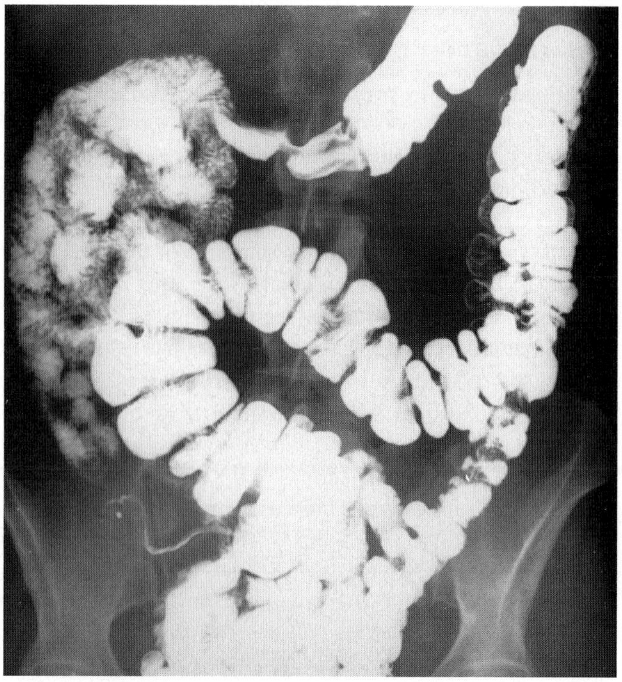

Figure 3-89 Small bowel loops are in the right upper quadrant in this patient with malrotation.

asymptomatic, but there is a predisposition for midgut volvulus and aberrant bands producing partial obstruction.

Internal Hernias

Intraabdominal hernias occur as the result of congenital or acquired defects in the mesenteries or peritoneal reflections. These defects can incarcerate the small bowel within them, being asymptomatic or producing obstruction and ischemia.

Paraduodenal hernias are the most common, caused by a defect in the parietal peritoneum at the ligament of Treitz. Left paraduodenal hernia is much more common than right-sided hernia. Radiographically, it can be recognized as a tightly bunched loop of bowel that remains fixed during the study.

Other internal hernias may be due to congenital developmental anomalies or surgically created defects in the mesentery. The diagnosis can be made by identifying several loops of bowel that appear in an unusual location and remain fairly fixed throughout the examination.

SUGGESTED READINGS

Balthazar EJ, Gordon R, Hulnick D: Ileocecal tuberculosis: CT and radiologic evaluation. AJR Am J Roentgenol 154:499-503, 1990.

Bartnicke BJ, Balfe DM: CT appearance of intestinal ischemia and intramural hemorrhage. Radiol Clin North Am 32:845, 1994.

Berk RN, Wall SD, McArdle CB, et al: Cryptosporidiosis of the stomach and small intestine in patients with AIDS. AJR Am J Roentgenol 143:549-554, 1984.

Bhatnagar A, Swaroop K, Behari V, et al: Scintigraphic detection of localized small bowel abnormality. Clin Nucl Med 20:367, 1995.

Buck JL, Sobin LH: Carcinoids of the gastrointestinal tract. Radiographics 10:1081-1095, 1990.

Carlson HC, Breen JF: Amyloidosis and plasma cell dyscrasias: gastrointestinal involvement. Semin Roentgenol 21:128-138, 1986.

Dudiak KM, Johnson CD, Stephens DH: Primary tumors of the small intestine: CT evaluation. AJR Am J Roentgenol 152:995-998, 1989.

Fanso A, Catassi C: Current approaches to diagnosis and treatment of celiac disease: an evolving spectrum. Gastroenterology 120:635-651, 2001.

Feczko PJ, Collins DD, Mezwa DG: Metastatic disease involving the gastrointestinal tract. Radiol Clin North Am 31:1359-1374, 1993.

Feczko PJ, Mezwa DG, Farah MC, et al: Clinical significance of pneumatosis of the bowel wall. Radiographics 12:1069-1078, 1992.

Frager D, Baer JW, Medwid SW, et al: Detection of intestinal ischemia in patients with acute small-bowel obstruction due to adhesions or hernia:efficacy of CT. AJR Am J Roentgenol 166: 67-71, 1996.

Frager D, Medwid SW, Baer JW, et al: CT of small-bowel obstruction: value in establishing the diagnosis and determining the degree and cause. AJR Am J Roentgenol 162:37-41, 1994.

Furukawa A, Saotome T, Yamaski M: Cross-sectional imaging in Crohn disease. Radiographics 24:689-702, 2004.

Ha AS, Levine MS, Rubesin SE, et al: Radiographic examination of the small bowel: survey of the practice patterns in the United States. Radiology 231:407-412, 2004.

Gazelle GS, Goldberg MA, Wittenberg J, et al: Efficacy of CT in distinguishing small-bowel obstruction from other causes of small bowel dilatation. AJR Am J Roentgenol 162:43-47, 1994.

Glick SN: Crohn's disease of the small intestine. Radiol Clin North Am 25:25-45, 1987.

Gramm HF, Vincent ME, Braver JM: Differential diagnosis of tubular small bowel. Curr Imaging 2:62-68, 1990.

Kalanteri BN, Mortele KJ, Cantisani V, et al: CT features with pathologic correlation of acute gastrointestinal graft-versus-host disease after bone marrow transplants in adults. AJR Am J Roentgenol 181:1621-1625, 2003.

Laurent F, Drouillard J, Lecesne R, et al: CT of small-bowel neoplasms. Semin Ultrasound CT MR 16:102, 1995.

Long FR, Kramer SS, Markowitz RI, et al: Radiographic patterns of intestinal malrotation in children. Radiographics 16:547, 1996.

Low RN, Chen SC, Barone R: Distinguishing benign from malignant bowel obstruction in patients with malignancy at MR imaging. Radiology 228:157-165, 2003.

Maglinte DDT, Kelvin FM, O'Connor K, et al: Current status of small bowel radiography. Abdomin Imaging 21:247, 1996.

Merine D, Fishman EK, Jones B, et al: Enteroenteric intussusception: CT findings in nine patients. AJR Am J Roentgenol 148: 1129-1132, 1987.

Meyers MA: Metastatic seeding along the small bowel mesentery: roentgen features. AJR Am J Roentgenol 123:67-73, 1975.

Raptospoulos V, Schwartz RK, McNicholas MMJ, et al: Mutiplanar helical CT enterography in patients with Crohn's disease. AJR Am J Roentgenol 169:1545-1550, 1997.

Rossi P, Gourtsoyiannis N, Bezzi M, et al: Meckel's diverticulum: imaging diagnosis. AJR Am J Roentgenol 166:567-573, 1996.

Rubesin SE, Gilchrist AM, Bronner M, et al: Non-Hodgkin lymphoma of the small intestine. Radiographics 10:985-998, 1990.

Rubesin SE, Herlinger H, Saul SH, et al: Adult celiac disease and its complications. Radiographics 9:1045-1066, 1989.

Scholz FJ: Ischemic bowel disease. Radiol Clin North Am 31: 1197-1218, 1993.

Smith C, Deziel DJ, Kubicka RA: Appearances of the postoperative alimentary tract. Radiol Clin North Am 31:1235-1254, 1993.

Szucs RA, Turner MA: Gastrointestinal tract involvement by gynecologic diseases. Radiographics 16:1251, 1996.

Teixidor HS, Honig CL, Norsoph E, et al: Cytomegalovirus infection of the alimentary canal: radiologic findings with pathologic correlation. Radiology 163:317-323, 1987.

Wall SD, Ominsky S, Altman DF, et al: Multifocal abnormalities of the gastrointestinal tract in AIDS. AJR Am J Roentgenol 146:1-5, 1986.

Zarvan NP, Lee FT Jr, Yandow DR, Unger JS: Abdominal hernias: CT findings. AJR Am J Roentgenol 164:1391-1395, 1995.

CHAPTER 4

Pancreas

EXAMINATION TECHNIQUES

The pancreas is a midline elongated retroperitoneal structure located diagonally in the upper abdomen. It consists of the head and uncinate process, body, and tail and lies in close proximity to the stomach, duodenal sweep, left kidney, spleen, aorta, inferior vena cava, portal and splenic veins, and superior mesenteric vessels. Its relationship with the stomach caused early anatomists to consider the pancreas as a "cushion" for the stomach. The head of the pancreas is "cradled" in the duodenal sweep, however. Langerhans described the unique histological structure of the pancreas in 1869. The main duct of the pancreas is the duct of Wirsung. The relationship of the main duct and the common bile duct at the level of the papillae varies. The ducts may open separately (approximately 20%) or have a common channel (approximately 80%). The accessory duct of Santorini is seen in about 75% of autopsy cases. It communicates with the main duct of Wirsung and drains via the minor papilla, which lies more proximally in the second portion of the duodenum than the major duct. The minor papilla is often difficult to detect, even with endoscopy.

The pancreas performs important exocrine and endocrine functions, and a detailed account of these secretory functions is beyond the scope of this book. Alkaline fluid secreted into the duodenum through the pancreatic duct neutralizes gastric acid, and the enzymes amylase and lipase aid in the digestion of carbohydrates and fats and several proteolytic enzymes. Various hormones, most importantly insulin, glucagon, and gastrin, are formed in the pancreatic islets of Langerhans and are secreted directly into the bloodstream to regulate glucose metabolism (insulin and glucagon) and gastric acid secretion (gastrin). Although the pancreas is not visible on plain film radiography, abdominal plain films are useful for showing pancreatic calcifications. An upper gastrointestinal (UGI) series may show deformity of the stomach and duodenum secondary to adjacent pancreatic inflammatory or neoplastic disease. Duodenal and proximal jejunal ulcers also may result from hypersecretion of gastric acid in response to a pancreatic gastrinoma (Zollinger-Ellison syndrome). Various methods of hypotonic duodenography have been developed for improved distention of the duodenum and visualization of ampullary, periampullary, and pancreatic head masses.

Cross-sectional computed tomography (CT) and, in particular, newer multitrack CT have revolutionized pancreatic imaging by allowing direct and detailed visualization of the pancreas and the peripancreatic structures. Percutaneous drainage of pancreatic or peripancreatic fluid collections and aspiration or biopsy of pancreatic masses also are widely performed using ultrasound guidance or computed tomographic guidance.

Ultrasound examination of the normal pancreas usually shows homogeneous echogenicity that equals or slightly exceeds that of the normal liver. Reported measurements of the normal pancreas vary, but currently accepted values are 2.6 cm for the anteroposterior diameter of the head, 2.2 cm for the anteroposterior diameter of the body, and 1.5 cm for the anteroposterior diameter of the tail. Advantages of ultrasonography compared with CT include lower cost, absence of ionizing radiation, and multiplanar imaging capabilities. The main disadvantage of ultrasonography is poor visualization of the pancreas secondary to obesity or overlying bowel gas. Interference by bowel gas may be overcome by having the patient ingest water, distending the stomach and duodenum and forming an acoustic window. Intravenous injection of glucagon may aid sonographic visualization of the pancreas by decreasing intestinal motility. Supplemental examination in prone, decubitus, upright, or oblique positions may be necessary to evaluate the pancreas completely.

Optimal computed tomographic demonstration of the pancreas requires a sufficient amount of oral contrast material to opacify the adjacent stomach, duodenum, and proximal jejunum. Rapid infusion of intravenous contrast material using a three-phase technique can allow clear definition of the peripancreatic arterial structures and the portal system and enhancement of the pancreatic parenchyma (Fig. 4-1). Multidetector CT allows rapid acquisition of contiguous axial images during peak vascular enhancement, and images can be reconstructed at thin slices in axial, coronal, or sagittal planes. CT is not limited by obesity or overlying bowel gas, and it provides excellent evaluation of associated peripancreatic and extrapancreatic extension of disease. Magnetic resonance imaging (MRI) of the pancreas continues to offer the advantages of multiplanar imaging capabilities, absence of ionizing radiation, and differentiation between tissue and flowing blood (Fig. 4-2). MRI is being used more frequently as the relative cost of the examination and image acquisition has decreased. Also, newer imaging sequences have been developed that further enhance the evaluation of pancreatic ductal structures and parenchyma. Intravenous injection of glucagon decreases motion artifacts caused by intestinal motility, and various negative and positive contrast agents are available for bowel opacification. With increasing advances in MRI, it is slowly becoming an important tool in the evaluation of pancreatic lesions.

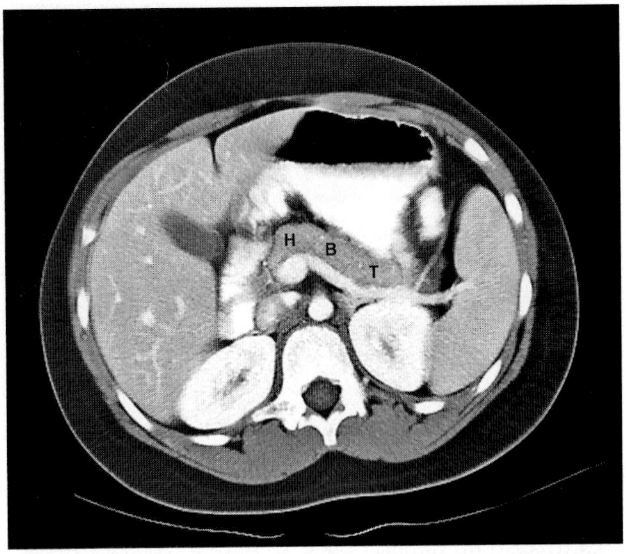

Figure 4-1 CT shows the normal pancreatic head *(H)*, body *(B)*, and tail *(T)*.

Endoscopic retrograde cholangiopancreatography (ERCP) remains the best of all choices for evaluating the pancreatic duct (Fig. 4-3). Coexistent disease of the biliary tree, such as common bile duct narrowing secondary to pancreatic carcinoma or choledocholithiasis causing pancreatitis, also can be evaluated by ERCP. ERCP is contraindicated in acute pancreatitis because overinjection of the pancreatic duct may cause parenchymal opacification (acinarization) and worsening of pancreatitis. Other disadvantages of ERCP relate to complications of

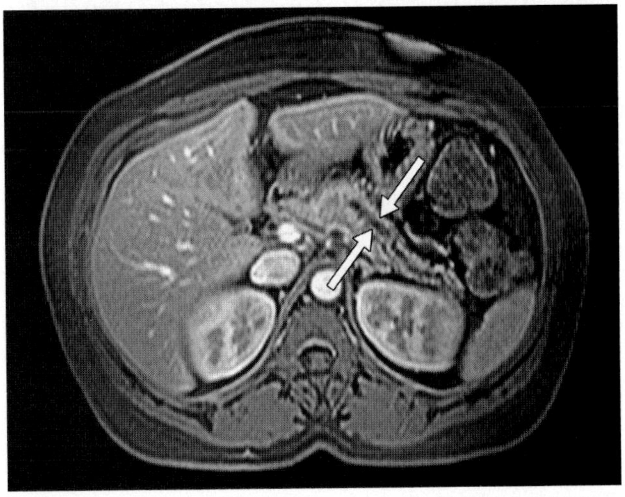

Figure 4-2 MRI through upper abdomen shows pancreas and dilated pancreatic duct *(arrows)*.

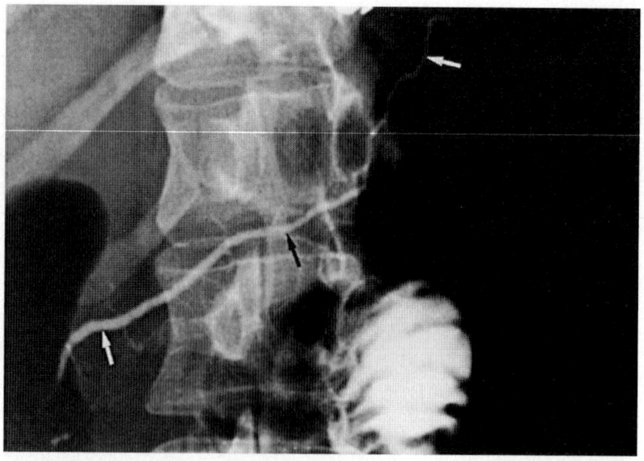

Figure 4-3 ERCP shows a normal pancreatic duct *(arrows)*.

endoscopy in general and potential trauma to the ampulla of Vater during duct cannulation. Also, the success rate varies and usually does not exceed 90%. The cost and length of the procedure, the use of relatively lengthy fluoroscopic times and radiation exposure, and the use of routine sedation prevent it from being a routine procedure.

Because of ERCP's disadvantages, magnetic resonance cholangiopancreatography (MRCP) is being used with more frequency as a noninvasive method of evaluating the ductal structures. Although at this time, the resolution of MRCP is slightly less than ERCP, it can provide useful information in a variety of circumstances (Fig. 4-4).

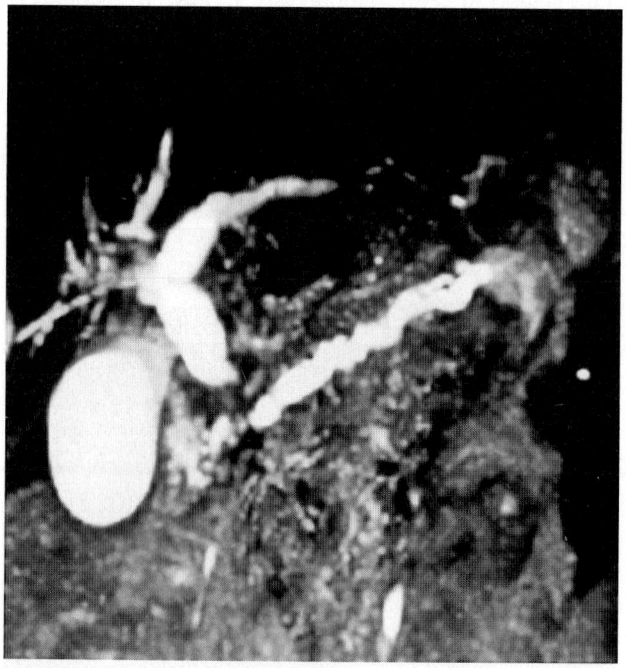

Figure 4-4 MRCP shows pancreatic and biliary systems on the same image. Note dilated pancreatic duct secondary to chronic pancreatitis.

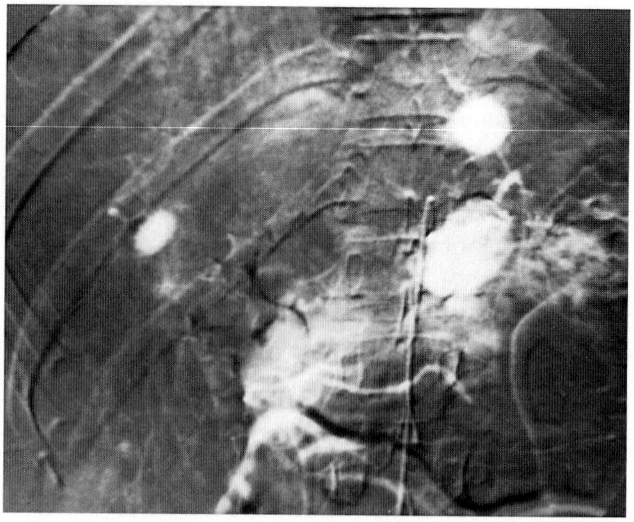

Figure 4-5 Arteriogram shows multiple hypervascular masses in the pancreas and both lobes of the liver. This is an islet cell tumor of the pancreas with liver metastases.

MRCP is performed using a heavily weighted T2 sequence. Its major advantages are that the ducts can be visualized in multiple planes, pancreatic and biliary ducts can be imaged simultaneously, success rate is not operator dependent, contrast agents or sedation is not routinely needed, and significant complications are rare. Additionally, MRCP can be performed on almost all patients, and the cost is considerably less than ERCP. Negative aspects include limited resolution; motion artifacts, particularly of side branches; and inability to perform therapeutic procedures. Nevertheless, it is likely that MRCP will supplant diagnostic ERCP in the near future.

Pancreatic angiography for evaluation of pancreatic carcinoma has been largely supplanted by ultrasound and multidetector CT. Superselective subtraction arteriography and venous sampling are still used, however, for localizing small insulinomas and other functioning islet cell tumors (Fig. 4-5).

Endoscopic ultrasound shows promising results in the detection of pancreatic head and body lesions and especially islet cell tumors. The instrument consists of an ultrasound transducer attached to the tip of an endoscope. After positioning of the transducer against the gastric or duodenal wall, images of the adjacent pancreas are obtained.

EMBRYOLOGY

Development of the pancreas in utero is a complex mechanism that results in a variety of anomalies and variants. Many of these are asymptomatic, but others can produce symptoms in either children or adults.

Box 4-1 Frequency of Pancreatic Anomalies

Dual drainage (accessory papilla) approximately 30%
Pancreas divisum <10%
Ectopic pancreatic tissue <10%
Hypoplasia/agenesis of a segment of pancreas
Annular pancreas

Understanding the complex nature of this embryological formation aids in the evaluation of the pancreas (Box 4-1).

The pancreas develops from the embryological fusion of dorsal and ventral buds of the foregut, which grow during week 4 of gestation. The ventral bud begins development to the right of the duodenum, whereas the dorsal bud develops from the left side of the duodenum (Fig. 4-6). The pancreas comes to occupy a position to the left of the duodenum by rotation of the ventral bud and by partial duodenal rotation, both of which occur at about week 6. The dorsal duct drains the body, tail, and superior portion of the head of the pancreas into the minor papilla, and the ventral duct drains the uncinate process and inferior portion of the pancreatic head (and the biliary system) into the major papilla. Under normal circumstances, the ventral duct (Wirsung) fuses with the dorsal duct (Santorini), usually around week 7. After fusion of the two ducts, the main duct of Wirsung, consisting of the ventral duct and the proximal segment of the dorsal duct, continues to drain into the major papilla. The distal segment of the dorsal duct, which drains into the minor papilla, partially regresses to form the accessory duct of Santorini.

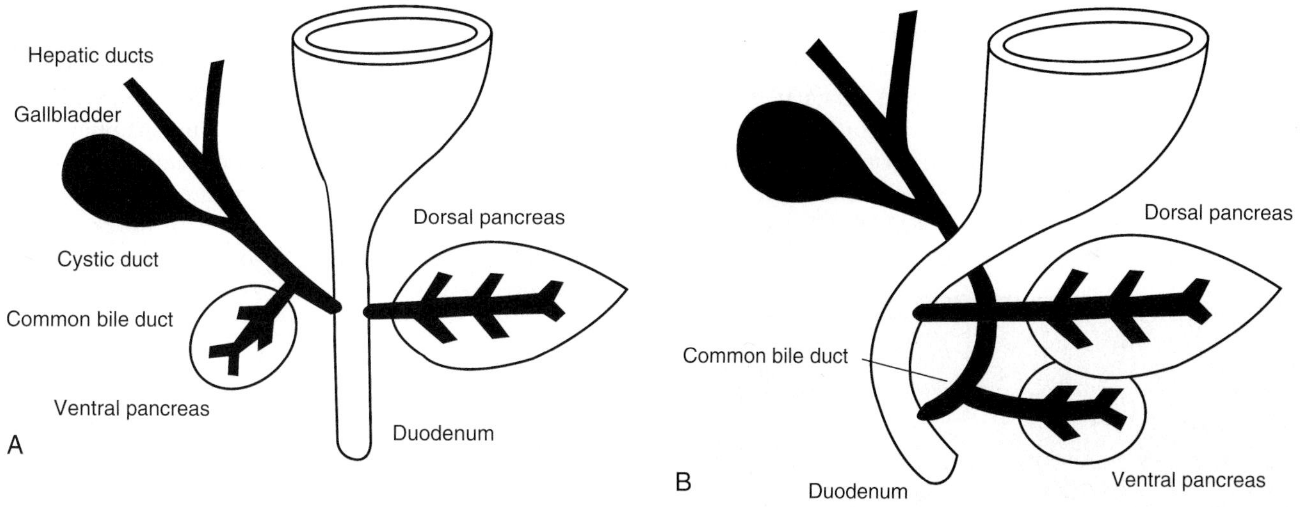

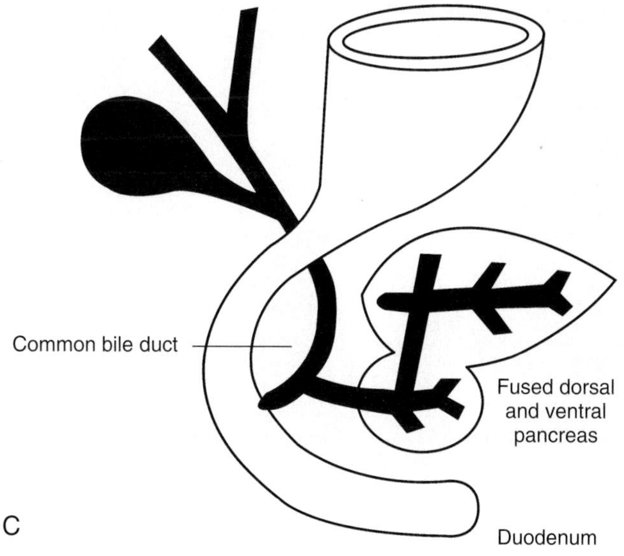

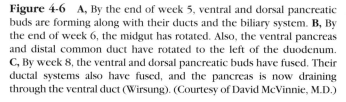

Figure 4-6 **A,** By the end of week 5, ventral and dorsal pancreatic buds are forming along with their ducts and the biliary system. **B,** By the end of week 6, the midgut has rotated. Also, the ventral pancreas and distal common duct have rotated to the left of the duodenum. **C,** By week 8, the ventral and dorsal pancreatic buds have fused. Their ductal systems also have fused, and the pancreas is now draining through the ventral duct (Wirsung). (Courtesy of David McVinnie, M.D.)

CONGENITAL ANOMALIES

Annular Pancreas

Annular pancreas is a rare congenital abnormality in which a ring of pancreatic tissue encircles the duodenum at or above the papilla of Vater. Its incidence has been estimated at 1:20,000. Normally, the ventral bud and the duodenum undergo rotation that places the ventral portion of the pancreas to the left of the duodenum. In annular pancreas, the ventral pancreas does not completely rotate, however, and there may be limited rotation of the duodenum. This limited rotation results in the ventral pancreas forming either a partial or a complete ring around the duodenum. Depending on the degree of obstruction, this condition may lead to an acute surgical condition in the newborn or be asymptomatic throughout life. Annular pancreas also may first become symptomatic in adulthood, producing epigastric pain, early satiety, and vomiting secondary to duodenal obstruction. Gastric and duodenal peptic ulcer disease and pancreatitis also occur with increased incidence in long-standing annular pancreas.

A typical finding of annular pancreas on UGI series is eccentric or concentric narrowing of the descending duodenum with associated mucosal effacement, but without ulceration or mucosal destruction (Fig. 4-7). The proximal duodenum may become dilated, and reversed peristalsis and dilatation of the duodenum distal to the annular narrowing have been described. CT shows the annulus surrounding and constricting the descending duodenum (Fig. 4-8). On ERCP, opacification of the ventral duct encircling the descending duodenum is diagnostic of annular pancreas. Recommended treatment of annular pancreas presenting in adulthood is surgical bypass of the narrowed segment of duodenum. Simple division of the pancreatic annulus is often insufficient for relief of symptoms because of the frequent association of duodenal stenosis and fibrosis at the site of long-standing narrowing. Division of the annulus with transection of the annular duct also may lead to pancreatitis and pancreatic fistula.

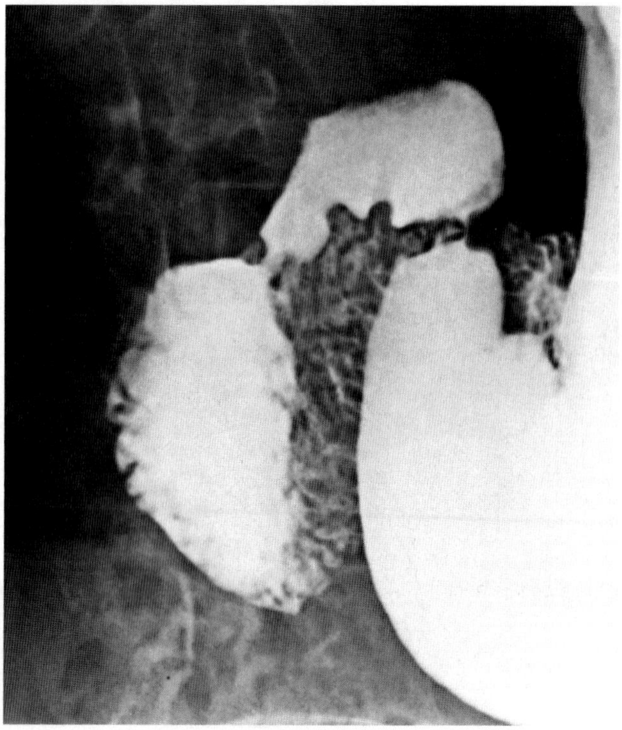

Figure 4-7 Bandlike narrowing of the duodenal sweep is due to an annular pancreas.

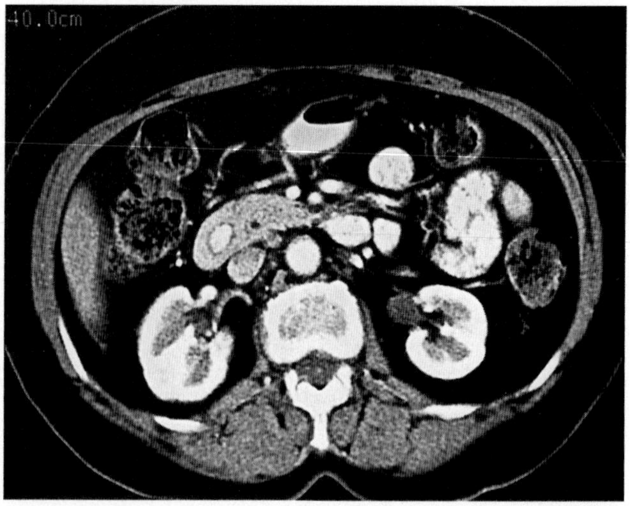

Figure 4-8 CT shows pancreatic tissue entirely surrounding the duodenum in a patient with annular pancreas.

Pancreas Divisum

Pancreas divisum is a common congenital abnormality of the pancreas, with an incidence of 11% recorded in an autopsy series. This anomaly results from failure of fusion of the embryological dorsal and ventral buds. Consequently, the dorsal and ventral ducts remain separate, with the dorsal duct draining the body, tail, and superior portion of the head of the pancreas into the minor papilla, and the ventral duct draining the uncinate process and inferior portion of the pancreatic head into the major papilla (Fig. 4-9).

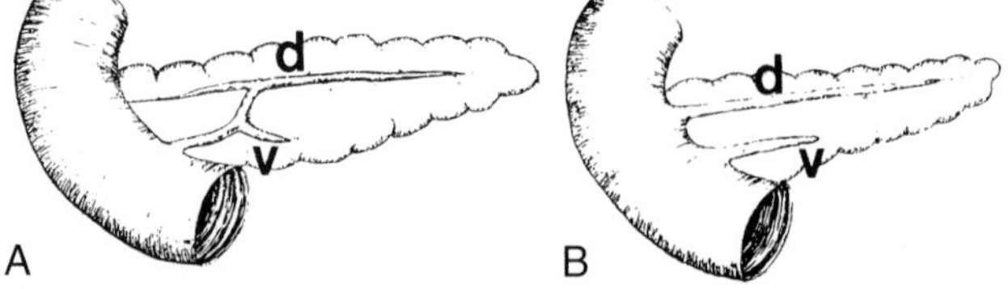

Figure 4-9 Diagrams illustrate the relationship of the ventral *(v)* and dorsal *(d)* pancreatic ducts, after fusion **(A)** and in pancreas divisum **(B)**.

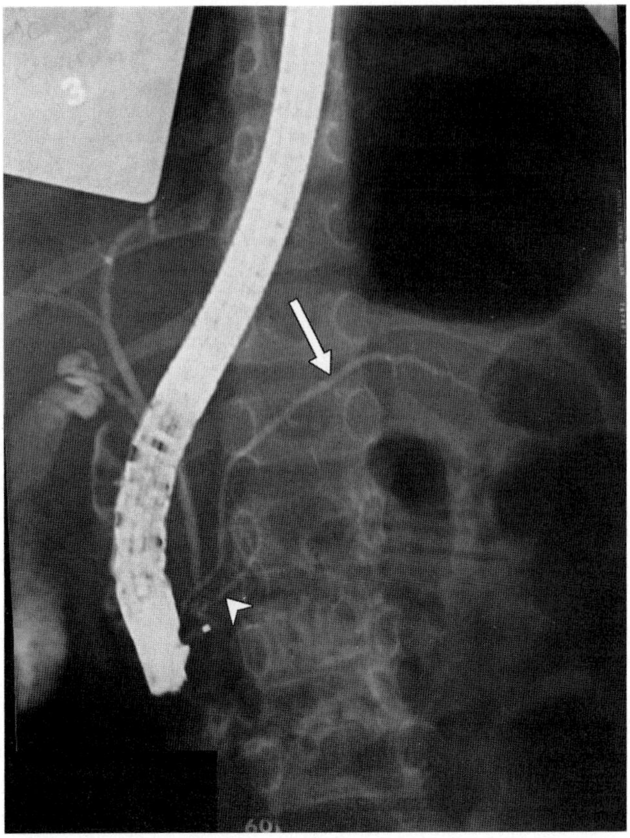

Figure 4-10 Pancreatic division. The major and minor papillae have been cannulated, and contrast material has been injected. The dorsal duct *(arrow)* and the short, arborizing ventral duct *(arrowhead)* are shown. (Courtesy of David McVinnie, M.D.)

On ERCP of pancreas divisum, injection of contrast material into the major papilla opacifies the short, tapering, arborizing ventral duct (Fig. 4-10). Visualization and cannulation of the minor papilla are often difficult because of its small size, but when accomplished show opacification of the long dorsal duct extending along the pancreatic body and tail. Thin-section CT may reveal lobulation of the pancreatic head, separation of the ventral and dorsal portions of the pancreas by a fat cleft, or failure of fusion of the ventral and dorsal ducts. Pancreatitis may occur with increased incidence in patients with pancreas divisum, possibly caused by impeded drainage of the bulk of the pancreatic parenchyma through the small minor papilla. The association of pancreatitis and pancreas divisum remains controversial, however.

Ductal Duplications

There are numerous variants of pancreatic divisum, in which the two ducts join but retain separate drainages to the duodenum (Fig. 4-11). Because of the complex nature of the joining of these ductal structures, there is no typical eventual appearance of the pancreatic ducts. Duplications of the ventral or dorsal pancreatic ducts represent rare embryological abnormalities that have been documented on ERCP (Fig. 4-12). There is no increased association of these anomalies with pancreatitis or other abnormalities.

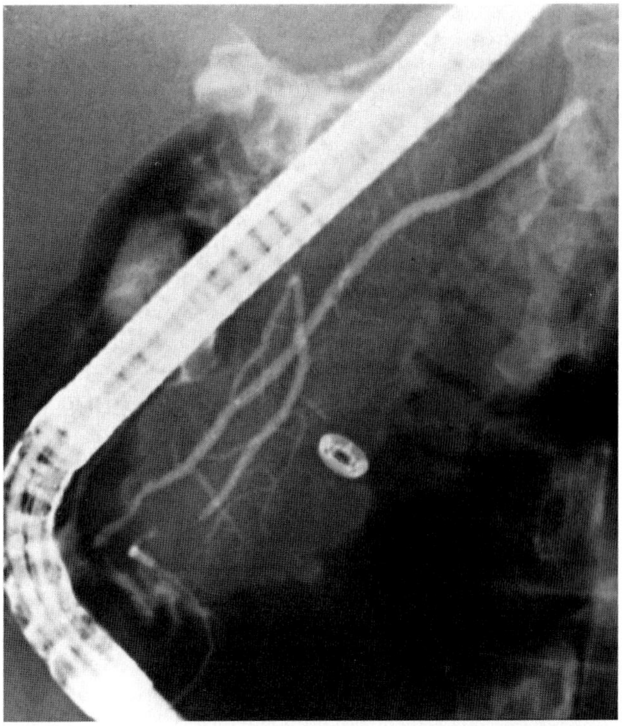

Figure 4-11 The dorsal and ventral ducts have maintained their normal size and have separate drainage paths into the duodenum. A small connecting channel is still present, however. This is a common variant of pancreas divisum.

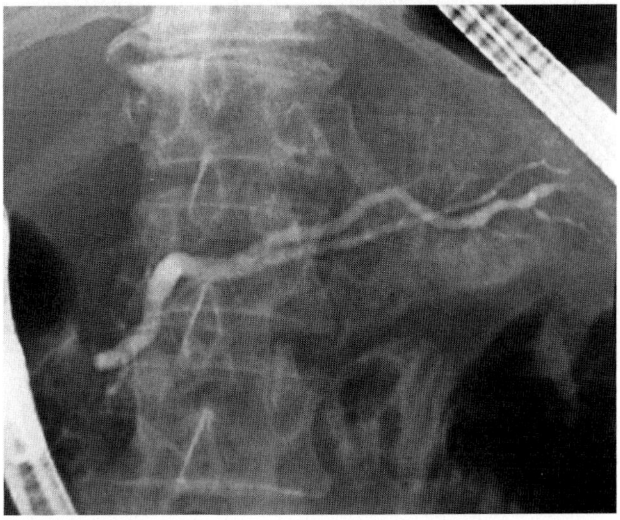

Figure 4-12 Two distinct ductal systems are seen in the body and tail because of a duplication of the pancreas.

Ectopic Pancreas

Ectopic or aberrant pancreas (pancreatic rest) represents pancreatic tissue occurring in extrapancreatic sites, most commonly along the greater curvature of the distal gastric antrum or in the periampullary portion of the descending duodenum. The ectopic tissue is typically small and submucosal in location. A tiny central umbilication that may represent a primitive pancreatic duct is sometimes noted. Ectopic pancreas, although usually asymptomatic, may cause gastrointestinal hemorrhage or obstruction, biliary obstruction, or small bowel intussusception. Rarely, inflammatory or neoplastic pancreatic lesions arise within ectopic pancreatic tissue.

Short Pancreas

Short pancreas is characterized by congenital absence of the pancreatic body and tail and a rounded appearance of the pancreatic head. This anomaly most likely results from agenesis of the dorsal pancreas and may occur as an isolated finding or in association with the polysplenia syndrome (Fig. 4-13).

Long Common Segment of Pancreatic and Common Bile Ducts

The pancreatic duct and the common bile duct normally enter the major papilla either separately or through a short common channel less than 1 cm in length. Abnormally high fusion of the ducts forms a long common channel, usually regarded as greater than 1 cm in length (Fig. 4-14). There is an increase in abnormalities of the bile ducts or pancreas when this occurs.

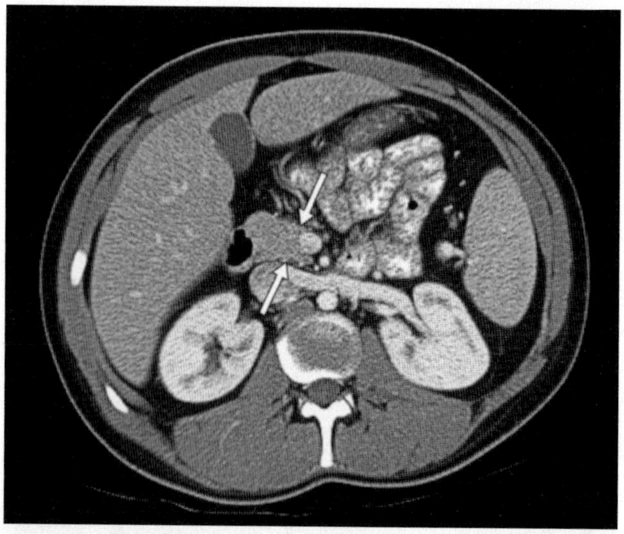

Figure 4-13 CT shows congenital absence of the body and tail of the pancreas. The spleen is in its normal location. Only the pancreatic head is seen *(arrows)*.

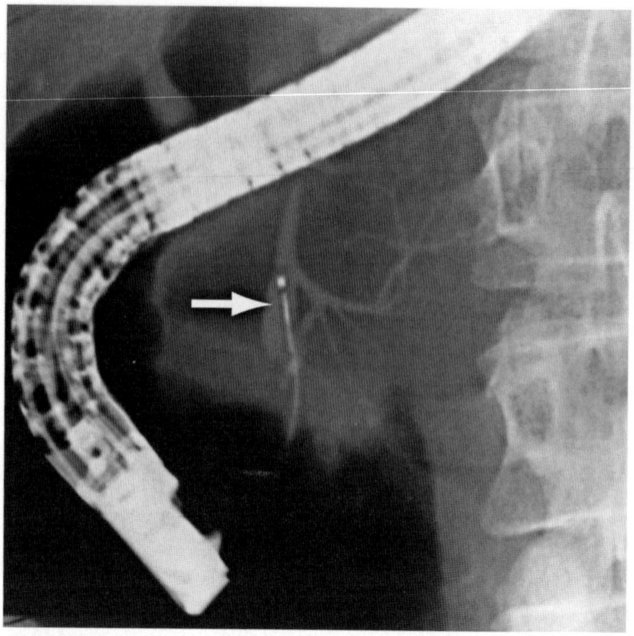

Figure 4-14 The ventral duct of the pancreas drains the head of the pancreas into the side of the common bile duct, resulting in a long common channel *(arrow)*. This patient also had pancreas divisum and a small choledochal cyst.

One theory is that reflux of pancreatic secretions into the common bile duct may lead to the development of a choledochal cyst, and a long common channel has been reported to be more common in patients with choledochal cysts. There is also an increased incidence of pancreatitis with this anomaly.

PANCREATIC SIZE

Enlarged

Pancreatitis

Acute

Acute pancreatitis often causes diffuse or focal enlargement of the pancreas secondary to inflammation and edema (Fig. 4-15). The disease is characterized by acinar damage, fat necrosis, and autodigestion. Acute pancreatitis is clinically characterized by abdominal pain radiating to the back. Serum amylase and lipase levels are elevated, and the serum calcium level is often reduced. Acute pancreatitis, although most often occurring secondary to alcohol ingestion or gallstone disease, also may result from various infections, medications, surgical or nonsurgical trauma, and metabolic or systemic disorders.

Abdominal plain films may show generalized or focal ileus (sentinel loop and colon cutoff sign) or abdominal fat necrosis in which hydrolyzed fat produces a mottled appearance (Fig. 4-16). Chest film findings at the left

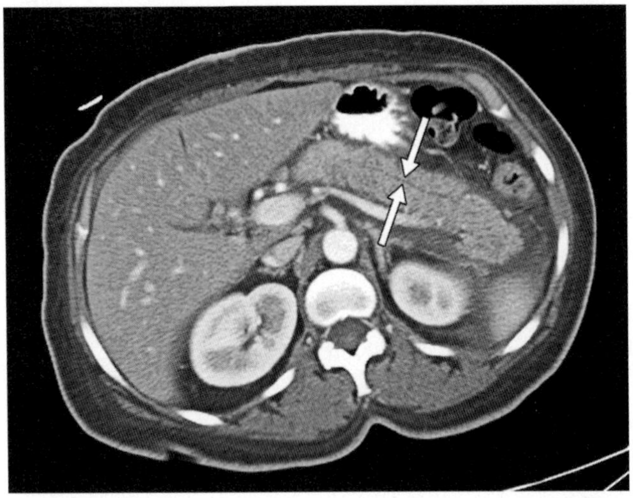

Figure 4-15 Acute pancreatitis with swelling and edema of the entire gland and hazy margins. Note the normal pancreatic duct *(arrows)*.

lung base are common and include basilar subsegmental atelectasis, pleural fluid, and elevation of the left hemidiaphragm. On UGI series, acute pancreatitis may cause widening of the duodenal sweep, thickening of duodenal folds, effacement of folds or a reverse figure 3 configuration as a result of duodenal fold tethering (Sellecks folds) along the inner aspect of the duodenal sweep, enlargement of the major papilla, or anterior displacement of the stomach as a result of organ enlargement and fluid in the lesser sac. These findings are not specific to acute pancreatitis and may be seen in chronic pancreatitis and to some extent in pancreatic carcinoma.

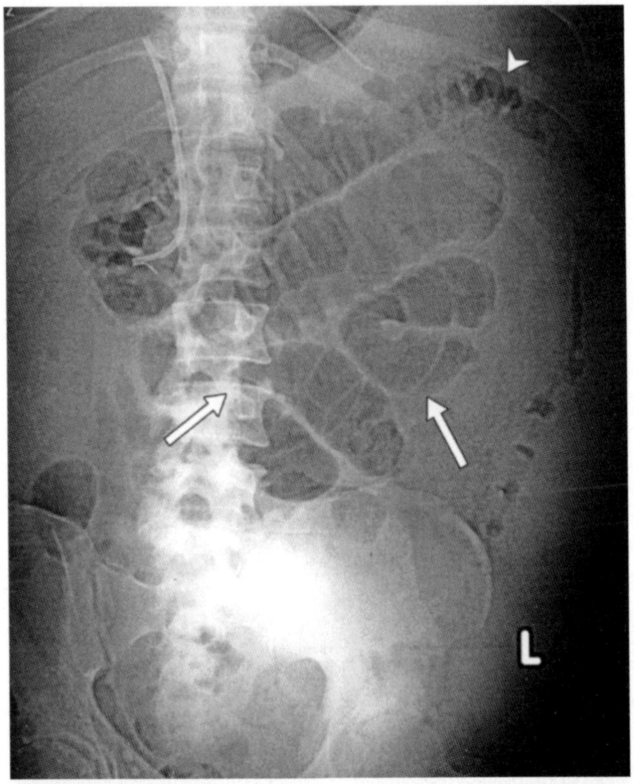

Figure 4-16 Plain film of patient with acute pancreatitis. Note collections of dilated small bowel in left upper quadrant *(arrows)* and colon cutoff *(arrowhead)*.

Ultrasound examination of acute pancreatitis typically shows diffuse or focal pancreatic enlargement, hypoechoic parenchyma, and poorly defined contour. Ultrasonography in these patients is frequently limited, however, by overlying bowel gas caused by intestinal ileus. Multidetector CT of acute pancreatitis, in addition to showing enlargement and poorly defined contour of the pancreas, may reveal inflammatory infiltration of peripancreatic and extrapancreatic fat and fascial planes. The pancreatic parenchyma usually shows decreased attenuation secondary to edema or necrosis, but on contrast-enhanced scans may appear diffusely hyperdense because of hyperemia. In acute hemorrhagic pancreatitis, a severe form of pancreatitis characterized by parenchymal hemorrhage, inflammation, and destruction, focal areas of increased attenuation are often seen on CT (Fig. 4-17). Ultrasonography and CT are useful for detecting various pancreatic and extrapancreatic fluid collections associated with acute pancreatitis. ERCP usually is contraindicated in the evaluation of acute pancreatitis because injection and manipulation of the pancreatic duct may worsen the pancreatitis. In any case in which ERCP is used as a diagnostic tool, the incidence of asympomatic laboratory pancreatitis is about 50%. Acute symptomatic pancreatitis is seen in about 3% of cases after diagnostic ERCP. The incidence increases in therapeutic ERCP.

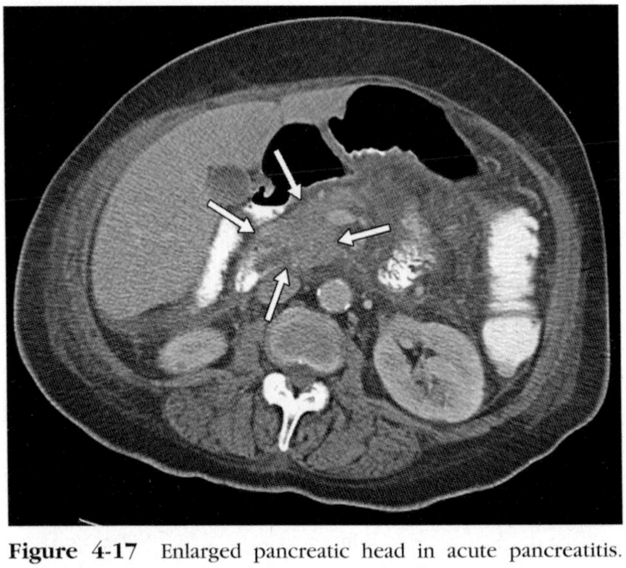

Figure 4-17 Enlarged pancreatic head in acute pancreatitis. Note swelling and edema of pancreatic head region *(arrows)*.

Chronic

Chronic pancreatitis is characterized by irreversible destruction of the pancreatic parenchyma. Similar to acute pancreatitis, chronic pancreatitis may cause focal or diffuse pancreatic enlargement. Common clinical manifestations include abdominal pain radiating to the back and severe diabetes mellitus. Amylase and lipase levels may be elevated, normal, or decreased. Chronic pancreatitis most often results from long-term alcohol ingestion, but also can be seen secondary to hereditary pancreatitis, trauma, hyperparathyroidism, and malnutrition.

Abdominal films commonly show focal or diffuse pancreatic ductal calculi. Most of the plain film and UGI findings seen in acute pancreatitis also may occur in chronic pancreatitis.

Ultrasonography and CT may show focal or diffuse pancreatic enlargement during acute relapses of chronic pancreatitis. With progression of the disease, diffuse parenchymal atrophy and ductal dilatation result (Fig. 4-18). Ultrasound may show irregular echogenicity with hyperechoic and hypoechoic areas secondary to fibrosis and edema. These alterations in parenchymal echo texture are a sensitive but nonspecific sign of chronic pancreatitis. Other findings of chronic pancreatitis seen on ultrasound examination and CT include ductal calculi, pseudocysts and other fluid collections, and biliary ductal dilatation (Figs. 4-19 and 4-20).

ERCP is useful in assessing severity and complications of chronic pancreatitis. Typical findings involving the pancreatic duct include dilatation, irregularity, and beading of the main duct; dilatation of side branches; periampullary ductal stenosis; and filling defects and obstruction caused by ductal calculi (Fig. 4-21). Opacification of the biliary tree during ERCP or percutaneous transhepatic cholangiography may reveal smooth stenosis or extrinsic displacement of the common bile duct.

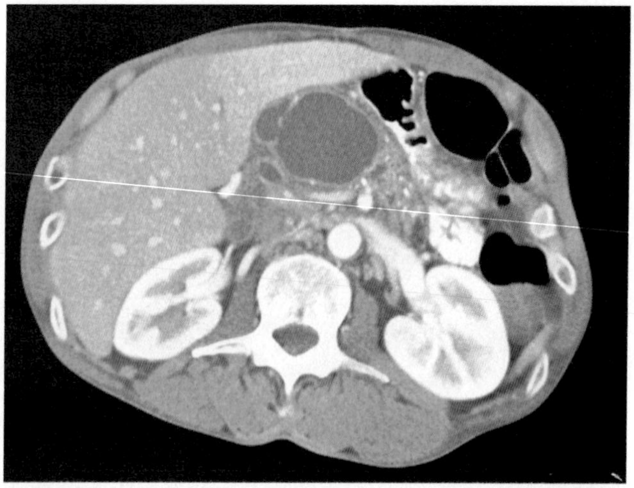

Figure 4-19 CT shows multiple pseudocysts in a patient with chronic pancreatitis.

Phlegmon and Abscess

In more severe forms of acute pancreatitis, the gland may undergo complete necrosis because of autodigestion. What may be left is a diffuse, necrotic area of tissue occupying the pancreatic bed region (Fig. 4-22). Typically, this area has low density, and strands of inflammatory changes can be seen extending into the peripancreatic areas. If this area becomes infected, an abscess can form. This type of pancreatitis is often encountered after trauma and sometimes as the result of instrumentation or surgery.

Hemorrhage

Hemorrhage into the pancreas is characterized by enlargement of the gland with either focal or diffuse areas of high attenuation (>60 HU). This increased

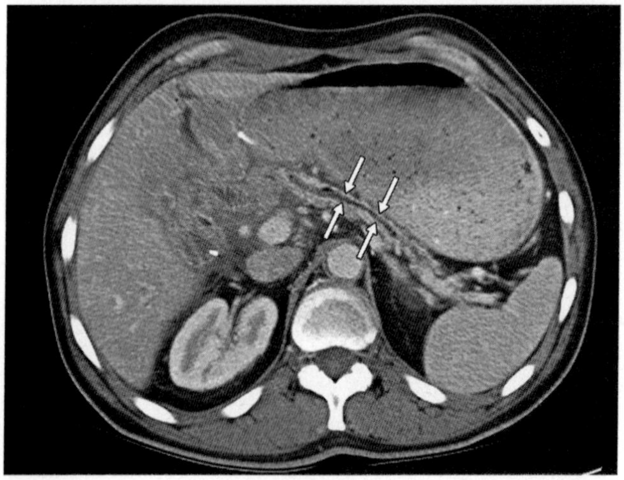

Figure 4-18 Patient with chronic pancreatitis. CT shows atrophy of the pancreas and dilated, irregular pancreatic duct *(arrows)*.

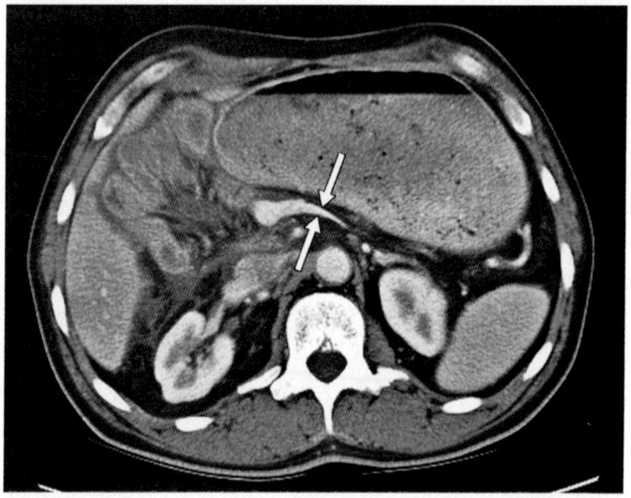

Figure 4-20 Chronic pancreatitis with atrophy of the pancreas and narrowing of the splenic vein *(arrows)* is seen.

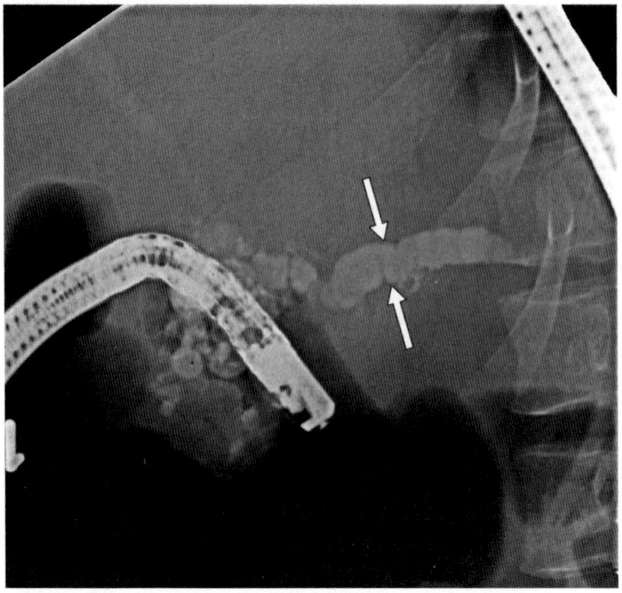

Figure 4-21 ERCP in a patient with chronic pancreatitis. The pancreatic duct is grossly dilated and beaded *(arrows)*.

density is distinctive and separates hemorrhage from other inflammatory conditions, which are typically low density.

Malignancy

Pancreatic carcinoma, islet cell tumors, and various other neoplasms may cause focal enlargement of the pancreas (Fig. 4-23). Involvement of peripancreatic nodes secondary to lymphoma or metastatic disease may mimic focal or diffuse enlargement of the pancreas itself (Fig. 4-24). Sometimes pancreatitis develops proximal to a tumor of the pancreas, which results in diffuse enlargement of the gland. In these circumstances, it may be difficult to separate the neoplastic tissue from the inflammatory changes. A distinguishing feature may be focal ductal dilatation proximal to the tumor.

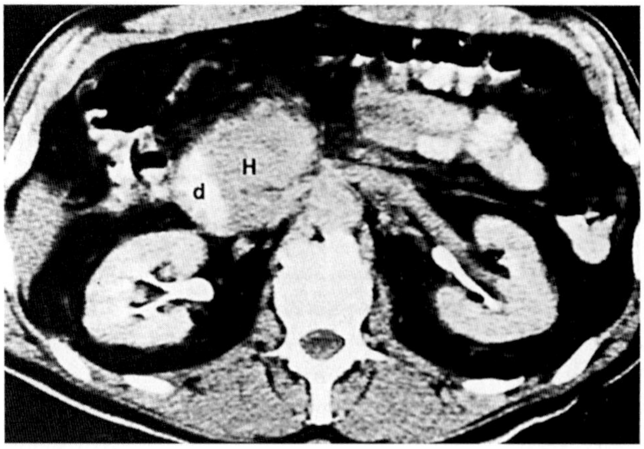

Figure 4-23 Enlargement of the pancreatic head *(H)* represents pancreatic adenocarcinoma. The adjacent duodenum *(d)* is opacified.

Fatty Infiltration

Pancreatic lipomatosis is a disorder in which the parenchyma of the exocrine pancreas is partially or completely replaced by fat. Rarely, massive pancreatic enlargement results from lipomatosis in the form of either diffuse fatty infiltration or multiple nodular fatty masses. This condition, known as lipomatous pseudohypertrophy of the pancreas, is of uncertain origin, but may result from various factors, including obesity, cystic fibrosis, diabetes mellitus, alcoholic cirrhosis, and chronic pancreatitis, as well as normal aging in older patients.

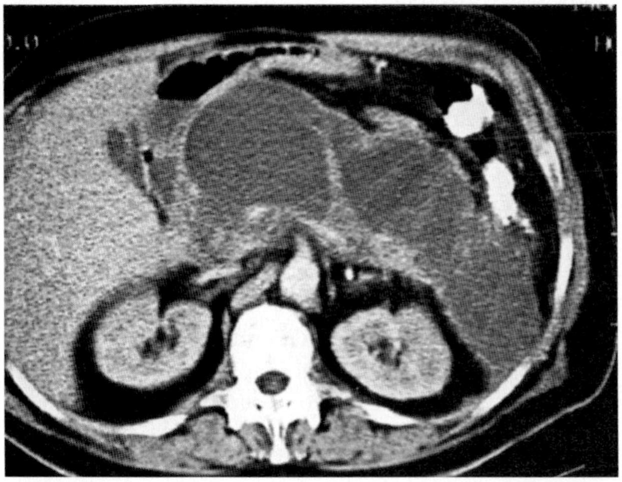

Figure 4-22 Diffusely enlarged pancreas with multiple low-density areas is due to pancreatic necrosis or phlegmon.

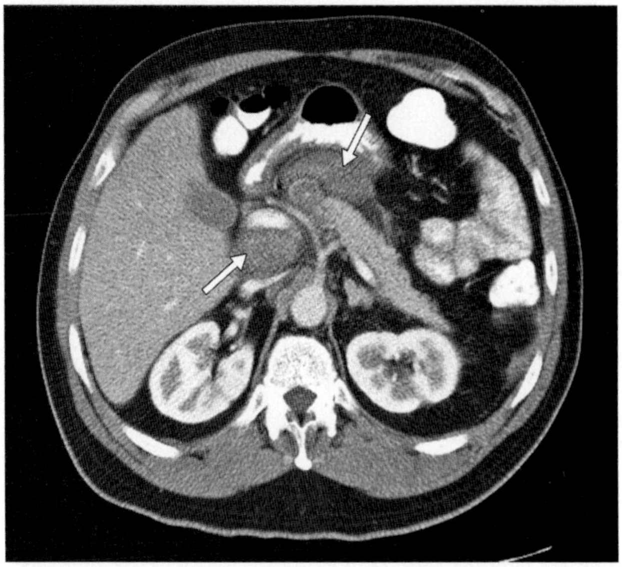

Figure 4-24 Enlargement of peripancreatic area secondary to peripancreatic nodes *(arrows)*.

Atrophic

Normal Aging

The pancreas normally decreases in size with aging and may appear atrophic in elderly patients (without a history of pancreatic disease). Associated findings include pancreatic ductal dilatation and fatty infiltration of the parenchyma. The amount of glandular tissue evident does not reflect the degree of function of the pancreas, and normal pancreatic function may persist despite apparent atrophy on imaging (Fig. 4-25).

Chronic Pancreatitis

Chronic pancreatitis often leads to diffuse atrophy of the pancreatic parenchyma. This condition is associated with parenchymal fibrosis, ductal dilatation, and ductal calculi.

Pancreatic Duct Obstruction

Long-standing obstruction of the pancreatic duct may result in parenchymal atrophy proximal to the obstructing process, involving the parenchyma surrounding the dilated segment of the duct. The obstruction may be the result of an impacted calculus or a benign or malignant tumor and may be located at the ampulla of Vater or anywhere along the course of the pancreatic duct.

Cystic Fibrosis

Cystic fibrosis (mucoviscidosis) is a common genetic (autosomal recessive) disorder in which abnormally thick mucous secretions lead to pulmonary, pancreatic, and gastrointestinal dysfunction. The disease may first become evident in a neonate as meconium ileus or in a child or young adult as recurrent pneumonia and progressive pulmonary or pancreatic insufficiency.

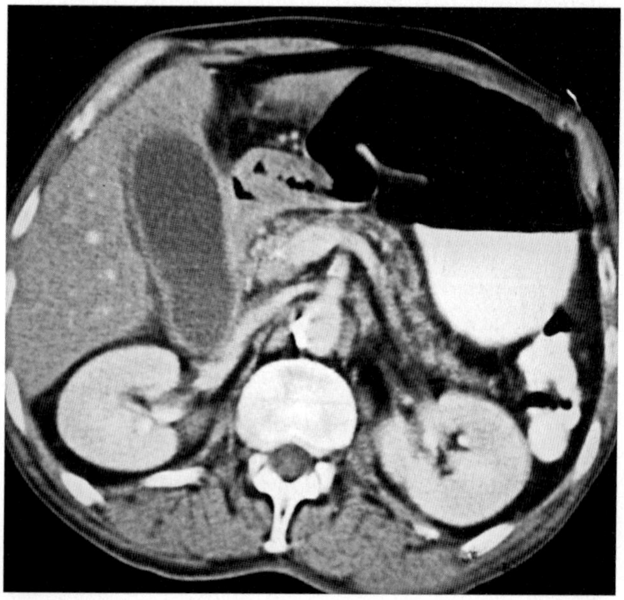

Figure 4-25 A diffusely thin pancreas is seen above the splenic vein. Atrophy is probably due to chronic pancreatitis.

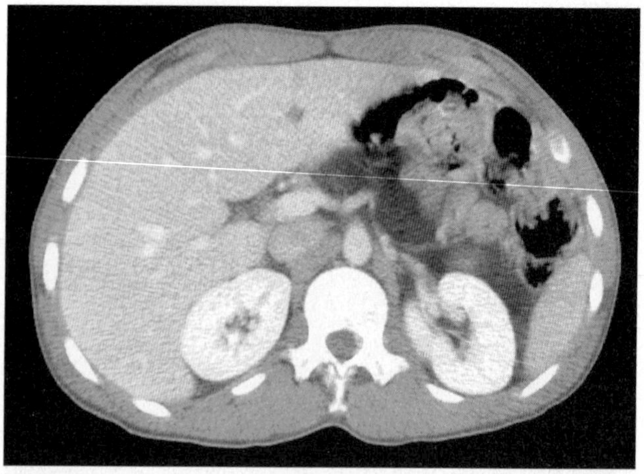

Figure 4-26 Patient with cystic fibrosis. Note the dramatic atrophic changes in the pancreatic bed with fatty replacement.

In the pancreas, mucus precipitates in the ducts and obstructs the secretion of pancreatic enzymes into the duodenum. This obstruction leads to intestinal malabsorption and steatorrhea and eventual fibrotic or fatty replacement of the exocrine pancreatic parenchyma. The pancreas may become diffusely atrophic with or without fatty replacement (Fig. 4-26).

Other Abnormalities

Congenital pancreatic hypoplasia (Shwachman's syndrome) is a rare genetic disorder characterized by abnormalities of the exocrine pancreas similar to the abnormalities seen in cystic fibrosis. In pancreatic hypoplasia, atrophy and fatty replacement of the pancreas are associated with various skeletal and hematological abnormalities. Viral infection, hemochromatosis, and malnutrition also may cause atrophy and fatty replacement of the pancreas.

PANCREATIC MASSES

Solid

Focal Acute Pancreatitis

Acute pancreatitis, although usually a diffuse process, may cause focal enlargement of any portion of the pancreas. The localized inflammatory mass may appear solid, cystic, or inhomogeneous on CT and hyperechoic, normal, or hypoechoic on ultrasonography. Focal pancreatic enlargement also may be seen in chronic pancreatitis.

Phlegmon

Pancreatic phlegmon represents diffuse pancreatic enlargement and peripancreatic inflammation secondary

Table 4-1 Epithelial Neoplasms

Tumor Type	Texture	Histology
Ductal adenocarcinoma	Solid	Malignant
Acinar cell carcinoma	Solid (partially necrotic)	Malignant
Microcystic adenoma	Cystic (numerous small cysts)	Benign
Mucinous cystic neoplasm	Cystic (fewer and larger cysts)	Premalignant or malignant
Solid and papillary epithelial neoplasm	Solid and cystic	Malignant (low grade)

to acute pancreatitis. It appears inhomogeneous on CT and ultrasonography and may resolve completely or worsen, leading to fluid collections, necrosis, or abscess formation.

Ductal Adenocarcinoma

Pancreatic ductal adenocarcinoma (pancreatic carcinoma) is the most common neoplasm of the pancreas (Table 4-1). It represents 80% to 90% of all tumors originating from the ductal epithelium of the exocrine pancreas. Approximately two thirds of pancreatic carcinomas arise in the head of the pancreas, and only 10% to 15% of the tumors are surgically resectable when first diagnosed. Even with improved methods of detection (multidetector CT), when surgical resection is performed, median postoperative survival is less than 20 months. The disease has been on the increase since the early 20th century, but has seemed to plateau in the last 25 years. It remains a serious diagnostic challenge, however, and there is some question as to whether improved conventional imaging would be the answer, or whether we must wait on microimaging of the gland in vivo, or possibly some specific screening serum marker that would indicate the presence of this deadly killer before symptoms or imaging findings.

Clinical signs and symptoms of pancreatic carcinoma are nonspecific and may include abdominal pain, weight loss, and jaundice. These signs are an indication of the advanced state of the disease. The lack of early symptoms is the major factor in the poor prognosis associated with the disease. Jaundice is present in at least half of patients at the time of diagnosis, resulting from obstruction of the extrahepatic bile ducts. The presence of a painless enlarged gallbladder in a jaundiced patient (Courvoisier's gallbladder) is highly suspicious of pancreatic adenocarcinoma or a primary bile duct lesion. UGI bleeding, thrombophlebitis (Trousseau's syndrome), and new onset of diabetes mellitus or pancreatitis also may be presenting clinical findings. Barium studies may show extrinsic compression or mural invasion of the adjacent stomach, duodenum, or transverse colon. Ultrasonography and CT have proved much more useful, however, for evaluating the pancreas, pancreatic and biliary ducts, liver parenchyma, and peripancreatic nodes, improving detection of pancreatic carcinoma and allowing determination of resectability (Fig. 4-27). These modalities also provide accurate guidance for percutaneous aspiration and biopsy of primary or metastatic pancreatic carcinoma.

Pancreatic carcinoma typically appears as a focal hypoechoic mass on ultrasound examination and a hypodense mass on CT (Fig. 4-28). Obstruction of the pancreatic duct by the mass often causes ductal dilatation and atrophy of the adjacent pancreatic parenchyma (Box 4-2). Coexistent obstruction of the intrapancreatic segment of the biliary duct also may be seen in cases of carcinoma involving the head of the pancreas. Dilatation of the pancreatic and biliary ducts is known as the double-duct sign. Although this dilatation also may result from intrapancreatic extension of cholangiocarcinoma, it is most commonly caused by carcinoma of the pancreatic head (Fig. 4-29).

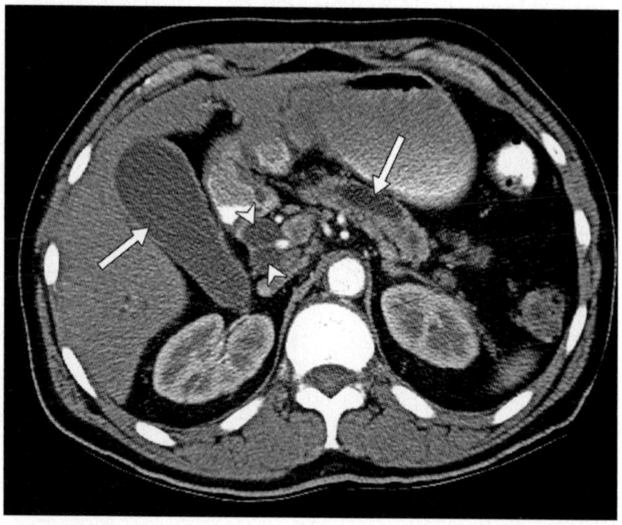

Figure 4-27 Patient with pancreatic head adenocarcinoma. Note the dilated pancreatic duct *(arrow)*, nodes in the peripancreatic region *(arrowheads)*, and Courvoisier's gallbladder *(arrow)*.

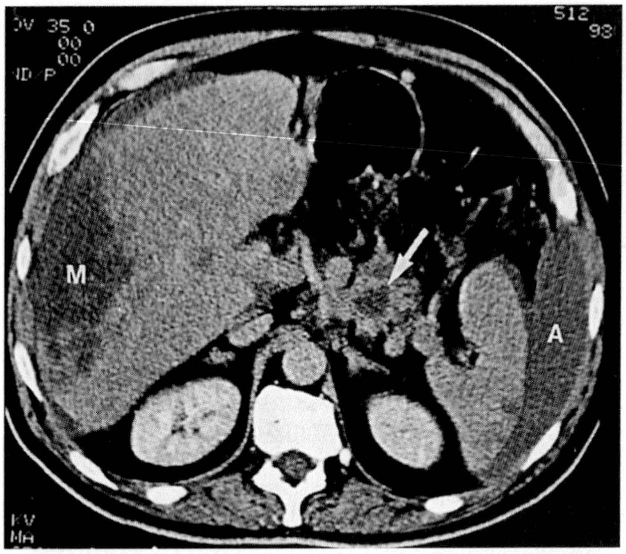

Figure 4-28 Irregular hypodense mass in the pancreatic tail *(arrow)* represents pancreatic adenocarcinoma. Hepatic metastasis *(M)* and ascites *(A)* indicate disseminated disease.

Box 4-2 Computed Tomographic Signs of Pancreatic Adenocarcinoma

Focal mass (low density)
Diffuse enlargement
Ductal dilatation
Proximal atrophy
Perivascular encasement

Box 4-3 Important Signs in Evaluating Resectability of Pancreatic Carcinoma

Liver metastases
Vascular encasement
Peritoneal implants
Peripancreatic extension
Size >3 cm
Adenopathy

Various CT criteria have been established for determining unresectability of pancreatic carcinoma (Box 4-3), including local extrapancreatic extension of tumor, invasion of contiguous organs, hepatic or regional nodal metastases, malignant ascites, and encasement or obstruction of major peripancreatic vessels. Obliteration of fat surrounding the celiac and superior mesenteric arteries, although usually secondary to vascular encasement by pancreatic carcinoma, has been reported in chronic pancreatitis and various nonpancreatic tumors, including metastatic disease and lymphoma. CT has proved to be highly effective in predicting unresectability of tumor. Of patients in whom CT findings suggest resectability of tumor, however, 20% to 40% are unresectable at surgical exploration.

An ERCP finding in pancreatic carcinoma is obstruction or encasement of the pancreatic duct (Fig. 4-30). Although involvement is usually irregular and abrupt, it occasionally appears smooth and tapering, mimicking

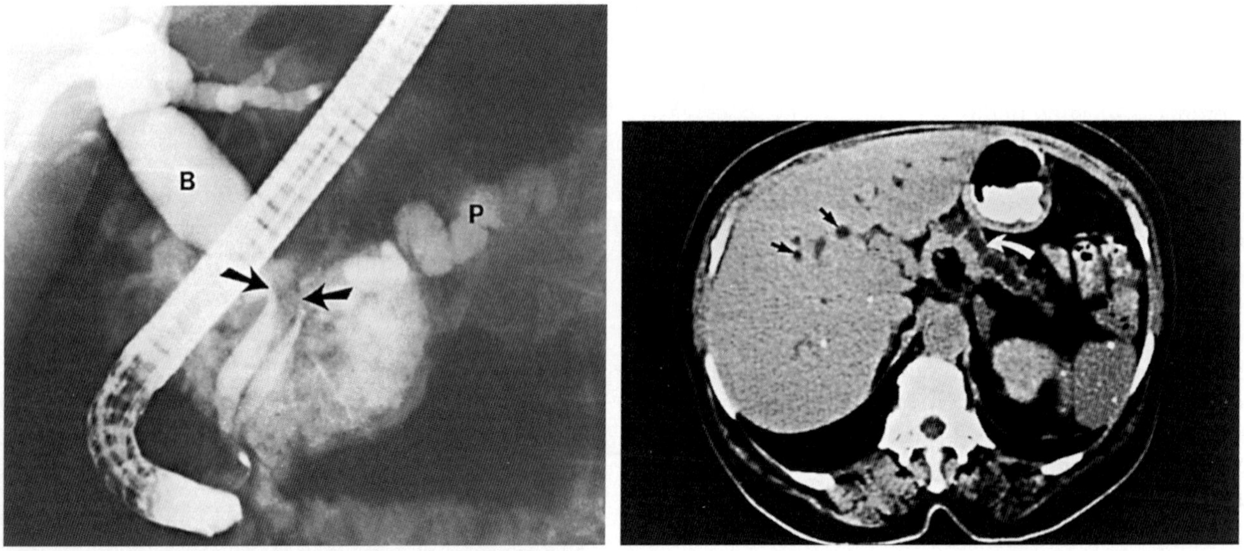

A B

Figure 4-29 **A,** ERCP shows adjacent narrowing *(arrows)* and proximal dilatation of the biliary *(B)* and pancreatic *(P)* ducts in a patient with pancreatic adenocarcinoma. **B,** CT shows dilatation of the biliary ducts *(arrows)* and pancreatic duct *(curved arrow)*.

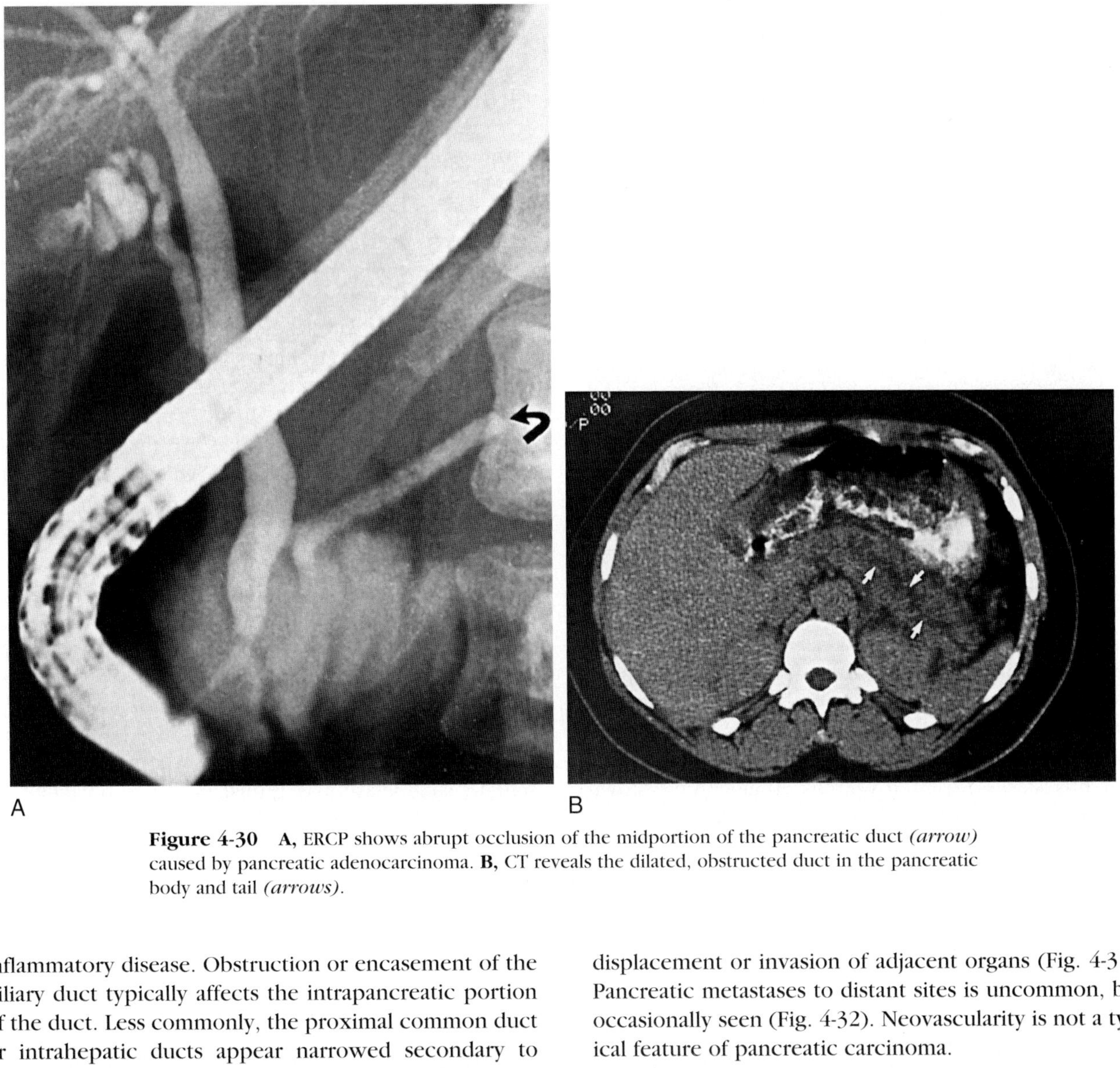

Figure 4-30 **A,** ERCP shows abrupt occlusion of the midportion of the pancreatic duct *(arrow)* caused by pancreatic adenocarcinoma. **B,** CT reveals the dilated, obstructed duct in the pancreatic body and tail *(arrows)*.

inflammatory disease. Obstruction or encasement of the biliary duct typically affects the intrapancreatic portion of the duct. Less commonly, the proximal common duct or intrahepatic ducts appear narrowed secondary to metastatic disease involving portal nodes or liver parenchyma. Opacification of an irregular cavity within the pancreas may result from tumor necrosis and subsequent communication between the tumor and the pancreatic duct. In cases of biliary duct obstruction, an internal biliary stent can be placed endoscopically during ERCP to achieve decompression.

Similarly, percutaneous transhepatic cholangiography may be performed to detect the level and degree of biliary duct obstruction secondary to pancreatic carcinoma. Pancreatic carcinoma may cause irregular or smooth narrowing of the biliary duct. Internal or external biliary drainage can be achieved by percutaneous stent placement immediately after percutaneous transhepatic cholangiography. The most common angiographic finding in pancreatic carcinoma is encasement of peripancreatic arteries or veins (Box 4-4). Less common findings include vascular occlusion, angulation, and displacement or invasion of adjacent organs (Fig. 4-31). Pancreatic metastases to distant sites is uncommon, but occasionally seen (Fig. 4-32). Neovascularity is not a typical feature of pancreatic carcinoma.

Box 4-4 Vascularity of Pancreatic Masses

HYPOVASCULAR

Adenocarcinoma
Lymphoma
Mucinous cystic neoplasms
Most metastases
Focal pancreatitis

HYPERVASCULAR

Islet cell tumors
Microcystic adenoma
Rare metastases (melanoma, hypernephroma)

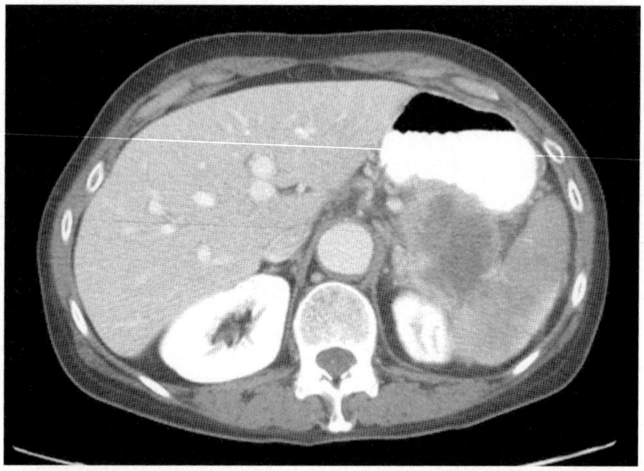

Figure 4-31 A large cystic carcinoma of the tail of the pancreas is seen invading the adjacent spleen and splenic vein.

Acinar Cell Carcinoma and Other Epithelial Tumors

Acinar cell carcinoma is a rare tumor arising from acinar cells of the exocrine pancreas (see Table 4-1). This tumor may be associated with elevated serum lipase levels and disseminated intraosseous and subcutaneous fat necrosis. Acinar cell carcinomas usually appear large, lobulated, and partially necrotic when first detected, and liver metastases are often present. Angiography shows moderate vascularity and vascular encasement and neovascularity.

Other rare pancreatic tumors of epithelial cell origin include pleomorphic carcinoma, adenosquamous carcinoma, and pancreatoblastoma. Radiographic findings are similar to those of pancreatic ductal adenocarcinoma.

Islet Cell Tumors

Tumors arising from the islet cells of the pancreas produce a variety of clinical and radiographic findings. Islet cells, classified as APUD cells because of their chemical properties of *a*mine *p*recursor *u*ptake and *d*ecarboxylation, elaborate various hormones, including insulin, glucagon, gastrin, and somatostatin (Table 4-2). APUD cells migrate from neural crest tissue during embryological development and are found not only in the pancreas, but also throughout the gastrointestinal tract and in endocrine organs, including the thyroid, parathyroid, and adrenal medulla.

Pancreatic islet cell tumors are divided into functioning and nonfunctioning types. The functioning types are hormonally active and are divided further according to the hormone that they produce and the subset of islet cells from which they arise (see Table 4-2). Functioning islet cell tumors may be associated with multiple endocrine neoplasia type I (MEN I or Wermer's syndrome), an autosomal dominant disease characterized by hyperplasia or neoplasia of the pituitary and parathyroid glands. Approximately 15% to 20% of patients with APUD tumors have MEN I syndrome. These tumors are usually multiple and may involve any subset of islet cells. Islet cell tumors also are found in approximately 20% of patients with von Hippel–Lindau disease, an autosomal dominant syndrome that includes central nervous system hemangioblastomas, retinal angiomas, renal cell carcinoma, and pheochromocytoma.

Insulinoma, the most common type of functioning islet cell tumor (about 75%), originates from the beta islet cell and produces insulin. Approximately 90% of these tumors are benign, solitary, and less than 2 cm in diameter at the time of diagnosis. They produce a symptom

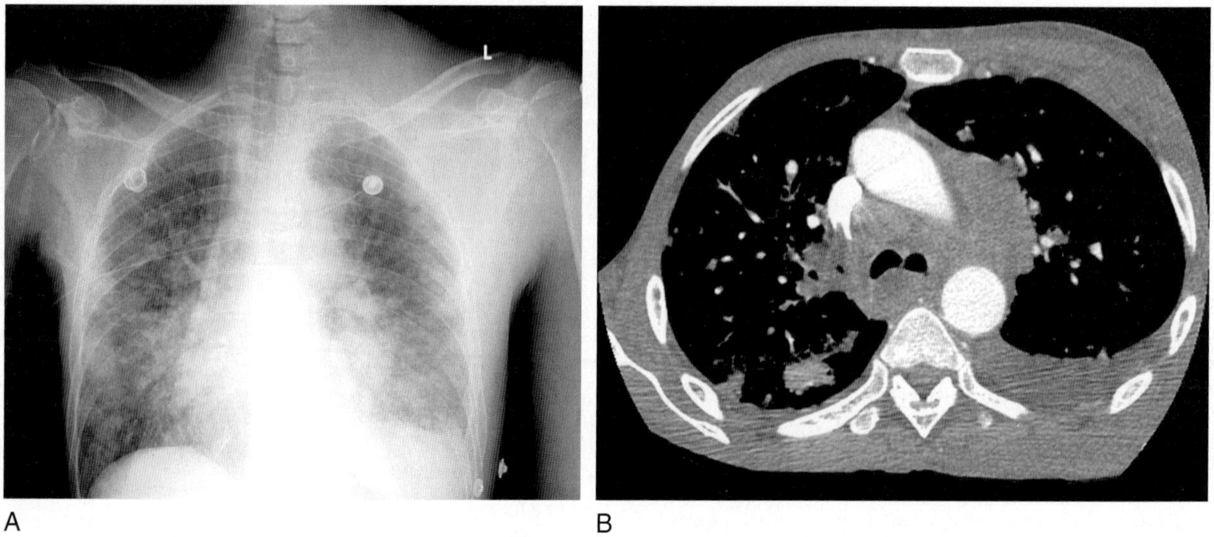

Figure 4-32 **A,** Metastatic spread of primary pancreatic adenocarcinoma to the lungs. **B,** Metastatic spread of pancreatic adenocarcinoma to the mediastinum and lungs in the same patient.

Table 4-2 Functioning Islet Cell Tumors

Tumor Type	Cell of Origin	Hormone Produced	Malignancy (% Cases)	Clinical Findings
Insulinoma	Beta	Insulin	10	Hypoglycemia
Gastrinoma	Alpha-1	Gastrin	60	Zollinger-Ellison syndrome
Glucagonoma	Alpha-2	Glucagon	80	Diabetes mellitus, necrolytic migratory erythema
Vipoma	Delta-1	VIP	50	WDHA syndrome
Somatostatinoma	Delta	Somatostatin	67 (4/6 reported cases)	Diarrhea, weight loss

VIP, vasoactive intestinal polypeptide; WDHA, watery diarrhea, hypokalemia, and achlorhydria.

complex known as Whipple's triad, which consists of hypoglycemia, central nervous system abnormalities related to hypoglycemia (including confusion, loss of consciousness, and seizures), and rapid response to oral or intravenous administration of glucose.

Clinical symptoms and laboratory evaluation usually lead to early diagnosis of insulinoma, and radiological studies are indicated primarily for localizing the tumor before surgical resection. Angiography using superselective injections can detect 80% to 90% of insulinomas and typically shows a well-defined hypervascular mass. CT typically shows a small enhancing mass that may or may not deform the pancreatic contour. Insulinomas also may be detected using radionuclide scans (Fig. 4-33). Ultrasound examination reveals a hypoechoic, solid mass. Because of the small size of most insulinomas, careful technique is essential for radiographic detection (CT with dynamic bolus and thin axial slices, real-time or

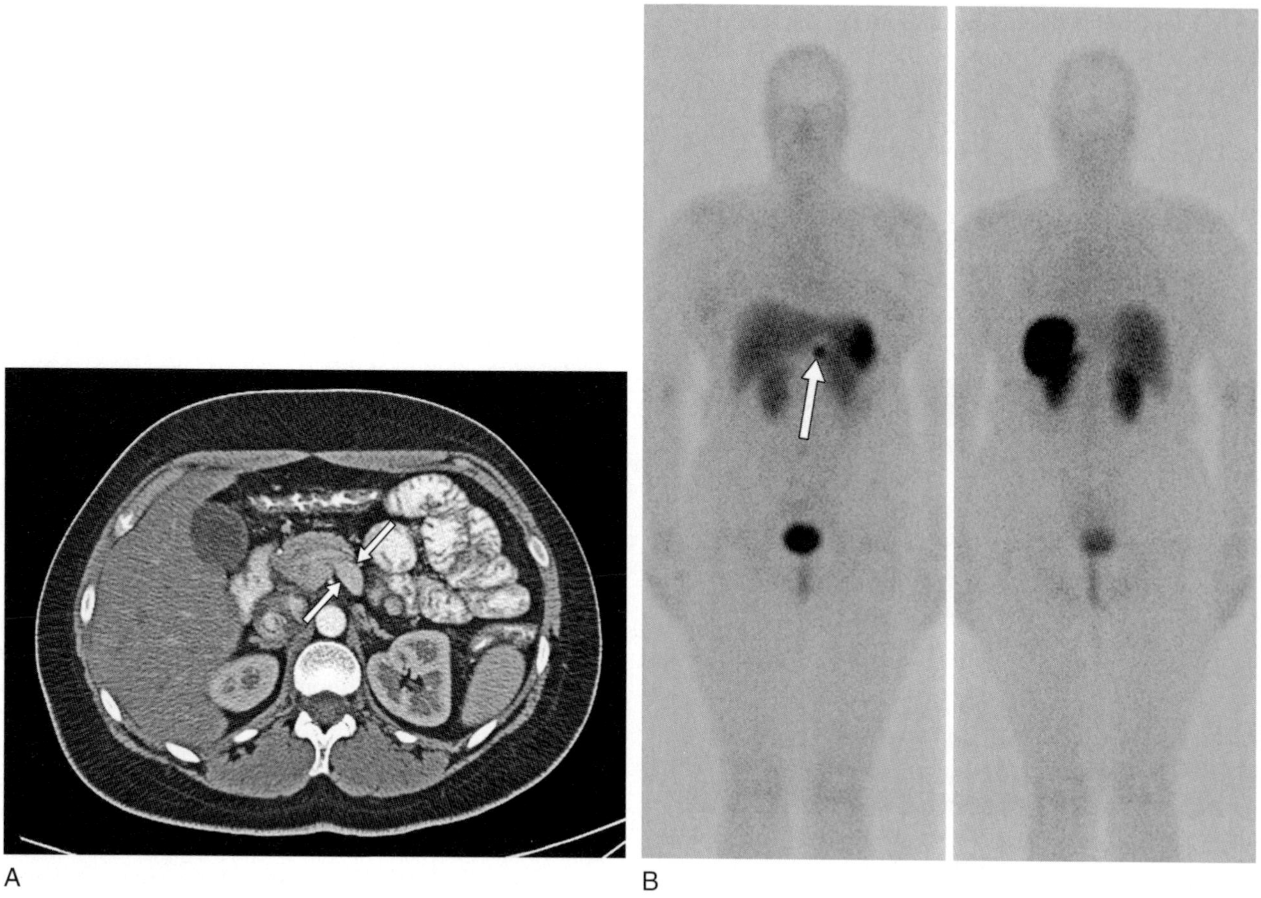

Figure 4-33 **A,** A 30-year-old woman with a small insulinoma at genu of pancreas *(arrows)*. **B,** Octreotide scan in same patient shows uptake in the epigastrium *(arrow)*.

high-frequency intraoperative ultrasound). Gastrinoma, the second most common type of functioning islet cell tumor, arises from the alpha-1 islet cell and produces gastrin. Approximately 60% of these tumors are malignant, and 50% to 66% have metastasized when diagnosed. Elevated serum gastrin levels produce Zollinger-Ellison syndrome, in which increased output of gastric acid in the stomach leads to an ulcer diathesis in the duodenum and proximal jejunum. In 10% to 40% of patients with Zollinger-Ellison syndrome, pancreatic gastrinomas are associated with MEN I.

As a result of the small size and sometimes ectopic location of primary gastrinomas, imaging studies have not proved reliable in their detection. Because gastrinomas frequently metastasize, CT and ultrasonography are useful for showing extrapancreatic disease, however, and determining an appropriate course of treatment. In the absence of metastases, surgical resection of the primary tumor is curative. If metastases are present, however, gastric acid hypersecretion can be controlled by either total gastrectomy or medical treatment with histamine H_2 receptor antagonists or omeprazole.

Glucagonomas are uncommon islet cell tumors and arise from the alpha-2 islet cell and produce glucagon. This slow-growing tumor is malignant in approximately 80% of cases and is often large and metastatic when first diagnosed. It usually occurs in the body or tail of the pancreas and metastasizes to the regional lymph nodes or liver (Fig. 4-34). Pancreatic glucagonomas and their liver metastases are typically hypervascular (see Fig. 4-5). Clinical findings include diabetes mellitus, anemia, weight loss, hypoaminoacidemia, and necrolytic migratory erythema (a recurrent skin rash that may blister and crust).

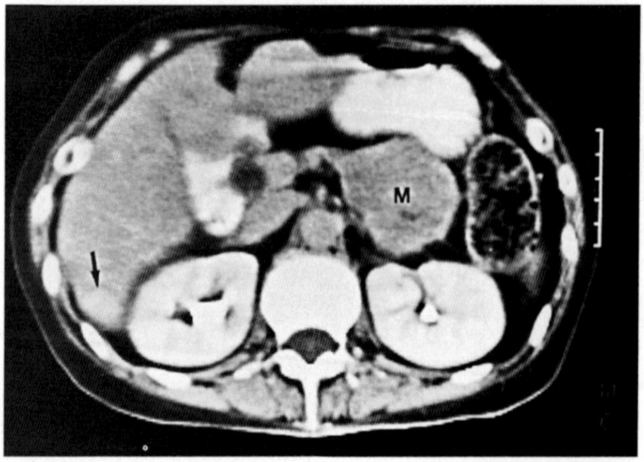

Figure 4-34 Contrast-enhanced CT shows a large soft tissue mass *(M)* in the pancreatic tail and an enhancing mass in the right lobe of the liver *(arrow)* in a patient with metastatic pancreatic glucagonoma. (From Goodman P, Kumar R: Diagnostic radiology case number 11. Intern Med 12:46, 1991.)

Vipoma (VIPoma) originates in the delta-1 islet cells and secretes vasoactive intestinal polypeptide (VIP). This tumor is malignant in 50% of cases and occurs most often in the pancreatic body and tail. Originally described by Verner and Morrison in 1958, vipoma produces a syndrome characterized by watery diarrhea, hypokalemia, achlorhydria, and hypovolemia (WDHA or WDHH syndrome). The primary tumor typically appears large and hypervascular on angiography.

Somatostatinoma, a rare tumor arising in the delta islet cell, produces somatostatin. Of the few reported cases of somatostatinoma, most were hypervascular, malignant, and associated with diarrhea and weight loss.

Nonfunctioning (or nonhyperfunctioning) islet cell tumors do not produce the clinical symptoms typical of their functioning counterparts. They constitute about 20% of all islet cell tumors. Only insulinomas and gastrinomas are more common. Although nonfunctioning tumors may secrete hormones, the type or amount of hormone produced cannot be detected or measured.

Nonfunctioning islet cell tumors are usually large and commonly are metastatic at the time of diagnosis. They cause nonspecific clinical symptoms related to focal mass effect, including abdominal pain, jaundice, and gastrointestinal bleeding or obstruction. Although typically hypervascular, nonfunctioning tumors may undergo focal necrosis because of their large size. Imaging studies are useful for showing the large primary tumor and local or distant metastases.

MRI shows islet cell tumors. The tumor has very high signal (white) on T2-weighted and short tau inversion recovery imaging. Gadolinium-enhanced MRI results in further hyperintensity of the tumor, especially during the hepatic artery phase. In comparison, pancreatic adenocarcinoma shows much less enhancement on T2-weighted studies and is much less vascular with gadolinium enhancement.

Lymphoma and Other Nonepithelial Tumors

Lymphoma rarely occurs as a primary tumor of the pancreas. More commonly, pancreatic involvement results from secondary spread of non-Hodgkin's lymphoma. Lymphoma may affect the pancreas, peripancreatic lymph nodes, or both (Fig. 4-35). Although typically large with solid, uniform texture, pancreatic lymphoma may appear cystic or inhomogeneous on cross-sectional imaging studies. Other radiographic findings of lymphoma include displacement of the pancreatic duct and vessels by the mass and displacement of the pancreas itself by adjacent peripancreatic adenopathy. Lymphoma may mimic pancreatic carcinoma, but is less likely to cause vascular or ductal encasement. Other rare pancreatic tumors of nonepithelial cell origin include hemangiomas, lymphangiomas, and sarcomas.

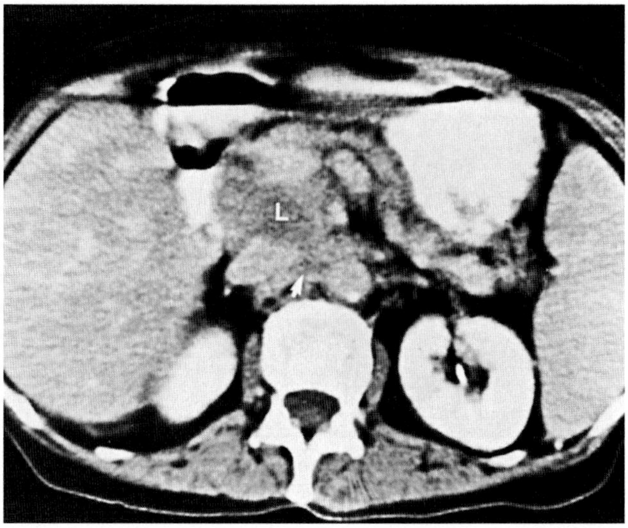

Figure 4-35 Hypodense masses occupying the peripancreatic *(L)* and interaortocaval regions *(arrow)* represent non-Hodgkin's lymphoma.

Metastases

Metastasis to the pancreas usually occurs through contiguous spread from adjacent organs, including the colon and stomach. Hematogenous metastases that may involve the pancreas include renal cell carcinoma; hepatoma; melanoma; leiomyosarcoma; and carcinoma of the breast, lung, ovary, or prostate. Pancreatic metastases are usually asymptomatic, but may cause recurrent acute pancreatitis (Fig. 4-36). Radiographically, pancreatic metastases may appear solid or cystic and show variable degrees of vascularity. Metastatic disease involving peripancreatic lymph nodes surrounding the head of the pancreas may mimic a primary pancreatic tumor. Rarely, metastatic tissue can infiltrate the interstitium of the pancreas without affecting the glandular substance itself (Fig. 4-37).

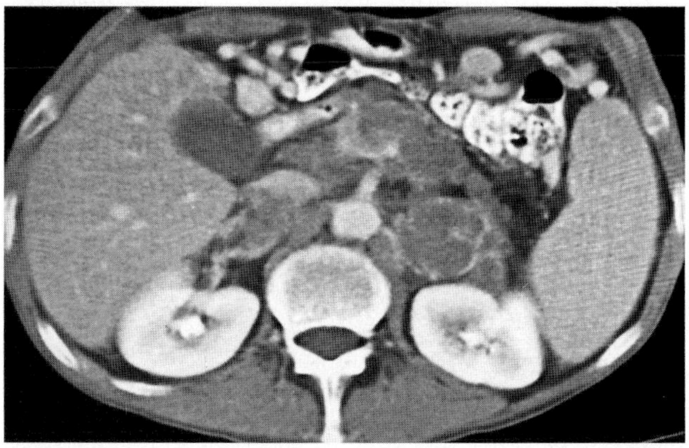

Figure 4-36 Multiple low-density solid lesions in the pancreas are from metastatic small cell carcinoma of the lung.

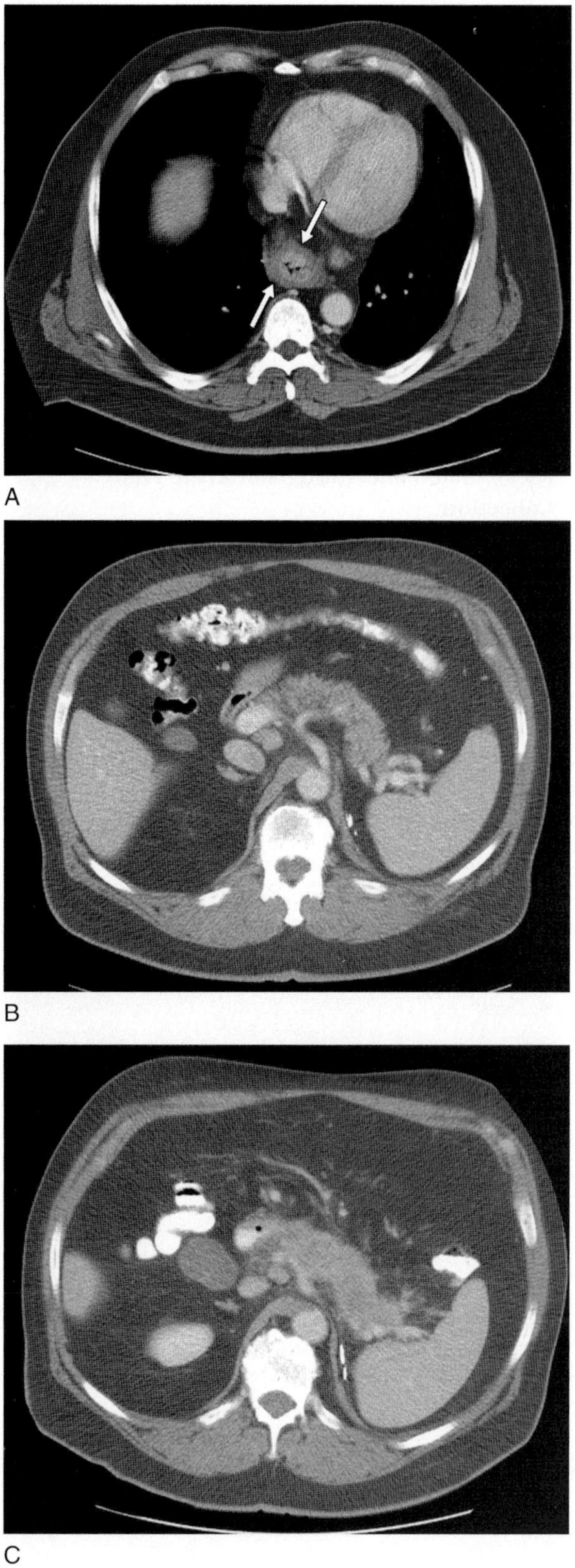

Figure 4-37 **A,** Carcinoma of the esophagus *(arrows)* is seen. **B,** The appearance is normal in this pancreas at the time of diagnosis of esophageal cancer. **C,** Same patient 6 months later. A biopsy specimen showed normal pancreatic tissue with esophageal metastatic disease in the pancreatic interstitium.

Cystic

Inflammatory pancreatic cystic lesions include focal acute pancreatitis, acute fluid collections, retention cysts, necrosis, and abscesses. A variety of neoplastic processes also may appear cystic on CT (Box 4-5). Pancreatic pseudocyst is a relatively common complication of pancreatitis. Pseudocysts can be of variable size and multiple and can be found not only in or around the pancreas, but also in sites more distant. Drainage of pseudocysts has been controversial. Most pseudocysts are sterile, however, and if asymptomatic probably should be left alone. Drainage, if necessary, is probably best effected with a percutaneous catheter technique.

Focal Acute Pancreatitis and Acute Fluid Collection

Focal acute pancreatitis may produce a cystic-appearing pancreatic mass resulting from localized edema. This mass appears hypoechoic on ultrasonography and shows low attenuation on CT. Acute fluid collections (phlegmon) occur secondary to release of pancreatic secretions from ruptured pancreatic ductules in acute pancreatitis. These collections may be confined to the pancreas or extend into the surrounding tissues. Acute fluid collections lack a fibrous capsule, but can be well defined or poorly marginated. Most resolve spontaneously over several weeks.

Pseudocysts

Pseudocysts are well-encapsulated collections of fluid that develop after pancreatitis. They begin as collections of necrotic tissue, secretions, and blood from one or more episodes of pancreatitis. In contrast to acute fluid collections, pseudocysts are surrounded by a fibrous capsule. They lack an epithelial lining, however, and are not considered true cysts. Pseudocysts occur in approximately 10% of patients with acute pancreatitis, but are more commonly associated with chronic pancreatitis (Figs. 4-38 and 4-39). Although usually located in the pancreas or peripancreatic region, pseudocysts may occur in areas distant from the pancreas (Fig. 4-40). Other causes of pseudocysts include trauma and surgery. Although uncomplicated pseudocysts appear cystic on CT and ultrasonography, superimposed hemorrhage or infection may cause the fluid contents to appear complex or inhomogeneous. As mentioned previously, asymptomatic pseudocysts are probably best left alone and observed.

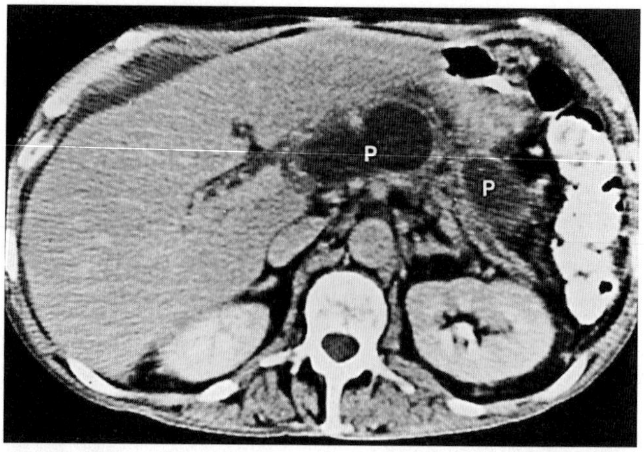

Figure 4-38 Cystic masses *(P)* represent pancreatic pseudocysts.

Box 4-5 Cystic Masses of the Pancreas

INFLAMMATORY

Pseudocysts and phlegmons
Abscess
Echinococcal cyst

TRUE CYSTS
Solitary
Multiple

Cystic fibrosis
Adult polycystic kidney disease
von Hippel-Lindau disease

NEOPLASTIC
Benign

Microcystic adenoma
Cystic teratoma

Malignant

Mucinous cystic adenocarcinoma
Papillary epithelial neoplasm
Cystic islet cell tumors (rare)

Retention Cysts

Retention cysts result from focal obstruction of pancreatic ductules. The cysts are usually small and lined with epithelium. Although most often seen in chronic

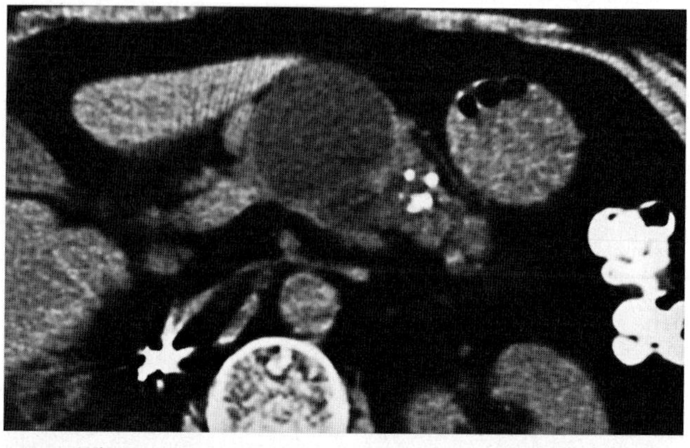

Figure 4-39 Large pancreatic pseudocyst is seen in the body. Note the pancreatic calcifications proximally, caused by chronic pancreatitis.

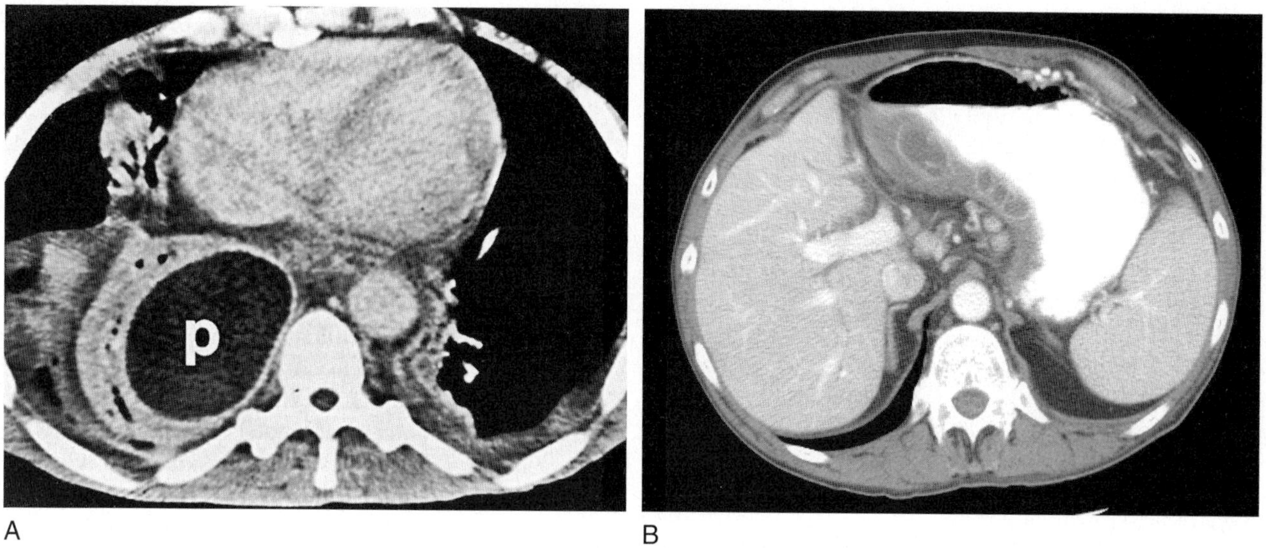

Figure 4-40 **A,** Fluid collection *(p)* in the posterior right hemithorax represents a pseudocyst surrounded by pulmonary consolidation. **B,** Pancreatic pseudocysts are seen within the medial wall of the stomach in a patient with chronic pancreatitis.

pancreatitis, retention cysts also may occur in pancreatic carcinoma, gallbladder disease, ampullary stenosis, acute pancreatitis, and various parasitic diseases associated with acute pancreatitis, including ascariasis and clonorchiasis. Hydatid disease of the pancreas may show multiseptated cysts that represent the echinococcal daughter cysts.

Necrosis and Abscess

Pancreatic necrosis (phlegmon) represents devitalized pancreatic tissue secondary to acute pancreatitis and resultant ischemia (Fig. 4-41). This devitalized tissue produces a diffuse or localized decrease in density of the pancreatic parenchyma on CT. Pancreatic abscess formation or fistulization to an adjacent hollow viscus may complicate pancreatic necrosis, forming gas collections within the pancreatic parenchyma in 25% of cases (Box 4-6). Pancreatic abscess develops in approximately 4% of patients with pancreatitis and may require prompt surgical débridement and drainage (Fig. 4-42).

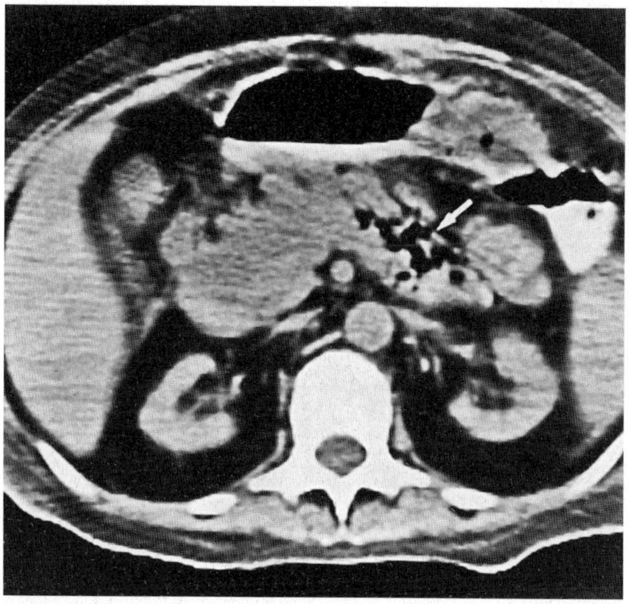

Figure 4-41 Numerous air bubbles *(arrow)* are seen in the pancreatic tail of a patient with pancreatitis and pancreatic necrosis.

Congenital Pancreatic Cysts

Congenital pancreatic cysts have an epithelial lining and are classified as true cysts. Solitary congenital cysts vary in size and may appear unilocular or multilocular.

Box 4-6 Computed Tomographic Differentiation of Inflammatory Cystic Lesions of the Pancreas

PSEUDOCYST

Low density
Well-defined wall
Possible calcification

PHLEGMON

Variable density
Poorly defined wall
Inflammatory changes present

ABSCESS

Variable density
Wall variable
Gas (approximately 30%)

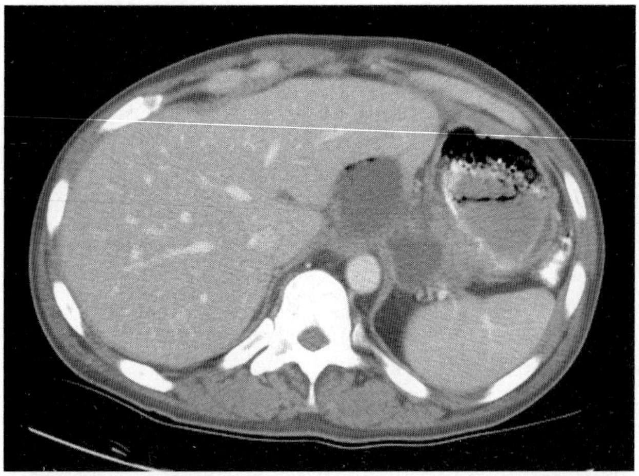

Figure 4-42 A large cavity with irregular walls is seen in the tail. This represents a pancreatic abscess.

They are seen mostly in neonates and result from abnormal segmentation of rudimentary pancreatic ducts. CT and ultrasound examination show their fluid content and thin wall.

Multiple congenital cysts are usually associated with adult polycystic kidney disease, von Hippel-Lindau disease, or cystic fibrosis. Multiple pancreatic cysts occur in 10% of patients with adult polycystic kidney disease and in 25% to 72% of patients with von Hippel-Lindau disease. The pancreatic cysts occurring in cystic fibrosis represent the sequelae of chronically dilated pancreatic ductal structures.

Intrapancreatic choledochal cysts and duodenal duplication cysts are other congenital lesions that can mimic true pancreatic cysts. Duplication or enterogenous cysts of the pancreas itself are extremely rare.

Microcystic Adenoma

Cystic tumors of the pancreas represent 5% to 15% of pancreatic cystic masses (see Table 4-1). Approximately half of these tumors are classified as microcystic adenoma (serous cystadenoma or glycogen-rich cystadenoma), and the other half are classified as macrocystic or mucinous cystic neoplasms (mucinous cystadenoma and cystadenocarcinoma). These tumors arise from ductal epithelium of the exocrine pancreas and together account for approximately 2% to 5% of nonfunctioning pancreatic neoplasms.

Microcystic adenomas can occur in any portion of the pancreas and are composed of numerous small cysts, each 0.1 to 2 cm in diameter. The cysts are lined by low cuboidal epithelium containing glycogen. These slow-growing tumors, although often discovered incidentally, may become large and produce symptoms of bowel or biliary duct obstruction. About 80% of cases are first detected after age 60, and the female-to-male ratio is 1.5:1. Microcystic adenoma occurs with increased incidence in patients with von Hippel-Lindau disease. Although microcystic adenoma is generally considered a benign lesion, a single case of malignancy has been reported.

CT of microcystic adenoma typically shows a low-attenuation mass on noncontrast scans and a honeycombed or spongy appearance on contrast-enhanced scans as a result of hypervascularity of the septa (Fig. 4-43). Overall, attenuation of the mass on contrast-enhanced scans varies from solid to cystic. A central scar with or without calcification is often present.

On ultrasound examination, microcystic adenoma appears primarily hyperechoic or hypoechoic, depending on the size of cysts and the number of fibrous septa. Angiography typically reveals hypervascularity and neovascularity, but hypovascular lesions also have been described.

Mucinous Cystic Neoplasms

Mucinous cystic neoplasms occur most often in the tail of the pancreas and are rarely seen in the pancreatic head. They typically are composed of no more than six cysts, with each cyst measuring more than 2 cm in diameter. The cysts are lined by tall columnar epithelium that produces mucin. The tumors are usually large and bulky when first detected. The mean age of patients with mucinous cystic neoplasms is 50 years old, and women are affected six to eight times more often than men. Mucinous cystadenoma, the benign form of mucinous cystic neoplasm, is generally considered premalignant.

CT and ultrasonography of mucinous cystic neoplasms show a multilocular or, less often, unilocular cystic lesion that may contain septations, papillary projections, or mural nodules (Figs. 4-44 and 4-45). Although contrast-enhanced CT may show enhancement of the septa and cyst wall, these areas are better visualized using ultrasound. Angiography reveals a hypovascular mass, and peripheral curvilinear calcifications are found in approximately 15% of cases. In the absence of metastatic

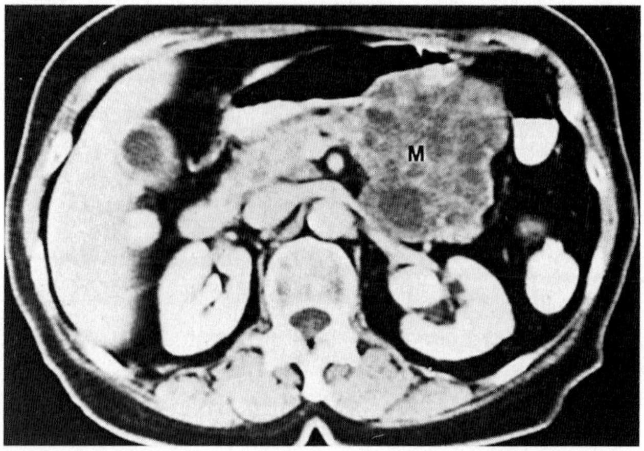

Figure 4-43 Large mass *(M)* composed of numerous small cysts represents a microcystic adenoma of the pancreatic tail.

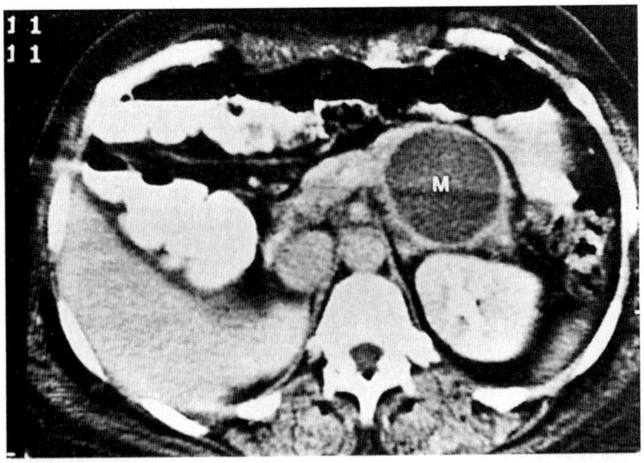

Figure 4-44 Large unilocular cystic mass *(M)* in the pancreatic tail represents a mucinous cystic neoplasm.

disease, benign and malignant lesions are difficult to distinguish radiographically.

Mucinous Pancreatic Duct Ectasia

Mucinous pancreatic duct ectasia (duct ectatic mucinous cystadenoma and cystadenocarcinoma) is a rare tumor of the pancreatic duct that has histological features similar to those of mucinous cystic neoplasms. This tumor consists of clusters of small, thin-walled cysts that cause dilatation of the side branches of the main pancreatic duct. This tumor occurs most often in the uncinate process of the pancreas and may undergo malignant transformation.

Solid and Papillary Epithelial Neoplasms

Solid and papillary epithelial neoplasms of the pancreas (papillary cystic tumors) are rare tumors arising from acinar cells (see Table 4-1). They most often affect young women and can arise in any portion of the pancreas. These large, well-circumscribed masses usually contain solid and cystic areas resulting from focal necrosis and hemorrhage (Fig. 4-46). Calcifications and septations rarely occur. These tumors are considered low-grade malignancies with a good prognosis after resection.

Other Pancreatic Cystic Tumors

Cystic islet cell tumors of the pancreas result from central necrosis of nonfunctioning or functioning islet cell tumors. These lesions are locally invasive and potentially or frankly malignant. A similar cystic appearance may be seen in necrotic pancreatic ductal adenocarcinoma and in metastatic lesions involving the pancreas (Fig. 4-47). Other rare pancreatic tumors that may appear cystic on radiographic studies include acinar cell carcinoma, cystic teratoma (Fig. 4-48), lymphoma, hemangioma, lymphangioma, sarcoma, and various types of anaplastic carcinoma.

PANCREATIC DUCT

The normal pancreatic duct size varies, but there are some guidelines by which to evaluate the duct. Typically, the duct is largest in the head, usually not exceeding 5 mm in diameter (Fig. 4-49). It gradually tapers towards the tail, and the distal duct is typically less than 3 mm in diameter. However, there are mild undulations in the course of the duct in normal individuals. Typically, these undulations have smooth margins and are not abrupt changes in caliber. Even subtle changes in caliber may indicate early disease, however.

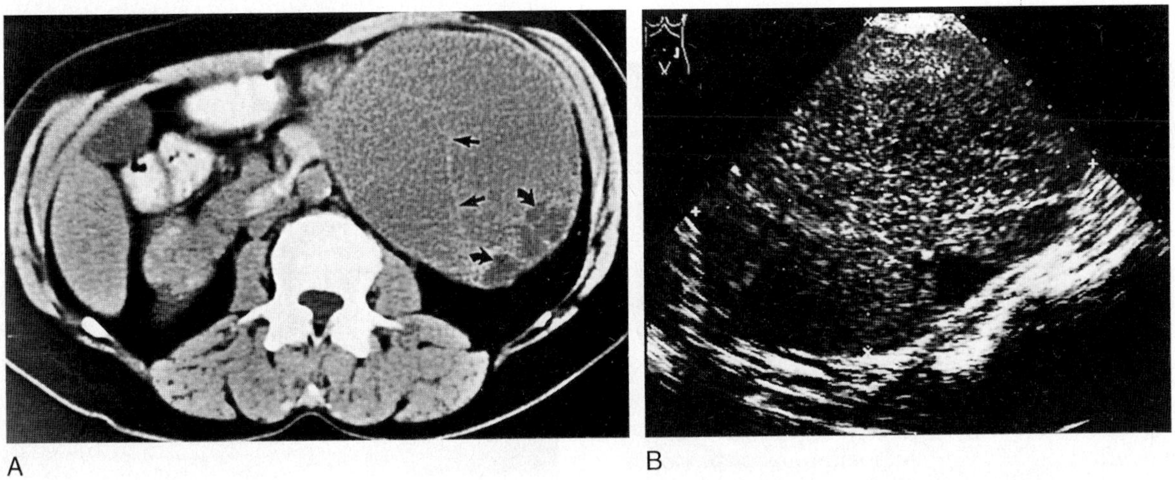

Figure 4-45 **A,** CT shows a large cystic mass containing septations *(arrows)* and mural nodules *(curved arrows)* in a patient with mucinous cystic neoplasm of the pancreas. **B,** Ultrasonogram shows numerous internal echoes throughout the mass.

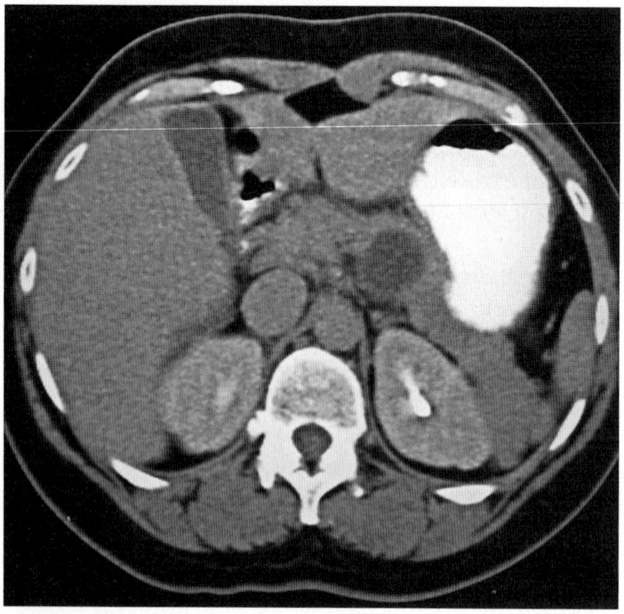

Figure 4-46 Small low-density cystic lesion in the body is a cystic adenoma.

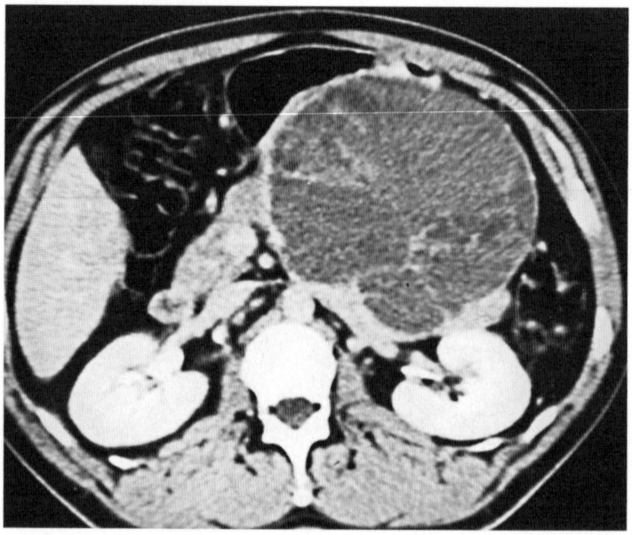

Figure 4-48 Large cystic mass with septations was found to be a cystic teratoma at surgery.

Dilated

Normal Aging

As individuals age, the pancreatic duct becomes slightly larger. This increase in size is probably the result of mild atrophy of the gland rather than any type of obstructive condition. It is not unusual with the newer CT scanners to identify the pancreatic duct in normal older individuals and even younger persons; this does not indicate disease. Distinguishing features of aging, particularly on ERCP, are that the duct shows diffuse enlargement, the changes are not focal, and the margins remain smooth.

Pancreatitis

Chronic pancreatitis (but not acute) also results in enlargement of the duct. This enlargement is the result of parenchymal loss and strictures that may develop as the result of repeated inflammation (Fig. 4-50). The changes of chronic pancreatitis include multifocal to diffuse areas of dilatation with scattered, bandlike areas of narrowing. The side branches of the pancreatic duct also are dilated or blunted and may show some clubbing. The degree of pancreatic duct change usually mirrors the severity of repeated inflammation and the degree of pancreatic dysfunction.

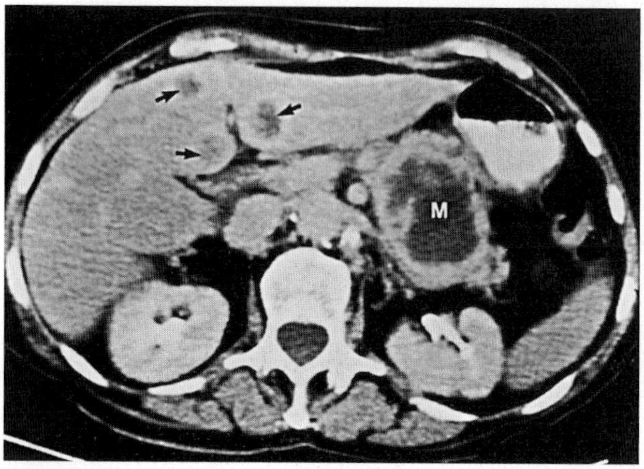

Figure 4-47 Irregular cystic mass *(M)* represents necrotic adenocarcinoma of the pancreatic tail. Hypodense hepatic lesions *(arrows)* indicate metastases.

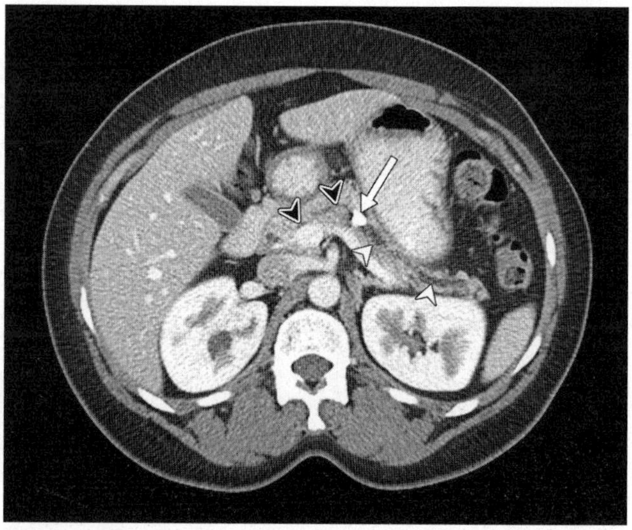

Figure 4-49 Ductal changes in a pancreatic duct obstructed by a stone *(arrow)*. Note the dilated duct distal to the stone *(white arrowheads)* and the normal-caliber duct proximal to the stone *(black arrowheads)*.

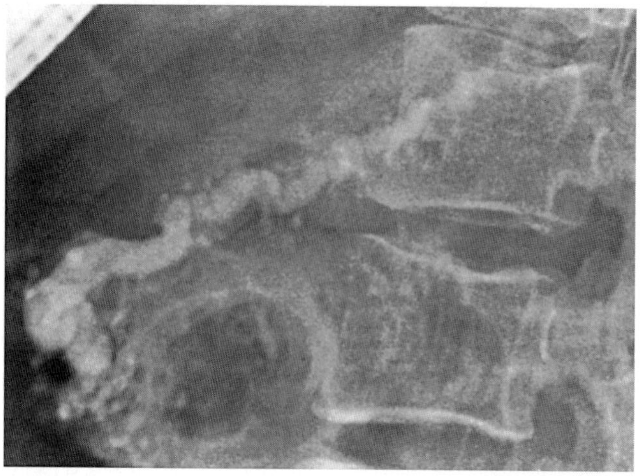

Figure 4-50 Dilated, tortuous main pancreatic duct and dilated side branches are seen in a patient with chronic pancreatitis.

Neoplasms

Neoplasms also produce pancreatic ductal dilatation; this is the result of dilatation proximal to the strictured area (Fig. 4-51). As the degree of neoplastic stricturing increases, the proximal dilatation worsens and begins to resemble chronic pancreatitis. There also is associated glandular atrophy in the areas proximal to the tumor. This dilatation is identifiable because it can be seen only proximal to the stricture. Typically, neoplastic strictures are much longer than the strictures seen with chronic pancreatitis.

Narrowed

Pancreatitis

The most common cause of narrowing of the pancreatic duct is prior inflammation, as from pancreatitis. Strictures secondary to pancreatitis can have a variety of appearances. Some features that are more typical of pancreatitis are multifocal, short, and bandlike (Fig. 4-52). Occasionally the strictures of pancreatitis are solitary or focal, which makes it much more difficult to distinguish from malignant strictures. If a pseudocyst is present, it may produce a focal compression of the pancreatic duct and may be difficult to distinguish from malignancy.

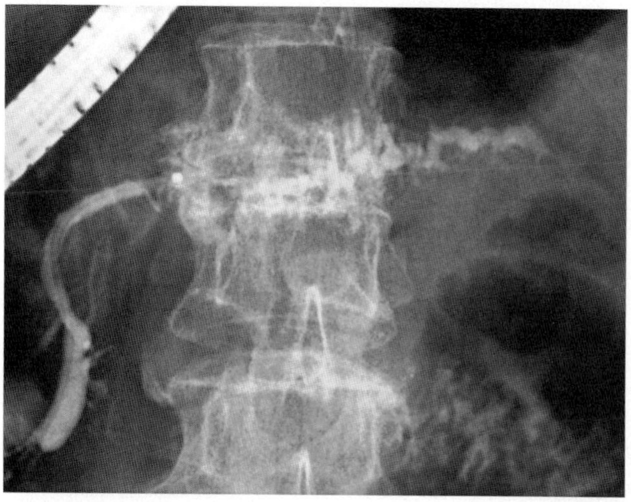

Figure 4-51 Dilated pancreatic duct is seen in the body and tail, with a normal duct in the head. This is due to a pancreatic carcinoma partially obstructing the duct and producing changes of pancreatitis proximally.

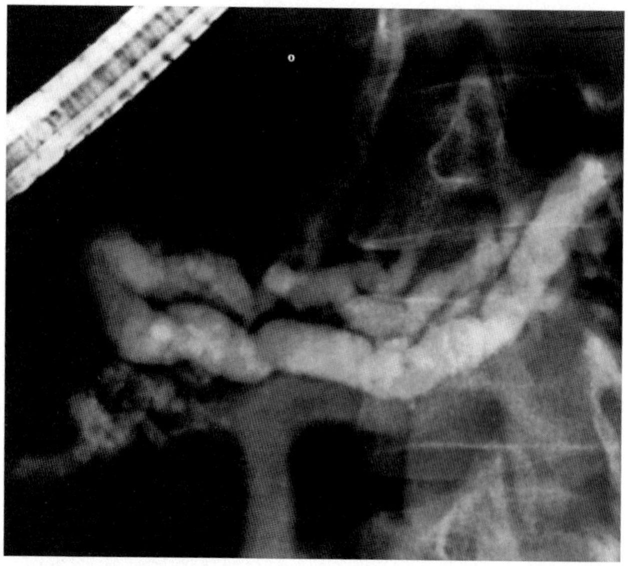

Figure 4-52 Bandlike areas across the ducts are a sequela of chronic pancreatitis. Note the duplication of the pancreatic ducts.

Neoplasms

Typical strictures produced by pancreatic malignancy are focal and have tapered margins; this is because pancreatic cancer infiltrates around the duct and produces circumferential narrowing. Because the process begins outside the lumen of the duct, the margins are tapered or smooth, not abrupt as in other gastrointestinal malignancies (Fig. 4-53).

Developmental Variation

In certain circumstances, there may be focal areas of narrowing of the pancreatic ducts in normal individuals. As mentioned previously, the pancreatic duct normally has mild undulations along its course. There may be a naturally occurring bend or narrowing where the ventral duct of Wirsung fuses with the dorsal duct of Santorini. To distinguish these physiological narrowings from pathological strictures, one must look for proximal dilatation and delayed emptying on the postdrainage film.

CALCIFICATIONS

Pancreatitis

Radiographically visible pancreatic calcifications occur in approximately 50% of patients with chronic pancreatitis secondary to alcohol ingestion. The calcifications

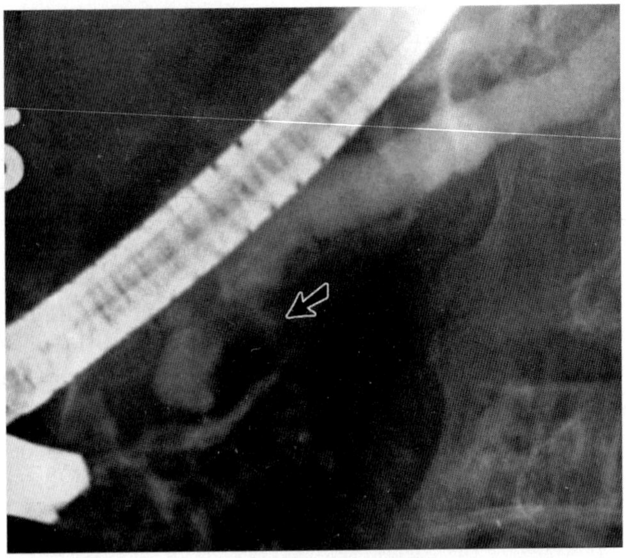

Figure 4-53 Area of narrowing *(arrow)* is due to pancreatic carcinoma.

Box 4-7 Differentiation of Pancreatic Calcifications

SMALL, PUNCTATE

Pancreatitis
Hyperparathyroidism
Cystic fibrosis

ROUND, LARGER

Hereditary pancreatitis
Ductal calculi

CURVILINEAR

Pseudocyst
Hematoma
Mucinous cystadenocarcinoma

STELLATE (STARBURST)

Microcystic adenoma

lie within the pancreatic ducts and vary in size, shape (Box 4-7), and distribution (Fig. 4-54).

Hereditary pancreatitis is an unusual form of chronic pancreatitis that shows autosomal dominant genetic transmission. The disease begins in childhood and recurs throughout adult life. It is characterized by a high incidence of pancreatic calculi. These calculi reside within the ducts and are much larger than calculi seen in conventional chronic pancreatitis (Fig. 4-55). Patients with hereditary pancreatitis have a 20% chance of developing pancreatic carcinoma.

Pseudocysts

Pancreatic pseudocysts sometimes have curvilinear calcification in the cyst wall (Fig. 4-56). These calcifications can be thick and diffuse and may involve the entire periphery of the pseudocyst. When they involve only a portion of the cyst, they are curvilinear and indistinguishable from calcifications seen in cystic neoplasms.

Neoplasms

Mucinous cystic neoplasms contain peripheral curvilinear calcifications in approximately 15% of cases (Fig. 4-57). Compared with pseudocysts, however, the calcification involves only a portion of the wall or septation and is curvilinear in appearance. Microcystic adenomas occasionally show stellate calcification within a central fibrous scar on plain films or CT.

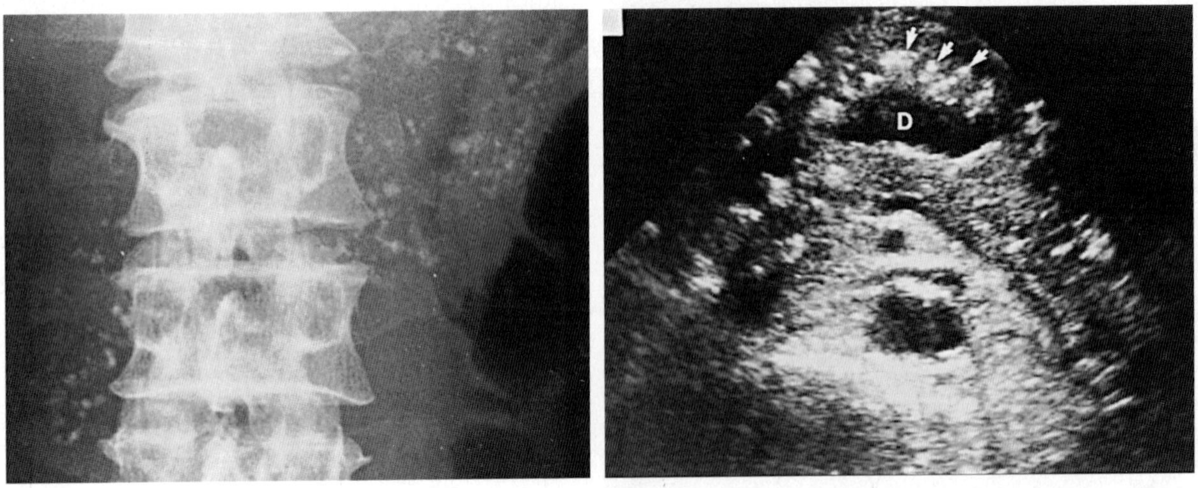

A B

Figure 4-54 **A,** Speckled calcifications in the midabdomen represent pancreatic calculi secondary to chronic pancreatitis. **B,** Ultrasonogram shows a markedly dilated pancreatic duct *(D)* and multiple pancreatic calcifications *(arrows)*.

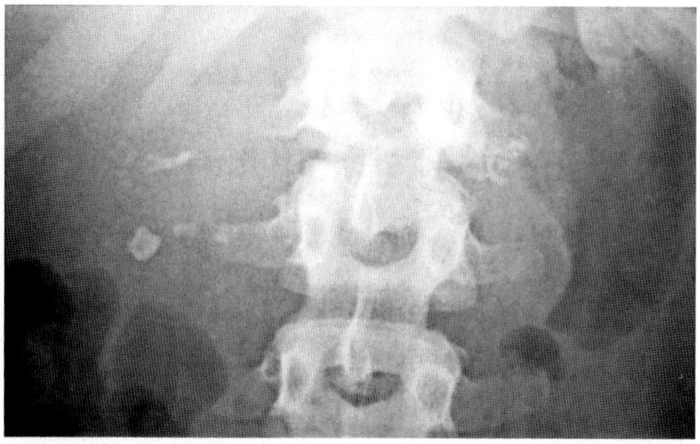

Figure 4-55 Large calculi reside in the head of the pancreas (actually in the main pancreatic duct) in a patient with congenital pancreatitis.

Dystrophic calcification may occur in solid and papillary epithelial neoplasms. Calcifications also have been reported in nonfunctioning islet cell tumors and rarely in gastrinomas associated with MEN I syndrome. Cavernous lymphangiomas of the pancreas are rare tumors that may contain calcifications in dilated lymphatic channels.

Hyperparathyroidism

Hyperparathyroidism may cause pancreatitis and pancreatic calcifications, most likely as a result of hypercalcemia.

Cystic Fibrosis

Pancreatic calcifications in cystic fibrosis typically appear granular and may be either focal or diffuse. Calcium precipitates within dilated pancreatic ductules secondary to obstruction by mucous plugs or within the pancreatic parenchyma secondary to extravasation of pancreatic enzymes from ruptured ductules and acini. Pancreatic calcifications in cystic fibrosis often are associated with marked pancreatic fibrosis and diabetes mellitus.

Malnutrition and Other Causes

In tropical countries, an idiopathic form of pancreatitis associated with pancreatic ductal calculi may result from malnutrition caused by a diet low in protein and high in

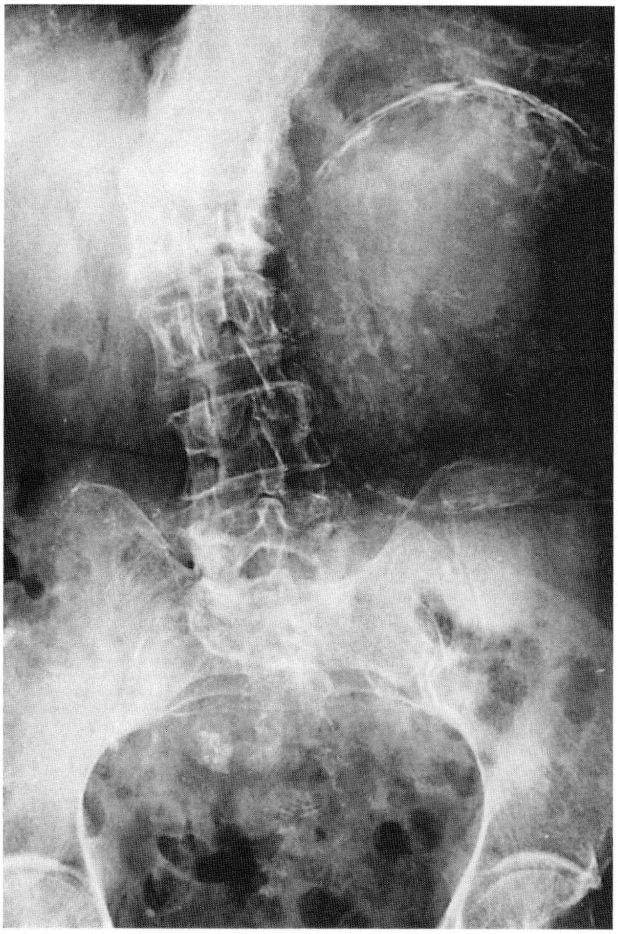

A

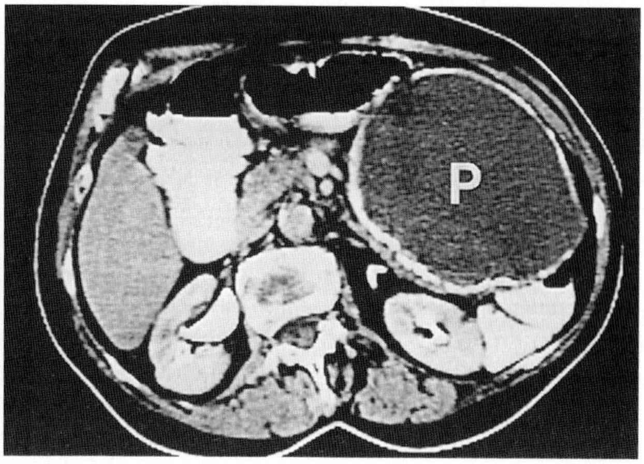

B

Figure 4-56 **A,** Large, peripherally calcified mass in the left upper quadrant represents a pancreatic pseudocyst. **B,** CT shows homogeneous cystic contents *(P)*.

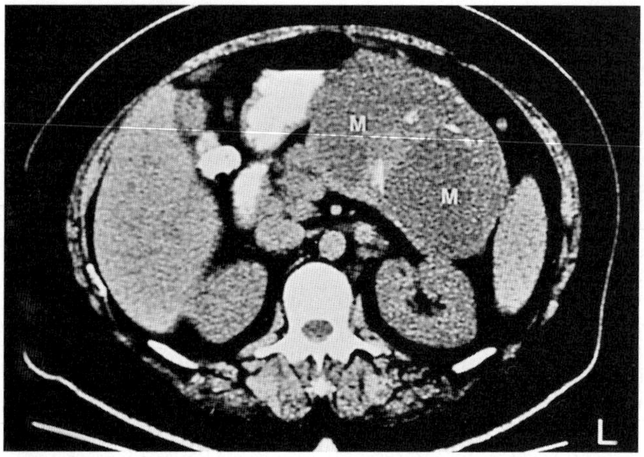

Figure 4-57 Large cystic mass *(M)* containing partially calcified septations represents mucinous cystic neoplasm of the pancreas.

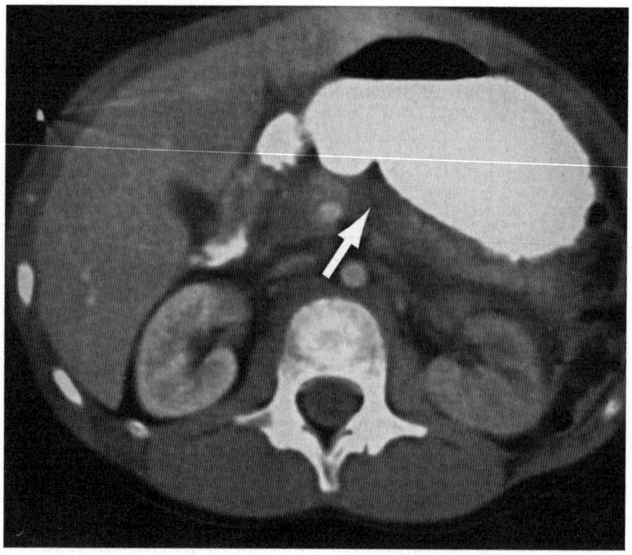

Figure 4-58 Low-density area *(arrow)* between the body and head of the pancreas is seen in an area of laceration following an automobile accident.

carbohydrates. Peripheral calcifications have been reported in congenital pancreatic cysts associated with von Hippel-Lindau disease. Hydatid cysts, although rarely occurring in the pancreas, also may calcify peripherally.

Other unusual causes of intraparenchymal pancreatic calcifications include previous trauma, hematoma, abscess, and infarction. A calcified aneurysm of the adjacent celiac or splenic artery may simulate an intrapancreatic mass.

TRAUMA

Pancreatic injury occurs in 3% to 12% of patients with blunt abdominal trauma, although it is frequently missed on imaging if not blatant. Patients with duodenal injury should be evaluated carefully on CT for pancreatic injury. The findings may be quite subtle, including a focal area of density change, minimal peripancreatic stranding, or minimal focal swelling of the gland. Clinical symptoms suggesting pancreatic injury are nonspecific. Elevated serum amylase levels are found in 90% of patients with blunt trauma to the pancreas, however. Pancreatic injuries include contusion, laceration, and transection (fracture) and most often result from compression of the pancreatic body against the spine. Thin-section, contrast-enhanced CT of the pancreas may show focal or diffuse pancreatic enlargement and extension of blood into the peripancreatic and retroperitoneal tissues. An area of decreased density perpendicular to the long axis of the pancreas may be seen immediately after trauma, suggesting a contusion or hematoma (Fig. 4-58). Within hours to days, a clear zone of disruption through the pancreatic parenchyma may become evident, indicating a laceration or transection. Ultrasound is sometimes able to show these findings, but frequently is limited by overlying bandages or by bowel gas secondary to intestinal ileus. Laceration of the pancreatic duct resulting from pancreatic transection is best evaluated by ERCP.

Pancreatic injury is accompanied by trauma to other visceral structures in 75% of cases and is fatal in 10% to 20% of cases. Surgical treatment of pancreatic transection usually consists of partial resection (when the body or tail is injured) or repair (when the head is injured). Complications of pancreatic trauma occur frequently and include chronic pancreatitis, pseudocysts, pancreaticoenteric fistulas, and abscesses.

POSTOPERATIVE PANCREAS

Resection

Surgical resection of the pancreas may be partial or complete. After resection of the tail or of the body and tail, the residual pancreas appears shortened.

The standard Whipple's procedure consists of resection of the pancreatic head and neck, subtotal gastrectomy, duodenectomy, gastrojejunostomy, pancreaticojejunostomy, and choledochojejunostomy. A total rather than a partial pancreatectomy is sometimes performed, leading to severe diabetes mellitus.

Cystogastrostomy

Cystogastrostomy or marsupialization represents a surgical anastomosis of a pancreatic pseudocyst to the adjacent gastric wall. This procedure allows the pseudocyst to drain internally and eventually resolve. A UGI series or CT using oral contrast material typically shows

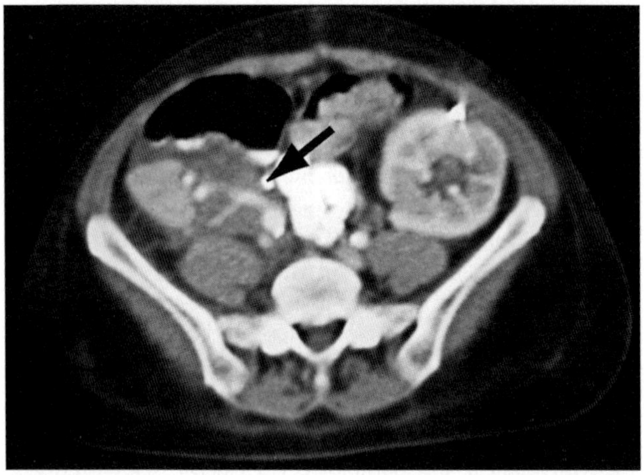

Figure 4-59 Note transplanted pancreas *(arrow)* on the right side of the pelvis and transplanted kidney on the left side in a patient with diabetes mellitus.

opacification of the pseudocyst through the patent anastomosis.

Puestow's Procedure

Puestow's procedure represents an end-to-end pancreaticojejunostomy. It is performed to allow drainage of the dilated, but nonobstructed pancreatic duct in chronic pancreatitis. It also may involve resecting portions of the pancreas. Puestow's procedure may be performed in instances of tumors in the head of the pancreas or ampullary region of the duodenum.

Pancreatic Transplantation

Pancreatic transplantation is an increasingly performed procedure for managing patients with severe diabetes mellitus. A cadaver donor pancreas and adjacent periampullary segment of duodenum are placed in the recipient's pelvis with vascular anastomoses to iliac vessels and duodenal anastomosis to the dome of the urinary bladder (Fig. 4-59). Complications include acute and chronic transplant rejection, intraperitoneal or

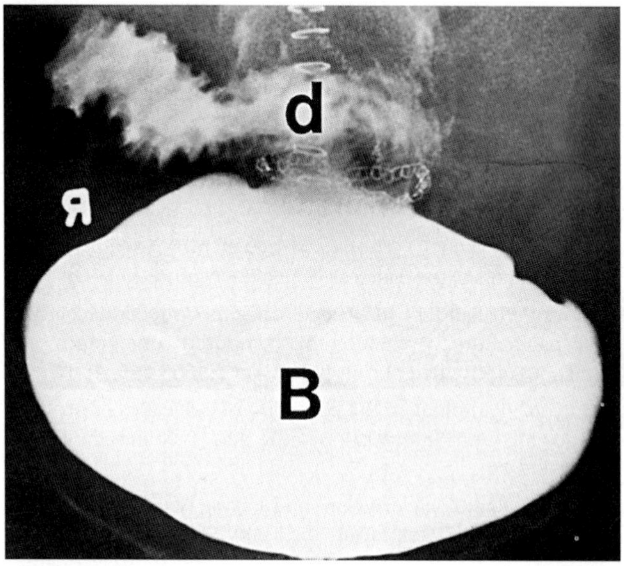

Figure 4-60 Cystogram after pancreatic and renal transplantation shows opacification of the urinary bladder *(B)* and transplanted duodenum *(d)*.

extraperitoneal leakage, fluid collections (hematomas, abscesses, and pseudocysts), fistulas, and various vascular abnormalities (Box 4-8).

Cystography has proved useful for detecting anastomotic leaks and fistulas by allowing opacification of the adjacent duodenal segment (Fig. 4-60). CT is useful for evaluating intraabdominal fluid collections and providing guidance for percutaneous drainage procedures and pancreatic biopsies. MRI has shown some promising results in detecting pancreatic transplant rejection.

Box 4-8 Complications of Pancreatic Transplantation

- Rejection
- Peripancreatic effusions (common after surgery)
- Ascites (usually indicates leakage)
- Leakage
- Ischemia/thrombosis
- Pancreatitis and pseudocysts
- Infection/abscess

SUGGESTED READINGS

Axon ATR: Endoscopic retrograde cholangiopancreatography in chronic pancreatitis: Cambridge classification. Radiol Clin North Am 27:39-50, 1989.

Balthazar E: CT diagnosis and staging of acute pancreatitis. Radiol Clin North Am 27:19-37, 1989.

Balthazar EJ, Robinson DL, Megibow AJ, et al: Acute pancreatitis: value of CT in establishing prognosis. Radiology 174: 331-336, 1990.

Bolondi L, LiBassi S, Gaiani S, et al: Sonography of chronic pancreatitis. Radiol Clin North Am 27:815-833, 1989.

Bret PM, Reinhold C, Taourel P, et al: Pancreas divisum: evaluation with MR cholangiopancreatography. Radiology 199:99, 1996.

Bronstein YL, Loyer EM, Kaur H, et al: Detection of small pancreatic tumors with multiphasic helical CT. AJR Am J Roentgenol 182:619-623, 2004.

Buck JL, Hayes WS: Microcystic adenoma of the pancreas. Radiographics 10:313-322, 1990.

Buetow PC, Miller DL, Parrino TV, et al: Islet cell tumors of the pancreas: clinical, radiologic, and pathologic correlation in diagnosis and localization. Radiographics 17:453-472, 1997.

Burdeny DA, Kroeker MA: CT appearance of the ventral pancreas. J Can Assoc Radiol 39:190-194, 1988.

Clark LR, Jaffe MH, Choyke PL, et al: Pancreatic imaging. Radiol Clin North Am 23:489-501, 1985.

Dodds WJ, Wilson SD, Thorsen MK, et al: MEN I syndrome and islet cell tumors of the pancreas. Semin Roentgenol 20:17-63, 1985.

Donovan PJ, Sanders RC, Siegelman SS: Collections of fluid after pancreatitis: evaluation by computed tomography and ultrasonography. Radiol Clin North Am 20:653-665, 1982.

Freeny PC: Radiology of the pancreas: two decades of progress in imaging and intervention. AJR Am J Roentgenol 150: 975-981, 1988.

Freeny PC: Radiologic diagnosis and staging of pancreatic ductal adenocarcinoma. Radiol Clin North Am 27:121-128, 1989.

Freeny PC, Marks WM, Ryan JA, et al: Pancreatic ductal adenocarcinoma: diagnosis and staging with dynamic CT. Radiology 166:125-133, 1988.

Friedman AC, Edmonds PR: Rare pancreatic malignancies. Radiol Clin North Am 27:177-190, 1989.

Fugazzola C, Procacci C, Bergamo Andreis IA, et al: Cystic tumors of the pancreas: evaluation by ultrasonography and computed tomography. Gastrointest Radiol 16:53-61, 1991.

Gunther RW: Ultrasound and CT in the assessment of suspected islet cell tumors of the pancreas. Semin Ultrasound CT MR 6:261-275, 1985.

Hill MC, Barkin J, Isikoff MB, et al: Acute pancreatitis: clinical vs. CT findings. AJR 139:263-269, 1982.

Jeffrey RB Jr: Sonography in acute pancreatitis. Radiol Clin North Am 27:5-17, 1989.

Jeffrey RB, Federle MP, Crass RA: Computed tomography of pancreatic trauma. Radiology 147:491-494, 1983.

Kettritz U, Semelka RC: Contrast-enhanced MR imaging of the pancreas. MRI Clin North Am 4:87, 1996.

Khrana B, Mortele KJ, Glickman J, et al: Macrocystic serous adenoma of the pancreas: radiologic-pathologic correlation. AJR Am J Roentgenol 181:119-123, 2003.

Kloppel G, Maillet B: Classification and staging of pancreatic nonendocrine tumors. Radiol Clin North Am 27:105-119, 1989.

Lane MJ, Mindelzun RE, Jeffrey RB: Diagnosis of pancreatic injury after blunt abdominal trauma. Semin Ultrasound CT MR 17:177, 1996.

Low RA, Kuni CC, Letourneau JG: Pancreas transplant imaging: an overview. AJR Am J Roentgenol 155:13-21, 1990.

Luetmer PH, Stephens DH, Ward EM: Chronic pancreatitis: reassessment with current CT. Radiology 171:353-357, 1989.

Mathiu D, Guigui B, Valette PJ, et al: Pancreatic cystic neoplasms. Radiol Clin North Am 27:163-176, 1989.

McNulty NJ, Francis IR, Platt JF, et al: Multi-detector row helical CT of the pancreas: effect of contrast-enhanced multiphasic imaging on enhancement of the pancreas, peripancreatic vasculature, and pancreatic adenocarcinoma. Radiology 220: 97-102, 2001.

Megibow AJ, Zhou XH, Rotterdam H, et al: Pancreatic adenocarcinoma: CT versus MR imaging in the evaluation of resectability. Radiology 195:327, 1995.

Mergo PJ, Helmberger TK, Buetow PC, et al: Pancreatic neoplasms: MR imaging and pathologic correlation. Radiographics 17:281-301, 1997.

Mitchell DG: MR imaging of the pancreas. MRI Clin North Am 3:51, 1995.

Moulton JS, Munda R, Weiss MA, et al: Pancreatic transplants: CT with clinical and pathologic correlation. Radiology 172: 21-26, 1989.

Op den Orth JO: Sonography of the pancreatic head aided by water and glucagon. Radiographics 7:85-100, 1987.

Reinhold C, Bret PM, Guibaud L, et al: MR cholangiopancreatography: potential clinical applications. Radiographics 16:309-320, 1996.

Rizzo RJ, Szucs RA, Turner MA: Congenital abnormalities of the pancreas and biliary tree in adults. Radiographics 15:49-68, 1995.

Ros P, Hamrick-Turner JE, Chiechi MV, et al: Cystic masses of the pancreas. Radiographics 12:673-686, 1992.

Rosch T, Lorenz R, Braig C, et al: Endoscopic ultrasound in pancreatic tumor diagnosis. Gastrointest Endosc 37:347-352, 1991.

Rossi P, Allison DJ, Bezzi M, et al: Endocrine tumors of the pancreas. Radiol Clin North Am 27:129-161, 1989.

Simeone JF, Edelman RR, Stark DD, et al: Surface coil MR imaging of abdominal viscera: the pancreas. Radiology 157:437-441, 1985.

Taylor AJ, Carmondy TJ, Schmalz MJ, et al: Filling defects in the pancreatic duct on endoscopic retrograde pancreatography. AJR Am J Roentgenol 159:1203-1208, 1992.

Tscholakoff D, Hricak H, Thoeni R, et al: MR imaging in the diagnosis of pancreatic disease. AJR Am J Roentgenol 148: 703-709, 1987.

White EM, Wittenberg J, Mueller PR, et al: Pancreatic necrosis: CT manifestations. Radiology 158:343-346, 1986.

Woolsey EJ, Tauscher JR, Dafoe DC: Pancreas transplantation with pancreato-duodeno-cystostomy for exocrine drainage: cystographic findings. AJR Am J Roentgenol 149:507-509, 1987.

Yu J, Fulcher AS, Turner MA, Halvorsen RA: Normal anatomy and disease process of the pancreaticduodenal groove: imaging features. AJR Am J Roentgenol 183:839-846, 2004.

Yuh WTC, Hunsicker LG, Nghiem DD, et al: Pancreatic transplants: evaluation with MR imaging. Radiology 170:171-177, 1989.

Zeman RK, McVay LV, Silverman PM, et al: Pancreas divisum: thin-section CT. Radiology 169:395-398, 1988.

CHAPTER 5

Liver and Spleen

LIVER

The liver is the largest organ in the abdomen, weighing about 1800 g in men and slightly less in women. Classically, the liver is divided into right and left lobes by the falciform ligament. Anatomical division with respect to vascular supply and biliary drainage differs, however, in that the division of the right and left lobes is to the right of the falciform ligament, along a plane of intralobar division that is determined by a line drawn from the inferior vena cava to the superior recess of the gallbladder fossa. Medial to this line is the medial segment of the left lobe, which is separated from the lateral segment by the vertical cleft in the surface of the left lobe, in which runs the ligamentum teres.

Segmental liver anatomy based on the internal vascular supply has a much more practical application with respect to hepatic surgical resection. With aggressive hepatic resection for limited metastatic disease becoming more common, segmental vascular anatomy has become more important. A numbering system developed by Couinaud divides the liver into eight segments, each of which has a major portal vein division and bile duct, drained by a distinct hepatic vein (Fig. 5-1).

The main blood supply to the liver is the portal vein, which receives almost all the blood from the digestive tract and accounts for almost 80% of blood supply to the liver parenchyma. The main arterial supply is the hepatic artery, which arises from the celiac axis and ascends anterior to the portal vein and behind the common bile duct to the porta hepatis region, where it divides into the right and left hepatic arteries. There are three main hepatic veins. In most individuals, the veins join before entering the vena cava. The middle hepatic vein is the segmental boundary between the right and left lobes of the liver. The caudate lobe (segment No. 1) has its own venous drainage directly into the inferior vena cava, and in some cases, the papillary process of the caudate lobe can extend between the portal vein and the inferior vena cava and is occasionally mistaken for disease (Fig. 5-2).

Examination Techniques

The standard of practice for liver imaging has undergone a significant change over the past two decades. The primary radiological evaluation of the liver using nuclear scintigraphy and angiography has given way to multidetector computed tomography (CT), ultrasonography, and magnetic resonance imaging (MRI).

The primary radiological technique for evaluating the liver is CT. Computed tomographic techniques for hepatic evaluation have evolved at a rapid pace. Helical multidetector fast computed tomographic scanning has markedly reduced scanning times, and resolution continues to improve with each generation of scanners introduced. Quality multiplanar image reconstruction and three-dimensional rendering make the newer generations of CT scanners exceptionally useful in the detection of disease and treatment planning. The continuous technical

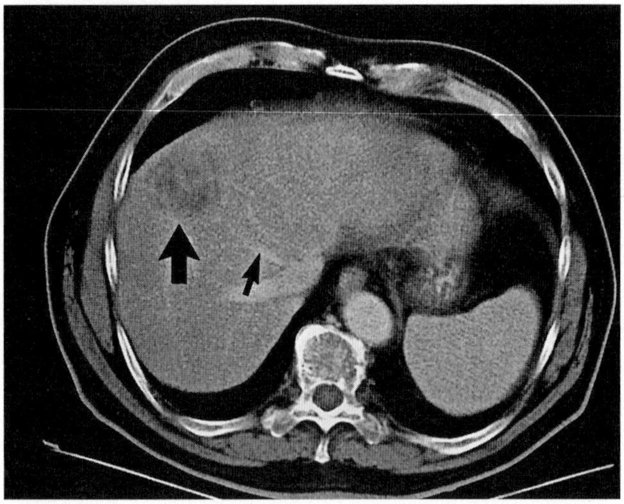

Figure 5-1 A 72-year-old patient with breast carcinoma and a solitary hepatic metastatic lesion. The lesion *(large arrow)* is located on the boundary between segment 4a (left lobe) and segment 8 (right lobe). The boundary between the segments is defined by the middle hepatic vein *(small arrow)*.

developments of CT being made available as diagnostic tools (e.g., subsecond scanning and CT fluoroscopy) will continue to make CT a modality of choice well into the future. Ultrasonography occupies a position just behind CT in liver evaluation, although some institutions have moved directly to MRI as the backup study if CT is not definitive. Ultrasonography does offer the benefits, however, of no ionizing radiation and the ability to evaluate the patency of the portal or hepatic veins.

MRI shows great promise for the detection of selected disease entities with excellent contrast and multiplanar examination, breath-hold imaging, and the use of gadolinium and newer contrast agents such as superparamagnetic iron oxide. There is no ionizing radiation involved, and MRI is preferred for patients with renal insufficiencies. Some difficulties remain, however, in bringing MRI to the forefront of liver disease detection. The length of the examination (compared with multidetector CT) is the most obvious difficulty, although we are seeing progress in that area. The usefulness of radionuclide imaging in evaluating hepatic disease has become more focused over the past few decades and tends now to be limited to evaluation of bile duct or cystic duct obstruction.

Computed Tomography

Multidetector CT is generally the acknowledged standard for liver tumor imaging. Meticulous attention to the technical aspects of the examination is required to fulfill its promise, however. In some instances (especially when evaluating for certain metastatic lesions, breast and colorectal tumors being the most common), unenhanced and enhanced evaluations of the liver are required (Fig. 5-3). The use of multiphase imaging (imaging during the arterial, early or late arterial portal, and delayed venous phases of opacification) has now become routine in many centers, with unenhanced images being obtained routinely before the triple-phase imaging. This approach is arguably the best in increasing the likelihood of detection of the three types of hepatic lesions: hyperdense, hypodense, and isodense lesions. In addition to considerations of vascular enhancements, attention to good opacification of the stomach and duodenum is one of the hallmarks of high-quality computed tomographic liver imaging. The contrast examination is almost uniformly performed

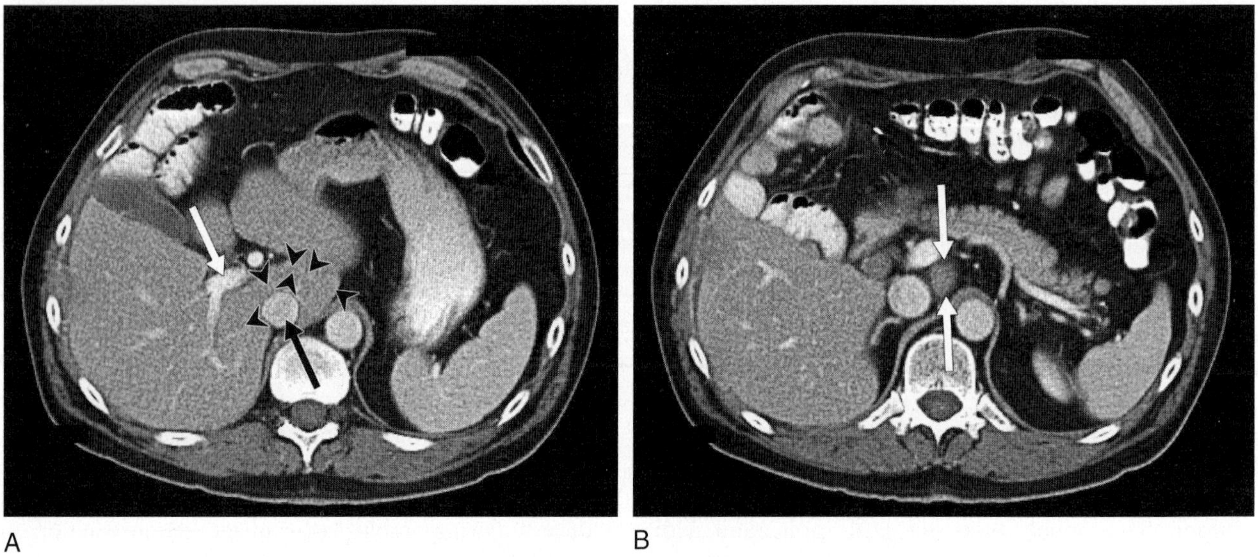

Figure 5-2 **A,** A long papillary process of the caudate lobe *(arrowheads)* is seen between the portal vein *(white arrow)* and the inferior vena cava *(black arrow)*. **B,** Lower extension of papillary process of caudate lobe *(arrows)* can be mistaken for adenopathy.

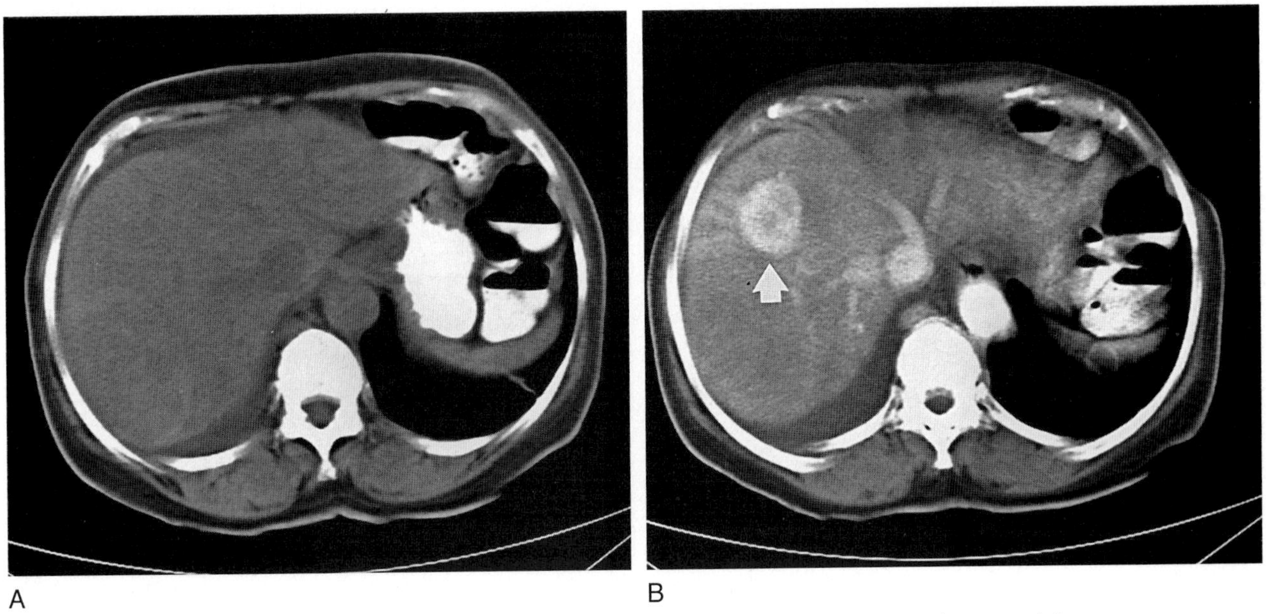

Figure 5-3 A patient with metastatic carcinoid. **A,** Unenhanced CT of liver shows no defects. **B,** Postenhancement image reveals a hypervascular liver metastatic lesion *(arrow)*.

using dynamic bolus technique and a power injector. With newer software, image reconstruction times have markedly lessened.

For the purposes of organizing this discussion of the liver, radiological problems related to the computed tomographic evaluation of liver abnormalities are the basis for discussion. The role of other imaging modalities is appropriately included whenever possible.

Ultrasonography

Ultrasonography is a relatively inexpensive and noninvasive method of evaluating the upper abdomen. It is especially useful in evaluating for the presence of bile duct obstruction and the presence or absence of gallstones. Because of the high incidence of gallstones throughout the population, some argument can be made for the primary use of ultrasonography in the evaluation of upper abdominal pain when gallstones are suspected. In addition, ultrasonography is especially useful in distinguishing between cystic and solid lesions. There are limitations, however. Although tumor masses can be detected, the false-negative rate for liver metastatic disease is higher than with CT, and findings and lack of findings necessitate additional evaluation, most likely by CT. For this reason, ultrasonography is generally not the primary screening technique in patients whose clinical presentation suggests something other than gallstone disease.

Magnetic Resonance Imaging

Although there continues to be considerable discussion in the literature of the comparative value of CT and MRI, multidetector CT remains the standard. This is not only for technical reasons, but also for practical ones because CT facilities are ubiquitous, whereas MRI facilities, although definitely on the increase, for the most part are still centered largely in major medical centers. The great bulk of the work being done in MRI is in the neuroradiological and musculoskeletal area. Much progress is being made in MRI abdominal technique, however, and with its capability of multiple imaging sequences and impressive multiplanar imaging, it is daily becoming a more important imaging tool for imaging the abdomen, particularly for liver disease. In the near future, MRI may well be the primary imaging tool for hepatic disease (Fig. 5-4).

Before MRI can assume a prominent role, some problems must be resolved. The issue of claustrophobia within the MRI gantry is real and affects about 10% to 15% of patients. The case for open MRI units is augmented further by the increasing size of patients. In addition, no generally acceptable intraluminal contrast material that is specific for MRI of the gastrointestinal tract has proved effective at this time. The examination is still lengthy compared with CT of the abdomen. Nevertheless, the potential of MRI becoming the primary imaging modality of the liver is great.

The basis of MRI image formation is much more complex than CT and involves many different factors, such as hydrogen ion tissue density, T1 and T2 relaxation times, vascular flow characteristics, and chemical shift. Various operator-dependent factors can be manipulated that also contribute to the image formation and contrast. The physics of MRI is beyond the scope of this book. Some elemental knowledge is necessary, however, to interpret the images appropriately, and readers are encouraged to

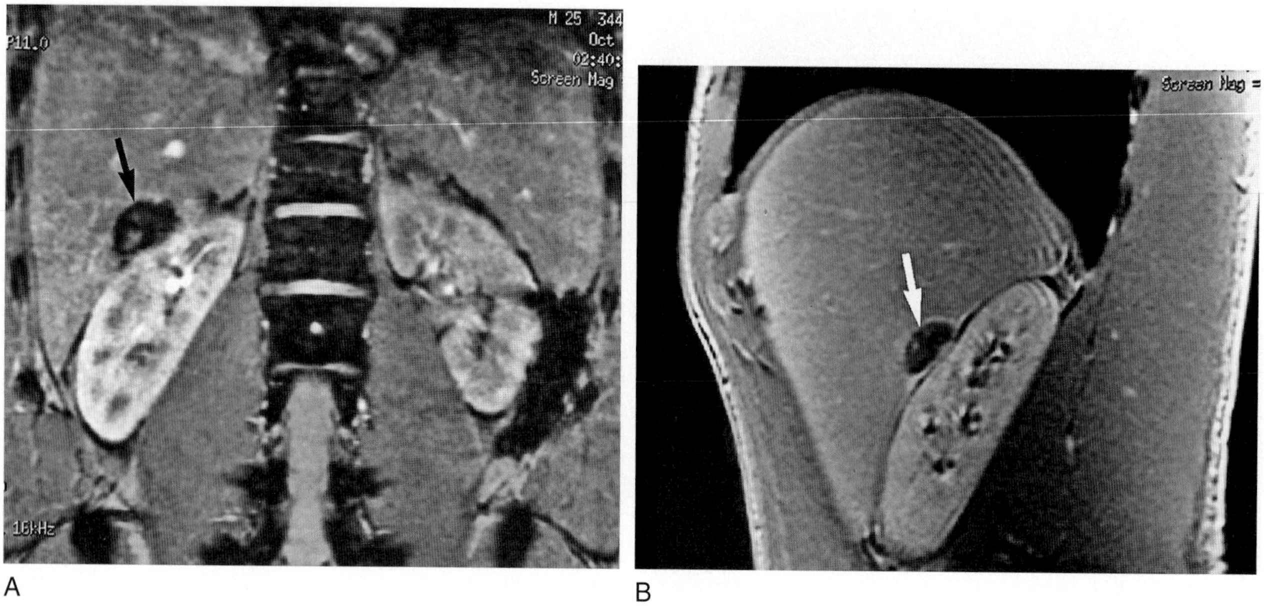

Figure 5-4 A patient with subcapsular hematoma. MRI in two planes shows hematoma to advantage. Hematoma seen on coronal **(A)** *(black arrow)* and sagittal oblique **(B)** *(white arrow)* images.

consult the many excellent books and courses that are currently being offered in this area.

Enlarged Liver without Focal Disease

Fatty Liver (Steatosis)

Diffuse fatty infiltration almost invariably results in an enlarged liver on cross-sectional imaging of the abdomen. The liver normally appears slightly denser than the spleen on CT (Fig. 5-5). The densities of the liver and spleen should not be compared on the arterial or portal phase, however, because the spleen almost always appears denser, which is a normal finding (Fig. 5-6). When the liver is fatty, it appears less dense on venous and unenhanced imaging. When present, the diffuse form of fatty infiltration can result in a relative increase in the contrast of the vascular structures of the liver, making them more prominent. Ultrasound examination of the fatty liver shows degrees of diffuse increased echotexture. Newer MRI techniques have been shown to be increasingly sensitive for the diagnosis of fatty infiltration of the liver (Fig. 5-7). Alternative techniques using the spectroscopic capabilities of MRI, as in proton spectroscopic imaging, also have been used to detect fatty infiltration.

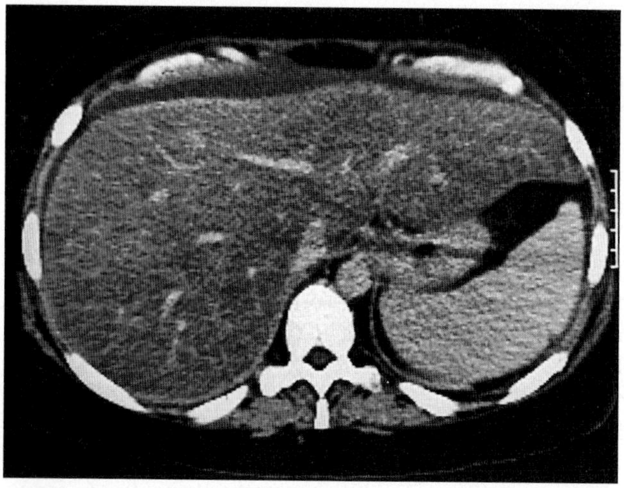

Figure 5-5 CT section through the liver and spleen shows hepatic enlargement and decreased density throughout the hepatic substance as a result of fatty infiltration.

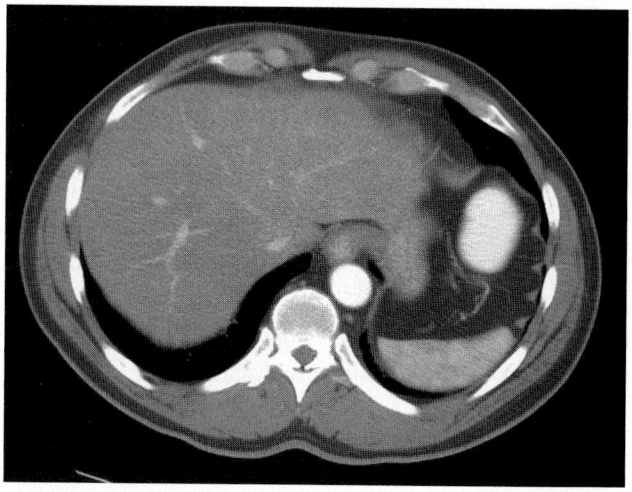

Figure 5-6 Liver and spleen seen on arterial phase commonly shows the liver less dense than the spleen.

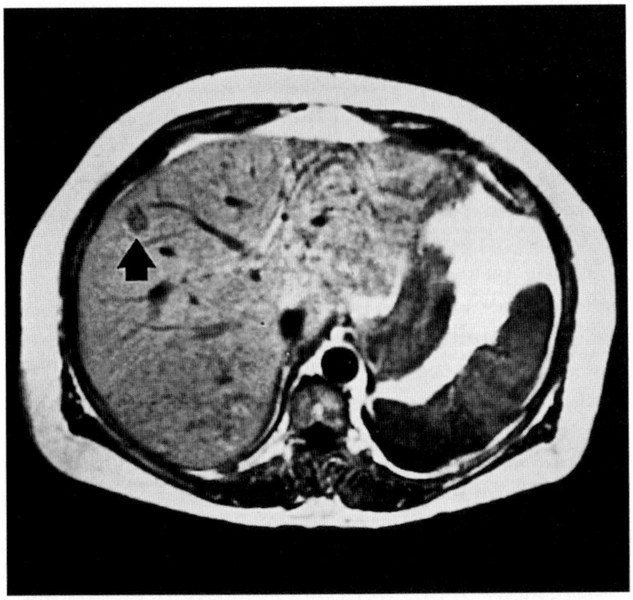

Figure 5-7 T1-weighted image through the liver in a patient with known fatty infiltration of the liver. Note the small, rounded metastatic lesion seen in the periphery of the right lobe of the liver *(arrow)*.

Fatty infiltration of the liver, although most commonly diffuse, can occur in focal form as either isolated or multiple focal lesions; this is especially true in the hilar part of the liver. Normally less than 5% of the liver is composed of fat. In diffuse fatty infiltration, 40% to 50% of the liver is composed of fat. Patients may be asymptomatic or may report vague abdominal pain. Jaundice is unusual, but has been reported in a few patients. A large liver can be detected clinically and radiologically, although splenomegaly is unusual.

The causes of fatty liver are numerous (Box 5-1) and generally can be divided into two categories, alcoholic and nonalcoholic. The histological, radiological, and clinical differences between these two are not discernible.

Most fatty livers result from chronic alcohol intake (80%). Relatively small amounts of alcohol can increase hepatic fat content over a short period; this probably represents the earliest of the toxic changes induced in the liver by alcohol. Ordinarily, these short-term changes in liver fat content are of no consequence, although they can precede more significant hepatotoxic changes of alcohol, progressing from fatty liver through alcoholic hepatitis and cirrhosis in a group of patients who either are genetically susceptible or indulge in regular high alcohol intake. The actual number of habitual drinkers in the United States is difficult to estimate, but is thought by some authors to be decreasing, as deaths from liver cirrhosis began to decline in the early 1970s. Women seem to be more at risk for alcoholic toxicity of the liver. The issue is complicated further by the presence of a 15% to 20% rate of infection with hepatitis C virus. Alcoholism is an important risk factor in the development of hepatocellular carcinoma worldwide, but it is considered less of a risk factor than viral hepatitis.

Numerous conditions can cause nonalcoholic fatty liver (20%). Viral hepatitis may produce mild fatty changes in the liver. Nutritional causes, such as starvation and prolonged hyperalimentation, also exist. Fatty liver has been described in Reye's syndrome in children. It is a common finding in patients undergoing chemotherapy and many other types of medication. Various metallic toxins, including antimony, thallium, and uranium compounds, also have been found to result in fatty deposition in the liver. Fatty liver has been shown in patients who have undergone intestinal bypass surgery or hyperalimentation. Some cases have been associated with inflammatory bowel disease. Fatty liver has been described in patients with diabetes mellitus and metabolic abnormalities, such as Cushing's disease, α_1-antitrypsin disease (Fig. 5-8), and certain types of porphyria. More recent data have suggested that metabolic nonalcoholic fatty liver changes may be more prevalent among the elderly.

Box 5-1 Some Common Causes of Fatty Changes in the Liver

Alcoholic hepatotoxicity
Toxicity from chemotherapy
Hepatitis
Hyperalimentation
α_1-Antitrypsin disease

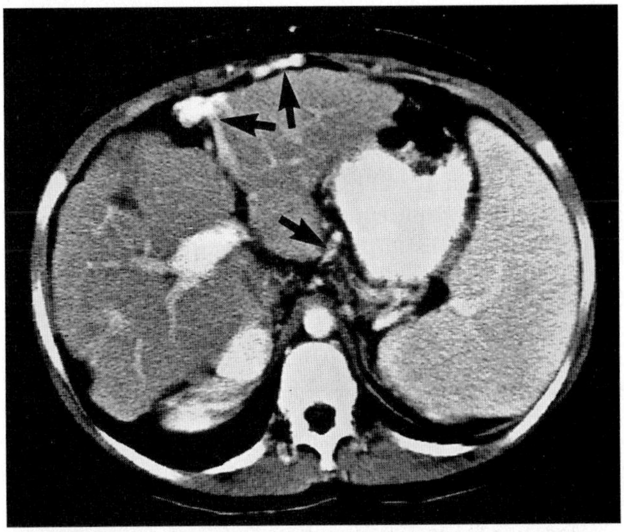

Figure 5-8 A patient with α_1-antitrypsin deficiency with fatty and cirrhotic liver. CT reveals marked collaterals with varices seen in the anterior abdominal wall, over the surface of the liver, and around the gastroesophageal junction *(arrows)*.

Administration of exogenous steroids is associated with fat deposition at several sites within the body, including the liver. Acute fatty liver of pregnancy is a relatively rare disorder in which diffuse fatty infiltration of the liver occurs during the latter part of pregnancy. This condition is distinct from preeclampsia or toxemia of pregnancy. It has serious prognostic implications and often results in hepatic failure and gastrointestinal bleeding.

Viral Hepatitis

Inflammation of the liver as a result of viral infection can be divided into hepatitis A and hepatitis B. When neither the A nor B viral cause can be identified, hepatitis is usually referred to as non-A/non-B type (hepatitis C). There are no specific clinical or radiological distinctions in the course of either hepatitis A or hepatitis B. Transmission for hepatitis A is known to be by the fecal-oral route, and the disease tends to be milder. Hepatitis A has worldwide distribution and is related to contaminated water supplies and undercooked foods, among other factors. About 85% of patients with hepatitis A have some degree of hepatomegaly, and about 15% have some splenomegaly. The incubation phase is about 2 weeks. The prodromal phase is characterized by fatigue, weakness, and possibly vague abdominal pain. Most infections are anicteric, especially in children. Most patients completely recover within 2 to 3 months, and the illness is generally benign and self-limiting.

Hepatitis B usually is transmitted parenterally, sexually, or by perinatal exposure. About 5% of the world population are said to be carriers. The incubation period is 60 to 120 days, and jaundice is more common than with the A type. Complications include the risk of chronicity (5%) or an acute, fulminant, often fatal, overwhelming infection (<1%). Patients with chronic disease are at increased risk for cirrhosis, portal hypertension, varices, and hepatocellular carcinoma. Approximately 90% of hepatocellular carcinomas result from chronic biological damage to the liver by hepatitis B or C or hepatitis B and C combined.

Hepatitis C is transmitted via blood route (transfusion, needle stick) or sexually. The prevalence of hepatitis C in intravenous drug abusers is 40% to 80%. Because of common transmission routes, hepatitis C and human immunodeficiency virus (HIV) occurring concomitantly is common. Transfusion risk has declined with more sensitive screening of donors and is expected to decline further as yet more sensitive screening tests are introduced. The overwhelming clinical presentation of chronic disease is marked fatigue, whereas acute disease is often asymptomatic. The incubation period for hepatitis C is probably between those of A and B.

Hepatitis C accounts for about 20% cases of acute hepatitis. At least 85% to 90% of these patients still have the virus at 6 months and progress to chronic disease and all its attendant complications. Hepatitis C has become an important factor in liver transplantation, partly because it is one of the primary indications for transplant (about 25% of liver transplants). Because these patients are universally viremic at transplantation, recurrence is almost entirely predictable. With advances in posttransplantation treatment, however, orthotopic transplantation is now common for patients with end-stage liver disease secondary to hepatitis B and C.

In the past 2 decades, viral hepatitis D and E types have been described. Hepatitis D is similar to hepatitis B and is often found as a coinfection in the same patient and carries the same risks as hepatitis B. Hepatitis E is a water-borne, fecal-oral infection not commonly seen in Western countries except in returning travelers. Its natural history is similar to hepatitis A.

Certain ultrasonographic patterns of accentuated brightness and prominence in the demonstration of the portal vein radicle walls, with generalized decrease in echogenicity of the liver (Fig. 5-9), have been described with acute hepatitis. The role of imaging in the diagnosis of viral hepatitis is limited, but imaging can be used to differentiate obstructive from nonobstructive jaundice. CT of the abdomen reveals nonspecific liver enlargement and possibly some mild fatty infiltration in the acute phase, but little else.

Liver and spleen imaging using technetium-99m sulfur colloid may be normal or show hepatic enlargement. If the hepatocellular disease is sufficiently severe, there may be patchy, inhomogeneous uptake and reversal of the normal pattern of greater liver activity than splenic activity.

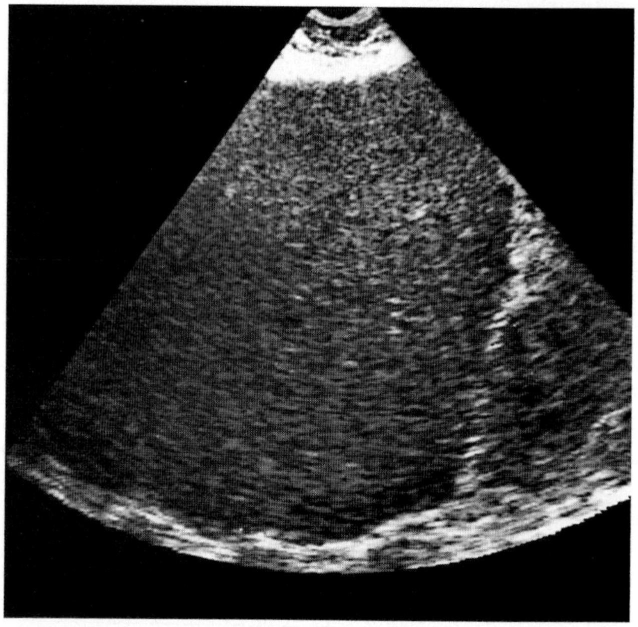

Figure 5-9 Ultrasonogram of the liver in a patient with acute hepatitis shows hepatomegaly and generalized decreased echogenicity of the liver.

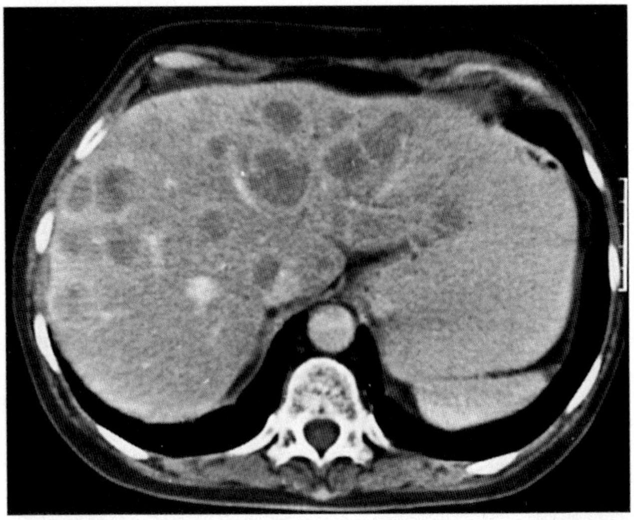

Figure 5-10 A patient with carcinoma of the lung. The patient has hepatic enlargement. Computed tomographic scan obtained through the liver shows multiple intrahepatic metastatic lesions.

Shift of the radionuclide to adjacent bone marrow or lungs also may be seen in severe cases.

Diffuse Metastatic Disease

The liver is the most common target for metatastic disease. Diffuse involvement of the liver by metastatic disease can result in an enlarged liver (Fig. 5-10). This type of metastatic involvement of the liver is most commonly encountered with breast and lung primary lesions and colorectal carcinomas. The prognosis depends on the degree of tumor burden, although multiple liver lesions generally have a poor prognosis, and survival, when symptoms appear, is usually measured in months.

Budd-Chiari Syndrome

The Budd-Chiari syndrome (hepatic venous occlusive disease) can result in hepatomegaly. There are many possible causes for hepatic vein occlusion, ranging from local disease, such as hepatocellular carcinoma, and adjacent disease, such as carcinoma of the pancreas and kidney, to more generalized causes, such as thrombosis secondary to polycythemia vera, and blood dyscrasias, such as leukemia and sickle cell disease (Fig. 5-11). There is an increasing suspicion that estrogen-containing birth control medication may be responsible for some cases. The imaging findings depend on the acuteness or chronicity of the condition. Acute hepatic vein occlusion often results in a dramatic presentation of symptoms with some cases presenting with severe abdominal pain and shock. In most chronic cases, patients present with ascites and hepatomegaly. This presentation is accompanied by abdominal pain in about half of the cases. Jaundice is much less common. Clinical findings center on intraperitoneal fluid and a large, tender liver.

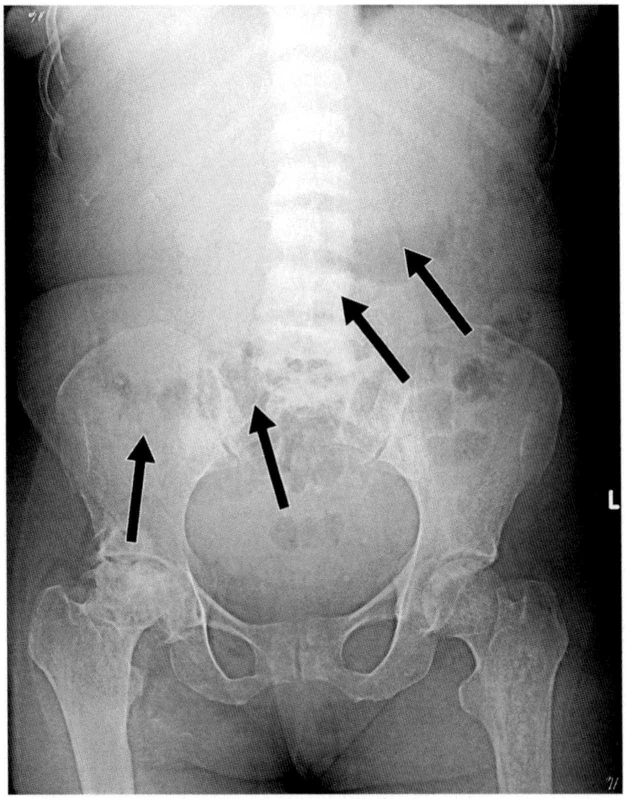

Figure 5-11 Plain film of the abdomen shows enlarged liver *(arrows)* in a patient with sickle cell disease.

The CT appearance of hepatic venous occlusion is that of hepatomegaly and accompanying ascites. During dynamic imaging of the liver, an inhomogeneous, patchy appearance may be observed, and the hepatic veins may not be seen clearly as a result of thrombosis and obliteration. In patients for whom the condition has been present for several weeks, the caudate lobe is enlarged (Fig. 5-12). This enlarged caudate lobe of the liver is readily detectable on CT and ultrasonography of the liver. MRI features of Budd-Chiari syndrome also include reduction of the size and number of hepatic veins. On CT and MRI, collateral circulation may be observed, particularly involving the azygos and hemiazygos veins in the retrocrural area (Fig. 5-13).

Other Uncommon Causes

Hepatomegaly can be seen when performing imaging on patients with numerous other, relatively uncommon conditions. Patients with congestive heart failure can experience hepatic enlargement and right upper quadrant tenderness as a result of capsular distention on the basis of chronic passive congestion (Fig. 5-14). Many hepatotoxic drugs sometimes can result in hepatomegaly, including methotrexate, methyldopa, isoniazid, acetaminophen, nitrofurantoin, tetracycline, and halothane.

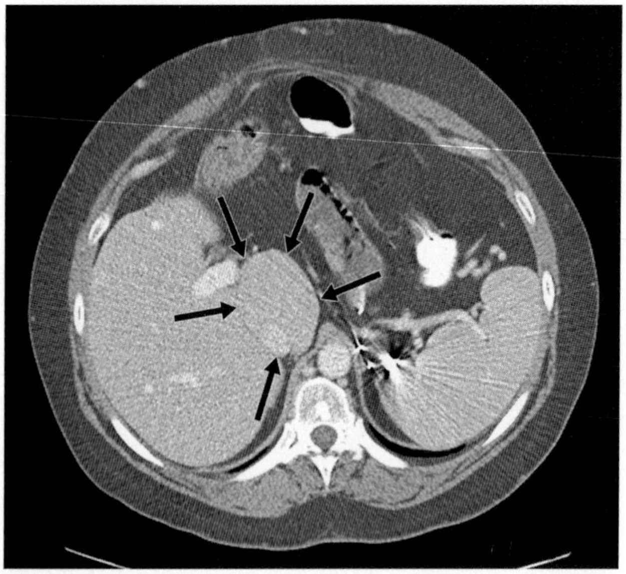

Figure 5-12 Caudate lobe enlargement *(arrows)* in a patient with inferior vena cava obstruction.

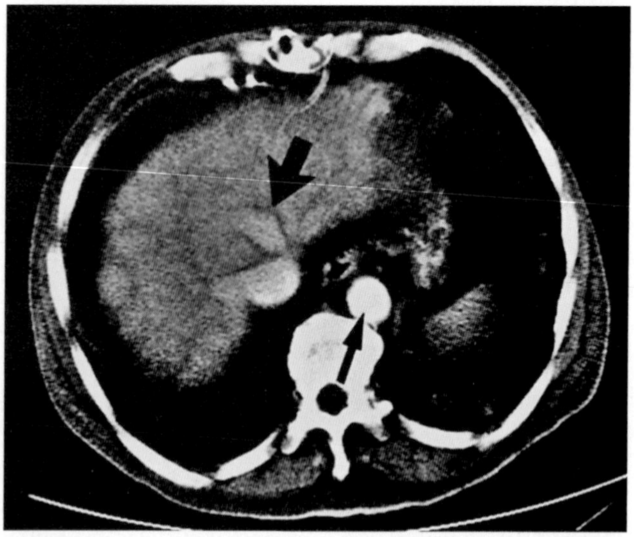

Figure 5-14 A patient with congestive heart failure. Note patchy appearance of liver and distention of the hepatic veins *(large arrow)*. The sluggishness of the circulation causes the aorta to remain quite bright *(smaller arrow)*.

In Weil's disease (leptospirosis), a common clinical presentation includes an enlarged liver and spleen. Leptospirosis is a spirochete infection that is spread to humans via animals. In addition to the enlarged liver and spleen, patients have constitutional symptoms of fever and generalized myalgias and varying degrees of central nervous system involvement.

Hepatic enlargement also may be seen as part of the clinical picture of abnormal iron deposition within the liver (hemochromatosis) and Wilson's disease (hepatolenticular degeneration), which is a hereditary disorder of copper metabolism and resultant copper deposition within the liver and brain. The striking computed tomographic finding in these diseases, particularly hemochromatosis, is not so much the enlarged liver, but the increased density of the liver seen on noncontrast studies. This increased density can be missed if the liver is studied only during contrast enhancement.

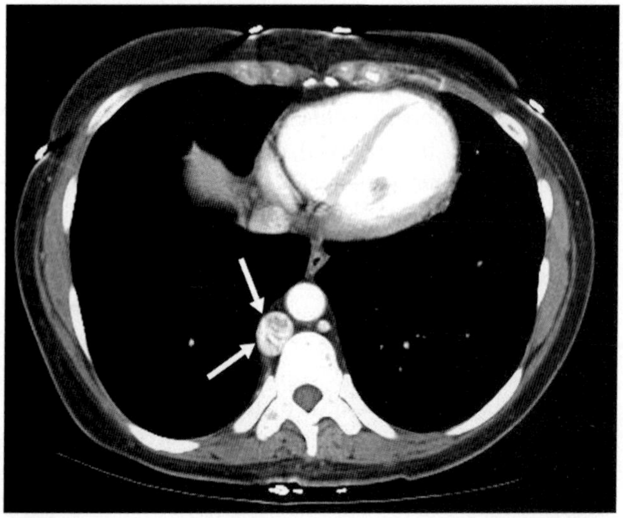

Figure 5-13 Distention of the azygos vein *(arrows)* in a patient with inferior vena cava obstruction.

Small or Shrunken Liver

Cirrhosis

Liver cirrhosis involves a chronic increase in fibrotic tissue throughout the liver, resulting in distortion of the normal liver architecture, fibrotic deposition around the portal vein tributaries, degrees of portal vein occlusion, portal vein hypertension, and redistribution of blood within the upper abdomen through collateral circulations. The ongoing fibrotic process results in decreasing liver size, although individual segments of the liver may maintain their size or even increase slightly. These latter changes are often seen in the lateral segment of the left lobe and the caudate lobe and may be related to blood supply of the areas. The liver margins become nodular and irregular. There is often evidence of fatty infiltration in the less severe cases. Other associated imaging findings include splenomegaly secondary to portal hypertension, ascites, and varices.

Generally, cirrhosis can be divided into Laënnec's and postnecrotic types. From an imaging perspective, there is little to distinguish between these two. A third type of cirrhosis associated with hemochromatosis and Wilson's disease is rare. In the United States, cirrhosis constitutes a relatively common cause of death in adults, with most cases secondary to alcoholic hepatitis (Laënnec's cirrhosis). A few cases may be attributed to the postnecrotic condition.

Primary biliary cirrhosis, which is a chronic progressive form of bile duct inflammation and fibrosis, also may be included in the discussion. The diagnostic designation is misleading because most of these patients present with an enlarged liver and spleen. In severe progressive disease, the typical appearance of cirrhosis may develop. This condition is seen mostly in women and usually has an insidious onset with patients often presenting with jaundice, pruritus, and constitutional symptoms, including vague abdominal pain.

CT of the upper abdomen of patients with advanced cirrhosis shows a small, shrunken liver (Fig. 5-15). Some relative increase in the size of the caudate lobe and lateral segment of the left lobe can be easily identified along with the accompanying findings of ascites, splenomegaly, and varices. CT also may show diffuse or focal fatty changes throughout the liver.

Superimposed disease is always a possibility, particularly hepatocellular carcinoma. The cirrhotic liver presents a potential imaging dilemma because the superimposed lesion may be masked by the cirrhotic changes, which can include areas of focal fatty changes, regenerating nodules, and fibrosis (Fig. 5-16).

Ultrasonography has been helpful in detecting the hepatic changes seen in cirrhosis along with the accompanying findings of ascites. The increased echogenicity of the liver is similar to the findings described for fatty liver, and differentiation cannot be made on the basis of echotexture alone. The cirrhotic liver may appear smaller, and there may be accompanying ascites. Regenerating nodules may be detected as areas of decreased echogenicity within the cirrhotic liver. Although ultrasound evaluation of the liver is sensitive in detecting the diffuse changes, it may not be able to differentiate between fatty infiltration and cirrhosis or other diffuse hepatocellular diseases.

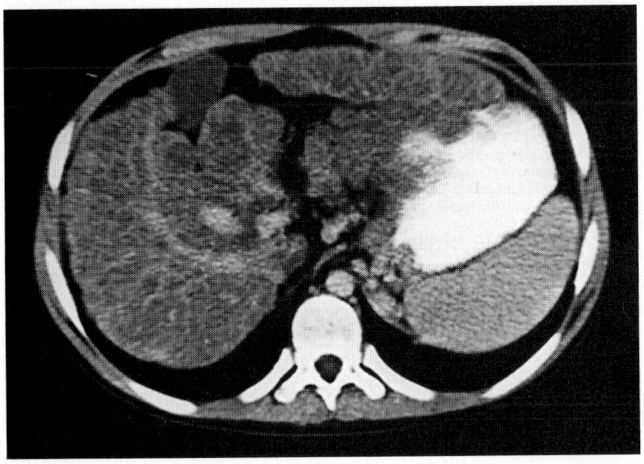

Figure 5-15 A patient with marked cirrhotic changes. The liver is shrunken and has fatty infiltration and lobular contours.

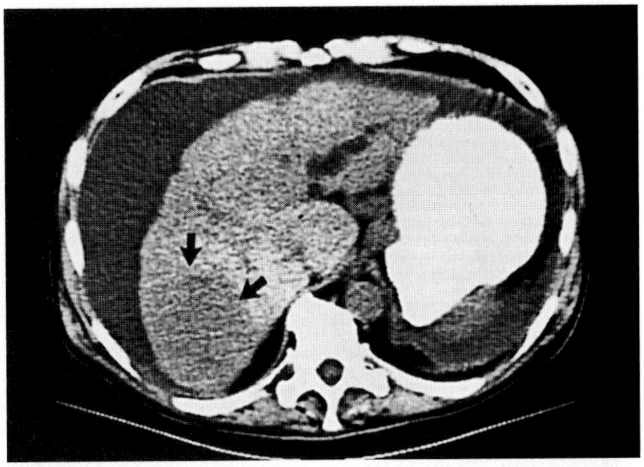

Figure 5-16 A patient with a small cirrhotic liver. A poorly defined, low-attenuation lesion *(arrows)* is seen on the posterior right lobe of the liver, representing hepatocellular carcinoma.

The radionuclide liver/spleen scan shows the changes typical of hepatocellular disease with inhomogeneous take-up and shift of colloid to bone marrow and lungs. The spleen appears enlarged. MRI evaluation of patients with cirrhotic liver shows morphological findings similar to those seen on CT. MRI often shows the portal venous system and its patency in addition to the presence of collateral circulation around the spleen and stomach.

Lobar Atrophy

Because the blood supply to the liver is rich and derived from the hepatic arterial and portal venous systems, hepatic infarction is highly unusual. Because the perfusion of normal hepatocytes is about 80% supplied from the portal venous system, however, prolonged obstruction of the portal vein may result in atrophy of the involved lobe (Fig. 5-17).

Other Causes of Contour Abnormalities

Most of the conditions that result in contour abnormalities of the liver are covered in the consideration of other radiological problems of the liver, in particular, parenchymal focal lesions that involve the edge of the liver, resulting in some focal bulging or deformity of the liver capsule. This includes all forms of liver masses, particularly adenomas and hepatic cysts. Hepatic trauma also can result in deformity of the hepatic margins as a result of blood either within or outside the hepatic capsule. The same may be said of subdiaphragmatic abscesses indenting the capsular surface of the dome of the liver (Fig. 5-18).

Dissemination of peritoneal metastatic disease can result in metastatic deposits along the peritoneal surface adjacent to the liver and along the capsular surface (Fig. 5-19). The most common of these lesions is ovarian cancer, although cancer of the pancreas, stomach, and colon can present with a similar pattern and appearance.

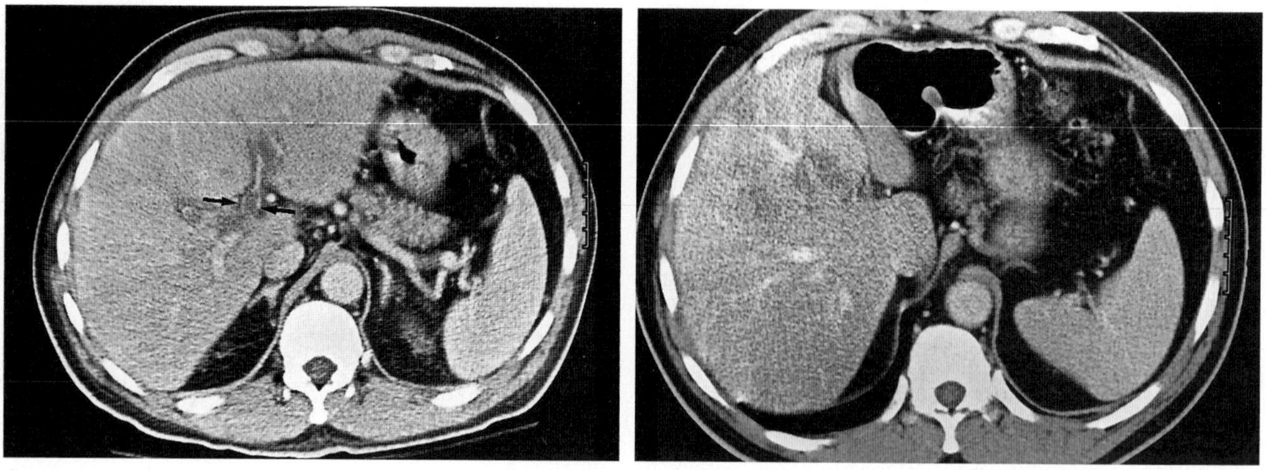

A B

Figure 5-17 **A,** A patient with thrombus of the left portal vein *(arrows).* **B,** Four months later, CT shows atrophy of the left lobe of the liver with the lateral segment almost completely absent.

Early diffuse peritoneal metastatic spread can be subtle and is often undetected by CT. Small peritoneal metastatic implants visualized along the peritoneal or visceral surface of liver or spleen may be the earliest sign. These may occur before the development of ascites and the more obvious mesenteric conglomerate masses known as *omental cakes.*

To some extent, hepatic venous occlusive disease (Budd-Chiari syndrome) can result in hepatic contour abnormalities. CT in such cases generally shows ascites and an enlarged liver. Hepatic veins may be poorly delineated. Because of the separate and direct drainage of the caudate lobe into the vena cava, the caudate lobe is spared and appears enlarged in chronic cases. Apart from the enlarged and apparently bulging caudate lobe, the hepatic contours should otherwise be smooth.

Solitary Defects

Hemangiomas

Although hepatic hemangiomas had been considered rare by clinicians, the experience of cross-sectional CT and ultrasonography over the past 3 decades has confirmed what pathologists have always maintained: This lesion is much more common than is clinically suspected (Box 5-2). It is thought to be the most common neoplastic lesion of the liver, with an incidence of 2% to 5%. It is more common in women, and some lesions may enlarge with age.

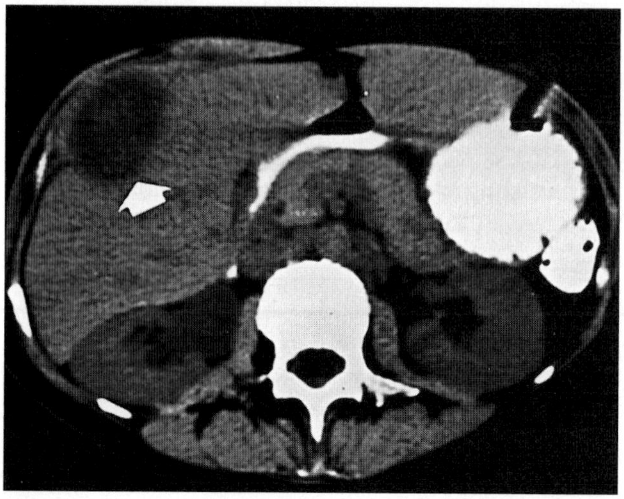

Figure 5-18 CT shows a low-density extrahepatic lesion *(arrow)* impressing the anterior lateral surface of the liver. This lesion proved to be actinomycosis.

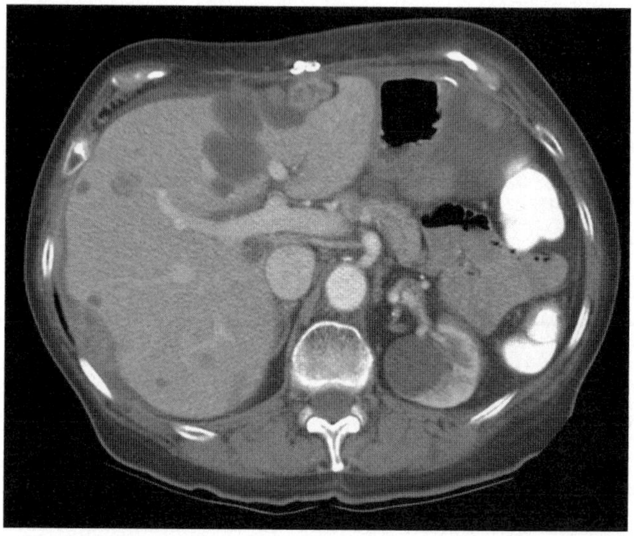

Figure 5-19 Contour deformity of the liver margin in this patient is secondary to metastatic gastrointestinal stromal tumor.

Box 5-2 Facts about Hemangiomas

Most common benign neoplastic lesion in the liver
Capillary or cavernous—capillary type most common
Usually asymptomatic
Most occur in the right lobe
Primary concern is possible confusion with other hepatic lesions (e.g., metastatic disease or hepatoma)

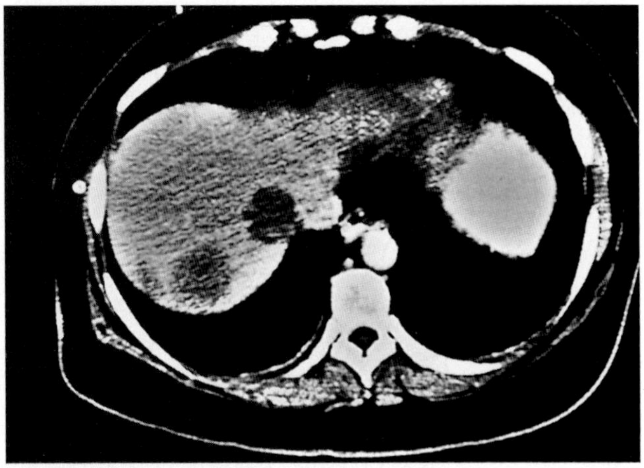

Figure 5-20 CT section through the dome of the liver shows multiple low-attenuation lesions in the right lobe, representing multiple hemangiomas.

This lesion shows a predilection for the posterior right lobe of the liver, and almost 70% of hepatic hemangiomas are subcapsular. They are mostly solitary, although multiple lesions sometimes occur.

Hemangiomas can be of the capillary or the cavernous variety, with the former being considerably more common. The capillary hemangioma is, as its name implies, a lesion composed of tiny capillary-like vessels. A cavernous hemangioma is composed of large cystic, blood-filled spaces lined with epithelium. The larger the lesion, the more likely that it is a cavernous hemangioma.

Virtually all hemangiomas are asymptomatic. Symptoms occur only when the lesion becomes quite large (> 4 to 5 cm). Symptoms are often nonspecific—usually vague right upper quadrant discomfort.

Although hepatic hemangiomas are rarely a clinical dilemma, they commonly result in a diagnostic dilemma for the radiologist. The appearance of hepatic hemangiomas can simulate other serious diseases, such as primary hepatic cancer or metastasis to the liver (Box 5-3). This diagnostic problem often can be resolved by obtaining computed tomographic images of the liver using dynamic-enhanced technique. A low-attenuation lesion with varying configuration and a zone of increased density along its margin is the initial finding (Fig. 5-20). Delayed images at the level of the lesion over the next 5 to 15 minutes show centripetal opacification of the lesion. A dynamic series of images at a predetermined level within the lesion, after a rapid bolus injection, shows similar findings with the initial enhancement at the margin and delayed enhancement centrally (Fig. 5-21).

Box 5-3 Methods of Differentiating Hemangiomas from Other Disease

Centripetal opacification on delayed CT
Radionuclide-tagged red blood cells
MRI
Characteristic ultrasound patterns
Direct aspiration
Angiography

A sizable percentage of cavernous hemangiomas do not show the classic findings during CT; this usually occurs when the lesions are quite small (< 2 cm) or quite large (> 5 to 6 cm). The extremely small lesions may fill in quickly, whereas the extremely large lesions may fill in incompletely or not at all. In the case of larger lesions, this problem is thought to result from the presence of thrombus and fibrosis and central scarring within the lesion (Fig. 5-22). This situation can cause considerable diagnostic confusion in attempting to differentiate correctly between a cavernous hemangioma and more serious disease, such as primary and secondary malignancies.

Characteristic acoustic patterns in the ultrasound evaluation of hemangiomas have been described. These have been shown to be well-defined, echogenic focal areas within the liver (Fig. 5-23). In small lesions (<1 cm) or extremely large lesions in which there are fibrotic, cystic changes or even thrombotic elements within the lesion, ultrasound examination of the liver is not definitive.

MRI of the liver can be useful in the diagnosis of hemangioma. On T2-weighted images, a high signal intensity is characteristically encountered (Fig. 5-24). Other lesions occasionally can give similar appearances, such as simple cysts or even some metastatic lesions. Although cysts usually have a long T1 value, this is not always the case in small lesions (Fig. 5-25). Gradient echo technique using in-phase and out-phase imaging is extremely helpful. Larger cavernous hemangiomas with fibrosis and thrombus formation also may give an atypical appearance on MRI and can be confused with other liver lesions. Gadolinuim-enhanced MRI protocols continue to show more promise in the specificity of hemangioma diagnosis by showing the same "filling-in" process seen on CT (Fig. 5-26).

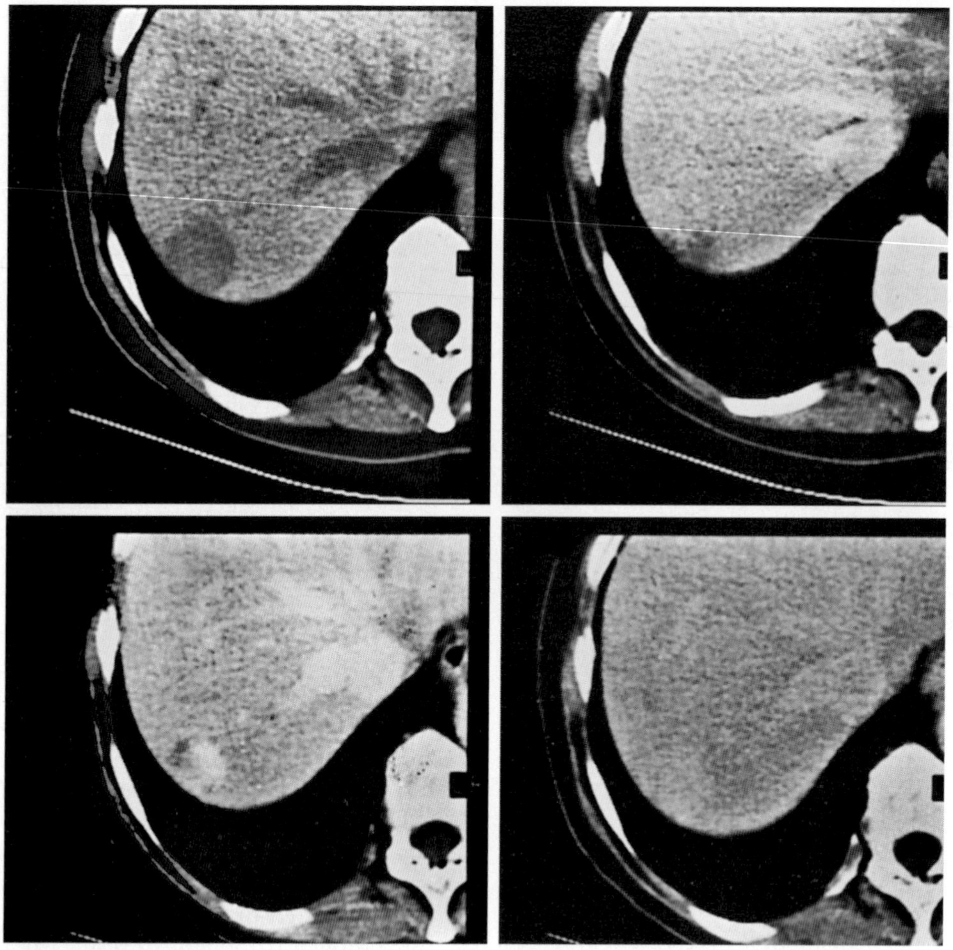

Figure 5-21 A patient with a rounded, low-attenuation lesion in the posterior right lobe of the liver *(upper left image)* undergoing dynamic scans during bolus injection at the level of the lesion. Progressive enhancement and fill-in of the lesion are seen on the subsequent three images, consistent with hemangioma.

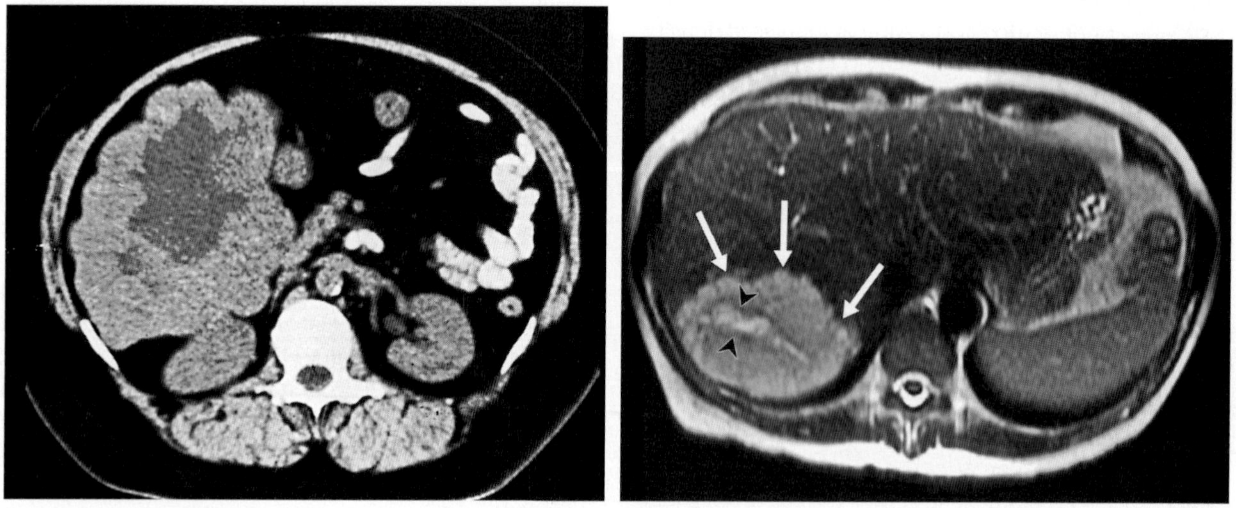

A B

Figure 5-22 **A,** Computed tomographic section through the inferior aspect of the liver shows a large lobulated mass that is arising from the inferior margin of the right lobe with central area of low density representing thrombus and fibrosis within this large cavernous hemangioma. **B,** MRI shows a large hemangioma in the posterior liver *(arrows)* along with a prominent central scar *(arrowheads)*.

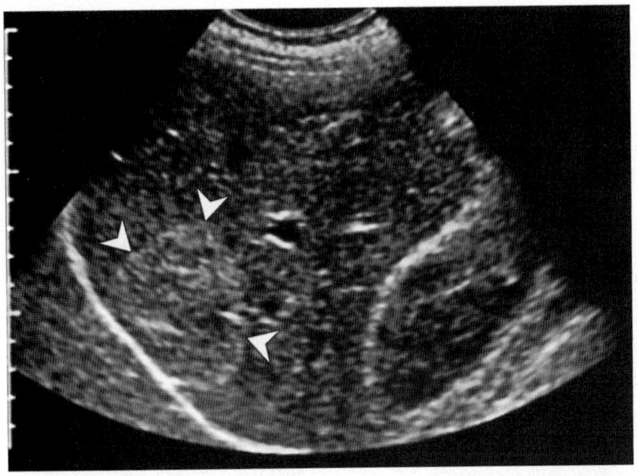

Figure 5-23 Ultrasonogram of the liver shows a well-defined echogenic lesion within the liver *(arrowheads)*, representing the most common ultrasound finding in small to moderate-sized hemangiomas.

Radionuclide imaging using tagged red blood cells has been used occasionally in an attempt to clarify a questionable hepatic lesion that may be a hemangioma (Fig. 5-27). In similar fashion, uptake is seen at the edge of the lesion, and delayed imaging shows gradual fill-in. The nuclear scan has exactly the same weaknesses as described for CT.

Although there has been a general hesitancy about performing direct aspiration biopsy on these questionable lesions, there is a slowly developing consensus that a thin-needle aspiration biopsy is the method of definitive clarification and diagnosis. Relative contraindications in this diagnostic approach are patients with coagulopathies and patients in whom the lesion is immediately subcapsular.

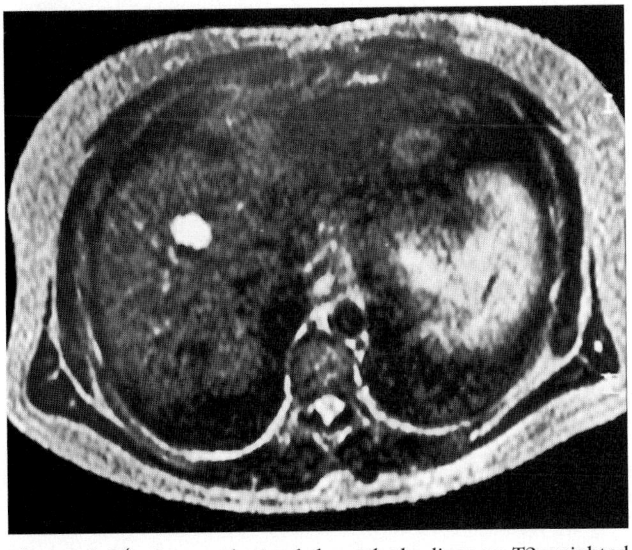

Figure 5-24 Image obtained through the liver on T2-weighted MRI shows a high signal intensity in a rounded hepatic hemangioma.

Metastatic Disease

Secondary metastatic lesions to the liver are common. Generally, the detection of such lesions is a grave prognostic indicator. In the past, it was observed that only about 5% of patients with liver metastatic disease survive 1 year beyond detection.

CT of liver metastatic lesions has shown that they come in all sizes, shapes, and numbers. The lesions can be focal or diffuse (Fig. 5-28). The most common appearance of hepatic metastatic disease on CT is a low-attenuation lesion with respect to the surrounding liver, although isodense and hyperdense lesions are encountered (Figs. 5-29 and 5-30). There may be degrees of peripheral ring enhancement similar to that observed in hemangioma, although the centripetal opacification is uncommon. The central portion of the lesion may be near fluid density in lesions large enough to undergo central necrosis. Calcifications are uncommon and tend to be seen in younger patients with aggressive primary lesions, such as mucinous adenocarcinomas of the colon, stomach, or ovary (Fig. 5-31).

In general, focal metastatic disease is not difficult to detect if the lesion is greater than 1 cm. Metastatic disease superimposed on a fatty liver can present a diagnostic dilemma, however.

The diffuse form of metastatic involvement of the liver occasionally occurs and can be especially difficult if intravenous contrast enhancement is not used. Certain types of diffuse metastatic disease that are hypervascular in nature, such as islet cell tumors and carcinoids (Fig. 5-32), may become isodense during the contrast enhancement of the liver. To confuse the issue further, occasionally a lesion is isodense on the enhanced images and well defined on only the postenhanced images (see Figs. 5-29 and 5-30). For this reason, preenhancement and postenhancement images of the liver are recommended routinely for the evaluation of the liver for possible metastatic disease.

In the late 1970s, interest in the possible resection of solitary metastatic liver lesions was revived. This approach has resulted in increased survival times in a select subgroup of patients.

Imaging techniques are not sufficiently sensitive to ensure that the liver is truly free from disease. At best, radiologists can attest to the fact that no metastatic disease is seen, or that there is disease apparently limited to one lobe. The presence of extrahepatic nodal disease negates the possibility of hepatic resection regardless of the state of the liver.

The increasing interest in the possibility of selective hepatic resection for metastatic disease has resulted in several attempts to refine the CT evaluation of the liver and its sensitivity for metastatic disease detection. For a time, the best approach seemed to be CT in arterial portography (CTAP). Most lesions are believed to be

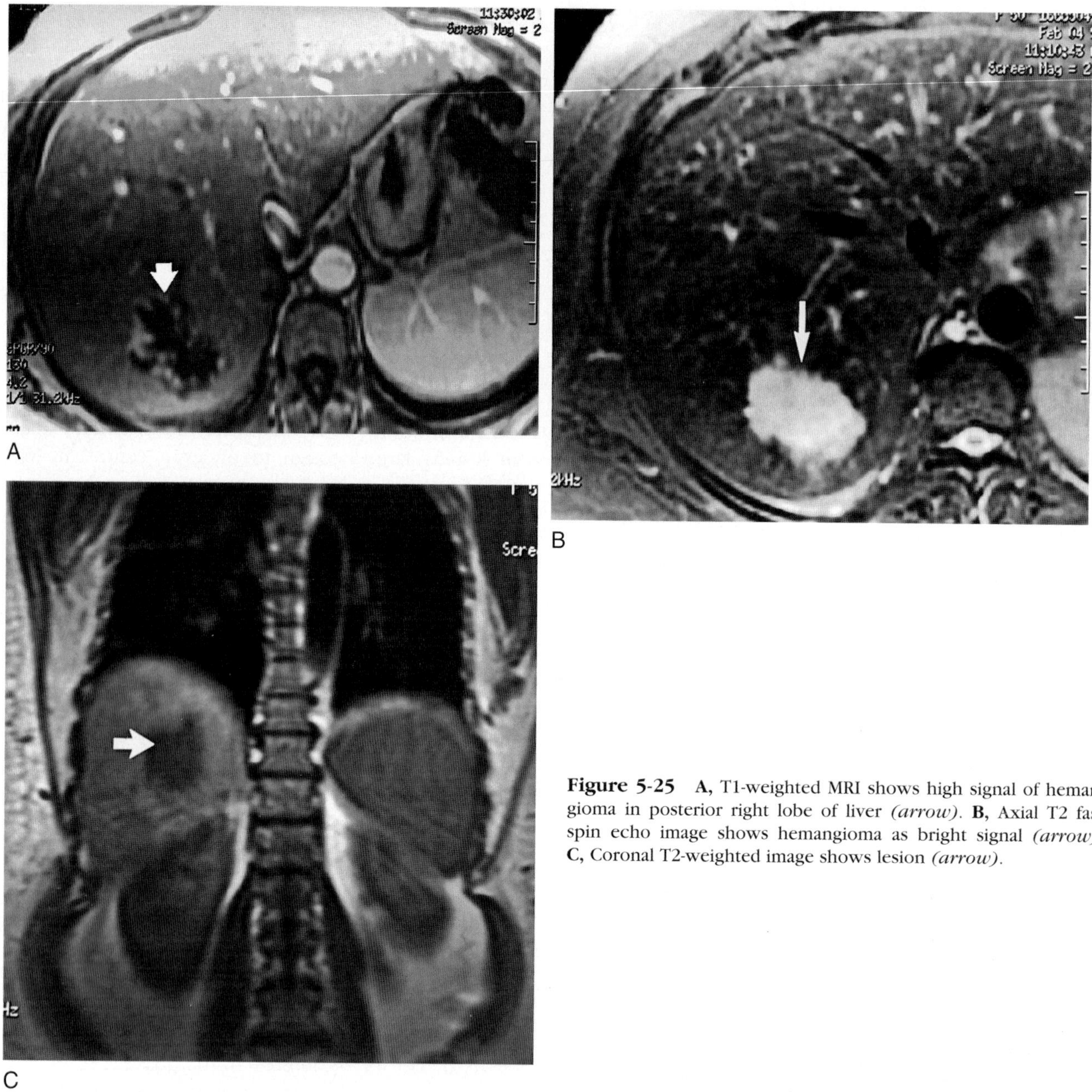

Figure 5-25 **A,** T1-weighted MRI shows high signal of hemangioma in posterior right lobe of liver *(arrow)*. **B,** Axial T2 fast spin echo image shows hemangioma as bright signal *(arrow)*. **C,** Coronal T2-weighted image shows lesion *(arrow)*.

supplied largely by blood drawn from the hepatic arterial system, whereas normal liver tissue derives most of its blood supply from the portal venous system. In CTAP, the portal system is flooded with contrast material while the liver is dynamically scanned; this results in increased contrast at the lesion-parenchymal interface and makes subtle, smaller, or otherwise invisible lesions more discernible.

CTAP requires arterial puncture and the advancement of a catheter tip to the celiac axis and subsequent selective catheterization of the splenic artery or superior mesenteric artery. The splenic artery may be preferred because of dilution factors and streaming artifacts associated with superior mesenteric artery injection portography. After placement of the catheter tip in the splenic artery, an injection bolus of 60 to 80 mL is given, followed by dynamic imaging of the liver (Fig. 5-33).

CTAP has resulted in improved sensitivity in the detection of liver metastatic disease during the prehelical single-tract scanning CT era. With multidetector CT

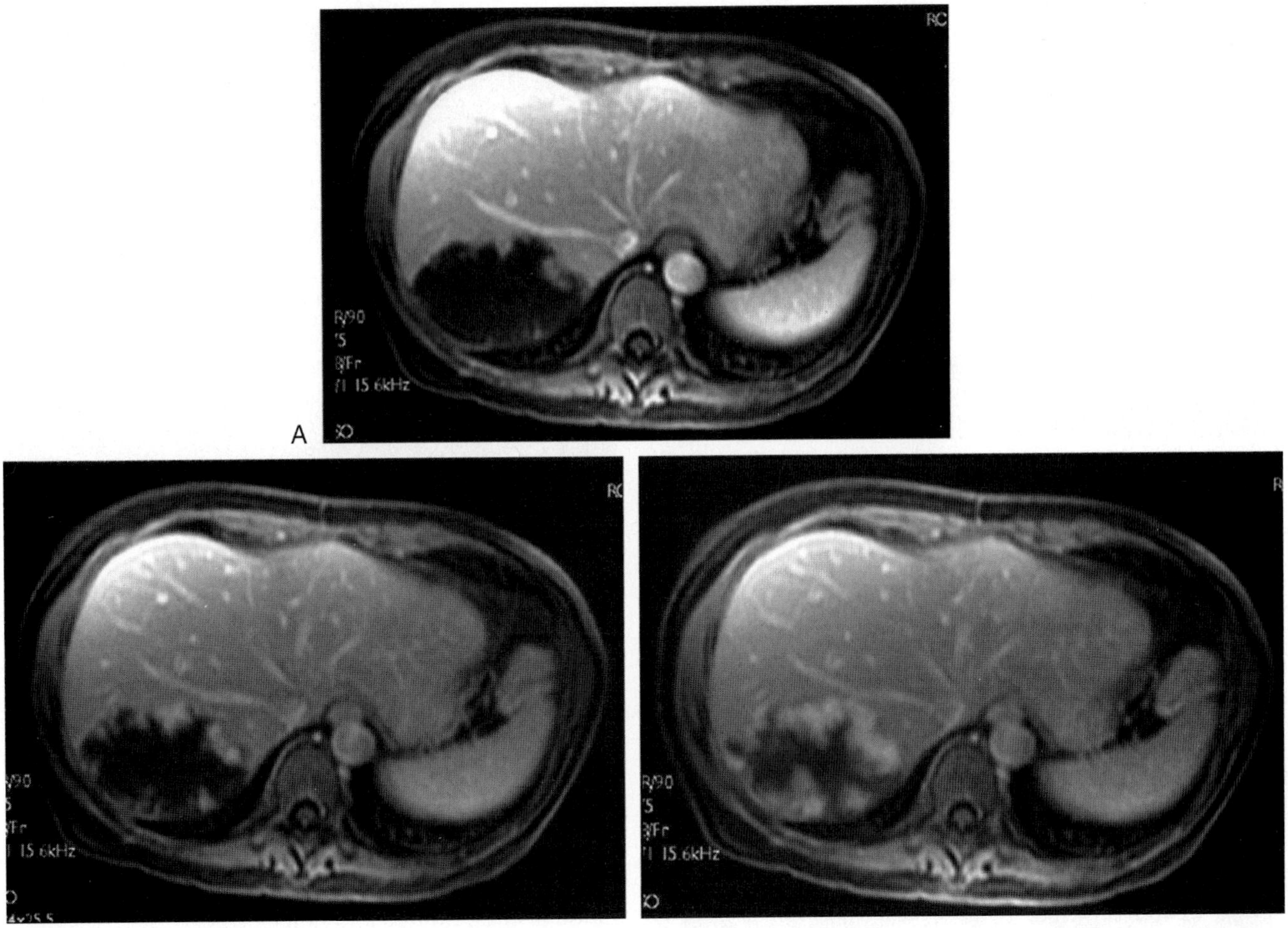

A

B

C

Figure 5-26 Gadolinium-enhanced MRI shows filling-in phenomenon, such as is common with CT of hemangioma.

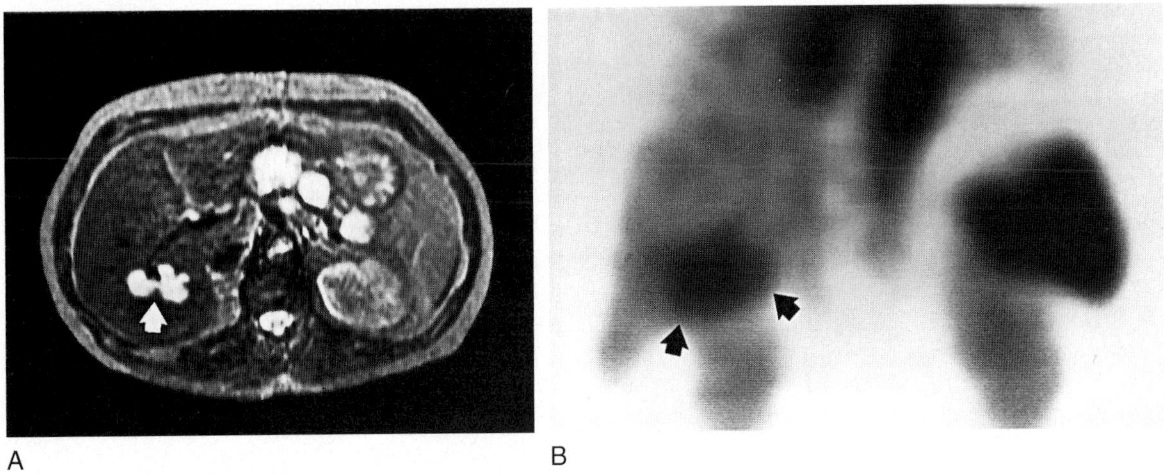

A

B

Figure 5-27 A patient with suspected hepatic hemangioma. **A,** MRI shows high-signal lobulated lesion in right lobe *(arrow)*. **B,** Radionuclide-tagged red blood cell scan confirms diagnosis of hemangioma *(arrows)*.

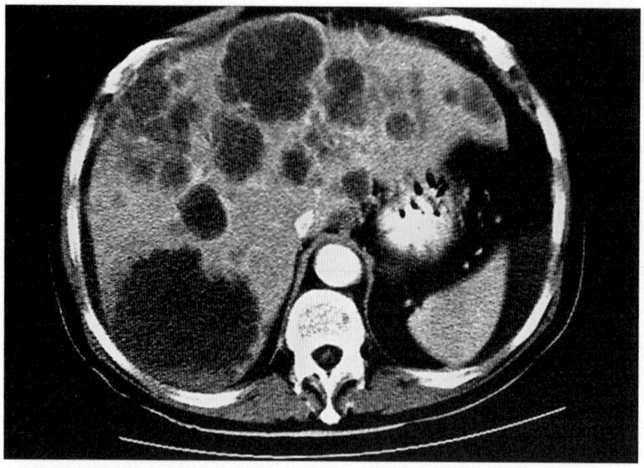

Figure 5-28 This patient has widespread metastatic lesions of the liver, with markedly varying sizes and resultant hepatomegaly.

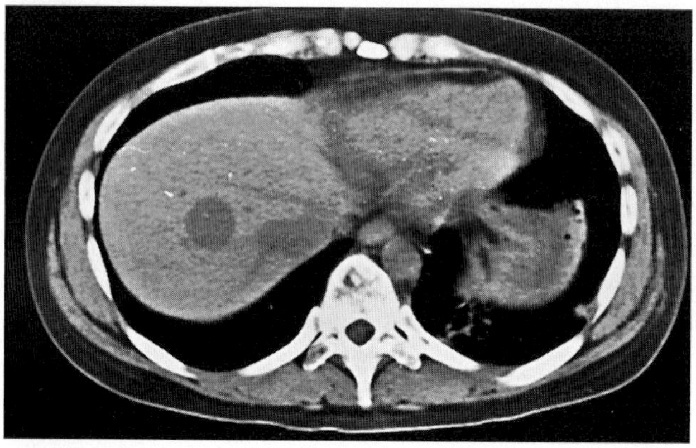

Figure 5-29 CT through the dome of the liver shows an isolated metastatic lesion.

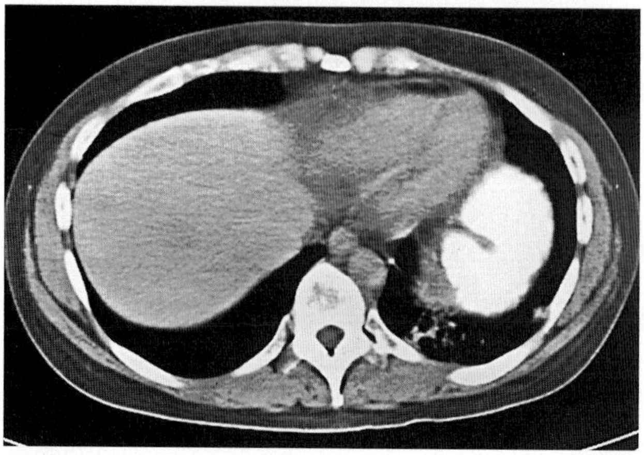

Figure 5-30 In the same patient as in Figure 5-29 after intravenous administration of contrast material, the well-defined lesion seen on the preenhancement scan has become isodense.

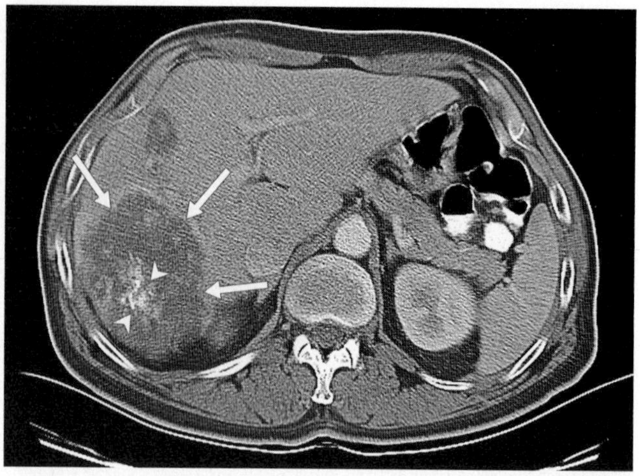

Figure 5-31 Hepatic metastatic lesion *(arrows)* from a mucinous adenocarcinoma of the rectum shows calcifications within the center *(arrowheads)*.

and the opportunity to acquire high-quality images in arterial, venous, and portal phases of the examination, however, the need for CTAP has diminished.

Sonography has not proved to be the diagnostic imaging method of choice for hepatic metastatic disease when CT or MRI capabilities are available. The false-negative rate is generally higher than with CT, and apart from distinguishing fluid from solid tissue, lesion characterization is often limited and nonspecific.

Currently, multidetector CT is the primary imaging modality for the detection of hepatic metastatic disease. Studies comparing multidetector CT and MRI sensitivity in the detection of hepatic metastatic lesions have been

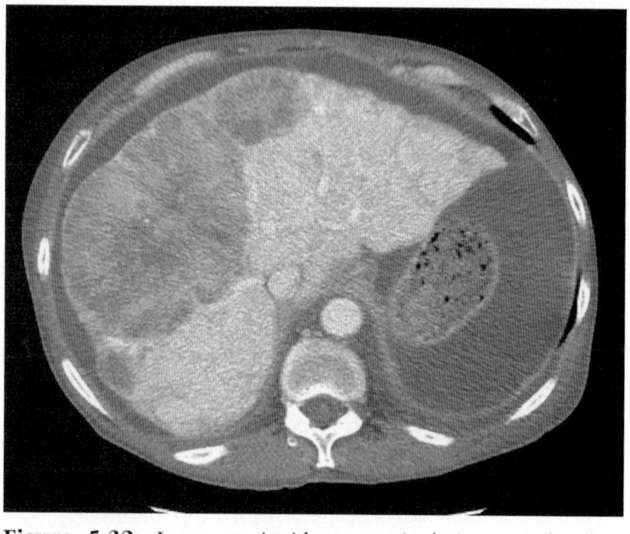

Figure 5-32 Large carcinoid metastatic lesions to the liver are seen.

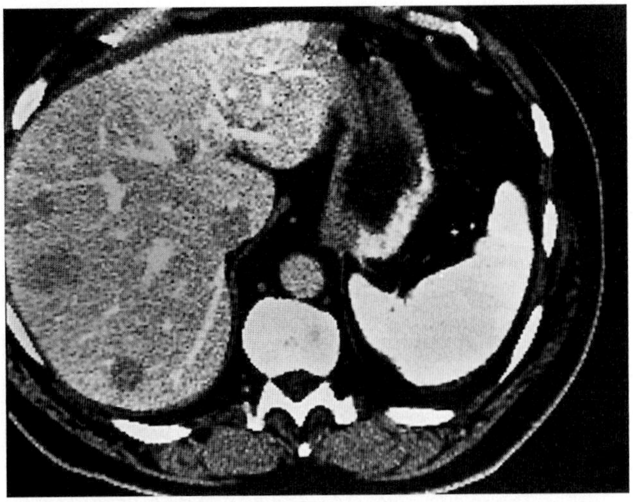

Figure 5-33 CTAP with injection of the splenic artery. Note the hyperdense appearance of the spleen and a portion of the gastric wall. Several defects are now clearly shown, predominantly in the right lobe of the liver.

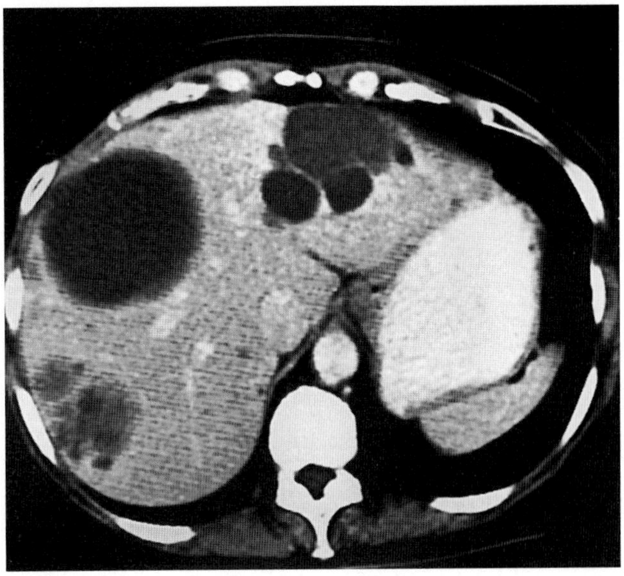

Figure 5-35 CT through the liver of a female patient shows multiple, benign hepatic cysts of varying size.

conflicting, but show an increasing ability to show smaller lesions using liver-specific contrast agents (Fig. 5-34).

Cysts

Simple congenital hepatic cysts are common. These lesions probably arise from defects in bile duct development in utero. They are rarely symptomatic, and liver function is usually unaffected. Cysts tend to be more common in women and more commonly localized to the right lobe of the liver. They range in size from 5 mm to 10 to 12 cm. Most congenital cysts have an epithelial lining and are filled with clear or cloudy fluid.

Cysts can occur as an isolated hepatic lesion or as multiple lesions involving both lobes of the liver. When the cysts are multiple, concomitant cystic disease of the kidneys, pancreas, and ovaries may be present. In 20% to 50% of patients with polycystic disease of the kidneys, hepatic cysts (usually asymptomatic) can be identified.

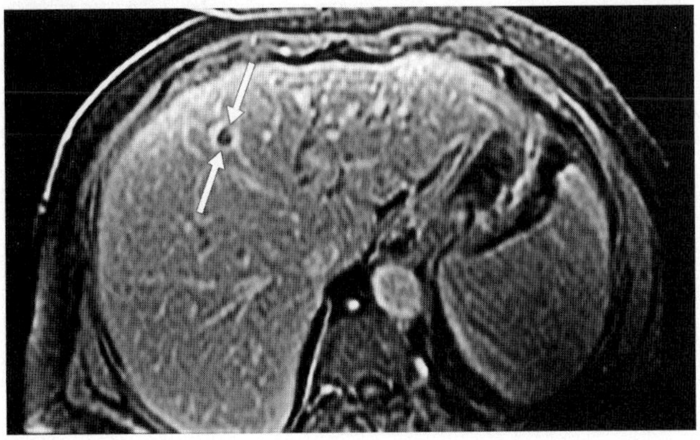

Figure 5-34 MRI of the liver shows a 1-cm hepatic metastatic lesion *(arrows)*.

CT of hepatic cysts discloses a sharp, well-circumscribed, low-attenuation lesion with extremely thin or no discernible walls (Fig. 5-35). Cysts are usually round. The internal content is homogeneous and low density, with Hounsfield numbers approaching those of water. Generally, no change occurs in the internal density of the cysts with intravenous contrast enhancement, although the cyst itself gives the appearance of being more lucent because of the increased density in the surrounding liver tissue. Extremely small cysts are difficult to evaluate and difficult to get a cursor on to obtain accurate density numbers (Fig. 5-36).

Ultrasonography is often helpful in distinguishing a simple cyst from a low-density solid lesion, such as an abscess, necrotic tumor, echinococcal cyst, or cystic neoplasm. The ultrasound characteristics are a focal, well-defined anechoic defect within the liver, through-transmission, and acoustic enhancement of the far wall (Fig. 5-37).

MRI characteristics of hepatic cysts also are characteristic, with a low signal on T1-weighted images and a very high signal on T2-weighted images. The relatively long T1 and T2 values are helpful in differentiating simple cysts from most hepatic neoplasms (Fig. 5-38). A hemangioma can give a similar signal pattern, however. In addition, difficulties may be encountered when imaging infected or bloody cysts.

Trauma

Contrast-enhanced multidetector CT is the modality of choice in the imaging evaluation of patients with

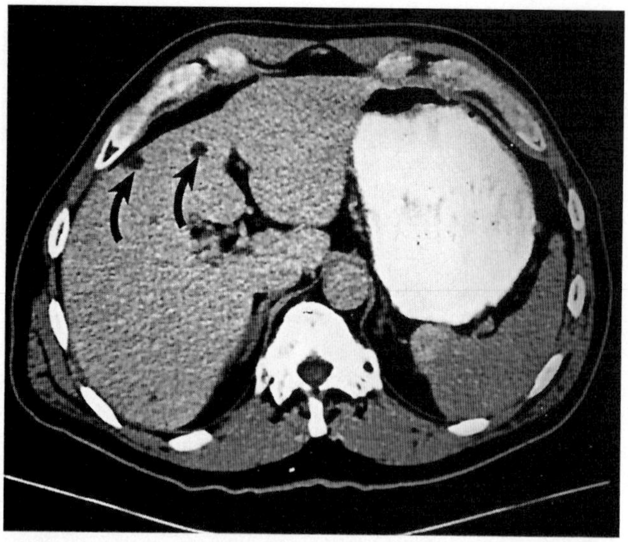

Figure 5-36 Two small cysts *(curved arrows)* are seen near the margin of the liver and measure approximately 1 cm. They were confirmed by ultrasound examination.

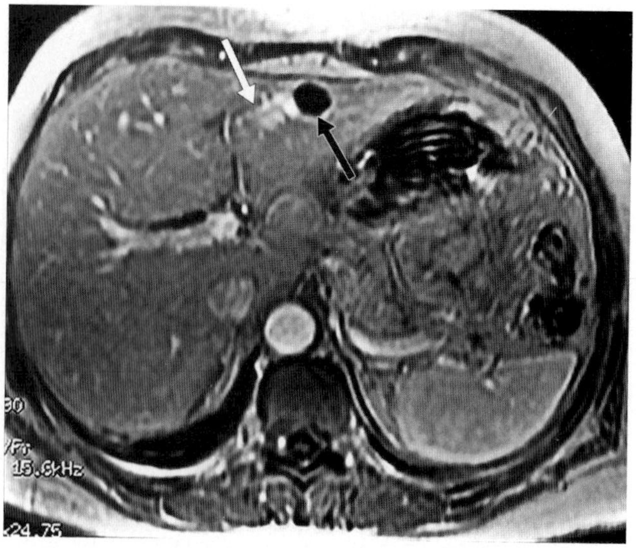

Figure 5-38 T1-weighted MRI shows high signal from a small hemangioma in the left lobe *(white arrow)* and low signal from an adjacent cyst *(black arrow)*.

blunt trauma to the abdomen. Blunt trauma to the abdomen resulting in hepatic laceration is most commonly seen as a solitary laceration or branching area of linear attenuation within the substance of the liver (Fig. 5-39). A fractured liver with multiple lacerations is uncommonly seen because these patients usually die before computed tomographic evaluation. In the uncommon event that patients do survive, their condition is usually unstable, and they are candidates for emergency exploratory surgery. Trauma can be contained within the liver capsule or result in capsular tear and intraperitoneal bleeding (Fig. 5-40). Longer term complications include infection, abscess, and chronic bile leak.

Hepatocellular Carcinoma

Hepatocellular carcinoma or hepatoma is a slow-growing, but nevertheless malignant, lesion originating

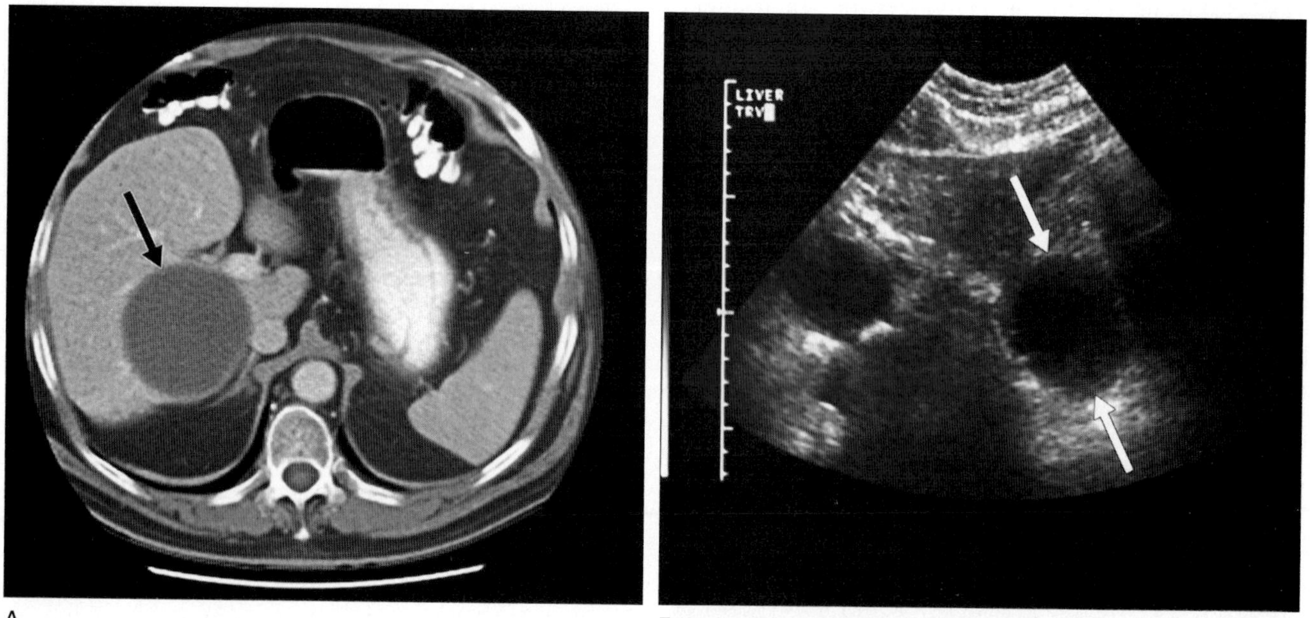

A B

Figure 5-37 **A,** Large circular cyst seen in liver on CT *(arrow)*. **B,** This is also well shown on ultrasound examination *(arrows)*.

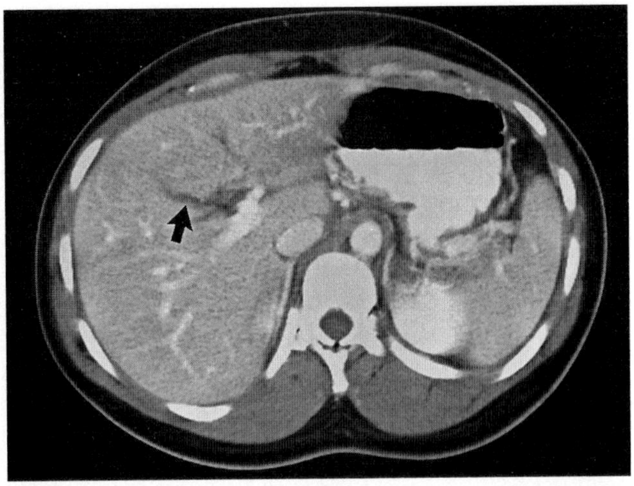

Figure 5-39 A patient with blunt trauma to the abdomen. CT of liver reveals an irregular linear defect *(arrow)*. No blood is seen around the liver.

in liver parenchymal cells (Box 5-4). It is the seventh most common tumor in men and the ninth in women and the most common primary hepatic malignancy. Distant metastatic involvement is unusual, but has been reported. Seventy-five percent of patients have contiguous or lymphatic extrahepatic spread of tumor at the time of diagnosis and are unresectable. In addition, portal vein thrombosis is seen in 50% of patients (Fig. 5-41). Invasion of the hepatic venous system can result in a Budd-Chiari–type picture. An elevated serum alpha-fetoprotein level is a good (but not absolute) serum indicator of the presence of hepatocellular carcinoma (or hepatoblastoma in children).

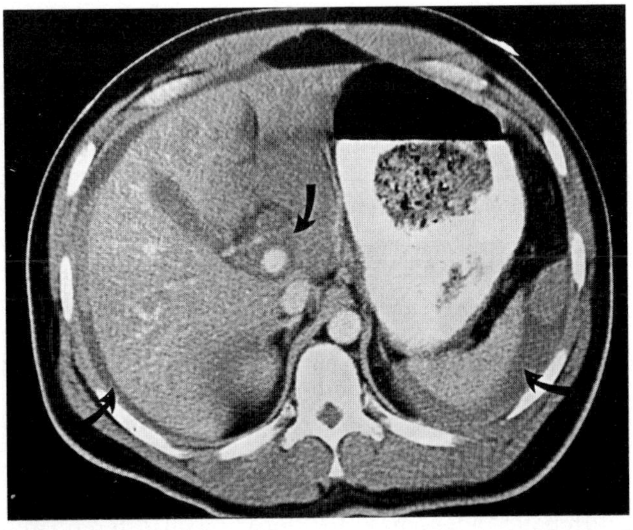

Figure 5-40 This patient was in a motor vehicle accident and sustained blunt trauma to the abdomen and lacerated liver. Blood is seen around the liver, around the spleen, and in the porta hepatis region *(curved arrows)*. Laceration is not shown on this image.

Box 5-4 Facts about Hepatoma

- Risk factors: hepatitis B infection, hepatitis C infection, cirrhosis, exposure to hepatocarcinogens
- Associated with elevated alpha fetoprotein
- Seen in the United States, but much more common in parts of Asia
- Imaging assessment by CT, CTAP, MRI, angiography
- Poor prognosis

The tumor seems to be more common in women and it is relatively common in the Far East, attributable to the presence of various parasites (especially liver flukes), diet, and a high incidence of hepatitis B or hepatitis C. In the West, the tumor is much less common. A definite relationship between hepatic cirrhosis and hepatocellular carcinoma exists, however. Almost 75% of patients with hepatocellular carcinoma have either cirrhosis or a history of cirrhosis. The risk of hepatocellular carcinoma is higher in patients with hemochromatosis of the liver.

Certain other risk factors have been described. Cirrhosis is the most common; 80% of hepatocellular carcinomas develop in cirrhotic livers secondary to hepatitis B and C and chronic alcoholism. In recent years, the use of anabolic steroids has been thought to place individuals at an increased risk for this disease.

Patients often present with cachexia, weakness, right upper quadrant pain, and weight loss. Clinically, an enlarged liver is commonly detected. Multidetector CT may show a solitary mass or multiple masses with a dominant lesion and multiple satellite lesions. The mass is usually of low attenuation (Fig. 5-42). A few patients (<10%) have some calcification within the lesion. In addition, the size of the lesion may be exaggerated on

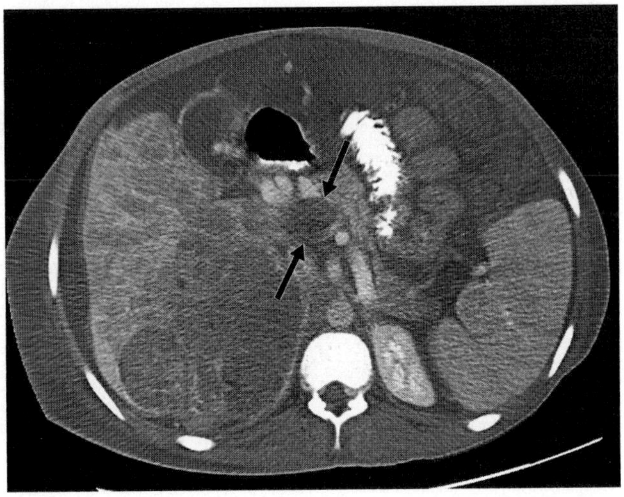

Figure 5-41 Large hepatocellular carcinoma involving most of the right lobe of the liver. Note thrombus in the portal vein *(arrows)*.

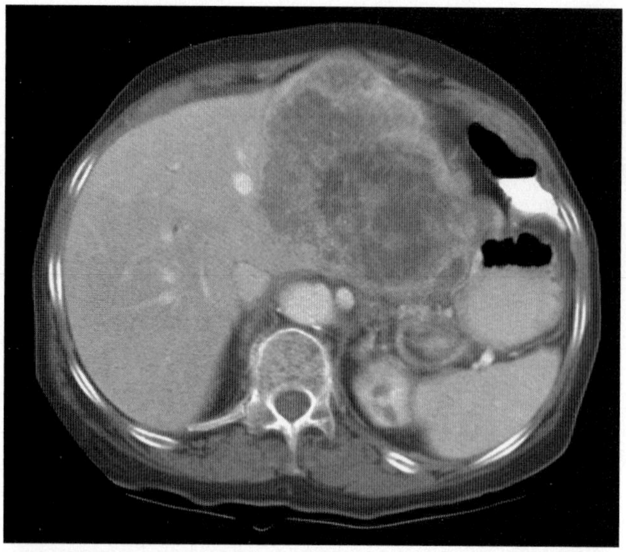

Figure 5-42 Large inhomogeneous lesion occupying and expanding most of the left lobe of the liver, representing a hepatocellular carcinoma.

CT by the presence of regional portal vein thrombosis in 50% of patients. Thrombosis may be seen on CT as regional wedgelike shapes of low density projecting peripherally. Extrahepatic bleeding sometimes occurs, and a positive peritoneal tap for blood in suspected cases of hepatoma in the pre-CT era was considered a strong diagnostic sign (Fig. 5-43).

In patients with a background of cirrhosis, involvement of the liver with hepatocellular carcinoma tends to be more diffuse and presents a diagnostic difficulty in differentiating among regenerating nodules, metastatic disease, and primary hepatic carcinoma. It is prudent to consider any low-attenuation lesion in the cirrhotic liver as a hepatocellular carcinoma until proved otherwise.

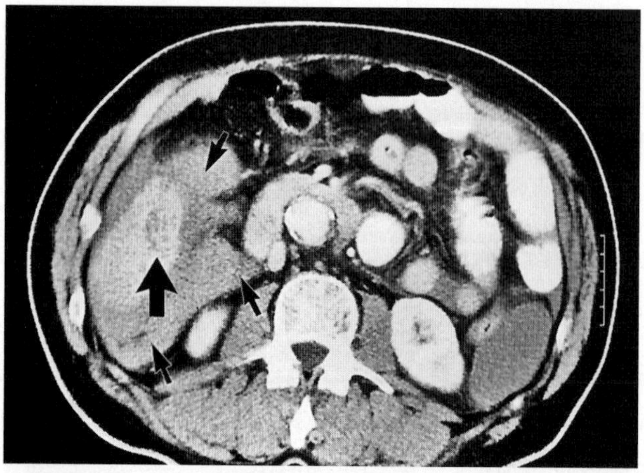

Figure 5-43 An 83-year-old man with hepatocellular carcinoma (hepatoma) presents with orthostatic hypotension. CT shows lesion in tip of liver *(large arrow)* and surrounding blood in lower perihepatic space *(small arrows)*.

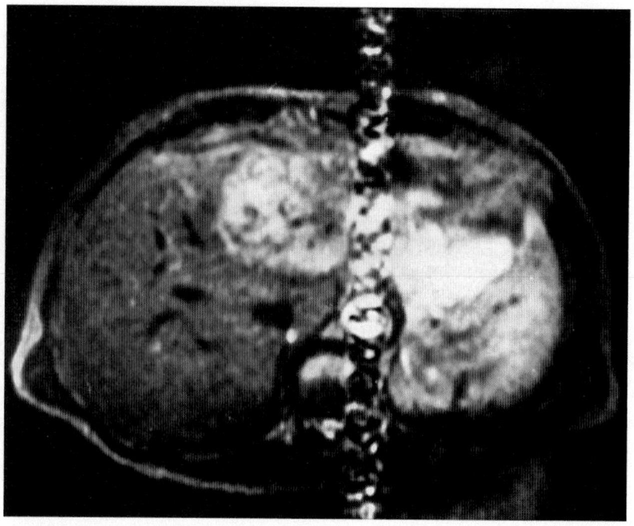

Figure 5-44 MRI in the same patient as in Figure 5-30 shows high signal within the lesion on T2-weighted image.

Multiple patterns have been described for the ultrasonographic presentations of this lesion. These range from discrete echogenic to relatively echo-free lesions. Lesions can have a mixed echo pattern, or there may be diffuse disease. MRI of hepatocellular carcinoma approaches CT in its accuracy. In large lesions, findings can be nonspecific and to some extent depend on the amount of fibrosis and necrosis within the lesion (Fig. 5-44). Generally, this lesion displays low signal intensity on T1-weighted images with an increase in signal intensity on T2-weighted images. MRI has proved to be quite superior, however, in showing vascular involvement by this tumor (Fig. 5-45).

Fibrolamellar hepatocellular carcinoma is a rare variety of hepatocellular carcinoma more commonly seen in younger patients with a roughly equal sex distribution. There is a tendency for intralesion calcification and central scar formation. There is a better prognosis with lesions being more amenable to surgical resection. Fibrolamellar hepatocellular carcinoma does not seem to respond any better to chemotherapy than conventional hepatocellular carcinoma. These lesions do not secrete alpha fetoprotein and are usually not associated with chronic hepatitis B or C. On computed tomographic examination, these lesions usually appear as large solitary hypoattenuating masses. In the arterial phase, there may be peripheral enhancement. In the portal and delayed phases, there is increased homogenicity possibly approaching isodensity (Fig. 5-46).

Adenomas

Hepatic adenomas are focal, well-differentiated benign lesions of the liver. They are usually solitary. More than 90% of these lesions are found in women. The lesions are generally well encapsulated. The incidence

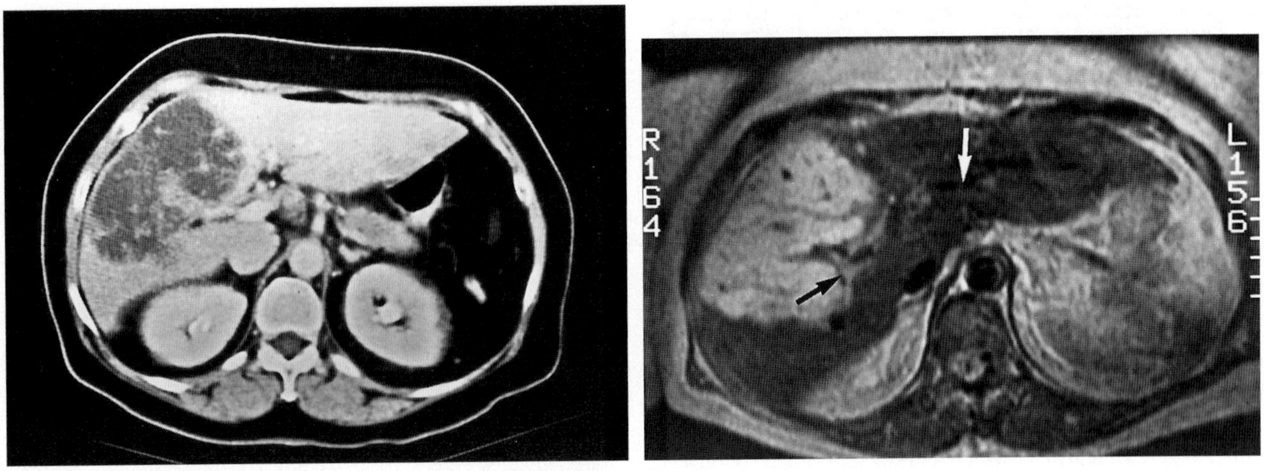

A B

Figure 5-45 **A,** CT in patient with hepatoma. The lesion is large and lobulated. **B,** Spin echo T2-weighted MRI shows lesion with tumor in portal veins *(black arrow)*. Uninvolved veins are seen distal to the lesion *(white arrow)*.

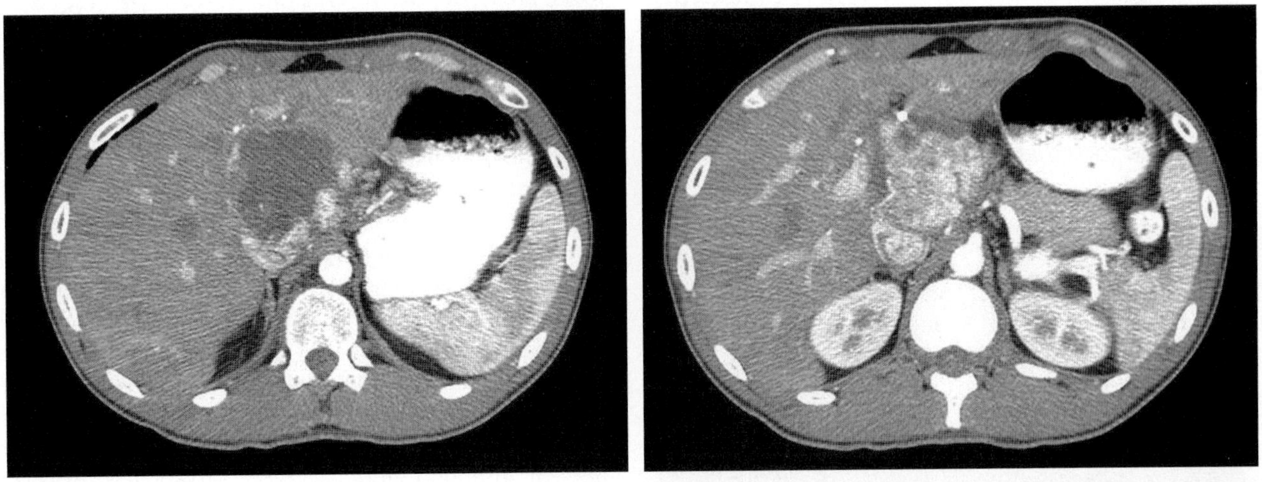

A B

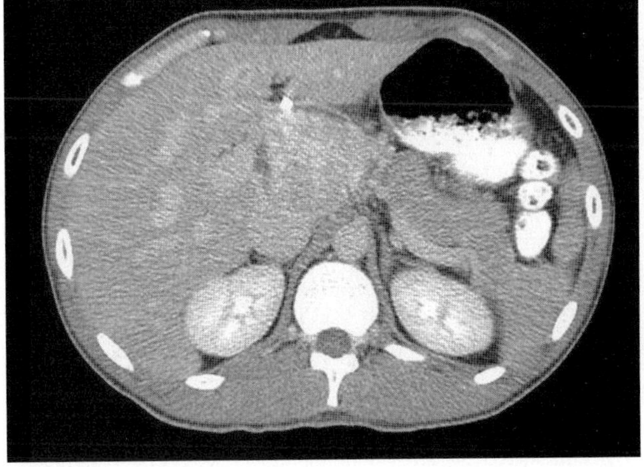

C

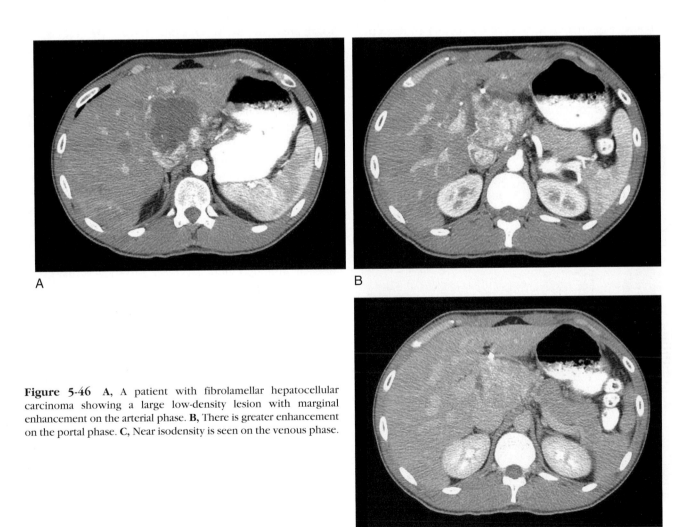

Figure 5-46 **A,** A patient with fibrolamellar hepatocellular carcinoma showing a large low-density lesion with marginal enhancement on the arterial phase. **B,** There is greater enhancement on the portal phase. **C,** Near isodensity is seen on the venous phase.

of hepatic adenomas has increased over the past four decades and is thought to be related to the increased use of oral contraceptive pills. Given the incidence of this lesion and the number of women using oral contraceptive pills, however, the risk seems exceedingly small, and it is possible there are other factors, such as genetics, to be considered. The incidence of hepatic adenomas in some glycogen storage diseases also has increased. Generally, the malignant potential of hepatic adenomas is considered low. Yet the suspected increased incidence of hepatocellular carcinoma in women taking oral contraceptive pills raises the question of some degree of malignant potential.

Adenomas tend to be hypervascular, and internal hemorrhage can lead to blood-filled cysts within the adenoma (Fig. 5-47). They are usually asymptomatic. Serum alpha-fetoprotein levels are normal. When symptoms do occur, they are usually acute and in 50% of the cases result from bleeding. The adenomas can be subcapsular or pedunculated on the edge of the liver, and bleeding can occur into the peritoneal cavity, resulting in a surgical emergency. The incidence of bleeding in hepatic adenomas is increased in women taking oral contraceptive pills.

Hepatic adenomas present as discrete masses, usually solitary on dynamic CT. They are commonly hyperdense. If hemorrhage or internal necrosis has occurred, the tumor can be heterogeneous in its appearance with focal areas of low attenuation (Figs. 5-48 and 5-49). Ultrasonography shows variable patterns, depending on the presence of intralesional bleeding. Bleeding results in a decreased echogenicity within the lesion. Otherwise, the adenoma is seen as a hyperechoic solid lesion (Fig. 5-50). Similar to hepatocellular carcinomas, hepatic adenomas are best shown on T2-weighted MRI.

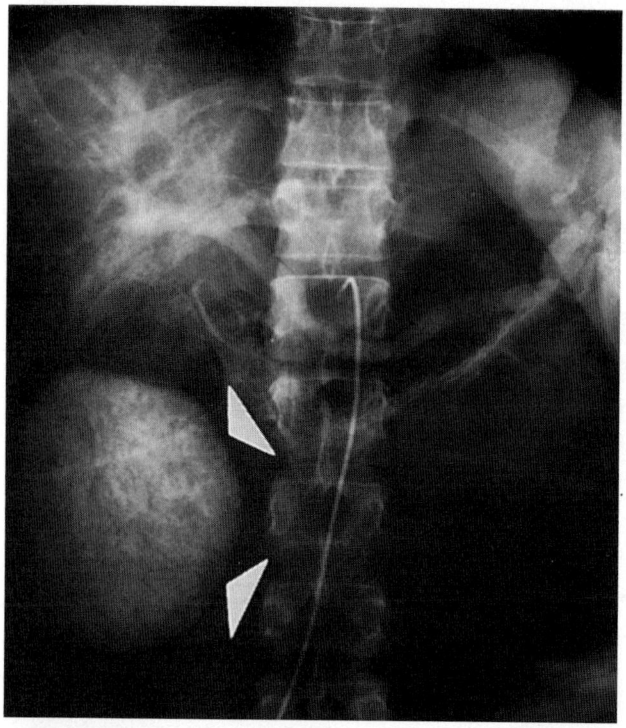

Figure 5-47 Vascular study during venous phase in a patient with pedunculated hepatic adenoma shows well-defined hypervascular lesion *(arrowheads)*.

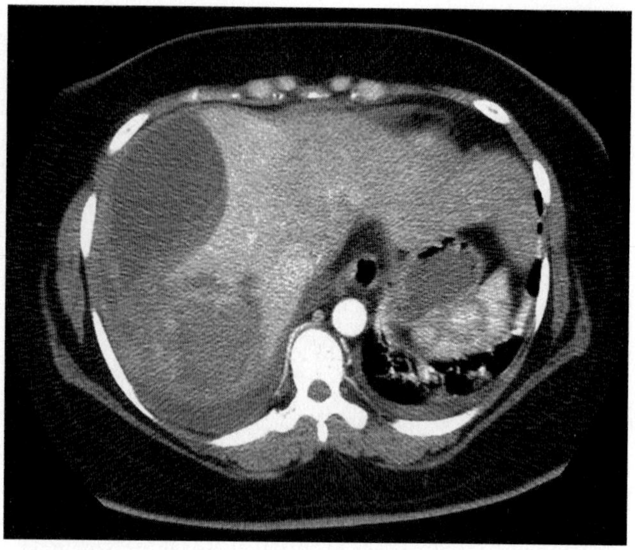

Figure 5-48 Large heterogeneous lesion involving the upper portion of the right lobe of the liver with perihepatic bleeding that proved to be a hepatic adenoma in a young woman.

Focal Nodular Hyperplasia

Focal nodular hyperplasia is the third most common benign tumor of the liver, but is nonetheless a relatively uncommon lesion. It is best described as a well-defined hepatic lesion, commonly solitary, composed of bundles of benign hyperplastic hepatocytes arranged around a stellate fibrous central scar. The etiological origins are unclear, although there is evidence to suggest that some degree of hormonal dependency is involved in either its origin or its growth. In contrast to hepatic adenomas (Table 5-1), differences in incidence between men and women are less striking, and there is a much smaller tendency for the lesion to bleed or rupture. Generally, focal nodular hyperplasia is asymptomatic. A few patients have vague right upper quadrant pain.

Most patients are women (70% to 80%) 30 to 40 years old. A relationship between focal nodular hyperplasia and the use of oral contraceptive pills has been postulated but not proved.

The lesions can be single or less commonly multiple. The mass is composed of hyperplastic liver parenchymal elements often partitioned into bundles by fibrous bands radiating from a large central scar. This configuration is seen in approximately 60% of patients with focal nodular hyperplasia. The size of the lesions varies from 1 to 20 cm.

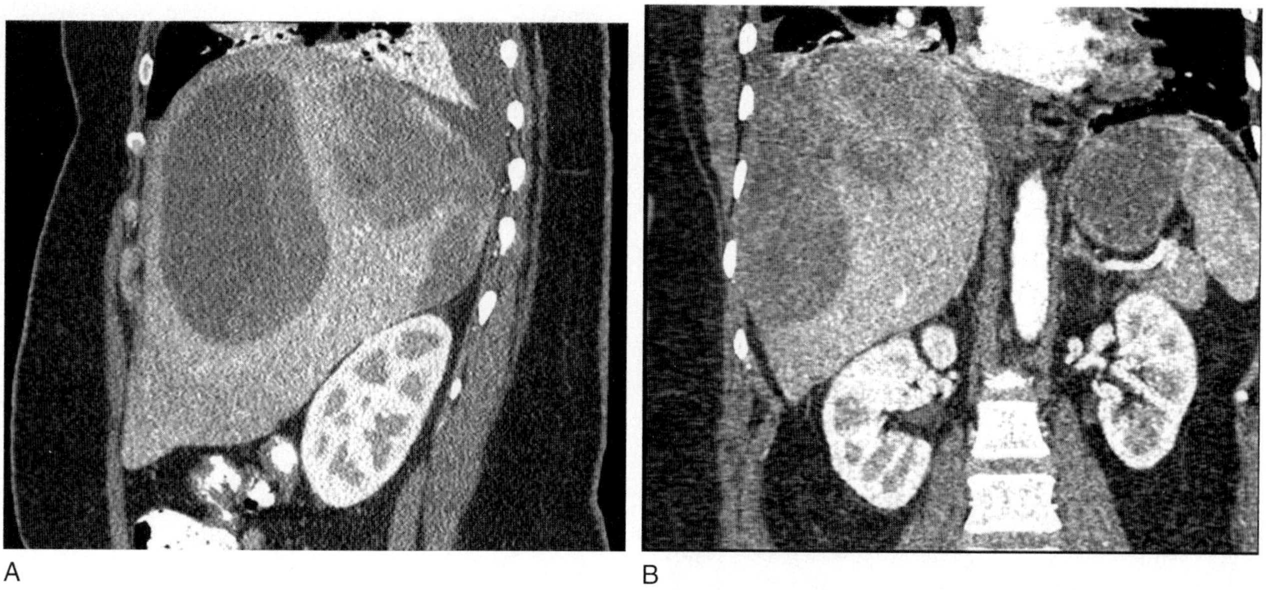

Figure 5-49 **A,** Sagittal reconstruction of a large hepatic adenoma with some perihepatic bleeding. **B,** Coronal oblique reconstruction of same patient shows the degree of extensive involvement.

They are seen most commonly in the right lobe of the liver.

CT may show an isodense or hypodense lesion on the unenhanced scans (Fig. 5-51). Similar to hepatic adenomas, the lesion shows an increase in homogeneous enhancement after intravenous contrast enhancement (Fig. 5-52). There may be an area of low attenuation in the center of the lesion if a central stellate area of scarring is present. It is sometimes difficult to differentiate between hepatic adenoma and focal nodular hyperplasia on CT.

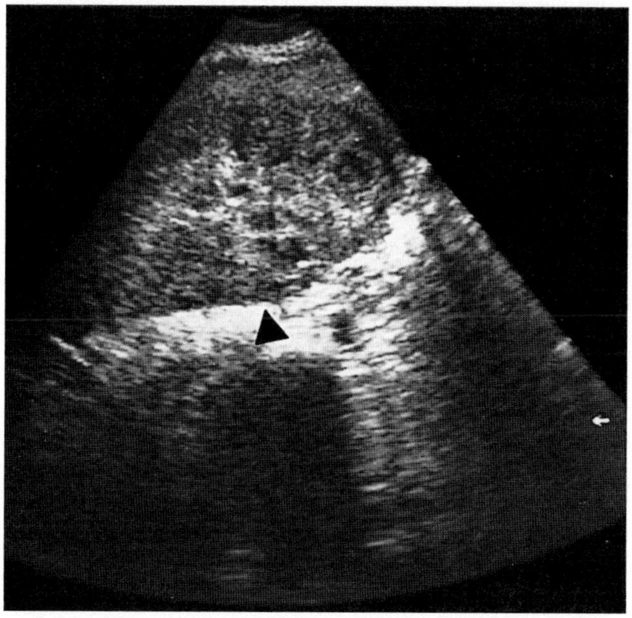

Figure 5-50 Ultrasonogram in a young woman with hepatic adenoma shows a large hyperechoic lesion *(arrowhead)*.

The ultrasound appearance is of a mass that may appear less echogenic than the surrounding normal liver. It also can appear isoechoic with the surrounding liver. Identification of the central scar may be helpful and is manifested by dense internal echoes.

MRI may be helpful. There is a tendency for the lesion to be isodense on all pulse sequences (Fig. 5-53). If the central scarring complex is present, this tends to have a low signal on T1-weighted images and a higher signal on T2-weighted images (Fig. 5-54). On technetium-99m sulfur colloid scans, focal nodular hyperplasia, because of the presence of Kupffer's cells, can show normal or near-normal uptake and may be indistinguishable from surrounding liver (60% to 70%) tissue, whereas a hepatic adenoma is almost always a cold defect.

Treatment is usually reserved for symptomatic cases in which the lesion is large and in which surgical resection would be curative.

Abscesses

Hepatic abscesses can be bacterial, parasitic, or mycotic. Bacterial or pyogenic abscesses are focal collections of pus within the liver. Most pyogenic abscesses occur as an extension of infection ascending through the biliary tree (ascending cholangitis). Hematogenous spread through the portal vein or the hepatic artery or direct contiguous spread from an adjacent site of infection also can cause hepatic abscess formation. Hepatic abscesses also can be seen in posttraumatic events involving the liver. Most commonly, a gram-negative organism

Table 5-1 Distinctions between Hepatic Adenoma and Focal Nodular Hyperplasia

	Hepatic Adenoma	Focal Nodular Hyperplasia
Sex distribution	Predominantly women	Predominantly women
Relationship to oral contraceptives	Related to long-term use of oral contraceptives	Relationship not well understood; may be no etiological relationship, but oral contraceptives may contribute to growth of lesion
Clinical presentation	50% bleed	Often asymptomatic; may complain of abdominal pain or mass
Pathology	Usually solitary adenomatous lesion	Proliferation of hepatocytes divided by fibrous septa
Radiology	Can be difficult to distinguish from FNH	Technetium-99m sulfur colloid liver scan can be helpful in 60%-70% of cases

FNH, focal nodular hyperplasia.

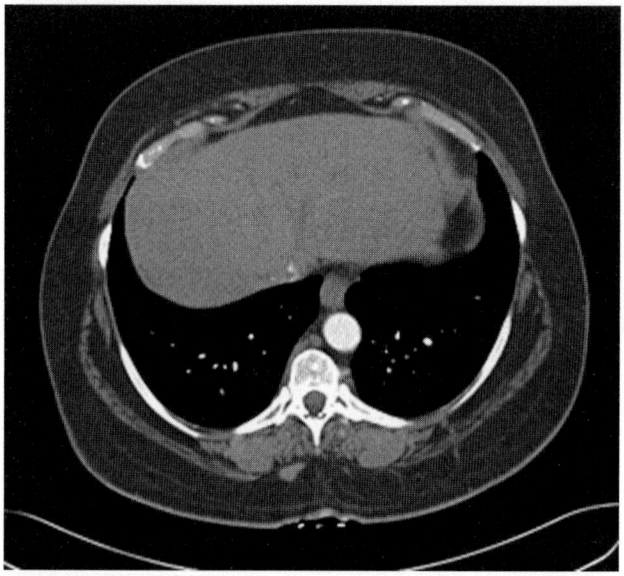

Figure 5-51 Focal nodular hyperplasia in a young woman in the dome of the liver is isodense in the arterial phase.

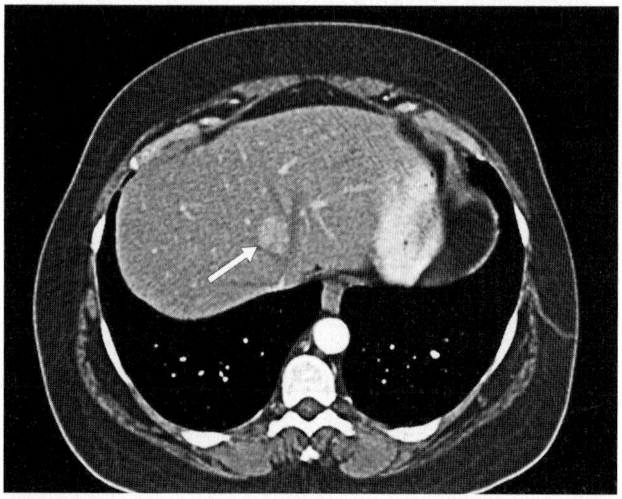

Figure 5-52 Same patient as in Figure 5-51. Focal nodular hyperplasia is now seen as a focal area of increased attenuation in the portal phase *(arrow)*.

is involved. The clinical course without therapeutic intervention is almost uniformly a rapid downhill decline and death.

Early symptoms vary and include fever, chills, sweating, right upper quadrant pain, pleuritic pain, nausea, and vomiting. Many patients have abnormal liver function tests, and one third of patients have some degree of jaundice. The size of the lesions varies, from 1 to 20 cm (Fig. 5-55). The smaller the abscess, the higher

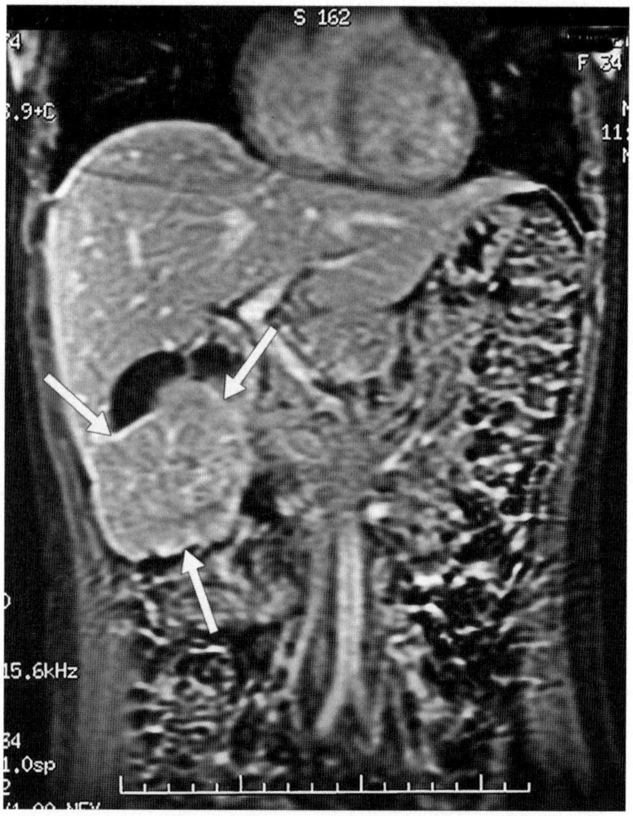

Figure 5-53 Coronal MRI shows pedunculated focal nodular hyperplasia *(arrows)* of the same density as the rest of the liver.

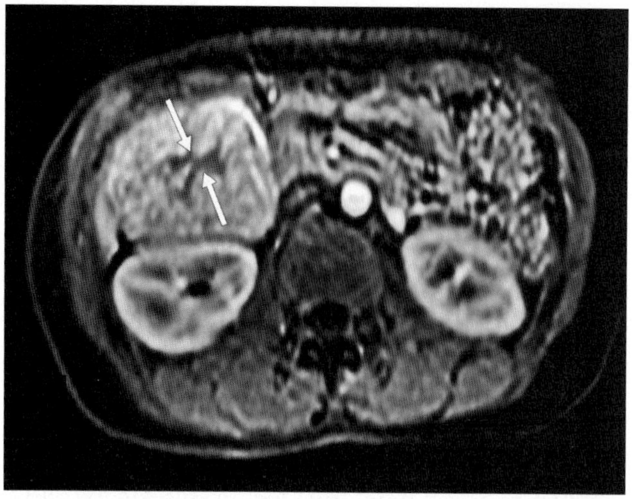

Figure 5-54 MRI through a pedunculated high-signal lesion at the lower margin of the liver. The lesion proved to be focal nodular hyperplasia. Note the central scar *(arrows)*.

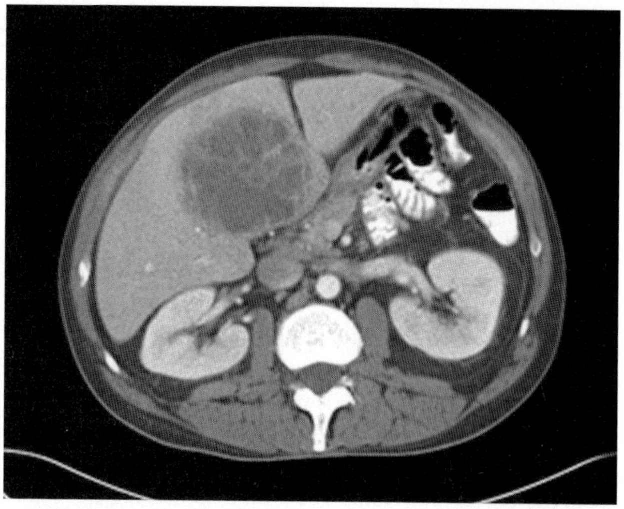

Figure 5-56 This patient has a large septated pyogenic abscess occupying the medial segment of the left lobe of the liver.

the probability of multiple sites within the liver. Approximately 50% to 70% of patients have multiple lesions. Of the lesions, 80% occur in the right lobe of the liver. CT of the liver generally discloses a low-attenuation lesion with a peripheral rim that usually enhances after intravenous contrast. Internally the liver may have septations or papillary projections (Fig. 5-56). In about one fifth of cases, gas bubbles can be detected. Air-fluid levels are identified occasionally. Lesions may be solitary or multiple, or there may be a grouping of lesions, generally in the right lobe with one large and several small adjacent lesions (Fig. 5-57). The computed tomographic appearance can be simulated by metastatic disease, although the clinical presentations are different. Needle aspiration is the most helpful method of differentiation. MRI of hepatic abscesses provides no additional specificity above CT. Ultrasonography generally shows a focal area of decreased echogenicity. If there is gas within the abscess or internal septations, internal echoes are generated.

Hepatic amebic abscesses, although common in many parts of the world, are rarely seen in the United States and Canada. It is thought that they are secondary to colonic amebiasis. Approximately 5% of these patients are estimated to have hepatic abscesses. Amebic abscesses

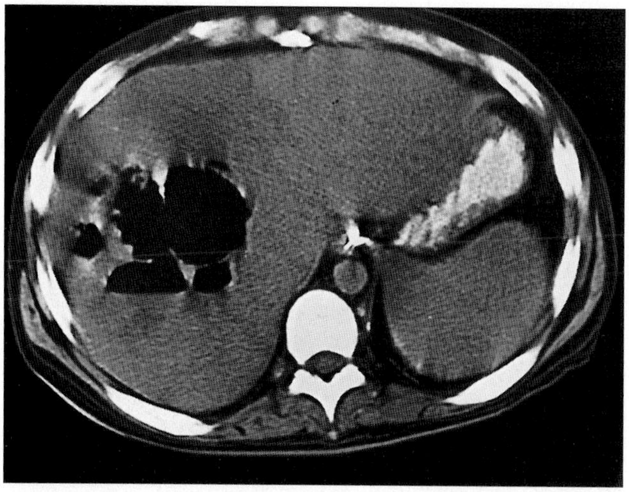

Figure 5-55 Large hepatic abscess occupying most of the right lobe of the liver. Note the internal septations, air-fluid levels, and wall irregularity of the lesion.

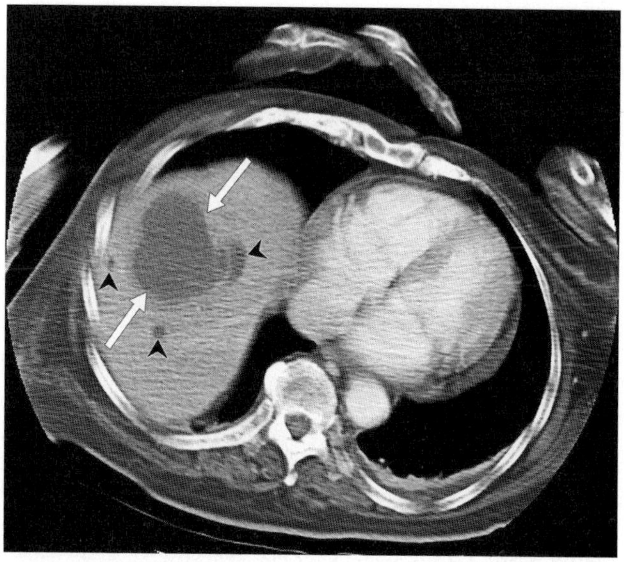

Figure 5-57 CT through dome of the liver shows a large abscess *(arrows)* with several small satellite abscesses *(arrowheads)*.

also can be seen within the lungs and brain. The organism, *Entamoeba histolytica,* is thought to enter the liver through the portal venous system. For that reason, the lesions tend to be peripheral in location. The classic "anchovy sauce" appearance of the contents of hepatic amebic abscess results from a combination of internal liquefaction, hepatonecrosis, and bleeding. The cysts are mostly solitary with thick, shaggy walls. Complications of these amebic abscesses include rupture upward through the diaphragm into the pleural or pericardial spaces or downward into the peritoneal cavity.

Patients almost always present with abdominal pain. Fever, weight loss, and symptoms relative to colonic involvement also may be present. Diagnosis is usually based on history, clinical presentation, and positive hemagglutination titers. Although considerable reluctance to perform needle aspiration of these lesions existed in the past, this procedure is being done today, with little or no occurrence of the catastrophic complications previously anticipated. The computed tomographic appearance of amebic abscesses in the liver is similar to that of pyogenic abscesses. Amebic abscesses tend to be unilocular, however (Fig. 5-58). Ultrasonography often shows ill-defined walls around a generally solitary ovoid lesion located near the liver capsule. Echogenicity within the lesion is decreased.

Echinococcal infection of the liver (hydatid cyst disease) can occur in two forms, *Echinococcus granulosus* or, less commonly, *Echinococcus multilocularis.* The former is more likely to involve the liver with large encapsulated cysts. The adult worm lives in the small bowel of the definitive hosts. Animals, particularly dogs, are the definitive hosts, whereas humans, sheep, cattle, and other animals become the intermediate hosts after contaminant ingestion of the parasitic eggs. The eggs hatch in the small bowel and colon of the intermediate host, and the larvae penetrate the bowel wall and primarily enter the portal blood system. In hydatid disease, 70% of the larvae are carried to the liver. The remaining larvae are carried to distant sites, such as lungs, spleen, and brain. In the liver, the larvae encyst, and for a long time the patient may be asymptomatic. Symptoms develop as the cyst grows and enlarges (usually >10 cm). Occasionally, the parasite dies, the fluid is absorbed, and an encapsulated, calcified lesion is all that remains. In cases of viable, long-standing cysts, calcification also may occur in the wall. The major clinical problems arise as a result of complications associated with the cysts. These complications can result from the pressure on the biliary system, raising the possibility of obstructive jaundice. The most significant complication is rupture into the peritoneal cavity, alimentary canal, or biliary tree. Cephalad development of the cysts could result in rupture into the pleural cavity or even the pericardial space. Rupture, especially into the peritoneum, is accompanied by profound shock, peritonitis, and possibly anaphylaxis. Prognosis after intraperitoneal rupture is poor.

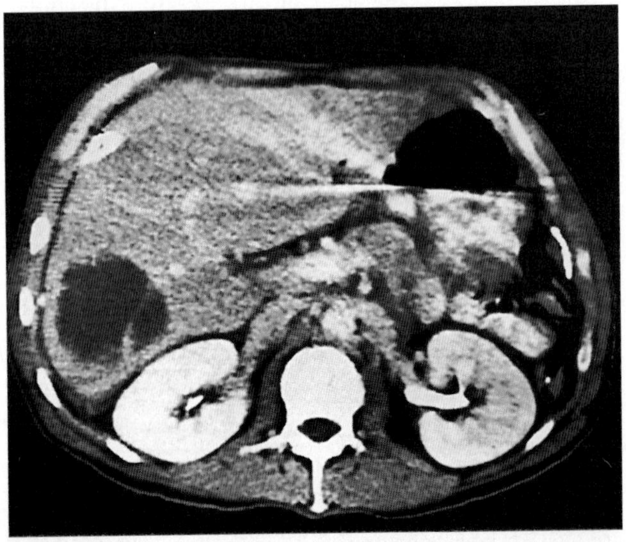

Figure 5-58 CT through the liver of a patient with known amebic abscess of the posterior right lobe. Note the well-defined margins of the abscess and the internal septation on this enhanced scan.

As would be expected, the disease is relatively common in sheep-raising areas in the world and to a lesser extent cattle-raising areas. With increased mobility and worldwide travel common today, however, the dissemination of this disease along with other diseases that were relatively confined to endemic regions of the world is now seen with more frequency in North America.

Hydatid cyst involvement of the liver is manifested by low-attenuation lesions on CT. Focal areas of additional attenuation within the cysts usually indicate daughter cysts. Calcification may be identified in the rims. Infection or bleeding can alter the CT appearance. Occasionally, the detached cyst membrane is seen on CT. This is analogous to the well-known "water lily" sign seen in the lungs of patients with pulmonary involvement. This finding has been described after cyst aspiration and is highly specific for hydatid disease. The ultrasound findings vary. Cyst wall calcification may be present. Otherwise, a well-defined mass with good through-transmission may be identified. Daughter cysts within the lesion are particularly helpful in making the diagnosis.

Mycotic abscesses of the liver are almost always multiple and small. These are commonly seen in immunocompromised patients and frequently are accompanied by multiple small abscesses within the spleen. The most common organism is *Candida albicans* (Fig. 5-59).

Angiosarcoma

Angiosarcoma (also known as Kupffer cell sarcoma and malignant hemangioendothelioma) is a rare tumor of

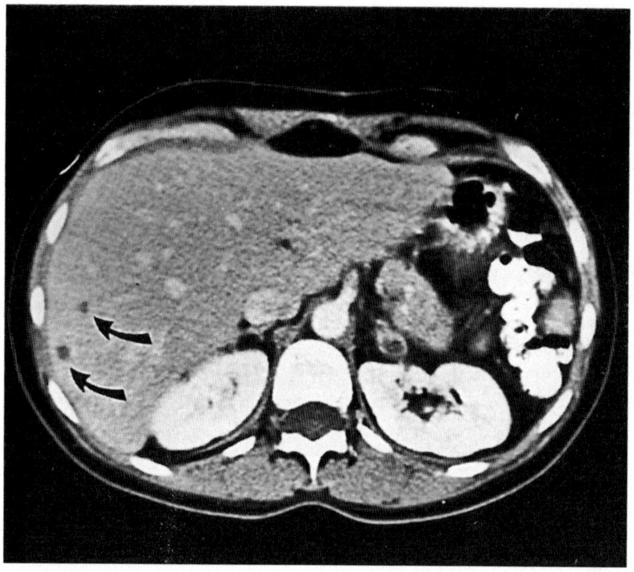

Figure 5-59 CT through the liver of a patient who has recently undergone bone marrow transplantation. At least two small abscesses are seen in the periphery of the right lobe of the liver *(curved arrows)*, representing hepatic candidiasis.

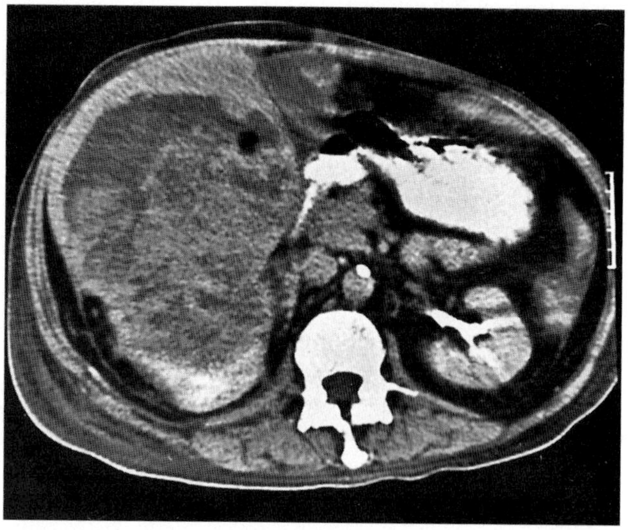

Figure 5-60 CT through the lower portion of the right lobe of the liver shows a huge inhomogeneous mass occupying and expanding most of the inferior portion of the right lobe of the liver, representing an angiosarcoma of the liver.

particular interest because of its association with Thorotrast and the industrial carcinogen vinyl chloride. During the 1940s and 1950s, a radioactive colloid suspension of thorium dioxide, called Thorotrast, was injected intravenously for hepatosplenic imaging. The radioactivity put the individual at high risk for malignant induction. Patients chronically exposed to arsenic or to vinyl chloride in the manufacture of plastics also are at risk for this tumor.

Generally, CT discloses a large, irregular, low-attenuation lesion within the liver that may manifest peripheral enhancement during the dynamic phase (Fig. 5-60). This tumor is rapid in its growth and generally unresponsive to treatment. Survival is usually limited to 6 months after diagnosis.

Other causes of solitary low-attenuation lesions of the liver include lipomas. These are unusual, but occur in about 10% of patients with renal angiomyolipomatosis. The computed tomographic appearance of this lesion is characteristic.

Biliary Cystadenoma and Cystadenocarcinoma

Biliary cystadenoma and cystadenocarcinoma are rare tumors arising from the bile ducts, but most commonly appearing as a liver lesion on CT; 80% are seen in middle-aged women. They are usually large, solitary lesions with low-attenuation characteristics on CT. They often show multiple loculations, which are lined with biliary epithelium.

Patients present with abdominal pain, upper abdominal mass, occasionally jaundice, and constitutional symptoms. The tumor tends to be slow growing. CT evaluation shows enhancement along the margin and the septum of the lesion. This unusual septal enhancement occurs as a result of papillary growth along the septum, which is seen in the cystadenocarcinoma. Lesser degrees of papillary growth can be seen in the cystadenoma. The cystadenoma usually shows a thin septum, however, and little or no enhancement. Absolute differentiation between the cystadenoma and the cystadenocarcinoma ultimately requires surgical removal and pathological evaluation of the lesion. Surgical resection of these lesions often yields excellent results.

Intrahepatic Cholangiocarcinoma

Intrahepatic cholangiocarcinoma arises from the epithelium of the bile ducts and is covered in more detail elsewhere. It is usually a sclerosing tumor with little or no mass effect. It is occasionally seen, however, as a solitary intrahepatic lesion. The lesion is usually central (Fig. 5-61).

Hepatic Pseudotumor

Focal fatty infiltration of the liver is a common finding on CT and can mimic other disease, such as primary or secondary malignancy of the liver. It most commonly is seen near the gallbladder fossa and porta hepatis area, but can occur anywhere in the liver. Ultrasound examination may not be conclusive, but various sequences of MRI of the liver that include T2-weighted images and gadolinium-enhanced studies may be more helpful.

Another pseudotumor seen in the liver that also can cause confusion is focal confluent fibrosis. These areas are hyperdense on CT. There may a wedge-shaped configuration and possibly distortion of the adjunct liver capsule. Other pseudotumors of the liver include

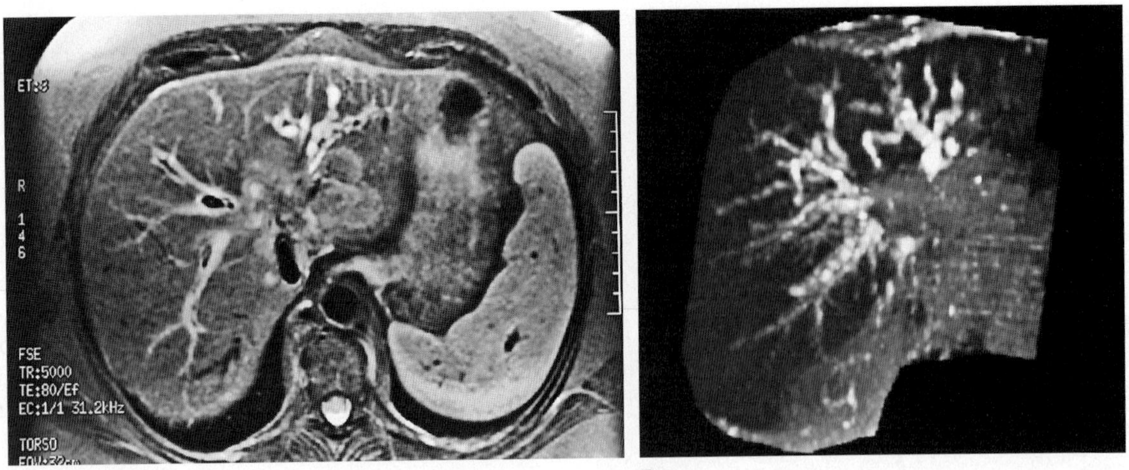

A B

Figure 5-61 **A,** T2-weighted axial MRI of the liver shows a large central lesion. **B,** MRI cholangiography (heavily weighted T2-imaging making bile appear white) shows the central nature of the lesion and suggests the origins of the lesion, which proved to be cholangiocarcinoma.

vascular lesions such as arteriovenous malformations and arterioportal shunting.

Multiple Defects

Many of the lesions that have been discussed previously and can present as a solitary lesion within the liver also may present as multiple lesions. To avoid redundancy, they are discussed only briefly here.

Metastatic Disease

Multiple bilobar metastatic involvement is a common presentation and results in the typical low-attenuation lesions previously described (Fig. 5-62). Hypervascular metastatic lesions are much less common, but include such malignancies as carcinoid, islet cell carcinomas, renal cell carcinomas, and some pancreatic cancers.

Lymphoma involves the liver in 20% to 50% of cases of Hodgkin's disease. Hepatic involvement is greater in non-Hodgkin's lymphomas. Lymphoma can be multiple and nodular, giving multiple, low-attenuation lesions on computed tomographic examination. Alternatively, the involvement may be diffuse, resulting in a homogeneous enlarged liver (Fig. 5-63). Primary hepatic lymphoma has been described in the literature, although the existence of such a lesion is disputed. Other lesions that rarely can involve the liver with focal nodular lesions include Burkitt's lymphoma and leukemia.

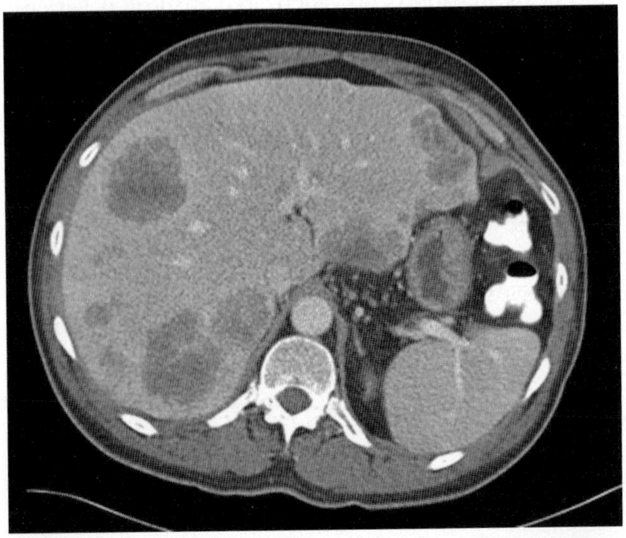

Figure 5-62 Typical presentation of diffuse hepatic metastatic disease. Low-attenuation lesions are seen in both lobes of the liver.

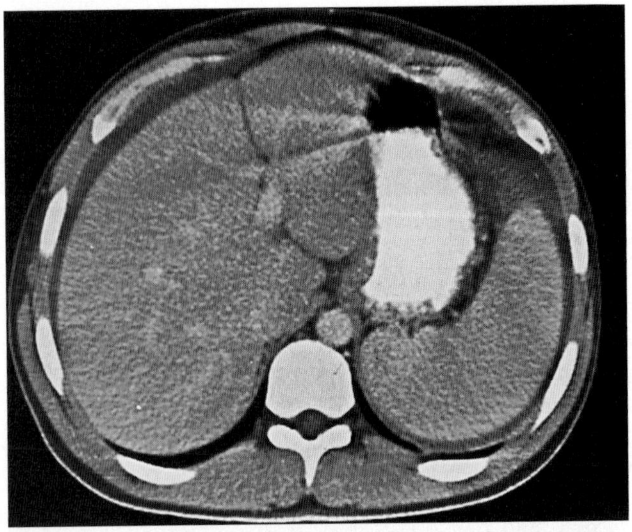

Figure 5-63 CT through the liver in a 27-year-old patient with lymphoma. The liver is diffusely and homogeneously infiltrated with lymphoma. Note the perihepatic fluid.

Focal Nodular Hyperplasia

Although usually solitary, focal nodular hyperplasia can present as multiple hepatic lesions.

Cysts

Hepatic cysts are commonly multiple. Along with hemangiomas, they represent the most common lesions incidentally encountered in CT and ultrasonography of the liver.

Abscesses

In about 50% to 70% of cases, abscesses are multiple in the liver. Most abscesses that result from bacteremia and the entrance of microorganisms through the hepatic artery are multiple and bilobar, although the right lobe is usually more involved. As previously mentioned, in adults, most pyogenic hepatic abscesses are associated with bile duct infections (Fig. 5-64).

Hemangiomas

In about 10% of patients, hemangiomas are multiple.

Caroli's Disease

Cavernous ectasia of the biliary tract (Caroli's disease) is an autosomal recessive disease of bile ducts in which cystic dilatation of the intrahepatic ducts occurs. In its severe form, it can look like multiple cystic lesions of the liver on CT and is included in the choledochal cyst classification as type V. A central dot sign within the apparent cystic lesions in the liver has been described on CT after intravenous contrast administration. This central dot is thought to represent portal vein surrounded by the dilated biliary ducts. When present, this finding may result in an increased degree of specificity for the diagnosis on CT. The liver is usually enlarged, and the disease has an association with polycystic disease of the kidney, despite differences in genetic expression. With the increase of biliary stasis in this condition, the risk for sepsis, stone formation, and ultimately cholangiocarcinoma is increased.

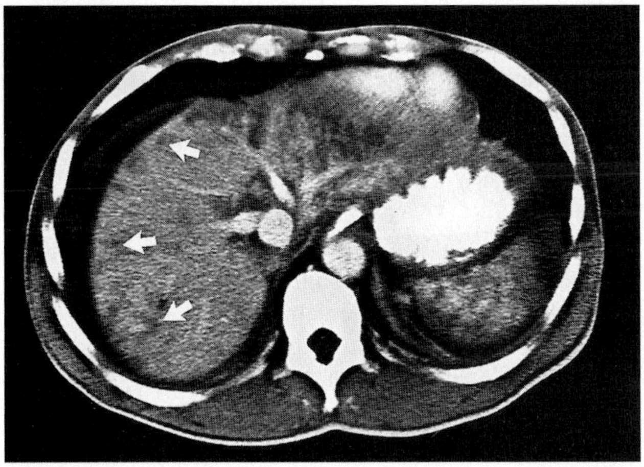

Figure 5-64 Multiple small hepatic abscesses *(arrows)* are seen in this immunosuppressed patient.

Epithelioid Hemangioendothelioma

Epithelioid hemangioendothelioma is a rare vascular tumor most commonly seen in adults. It often starts as a multinodular lesion of the liver and may progress to a more diffuse pattern. The usual computed tomographic finding is multiple low-attenuation lesions with a low-attenuation halo around all the lesions. These are slow-growing, indolent, but progressive lesions.

Regenerating Nodules

Regenerating nodules, seen in cirrhotic livers, also are referred to as adenomatous hyperplasia or nodular hyperplasia of the liver. There is no definite capsule or fibrous scarring in or around the lesion. They generally are considered precancerous lesions in cirrhotic livers. Often these nodules contain malignant foci. A small, well-differentiated hepatocellular carcinoma is extremely difficult to distinguish from a regenerating nodule. Multidetector CT multiphase examination might be an acceptable method to differentiate the two at this time. Because regenerating nodules tend to have an abundance of portal blood supply, as opposed to diminished portal blood supply for hepatocellular carcinomas, CTAP provides a helpful method in distinguishing them. MRI of regenerating nodules tends to show a low signal on T2-weighted images, as opposed to hepatocellular carcinoma, which tends to have a high signal on T2-weighted images.

Peliosis Hepatis

Peliosis hepatis is considered a rare lesion but has been seen with increasing frequency over the past decade. This increased incidence is thought to relate to the increasing use of androgenic anabolic steroids. The condition is manifested as multiple, blood-filled cysts throughout the liver. The earliest cases were thought to be a result of advanced tuberculosis or cancer. More recently, peliosis hepatis in HIV-infected patients with associated cutaneous bacillary angiomatosis, a pseudoneoplastic vascular proliferation containing bacteria, has been reported. Peliosis involving the spleen also has been reported. Multiple small intrahepatic cystic lesions may be seen on CT and ultrasonography of the liver.

Biliary Dilatation

Dilated bile ducts sometimes give the appearance of multiple hepatic defects (Fig. 5-65); this is usually the case if the obstruction is at the level of the major

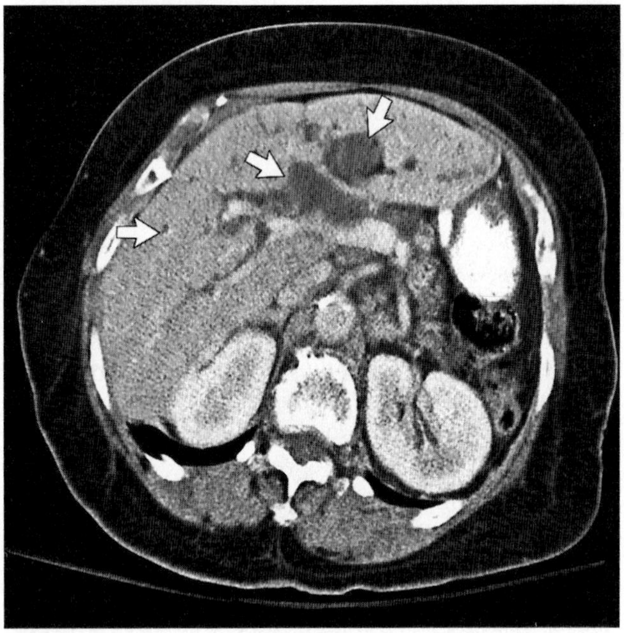

Figure 5-65 This patient has obstruction of the common bile duct from a pancreatic lesion as well as multiple defects in the liver *(arrows)* representing dilated bile ducts. Note how the left biliary system tends to dilate before the right *(upper arrows)*.

bifurcation of the common hepatic duct in the porta hepatis. Enhanced views and a branching pattern usually suggest the nature of the defects. Otherwise the identification of a dilated common bile duct or dilated gallbladder (Courvoisier's sign) confirms the biliary obstruction (Fig. 5-66).

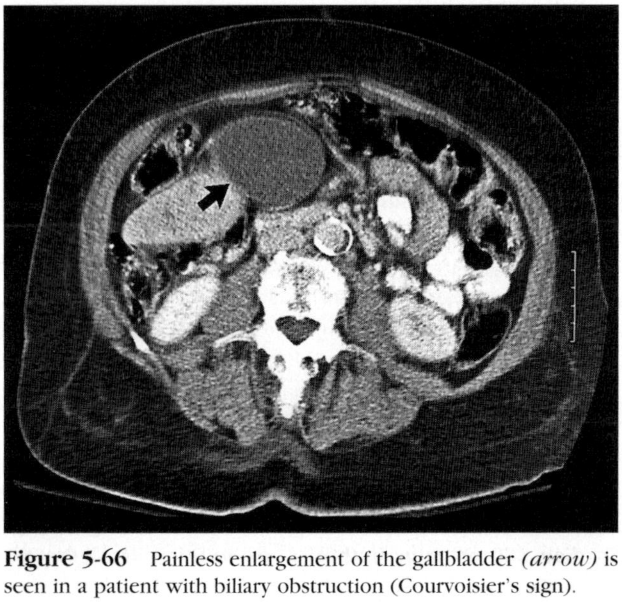

Figure 5-66 Painless enlargement of the gallbladder *(arrow)* is seen in a patient with biliary obstruction (Courvoisier's sign).

Calcifications

Granulomatous Diseases

Granulomatous diseases excite the immune system in a specific manner that results in a characteristic inflammatory response. The particular response results in the formation of a granuloma that commonly calcifies after a time. Granulomatous inflammatory responses, especially without caseation, are nonspecific, and frequently the offending organism cannot be identified unless associated with other systemic or laboratory findings.

The most common granulomatous disease seen in North America is histoplasmosis, which is endemic in certain regions of the United States. In its postinfectious state, it is seen as tiny punctate calcifications scattered throughout the liver and possibly the spleen. Tuberculosis; rickettsial infection; and bacterial, viral, fungal, and parasitic involvement of the liver can give a similar pattern. Patients with sarcoid may have liver involvement in a similar pattern. The liver is the third most common site of involvement of sarcoidosis after the lungs and lymphatics.

Primary hepatic granulomatous disease is uncommon and represents only about 5% of cases and tends to have little or no calcification associated with it. At least 60 drugs have been implicated in "drug induced" granulomatous hepatitis. Withdrawal of the offending agent is curative.

Metastatic Disease

Calcifications within hepatic metastatic lesions are unusual. They have been described in association with mucinous (colloid) lesions of the colon or stomach. These are typically tiny stippling calcifications seen focally within the liver (Fig. 5-67).

Hepatocellular Carcinoma

Calcification within hepatocellular carcinoma is unusual, and less than 10% of these lesions are said to calcify. If the calcification is present in the right clinical circumstances (younger patients, absence of alpha fetoprotein), the possibility of a fibrolamellar hepatocellular carcinoma may be considered because these lesions more frequently (30%) show calcification.

Abscesses

Calcification may be seen in the wall of old pyogenic or amebic abscesses. Often this condition is a result of chronic, organized inflammation; secondary infection; or bleeding into the wall of the lesion (Fig. 5-68).

Cysts

Simple hepatic cysts do not calcify. Echinococcal cysts (hydatid disease) commonly develop wall calcifications

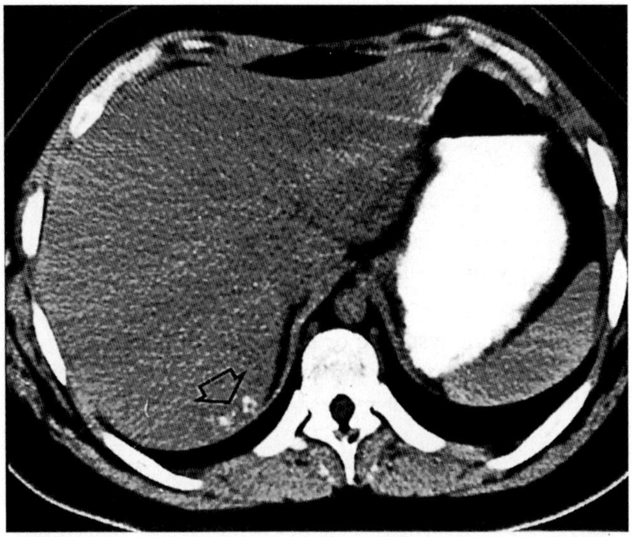

Figure 5-67 Calcifications seen in a small metastatic lesion in the posterior aspect of the right lobe of the liver *(arrow)*. The primary tumor was a mucinous carcinoma of the colon.

over several years. This development occurs whether the cyst is viable or nonviable. The calcification tends to be denser in nonviable cysts. A typical ring of calcification of varying thickness is seen within the liver, and lesions range from 2 to 15 cm.

Hemangiomas

Although hemangioma is a common hepatic lesion, it only rarely calcifies. A large cavernous hemangioma may sometimes calcify centrally in its fibrotic component, and there may be some calcification along the radiating strands of fibrosis. This is a typical sunburst pattern seen in hemangiomas elsewhere in the body. The typical phlebolith-like calcification seen in hemangiomas elsewhere in the body is exceedingly rare in the liver.

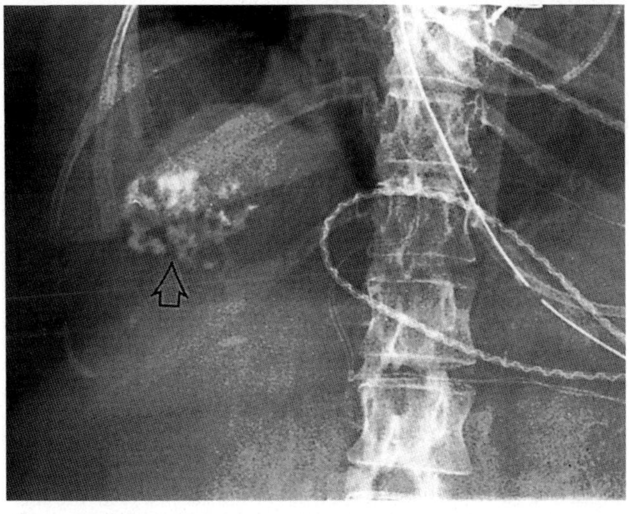

Figure 5-68 Plain film of the abdomen shows flocculent calcification *(arrow)* in an old intrahepatic abscess.

Hematomas

Old subcapsular hematomas may calcify on the liver margin, giving linear or coarse focal areas of calcification.

Tertiary Syphilis

Tertiary syphilis lesions are only rarely seen today. Medical practitioners in the tropics or developing countries are increasingly likely, however, to encounter a hepatic gumma, known to an earlier generation of physicians as hepar lobatum. This condition is a manifestation of late or tertiary syphilis that may calcify.

Parasites

An uncommon cause of hepatic calcification rarely encountered in the West is parasitic infestation. Parasites, such as the tongue worm *(Armillifer armillatus)*, can involve the liver and result in numerous tiny, comma-shaped hepatic calcifications.

Increased Density

Hemochromatosis

Hemochromatosis is an uncommon disorder in which the total iron deposition within the liver and other organs progressively increases. It can be regarded as either a primary idiopathic disease or a secondary disorder. The primary condition is autosomal recessive in its genetic manifestation and is characterized by excessive iron absorption from the small bowel, which is transported to the liver. Secondary forms are seen in patients with a history of multiple blood transfusions, chronic anemia, and erythroid hyperplasia, such as in thalassemia or sideroblastic anemia. Secondary hemochromatosis also can occur as a consequence of high dietary intake of iron.

From whatever cause, excessive iron deposition in the liver over many years results in an enlarged liver with evidence of cirrhosis. Hemosiderin is found in the hepatic cells and Kupffer's cells and within the fibrous matrix of the liver.

CT shows varying degrees of diffuse homogeneous high attenuation throughout the liver (Fig. 5-69). The effects of hemochromatosis are systemic and involve other organs, including the pancreas and the heart (Fig. 5-70). As a result, in addition to impairment of hepatic function, cirrhosis, and possible portal hypertension, patients manifest symptoms secondary to disease in other organ systems. These patients also are at increased risk for hepatocellular carcinoma (Fig. 5-71). Cardiac failure or arrhythmias, in addition to diabetes, are not unusual.

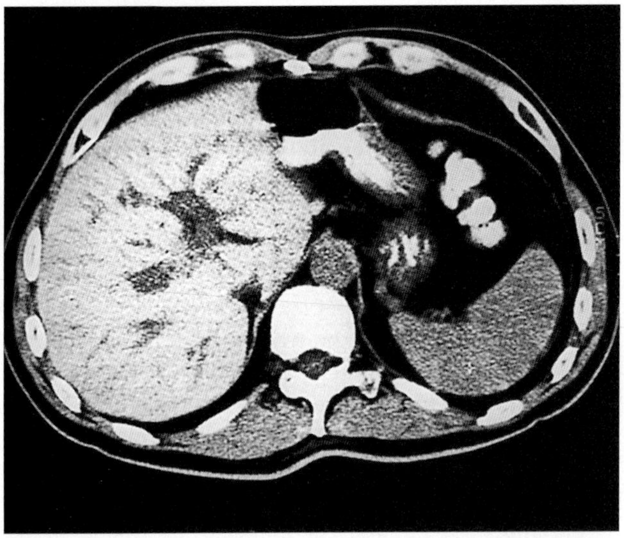

Figure 5-69 CT of the liver in a patient with hemochromatosis during the preenhancement phase. Note the marked density of the liver parenchyma.

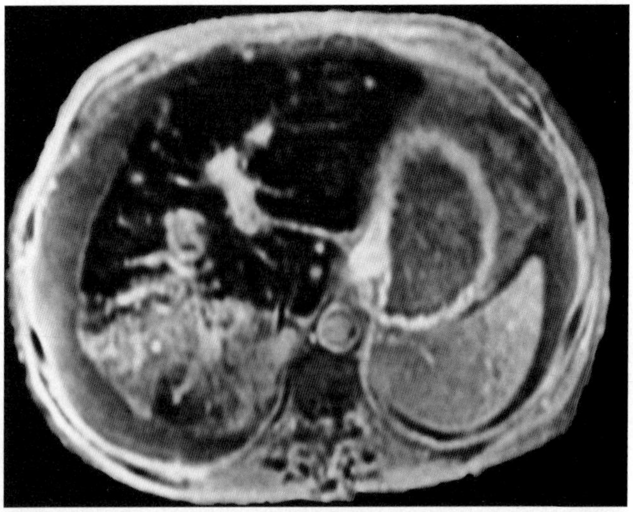

Figure 5-71 A patient with hemochromatosis and cirrhosis complicated by hepatoma. T1-weighted spin echo MRI shows low signal in the anterior liver and brighter signal at the site of hepatocellular cancer (hepatoma) in the posterior liver.

Chronic Cirrhotic Liver Disease

In severe chronic cirrhosis, the liver may appear small and contracted and show density above the normal expectations on unenhanced CT. Conversely, because of the distortion and redistribution of the intrahepatic vascular system in these patients, enhanced computed tomographic scans may show little increase in density compared with unenhanced scans (Fig. 5-72). The relative increase in density on unenhanced scans may be explained on the basis of increased diffuse fibrosis throughout the liver and decreased fat content.

Thorotrast

The radioactive colloid suspension of thorium dioxide, injected intravenously and used during the 1940s and 1950s, was taken up primarily in the reticuloendothelial cells of the liver, spleen, and lymph nodes. This agent was administered for imaging of the liver and spleen. The radionuclide is a long-term, alpha-emitting agent, resulting in many patients' developing bone marrow dyscrasias, neoplasms, or local malignancy in the liver. This agent has not been used in many years, and patients with high-density liver and spleen secondary to Thorotrast injection are becoming rare.

Drug-Induced Causes

Certain drugs increase hepatic density. The use of parenteral gold injections for the treatment of rheumatoid

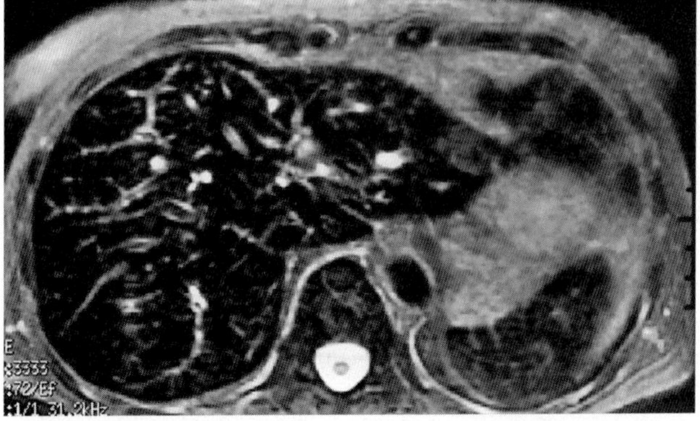

Figure 5-70 A patient with hemochromatosis secondary to hemosiderosis. MRI (T2 fast spin echo) shows low signal in liver, marrow, and spleen typical of hemosiderosis. Low signal would be confined to the liver in hemochromatosis of other causes.

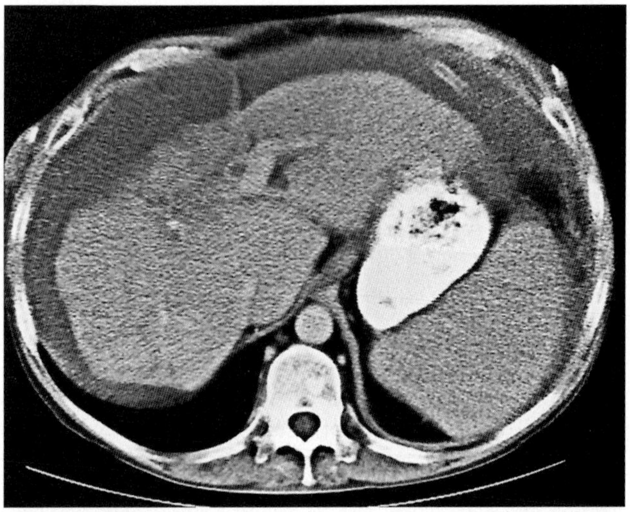

Figure 5-72 A patient with cirrhosis and ascites. Note the small liver with nodular margins and the free fluid in the perihepatic spaces.

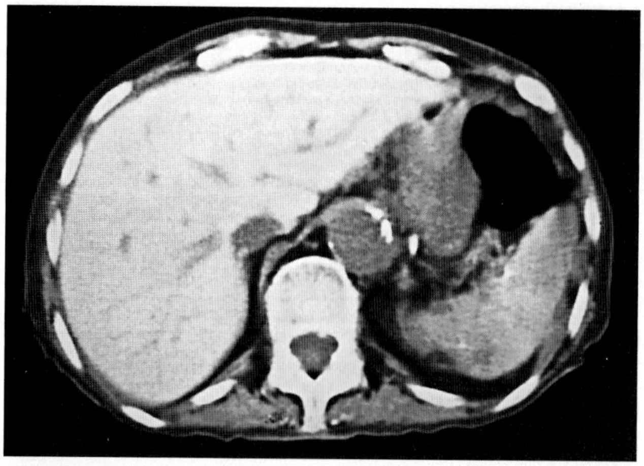

Figure 5-73 CT of the liver in a patient being treated for cardiac dysrhythmia with amiodarone, resulting in increased density throughout the liver.

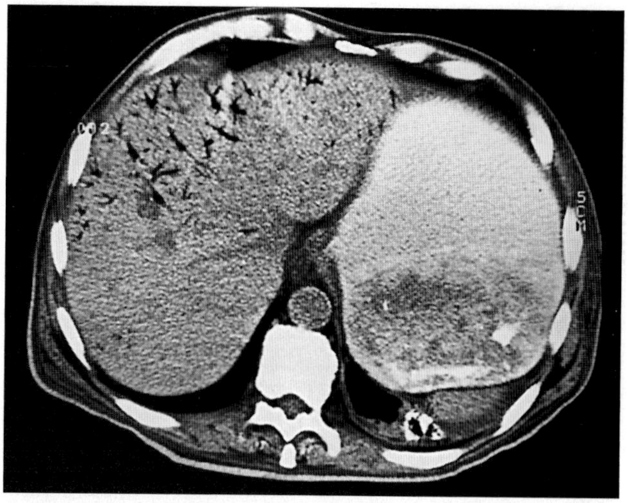

Figure 5-74 CT shows air in the portal venous system of the liver in a postoperative patient. This was not related to bowel necrosis, and the patient had an uneventful recovery.

arthritis over a prolonged period may lead to hepatic deposition and an increase in liver density.

Many drugs can result in hepatic toxicity or cholestasis. It is extremely unusual, however, for a drug or its metabolites to accumulate in the liver and result in increased liver density. One such drug is amiodarone (Fig. 5-73). This is an effective antidysrhythmic drug containing 40% iodine by weight. Because of its prolonged half-life, the significance of serum therapeutic levels is difficult to interpret. In response to this, it has been suggested that the density of the liver be evaluated in patients who are receiving this medication and still experiencing cardiac dysrhythmias in an attempt to determine whether insufficient medication or a toxic side effect of the medication is the basis of the dysrhythmia. It is postulated that normal liver densities during the administration of the drug and continuing dysrhythmias may indicate insufficient therapeutic levels of the medication, whereas increased liver density suggests adequate to toxic levels of the drug.

Portal Venous Air

Air in the portal venous system is an occasional dramatic finding on plain films or CT of the abdomen (Fig. 5-74). It can be benign in a distinct minority of patients, secondary to recent gastrointestinal surgery, gastric or duodenal ulcers, or instrumentation associated with mucosal tears. Occasionally, portal venous air also is benign in a patient with severe gastric outlet obstruction who develops mucosal defects as a result of the gross acute distention. It has been reported in some patients who have undergone recent barium enemas. Many gastrointestinal radiologists have not seen this phenomenon in their entire careers, however. Given that the risk of bowel perforation is 10 times or more increased in colonoscopy, one would expect the incidence of this side effect to be much higher in that procedure. Even there, it remains relatively uncommon.

When making the diagnosis of portal venous air, the radiologist should expect the worst and hope for the best. A proper clinical history is invaluable in deciding how much concern and activity the finding should generate. The finding in most cases carries grave prognostic implications, most commonly associated with bowel infarction, breakdown of the mucosal barrier, and leakage of air and toxins into the portal venous system. There it eventually percolates into the liver. These patients are usually toxic and obviously ill, although in older patients the symptoms initially may not be pronounced. The findings must be correlated to the clinical situation. In a patient with minimal or no abdominal findings, this radiological finding may be benign, and close observation and monitoring are the appropriate actions.

This particular radiological problem, with its emphasis on clinical correlation, as in so many other conditions, is another example of how the historical and expected role of the radiologist as a physician, practicing the specialty of radiology, must be defended. No physician would attempt a physical examination without a clinical history, and it seems equally foolish for a radiologist to undertake an examination or interpretation without an appropriate medical history. Radiologists who do otherwise are doing themselves and the patient an injustice. Clinicians who expect radiologists to practice in such a manner have misguided and foolish perceptions of the role of the imaging and the radiologist.

The most important initial task for the radiologist when linear branching collections of air are seen in the liver is to distinguish between portal venous air and air

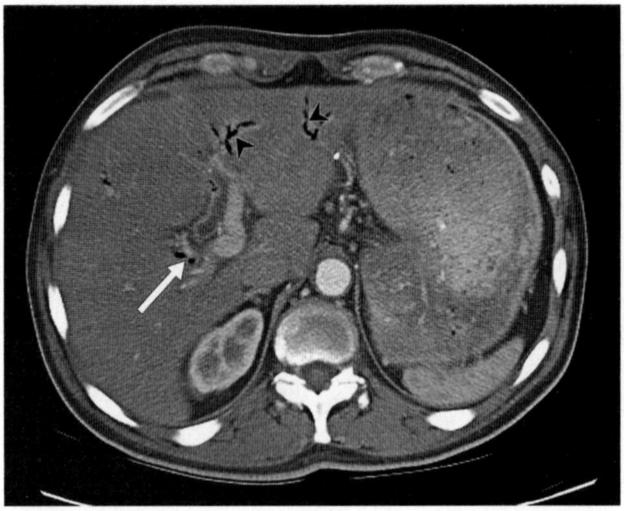

Figure 5-75 CT shows air in the biliary system. Note some air centrally *(arrow)* and in the segmental bile ducts *(arrowheads)*.

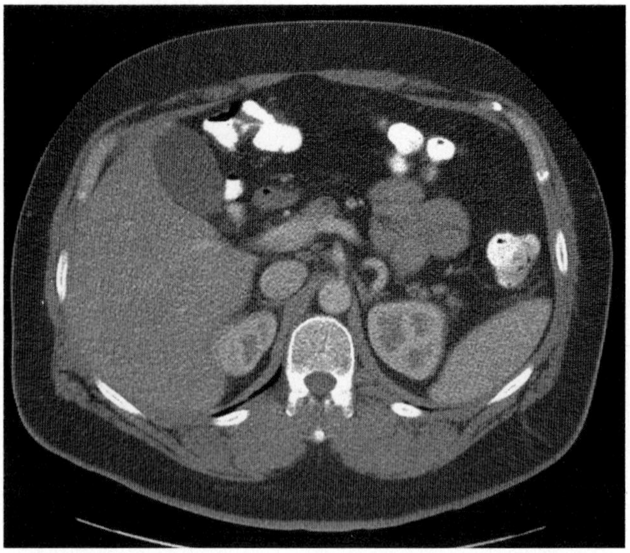

Figure 5-76 Normal appearance of the spleen on CT through the upper abdomen.

in the hepatic biliary system, which is almost always benign (Fig. 5-75). The difference is based on the physiological flow characteristics of the two systems. Bile flows in a centripetal pattern from the liver periphery to the liver hilum, and as a result, air collections in the biliary system tend to be central in the common hepatic and main hepatic ducts. Conversely, portal venous flow is centrifugal from hilum to periphery, and air in the portal venous system is found in the periphery along the margins of the liver (Table 5-2). If sufficient air has leaked into the portal system, however, it also can be seen in the liver hilum, within the portal vein, or even backed up into the splenic pulp. Air also is seen occasionally within the superior mesenteric vein on CT. Additionally, a careful search of the abdominal plain films or computed tomographic scans is warranted to identify intramural air collections in the bowel.

SPLEEN

The spleen is the largest component of the reticuloendothelial system, comprising white pulp (lymphoid tissue) and red pulp (vascular sinuses and end arterial vessels) contained within a thin fibrous capsule. It is located in the left upper quadrant and may be found in considerable variations of size and shape in normal individuals (Fig. 5-76). The normal dimensions given for the spleen in various textbooks are of relatively little use in evaluating for splenomegaly because of the marked variation from person to person in the size and configuration of the spleen. In imaging of the spleen, the most accurate method for evaluating the possibility of splenomegaly may be the observations of an experienced radiologist or, even better, a previous study. In general, the normal spleen occupies approximately 15% to 25% of the volume of a normal liver and weighs between 100 and 250 g (Fig. 5-77).

Accessory spleens are a common computed tomographic finding and most often are seen in the region of the splenic hilum around or near the tail of the pancreas. Approximately 20% of patients undergoing CT of the abdomen have this finding.

Table 5-2 Air within a Branching Pattern in the Liver

Portal Venous	Bile Ducts
Peripheral in location owing to centrifugal flow of portal blood	Usually centrally located owing to centripetal flow of bile
Can be benign secondary to surgery, ulceration, or instrumentation	Usually benign
Most frequently associated with sick bowel, ischemia, or necrosis	May be result of fistulous communication, surgical, or developmental. May be seen in patients with history of papillotomy

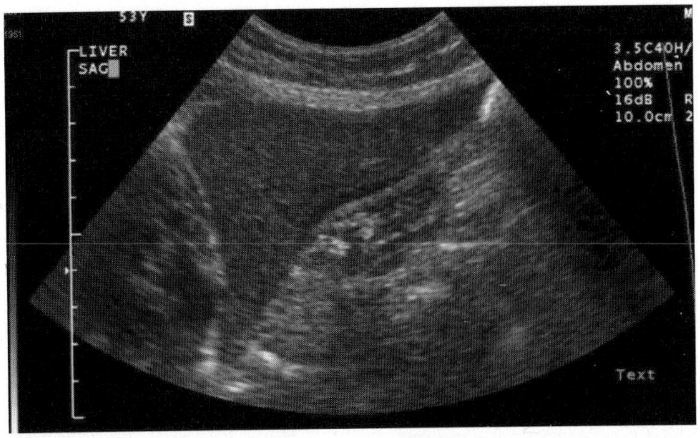

Figure 5-77 Normal spleen seen on ultrasonogram. Note the homogeneous appearance and well-defined margins.

Enlarged Spleen

Common causes of an enlarged spleen are summarized in Box 5-5.

Passive Congestion

Although chronic right-sided congestive heart failure occasionally results in some degree of splenomegaly, the most common cause of splenomegaly is congestion within the portal venous system secondary to cirrhotic changes within the liver. Portal hypertension secondary to hepatic cirrhosis of any cause, most commonly alcoholic, almost always results in some degree of splenic enlargement. Fifty percent of patients with portal hypertension have a palpable spleen. It is an even more common finding on CT. The splenic enlargement is secondary to obstructive and congestive changes within the spleen, particularly the red pulp. The term *Banti's syndrome* is occasionally used in describing passive congestion of the spleen secondary to portal hypertension and hepatic cirrhosis. The original description of this syndrome postulated a splenomegaly that preceded the cirrhotic changes within the liver, however, and is the reverse of the sequence of events seen in portal hypertension. Any condition that can result in intrahepatic vascular congestion can secondarily cause splenomegaly; this includes not only any cause of cirrhosis, but also any cause of hepatic or portal venous occlusive disease and congenital hepatic fibrosis. Splenic vein thrombosis may cause acute congestive splenomegaly, as can Budd-Chiari syndrome. Chronic passive congestion can result in a spleen that is many times its original size and can weigh 1000 g and can at times compress the left kidney (Fig. 5-78).

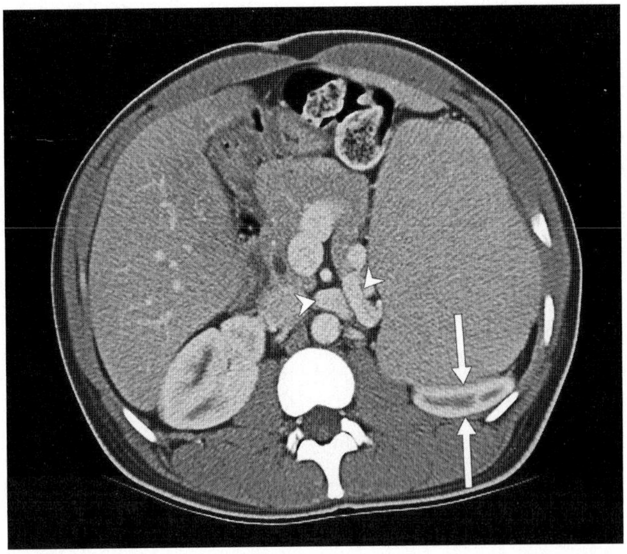

Figure 5-78 Markedly enlarged spleen is seen compressing the left kidney *(arrows)*. Also note large varices *(arrowheads)*.

Box 5-5 Some Common Causes of Oversized Spleen

- Portal hypertension
- Trauma
- Lymphoma
- Leukemia
- Infection
- Hemolytic anemias
- Metabolic storage diseases

Computed tomographic findings in cirrhotic patients with splenomegaly as a result of portal hypertension show characteristic changes within the liver and prominence of the collateral vascular (varices) structures in the region of the splenic hilum, the gastrohepatic ligament, and around the gastroesophageal junction and cavernous transformation of the portal vein in patients with chronic portal vein occlusion (Fig. 5-79). Ultrasound scans of such a spleen may show an isoechoic or hypoechoic pattern. Liver and spleen radionuclide scans show a relative increase in the uptake of the radionuclide in the spleen compared with the liver (colloid shift). Uptake in bone marrow also may be shown.

Trauma

Posttraumatic splenic injury with an intact capsule or tamponaded splenic capsule also can result in transitory splenic enlargement. This is often associated with lower left rib injuries, although this associated finding need not be present (Fig. 5-80).

Hodgkin's Lymphoma

Outside of the usual nodal sites, the spleen is the organ most commonly involved with Hodgkin's disease. Splenic involvement is shown in approximately one third of patients undergoing staging laparotomies.

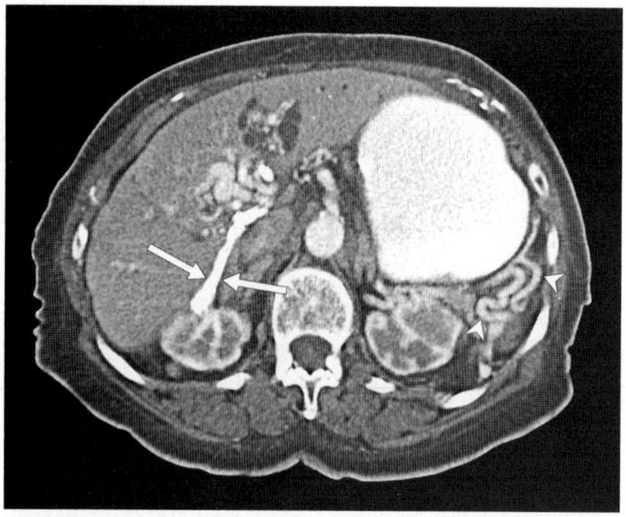

Figure 5-79 Chronic portal vein occlusion with the development of cavernous transformation of the portal vein with a spontaneous portorenal shunt on the right *(arrows)*. Note varices on the left *(arrowheads)* and absence of portal vein.

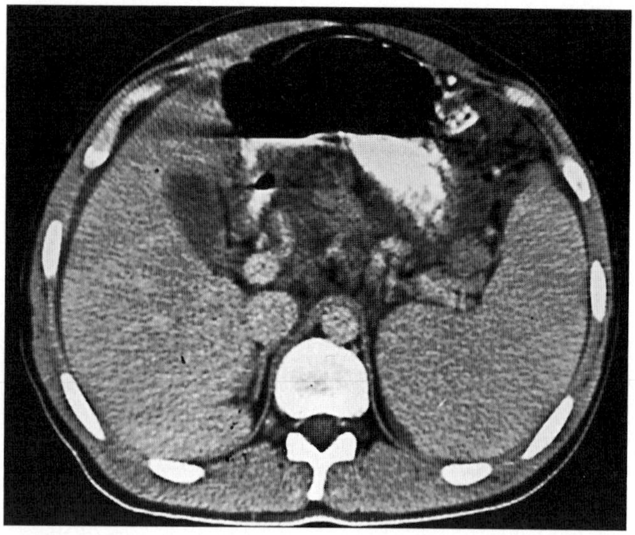

Figure 5-81 CT of the hepatosplenic area in a patient with Hodgkin's lymphoma and known splenic involvement shows diffuse homogeneous enlargement of the spleen.

Although CT can be extremely helpful in evaluating the possibility of splenic involvement (particularly with focal disease), the definitive assessment for splenic involvement is splenectomy. Splenic enlargement in most cases signifies splenic involvement, whereas a normal spleen size in most cases suggests noninvolvement. The incidence of false-positive and false-negative results, based on size criteria alone, is significant.

Computed tomographic evaluation of splenic involvement with Hodgkin's disease can include many presentations, ranging from numerous small nodules to a solitary splenic tumor mass to diffuse enlargement without focal defects (Fig. 5-81). Because involvement of the spleen with Hodgkin's disease has significant therapeutic and prognostic implications, the determination of splenic involvement is crucial, hence the necessity of splenectomy in the staging process.

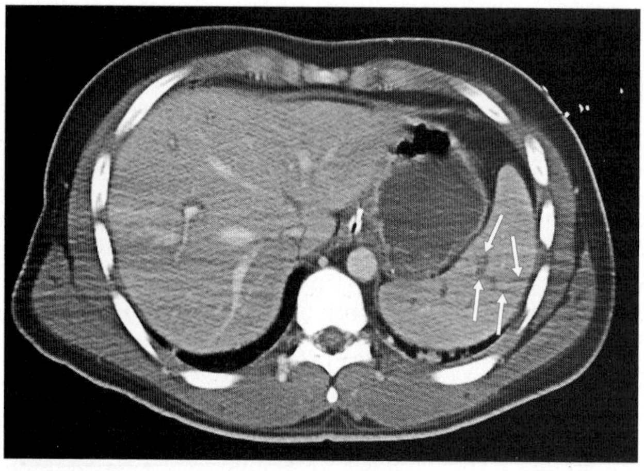

Figure 5-80 Linear lucencies in the spleen *(arrows)*, representing splenic lacerations, are seen in a 17-year-old boy after a motor vehicle accident.

Non-Hodgkin's Lymphomas

Involvement of the spleen with non-Hodgkin's-type lymphomas is more common than with Hodgkin's disease and occurs in more than 50% of patients. The lymphomatous involvement of the spleen may present as diffuse enlargement without focal disease, as a round tumor mass, or as multiple, small nodules. In contrast to Hodgkin's disease, splenomegaly usually is a more accurate indication of tumor involvement. Discrete lymphomatous lesions often show increased signal on T2-weighted MRI. Focal lesions also can be detected with ultrasound and are shown as hypoechoic foci.

Leukemia

Splenomegaly is a relatively common occurrence in leukemia, but its presence and severity depend on the type and duration of the leukemia. Although a common presenting finding in hairy cell leukemia, it is rare in acute lymphoblastic leukemia. The presence of splenomegaly does give rise to the possibility of splenic rupture as a complication of some of the chronic leukemias.

Chronic myeloid leukemia is associated with significant splenomegaly that often can reach massive proportions. In patients with chronic lymphocytic leukemia, splenomegaly also may be a prominent feature, although the size of the spleen is less striking than that seen in chronic myeloid disease. Generally, splenomegaly is more commonly associated with the chronic forms of leukemia and is probably a poor prognostic sign.

CT generally shows an enlarged spleen with a homogeneous appearance. Enlargement of the spleen in leukemia is almost always associated with disease involvement. Often, the involved spleen shows an isoechoic ultrasound pattern.

Chronic Myeloproliferative Disorders

The chronic myeloproliferative disorders represent a group of related disease processes that are thought to be clonal disorders of the hematopoietic stem cell. They include such entities as polycythemia vera, myeloid metaplasia, essential thrombocythemia, and chronic myeloid leukemia. Various authors overlap the myeloproliferative disorders and the leukemic disorders, and some include the acute nonlymphocytic leukemias in the myeloproliferative group.

Splenomegaly is common in chronic proliferative conditions, with the degree varying from condition to condition. The most prominent example of splenomegaly in this group tends to occur in myeloid metaplasia. Lesser degrees of splenomegaly are seen in polycythemia vera and essential thrombocythemia. Imaging generally shows an obviously enlarged, homogeneous-appearing spleen (Fig. 5-82).

Protozoan Infection

Splenomegaly is characteristically associated with malaria. In the acute presentations, the spleen may become grossly enlarged, reaching gigantic proportions. With chronic disease and gradual development of fibrosis and scarring, the degree of splenomegaly is diminished.

Systemic Infections

Mild to moderate degrees of splenic enlargement may be seen in patients with mononucleosis, and splenic rupture is a rare but known complication of infectious mononucleosis. Splenomegaly is a relatively common finding in patients with subacute bacterial endocarditis, and the enlargement usually is secondary to multiple, small septic foci within the spleen. Degrees of splenic enlargement may be seen in the miliary stage of tuberculosis (Fig. 5-83). Disseminated fungal infections, including candidiasis and histoplasmosis, also may produce splenic enlargement. Splenomegaly is a common finding in patients with typhoid fever.

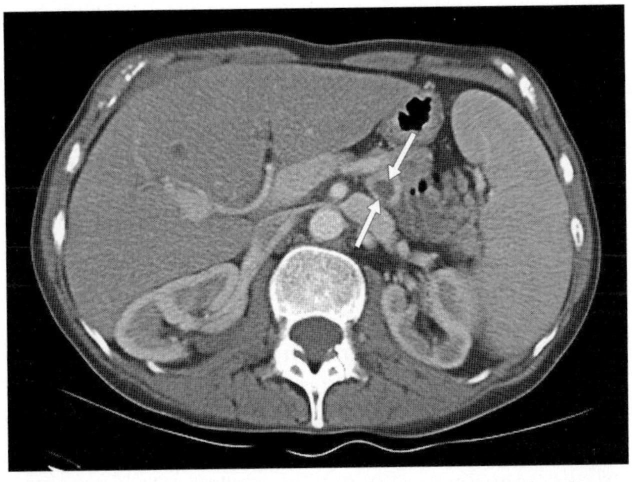

Figure 5-82 A patient with polycythemia vera with a homogeneous enlarged spleen. Note thrombus in the splenic vein *(arrows)*.

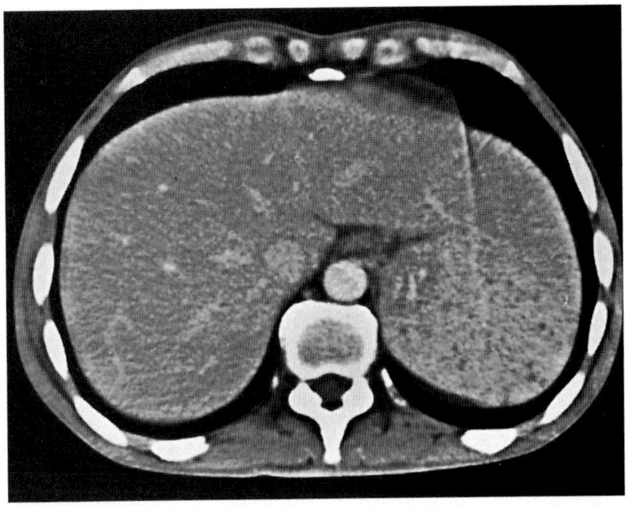

Figure 5-83 CT of the splenic region in a patient with AIDS and tuberculosis. The spleen is enlarged, and there are multiple, tiny splenic abscesses.

Erythropoietic Disorders

Hereditary spherocytosis is the best known of the erythropoietic disorders. This condition is inherited as an autosomal dominant trait and results in spherocytic changes in the affected individual's red blood cells. Splenomegaly is almost always present and of a mild to moderate degree. Splenomegaly is usually therapeutic in the treatment of this disorder because of the important role of the spleen in erythrocyte destruction.

Splenomegaly may be a prominent early childhood manifestation of sickle cell disease. The older the patient, the less prominent the spleen as a result of progressive atrophy and fibrosis secondary to repeated infarctions.

The thalassemia syndromes, representing an abnormality of hemoglobin production, can result in mild to moderate degrees of splenomegaly. Similar findings are present in patients with autoimmune hemolytic anemias and idiopathic thrombocytopenic purpura.

Felty's syndrome, although an abnormality of granulocytes rather than erythrocytes, may be included here as an additional example of splenomegaly associated with blood cell abnormalities. The syndrome consists of the triad of rheumatoid arthritis, splenomegaly, and neutropenia.

It is most commonly seen in patients with long-standing rheumatoid arthritis. The spleen may be markedly enlarged, possibly relating to the ongoing selective granulocytic destruction occurring within the spleen.

Infiltrative and Storage Diseases

Lipogenic storage disorders, such as all forms of Gaucher's disease and Niemann-Pick disease, are associated with moderate to massive splenomegaly. Increased splenic size also may be a feature of the mucopolysaccharidoses, the best known being Hurler's and Hunter's syndromes. Patients with histiocytosis X, particularly with Letterer-Siwe disease, occasionally have splenomegaly as part of the presenting picture. Although primary and secondary amyloidosis can involve the spleen, it is more common in the secondary form and frequently causes splenomegaly.

Small or Shrunken Spleen

Sickle Cell Disease

Sickle cell disease is a common cause of diminished splenic size. In the advanced stages, fibrotic changes as a result of chronic recurrent infarctions lead to a small, shrunken, and often calcified spleen. The extensive fibrosis coupled with diffuse occlusion of the splenic microvasculature results in nonfunction and autosplenectomy.

Essential Thrombocythemia

Splenic atrophy also may be seen during the chronic course of essential thrombocythemia. The resultant infarctions are most likely secondary to stagnated aggregates of platelets within the splenic circulation.

Congenital Causes

Congenital hypoplasia of the spleen is relatively uncommon, but has been seen and described in cases of Fanconi's anemia with associated marrow hypoplasia.

Irradiation

Radiation to the upper abdomen and splenic bed can result in a small, shrunken fibrotic spleen with thickened capsule. Usually this is a delayed response to radiation-induced vascular damage of the spleen.

Thorotrast

Thorotrast, a radioactive contrast agent emitting alpha rays, which had been formerly used as an angiographic contrast agent, is retained within the reticuloendothelial system and may be seen within the liver or spleen (Fig. 5-84). In the spleen, over a period of years, splenic atrophy and fibrosis develop. Although these changes within the liver put patients at a higher risk for malignant disease, the same malignant potential has not been reported for the spleen.

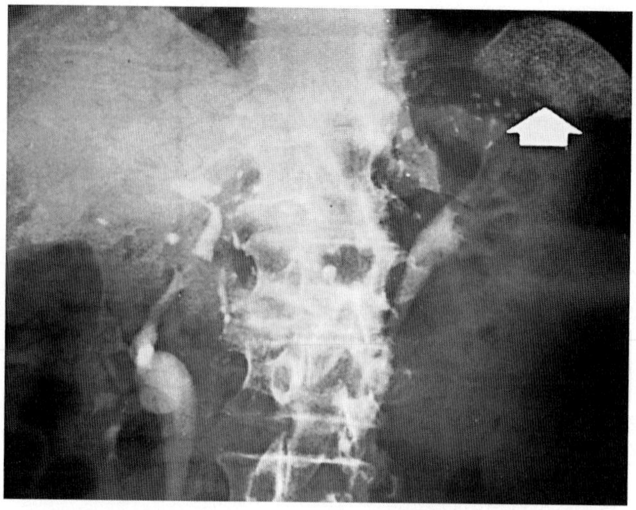

Figure 5-84 Film obtained during an intravenous pyelogram in patient who had previously received Thorotrast for hepatosplenic imaging. The spleen is small *(arrow)*, with fine, nodular, calcium-like density throughout the spleen.

Malabsorption Syndromes

Degrees of atrophy of the spleen are rarely seen as a complication of some malabsorption syndromes. Splenic atrophy has been reported in inflammatory bowel disease, particularly ulcerative colitis, and to a lesser extent in Crohn's disease. It also is associated with celiac disease. This complication of malabsorption syndromes is relatively uncommon and something of a curiosity. It cannot be related directly to malnutrition because hyposplenism is not seen in starvation. The exact causes of this complication are unknown.

Focal Defects

Cystic Lesions

The most common type of splenic cyst is the pseudocyst or so-called acquired cyst of the spleen. These cysts are found most commonly in adults and are presumed to be of traumatic origin. The cyst wall may be calcified and without an epithelial lining. These account for approximately 80% of splenic cysts. True epidermoid cysts are less common (approximately 20%) and are lined by stratified squamous epithelium. These cysts are believed to be congenital in origin (Figs. 5-85 and 5-86). Calcification can be seen in the wall of acquired and congenital types of splenic cysts. The cysts vary in size and generally contain clear fluid, although turbid or bloody contents also may be present. There is no gender predilection for the congenital type of cyst. Congenital splenic cysts are not thought to represent part of the spectrum of more widespread cystic disease involving

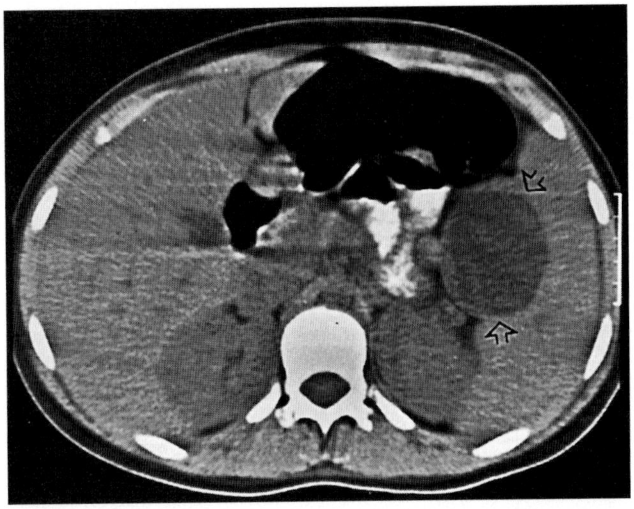

Figure 5-85 A large splenic epithelial cyst *(arrows)* is seen during a computed tomographic examination in a patient with a diagnosis of appendicitis.

the pancreas, kidney, and liver. These usually occur as incidental findings within the spleen of asymptomatic patients. Rarely, splenic cysts may be complicated by hemorrhage, rupture, or even infection.

Pancreatic pseudocysts involving the tail of the pancreas occasionally give the appearance of splenic cysts on CT. The cyst may adhere to and indent the splenic capsule or invade the substance of the spleen.

Echinococcal cysts involving the spleen are uncommon. Less than one third of cases of hydatid disease have splenic involvement.

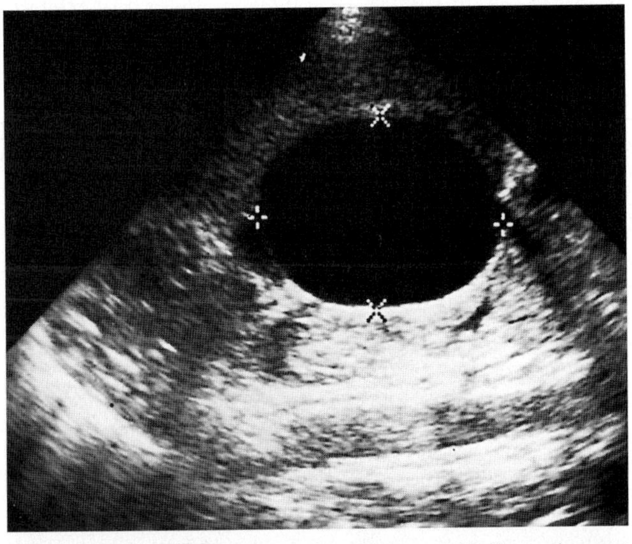

Figure 5-86 The same patient as in Figure 5-85 also underwent ultrasound examination of the spleen, which showed the typical appearance of a large, well-defined splenic cyst.

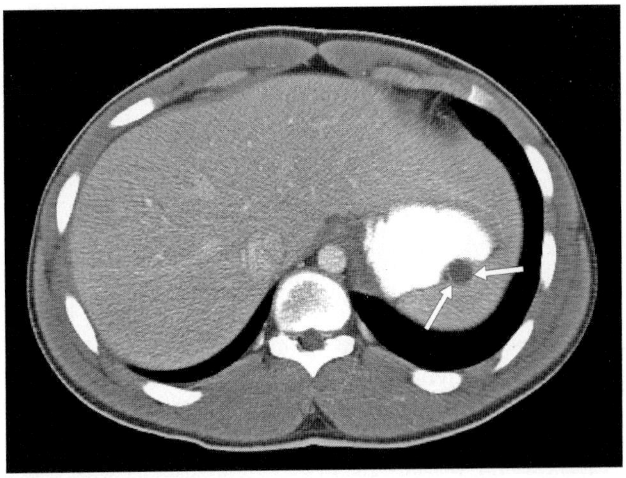

Figure 5-87 Small hemangioma of the spleen *(arrows)* is seen.

Primary Neoplastic Lesions

Hemangiomas are the most common benign neoplasms of the spleen. These are almost always asymptomatic and are incidental findings (Fig. 5-87). It is possible that a large splenic hemangioma or diffuse splenic hemangiomas could lead to splenomegaly, although this is rare. The lesions are usually solitary. Lymphangiomas occur in the spleen and are less common than hemangiomas. Distinguishing between the two can be impossible. It has been suggested that lymphangiomas occur more commonly in the subcapsular region than hemangiomas.

Splenic hamartomas are uncommon and are almost always asymptomatic. Most are solitary. CT may show a well-defined, solitary splenic lesion with homogeneous or mixed cystic components.

Primary malignant lesions of the spleen are rare. These are generally angiosarcomas, and in contrast to those in the liver, there seems to be no direct relationship between Thorotrast and development of splenic angiosarcomas. Patients with these tumors carry a poor prognosis, often having widespread metastatic disease at the time of diagnosis. Primary malignant fibrous histiocytomas of the spleen have been reported but are extremely rare.

Metastatic Disease

Apart from lymphomatous involvement, secondary hematogenous metastatic lesions to the spleen are unusual (Fig. 5-88). Many different theories have been put forward to explain this scarcity of splenic metastatic disease, although none is fully satisfying. Metastatic lesions to the spleen, although rare, do tend to occur when there is a widespread dissemination of tumor throughout the body. In such patients, splenic involvement is found in less than 4% at autopsy. Metastatic spread from contiguous organs can occur (Fig. 5-89).

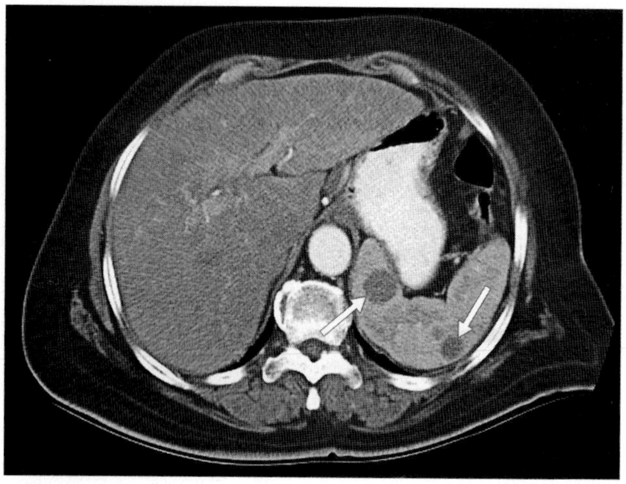

Figure 5-88 This patient had known pancreatic carcinoma with metastatic disease involving the spleen *(arrows)*.

Lymphoma

As previously discussed, Hodgkin's and non-Hodgkin's lymphoma can involve the spleen. The involvement can be diffuse or focal. The focal lesions can be solitary or more commonly multiple. These are usually shown on CT as low-density lesions or on MRI as high-signal lesions on T2-weighted images.

Abscesses

Large solitary focal abscesses of the spleen are an uncommon condition because they generally are associated with high mortality. These lesions tend to be poorly encapsulated and have intermediate densities on CT. There is often enhancement of the rim during the contrast phase of computed tomographic examination.

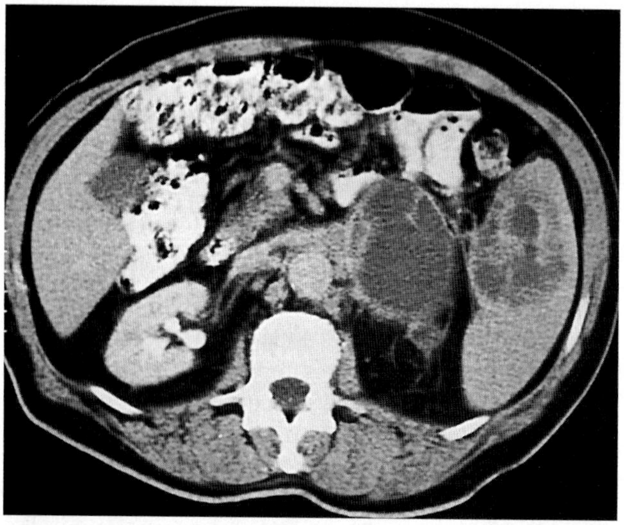

Figure 5-89 CT through the midabdomen shows a cystic neoplastic lesion of the tail of the pancreas. There also has been metastatic spread of the lesion to the spleen.

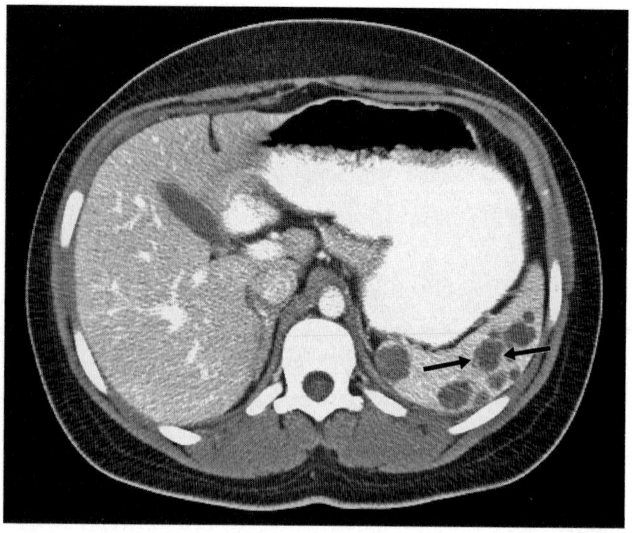

Figure 5-90 Multiple splenic abscesses are seen in the spleen with rim enhancement *(arrows)*.

Widespread disseminated microabscesses occur in the liver and spleen and are seen predominantly in immunosuppressed patients (Fig. 5-90). They are commonly due to *Candida albicans* and occasionally tuberculosis. CT shows multiple areas of low attenuation within the spleen and commonly in the liver as well. Rarely, abscesses of the spleen may be associated with bacterial endocarditis or mycotic aneurysms of the aorta (Fig. 5-91).

Focal Infarctions

In any condition in which systemic emboli may occur, such as in cardiac valvular disease, emboli can become lodged within the vasculature of the spleen and result in splenic infarctions. In the early stage, these are hemorrhagic in their appearance. A squared or triangular area or area of low attenuation with its base on the

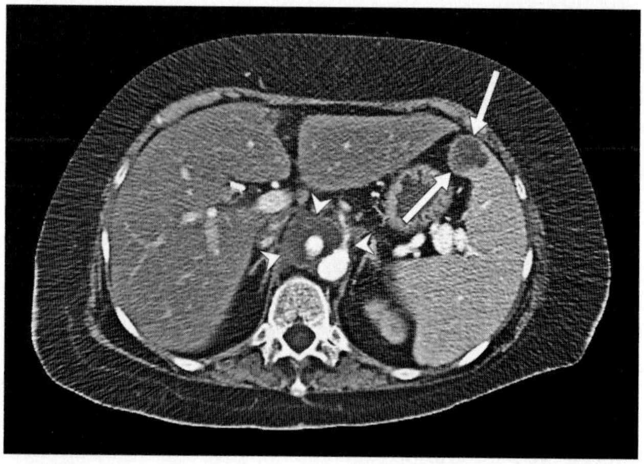

Figure 5-91 An abscess is seen in the anterior tip of the spleen *(arrow)*. Note mycotic abdominal aortic aneurysm *(arrowheads)*.

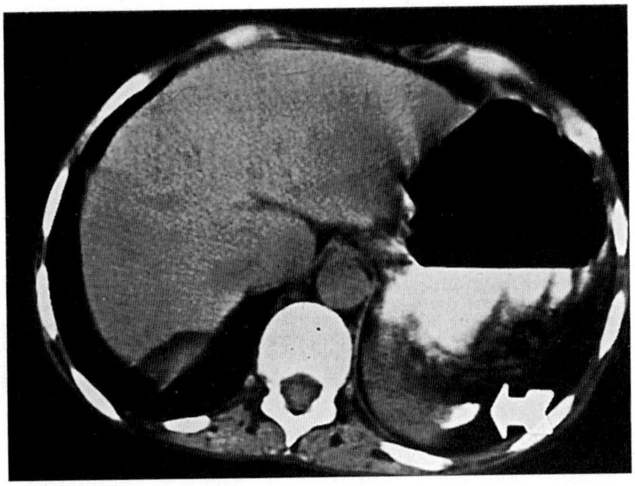

Figure 5-92 CT shows a tiny, calcified, shrunken spleen posterior to the stomach *(arrow)* in this patient with sickle cell anemia. The spleen has undergone autoamputation.

splenic capsule is the usual finding on CT. Eventually, these infarctions become smaller, fibrotic, and more dense. Often, in the acute stage, they are associated with left upper quadrant pain, and initially there may be some mild splenomegaly. Vascular thrombosis within the spleen and resultant infarctions also may be seen in disease processes such as leukemia, particularly of the chronic myelogenous variety, and are commonly encountered in patients with sickle cell disease, eventually leading to splenic atrophy. Splenic infarcts secondary to septic emboli also may be encountered as a result of bacterial endocarditis.

Increased Density

On routine CT of the abdomen (particularly unenhanced), the tissue density of the spleen is slightly less than that of the liver. There are relatively few conditions that result in true increased splenic density. The use of the contrast agent Thorotrast in earlier decades was discussed previously. It is possible for the spleen to show increased density in cases of hemochromatosis. In a small, shrunken, nonfunctioning spleen having undergone autoamputation, the spleen may appear increased in density (Fig. 5-92). This increased density most commonly occurs as a chronic sequela of sickle cell disease. Splenic trauma with diffuse bleeding throughout the spleen in the acute stage results in increased density in the subcapsular region or possibly diffusely throughout the spleen (Fig. 5-93).

Calcifications

The most common cause of calcification in the spleen is previous histoplasmosis in which small punctate calcifications are identified within a normal-sized spleen (Fig. 5-94).

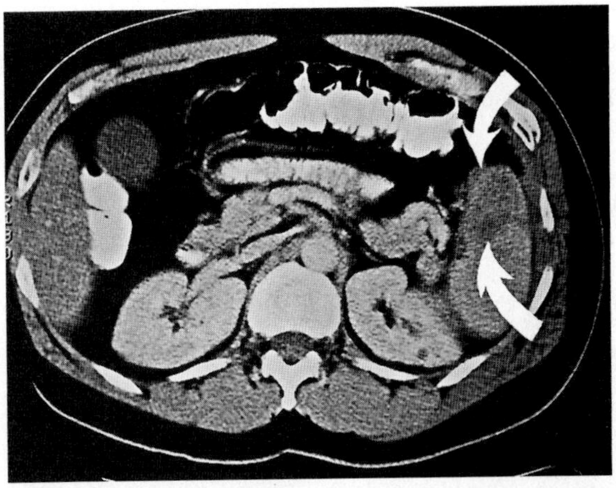

A

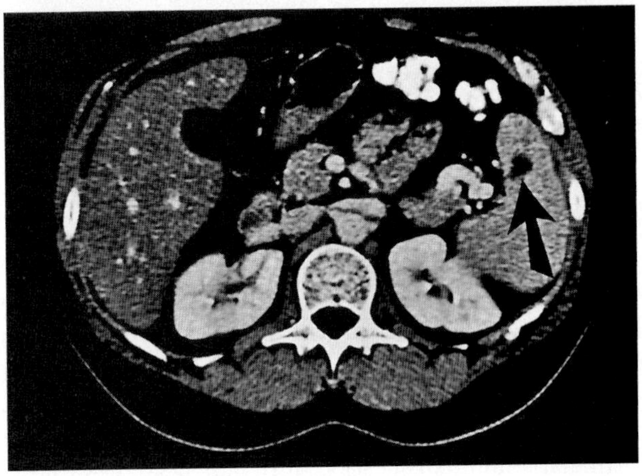

B

Figure 5-93 This 50-year-old man fell off a ladder and injured the left ribs. **A,** CT at the time of injury shows an ill-defined splenic defect with hazy margins representing a splenic hematoma *(arrows)*. **B,** Images obtained 1 month later show marked interval improvement. Only a small, well-defined cyst remains *(arrow)*.

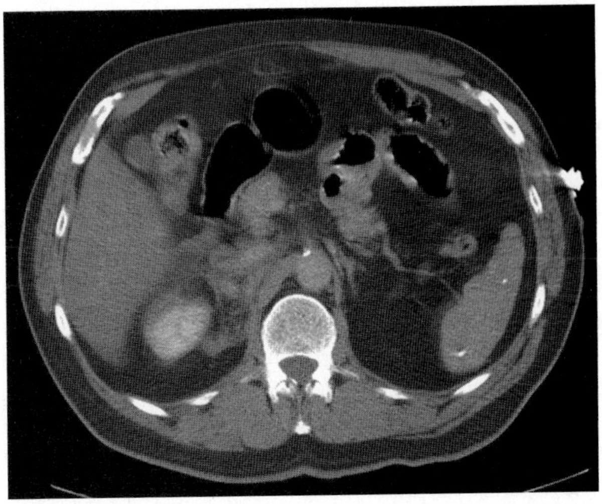

Figure 5-94 Small punctate calcifications in a normal-sized spleen is a fairly routine finding on CT.

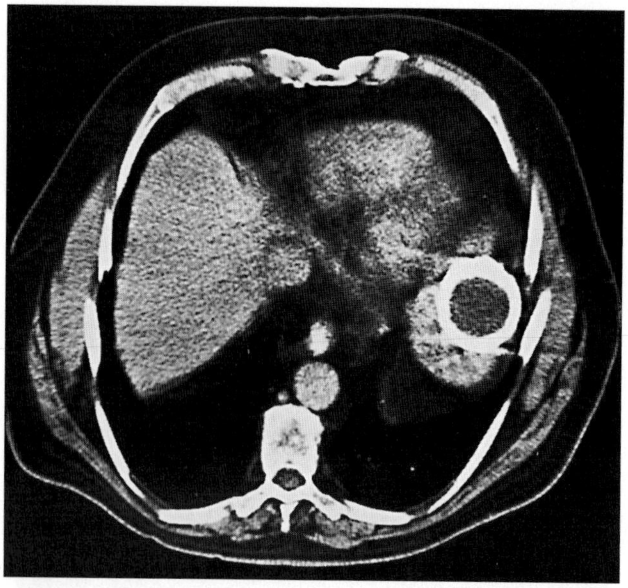

Figure 5-95 CT shows an old splenic abscess that is densely calcified in the wall.

Tuberculosis and brucellosis also may result in calcifications. Phlebolith formation within the spleen with calcification is rare but can occur. The possibility that old focal areas of infarction will calcify also must be a consideration. Old healed abscesses within the spleen, particularly microabscesses, also may lead to residual calcification (Fig. 5-95). Old hematomas readily calcify. Calcification can be seen in the walls of acquired and congenital cysts. In addition, focal calcifications in abdominal organs, including the spleen, have been described in acquired immunodeficiency syndrome (AIDS) patients with disseminated *Pneumocystis carinii* infections.

SUGGESTED READINGS

Liver

Acunas B, Rozanes I, Acunas G, et al: Hydatid cyst of the liver: identification of detached cyst lining on CT scans obtained after cyst puncture. AJR 156:751-752, 1991.

Baker ME, Silverman PM: Nodular focal fatty infiltration of the liver: CT appearance. AJR 145:79-80, 1985.

Beggs I: The radiology of hydatid disease. AJR 145:639-648, 1985.

Bonaldi VM, Bret PM, Reinhold C, et al: Helical CT of the liver: value of an early hepatic arterial phase. Radiology 197:357-363, 1995.

Bradley DW, Maynard JE: Etiological and natural history of post-transfusion and enterically transmitted non-A, non-B hepatitis. Semin Liver Dis 6:56-63, 1986.

Brown JJ, Naylor MJ, Yagan N: Imaging of hepatic cirrhosis. Radiology 202:1-16, 1997.

Choi BI, Han MC, Kim CW: Small hepatocellular carcinoma versus small cavernous hemangioma: differentiation with MR imaging at 2.0 T. Radiology 176:103-106, 1990.

Choi BI, Yeon KM, Kim SH, et al: Caroli disease: central dot sign in CT. Radiology 174:161-163, 1990.

Dodds WJ, Erickson SJ, Taylor AJ, et al: Caudate lobe of the liver: anatomy, embryology, and pathology. AJR 154:87-93, 1990.

Egglin TK, Rummeny E, Stark DD, et al: Hepatic tumors: quantitative tissue characterization with MR imaging. Radiology 176:107-110, 1990.

Faria, SC, Iyer RB, Rashid A, Whitman GJ: Hepatic adenoma. AJR 182:1520, 2004.

Fasel JH, Selle D, Evertsz CJ, et al: Segmental anatomy of the liver: poor correlation with CT. Radiology 206:151-156, 1998.

Ferlicot S, Kobeiter H, Nhieu JTV, et al: MRI of atypical focal nodular hyperplasia of the liver: radiology-pathology correlation. AJR 182:1227-1231, 2004.

Ferrucci JT: Liver tumor imaging: current concepts. AJR 155: 473-484, 1990.

Furata A, Ito K, Fujita T, et al: Hepatic enhancement in multiphasic contrast-enhanced MDC. AJR 183:157-162, 2004.

Furui S, Itai Y, Ohtomo K, et al: Hepatic epithelioid hemangioendothelioma: report of five cases. Radiology 171:63-68, 1989.

Grace ND, Powell LW: Iron storage disorders of the liver. Gastroenterology 67:1257-1283, 1974.

Han JK, Choi BI, Kim TK, et al: Hilar cholangiocarcinoma: thin-section spiral CT findings with cholangiographic correlation. Radiographics 17:1475-1485, 1997.

Heiken JP, Weyman PJ, Lee JK, et al: Detection of focal hepatic masses: prospective evaluation with CT, delayed CT, CT during arterial portography, and MR imaging. Radiology 171:47-51, 1989.

Holley HC, Koslin DB, Berland LL, et al: Inhomogeneous enhancement of liver parenchyma secondary to passive congestion: contrast-enhanced CT. Radiology 170:795-800, 1989.

Hussain SM, Terkivatan T, Zondervan PE, et al: Focal nodular hyperplasia: findings at state-of-the-art MRI Imaging, US, CT and pathologic analysis. Radiographics 24:3-19, 2004.

Kamel IR, Lawler LP, Fishman EK: Comprehensive analysis of hypervascular liver lesions using 16-MDCT and advanced image processing. AJR 183:443-452, 2004.

Khuroo MS, Zarger SA, Mahajan R: *Echinococcus granulosus* cysts in the liver: management with percutaneous drainage. Radiology 180:141-145, 1991.

Kim HC, Kim TK, Sung KB, et al: Preoperative evaluation of hepatocellular carcinoma: combined use of CT with arterial portography and hepatic arteriography. AJR 180:1593-1599, 2003.

Landay MJ, Setaiwan H, Hirsh G, et al: Hepatic and thoracic amoebiasis. AJR 135:449-454, 1980.

Langer JC, Rose DB, Keystone JS, et al: Diagnosis and management of hydatid disease of the liver. Ann Surg 199:412-417, 1984.

Lee KH, O'Malley ME, Haider MA, Hanbidge A: Triple phase MDCT of heptocellular carcinoma. AJR 182:643-649, 2004.

Lee MJ, Saini S, Hamm B, et al: Focal nodular hyperplasia of the liver: MR findings in 35 proved cases. AJR 156:317-320, 1991.

Ludwig J: Drug effects on the liver. Dig Dis Sci 24:785-796, 1979.

Markos J, Veronese ME, Nicholson MR, et al: Value of hepatic computerized tomographic scanning during amiodarone therapy. Am J Cardiol 56:89-92, 1985.

Matsui O, Kadoya M, Kameyama T, et al: Adenomatous hyperplastic nodules in the cirrhotic liver: differentiation from hepatocellular carcinoma with MR imaging. Radiology 173: 123-126, 1989.

Matsui O, Kadoya M, Kameyama T, et al: Benign and malignant nodules in cirrhotic livers: distinction based on blood supply. Radiology 178:493-497, 1991.

Matsui O, Takashima T, Kadoya M, et al: Liver metastases from colorectal cancers: detection with CT during arterial portography. Radiology 165:65-69, 1987.

Mergo PJ, Ros PR, Buetow PC, et al: Diffuse disease of the liver: radiologic-pathologic correlation. Radiographics 14:1291-1307, 1994.

Miller WJ, Baron RL, Dodd GD, et al: Malignancies in patients with cirrhosis: CT sensitivity and specificity in 200 consecutive transplant patients. Radiology 193:645-650, 1994.

Mitchell MC, Biotnott JK, Kaufman S, et al: Budd-Chiari syndrome: etiology, diagnosis and management. Medicine 61: 199-218, 1982.

Murphy BJ, Casillas J, Ros PR, et al: The CT appearance of cystic masses of the liver. Radiographics 9:307-322, 1989.

Nadell J, Kosek J: Peliosis hepatis: twelve cases associated with oral androgen therapy. Arch Pathol Lab Med 101:405-410, 1977.

Nakeeb A, Pitt HA, Sohn TA, et al: Cholangiocarcinoma: a spectrum of intrahepatic, perihepatic and distal tumors. Ann Surg 224:463-475, 1996.

Nelson RC, Chezmar JL: Diagnostic approach to hepatic hemangiomas. Radiology 176:11-13, 1990.

Nelson RC, Chezmar JL, Sugarbaker PH, et al: Preoperative localization of focal liver lesions to specific liver segments: utility of CT during arterial portography. Radiology 176:89-94, 1990.

Perkocha LA, Geaghan SM, Yen TSB, et al: Clinical and pathological features of bacillary peliosis hepatis in association with human immunodeficiency virus infection. N Engl J Med 323: 1581-1586, 1990.

Proietti S, Abedlmoumene A, Genevay M, Denys A: Echinococcal cyst. Radiographics 24:861-865, 2004.

Rao BK, Brodell GK, Haaga JR, et al: Visceral CT findings associated with Thorotrast. J Comput Assist Tomogr 10:57-61, 1986.

Rummeny E, Weissleder R, Stark DD, et al: Primary liver tumors: diagnosis by MR imaging. AJR 152:63-72, 1989.

Siegelman ES, Mitchell DG, Semelka RC: Abdominal iron deposition: metabolism, MR findings, and clinical importance. Radiology 199:13-22, 1996.

Silverman PM, Kohan L, Ducic I, et al: Imaging of the liver with helical CT: a survey of scanning techniques. AJR 170:149-152, 1998.

Soto JA, Barish MA, Yucel EK, et al: Magnetic resonance cholangiography: comparison with endoscopic retrograde cholangiopancreatography. Gastroenterology 110:589-597, 1996.

Soyer P, Poccard M, Boudiaf M, et al: Detection of hypovascular hepatic metastases at triple-phase helical CT: sensitivity of phases and comparison with surgical and histopathologic findings. Radiology 231:413-420, 2004.

Terrier F, Becker CD, Triller JK: Morphologic aspects of hepatic abscesses at computed tomography and ultrasound. Acta Radiol Diagn 24:129-137, 1983.

Torres WE, Whitmire LF, Gedgaudas-McClees K, et al: Computed tomography of the hepatic morphologic changes in cirrhosis of the liver. J Comput Assist Tomogr 10:47-50, 1986.

Vasile N, Lardé D, Zafrani ES, et al: Hepatic angiosarcoma. J Comput Assist Tomogr 7:899-901, 1983.

Yang PJ, Glazer GM, Bowerman RA: Budd-Chiari syndrome: computed tomographic and ultrasonographic findings. J Comput Assist Tomogr 7:148-150, 1983.

Yoon W, Jeong YY, Kim JK, et al: CT in blunt liver trauma. Radiographics 25:87-104, 2005.

Ward J, Guthrie JA, Wilson D, et al: Colorectal hepatic metastases: detection with SPIO-enhanced breath-hold MR imaging—comparison of optimized sequences. Radiology 228:709-718, 2003.

Spleen

Amorosi EL: Hypersplenism. Semin Hematol 2:249-285, 1965.

Baron JM, Weinshelbaum EI, Block GE: Splenic rupture associated with bacterial endocarditis and sickle cell trait. JAMA 205:112-114, 1968.

Bensinger TA, Keller AR, Merrell LF, et al: Thorotrast-induced reticuloendothelial blockage in man. Am J Med 51:663-668, 1971.

Castellino RA: Hodgkin disease: practical concepts for the diagnostic radiologist. Radiology 159:305-310, 1986.

Dachman AH, Ros PR, Murari PJ, et al: Nonparasitic splenic cysts: a report of 52 cases with radiologic-pathologic correlation. AJR 147:537-542, 1986.

Dodds WJ, Taylor AJ, Erickson SJ, et al: Radiologic imaging of splenic anomalies. AJR 155:805-810, 1990.

Gill PG, Souter RG, Morris PJ: Splenectomy for hypersplenism in malignant lymphomas. Br J Surg 68:29-33, 1981.

Louie JS, Pearson CM: Felty's syndrome. Semin Hematol 8: 216-220, 1971.

Peters SP, Lee RE, Glew RH: Gaucher's disease: a review. Medicine 56:425-442, 1977.

Radin DR, Baker EL, Klatt EC, et al: Visceral and nodal calcification in patients with AIDS-related *Pneumocystis carinii* infection. AJR 154:27-31, 1990.

Strijk SP, Wagener DJT, Bogman MJ, et al: The spleen in Hodgkin disease: diagnostic value of CT. Radiology 154: 753-757, 1985.

Svartholm EG, Haglund U: Splenic resection for benign cyst. Acta Chir Scand 151:491-494, 1985.

CHAPTER 6 Biliary System and Gallbladder

DUCTAL ANATOMY

The adult liver is said to contain almost 2 km of bile ducts and ductules. The smallest of these ductules, the biliary canaliculi, have a membranous connection to adjacent hepatocytes across which bile passes through membranous channels from hepatocyte to the biliary system. These interlobar ductules form an anastomosing network around the branches of the portal vein. As the ductules increase in diameter, they develop a smooth muscular layer in the walls.

Eventually, the ducts combine to form the main right and left hepatic ducts at the hilum of the liver and, in most cases, just outside of the liver parenchyma. The joining of the main intrahepatic ducts gives rise to the common hepatic duct, which becomes the common bile duct below the level of the cystic duct connection. The connection of the cystic duct with the common bile duct can vary. About 75% of the time, the cystic duct enters the main extrahepatic duct at the expected location, approximately 3 cm from the union of the right and left hepatic ducts. Union with the cystic duct also can be seen much more distally and medially, however, within a few centimeters of the duodenal ampulla of Vater. Normally, the common bile duct is 5 to 7 cm long and has a diameter of 5 to 15 mm.

The gallbladder is a bile reservoir that concentrates the bile and delivers it to the digestive tract in a controlled manner as needed, by hormonal control, which depends largely on the composition of ingested materials. Because bile is necessary for the absorption of fat, the ingestion of fatty meals stimulates the gallbladder to contract and expel bile into the duodenum. The gallbladder resides in a fossa on the underside of the right lobe of the liver. It is pear-shaped; measures 3 to 4 cm wide and 7 to 8 cm long; and may be divided into the fundus, body, and neck. The posterior fundal portion of the gallbladder is in close proximity with the transverse colon, duodenum, and rarely the antrum of the stomach. This relationship gives rises to gallstones eroding into these adjacent structures. A gallstone eroding into the gastric antrum, impacting in the pyloric channel and causing outlet obstruction, gives rise to Bouveret's syndrome. A gallstone eroding into the bowel (usually duodenum) that is large enough to impact in the narrowest portion of the small bowel (distal ileum) gives rises to a small bowel–obstructing process that has been given the misnomer "gallstone ileus." The neck of the gallbladder sometimes is referred to as Hartmann's pouch and can be a place in which large gallstones may become impacted, resulting in cystic duct obstruction. The neck of the gallbladder devolves into the cystic duct, which is normally 4 cm in length. The length of the cystic duct is noteworthy by the presence of the spiral valves of Heister.

The gallbladder is lined by a mucosal surface of numerous folds and ridges, and the wall itself comprises the layers of mucosa, lamina propria, muscle layer, and serosa. Invaginations or sinuses in the mucosa and the lamina are the Rokitansky-Aschoff sinuses, which become prominent and may be seen in adenomyomatosis of the gallbladder.

BILIARY SYSTEM

Examination Techniques

The gallbladder and biliary tree are separated into two sections in this chapter. To avoid redundancy caused by overlaps in discussion of imaging techniques applicable to both, ultrasonography, magnetic resonance imaging (MRI), computed tomography (CT), and radioisotope scanning are discussed here in the biliary system section. The role of ultrasonography in imaging of the gallbladder is discussed and amplified at the beginning of the gallbladder section, along with the declining use of the oral cholecystogram (OCG).

For purposes of discussing radiological problems associated with the biliary tree, the radiological problems are based on conventional imaging of the biliary tree after luminal filling with contrast material, such as in endoscopic retrograde cholangiopancreatography (ERCP), percutaneous transhepatic cholangiography, operative cholangiography, or T tube injections. Although these examinations have been among the standard imaging studies for biliary diagnosis for decades, the impact of ultrasonography and especially of CT and multidetector CT in the last 3 decades has moved these modalities to the forefront of biliary imaging. The continued progress in magnetic resonance cholangiopancreatography (MRCP) is the most exciting of all advances in imaging the biliary system. Ongoing technical improvements that result in better resolution of the smaller ducts and the use of pharmacological aids to increase contraction at the sphincter of Oddi are expected to result in further improved imaging of the biliary system using MRCP. MRCP is likely eventually to replace diagnostic ERCP and percutaneous transhepatic cholangiography (PTC).

Endoscopic Retrograde Cholangiopancreatography

ERCP remains the most common invasive examination performed, in which the papilla of Vater is endoscopically cannulized and contrast material is injected. Depending on the clinical indication, the examination usually requires filling of the pancreatic duct and the biliary system. The success rate for cannulation ranges from 75% to 90%, with the chief determining factor seeming to be the expertise and experience of the endoscopist. Other causes of failure, such as papillary stenosis, peripapillary duodenal fibrosis and deformity, previous gastric surgery, severe duodenal inflammatory disease, and duodenal diverticula in the area of the papilla, also may result in unsuccessful cannulation. ERCP is a staple of the workup of a jaundiced patient when obstructive causes are suspected. The examination can be done regardless of the degree of jaundice or hepatic disease. The common bile duct and gallbladder are usually easily shown. The pancreatic aspect of the examination is discussed in Chapter 4.

The varying length of fluoroscopic times that these examinations require makes exposure of the patient and involved medical and support staff in the room to ionizing radiation a major safety consideration with ERCP. The complication rate of ERCP is around 5%, and the mortality rate is 0.1% to 0.2%. The most common complication is cholangitis. Bacteremia is reported in a small percentage of patients. Elevations in the serum amylase level and clinical pancreatitis are reported in 1% to 8% of patients.

Percutaneous Transhepatic Cholangiography

PTC involves the direct percutaneous injection of contrast material into bile ducts within the liver. PTC is reported to have been performed first in Hanoi in the 1930s. The procedure usually involved the use of the Chiba (named after the Japanese university) skinny needle. Numerous other types of needles are now used, however. Ultrasound, computed tomographic, or fluoroscopic guidance is used in this procedure. The success of injecting a bile duct increases in the presence of biliary dilatation, reaching almost 100% when the ducts are significantly dilated. With nondilated ducts or strictured ducts, the success rate decreases to less than 90%.

Operative Cholangiography

Transcystic duct cholangiography performed intraoperatively after cholecystectomy allows radiological demonstration of the common bile duct in the search for residual stones, confirmation of ductal patency, and exclusion of ductal injury. Contrast material is injected through the cystic duct stump, and filling of the biliary tree is attempted. Because of positioning of the patient and the less than optimal situation of obtaining a radiograph on the operating room table, these examinations leave much to be desired technically. Often there is incomplete filling of the biliary system. Injected air bubbles also cause interpretive difficulties, and leakage around the cystic duct stump is common. Reflux into the pancreatic duct is frequent.

Computed Tomography

CT of the liver has emerged since the 1980s as a highly sensitive and noninvasive method of detecting biliary ductal distention. In some cases, mild to moderate degrees of distention can be observed before the patient presents with obstructive jaundice. The evaluation of the common bile duct in the region of the pancreatic head is relatively easy, and a fairly accurate measurement usually can be obtained. The usual cause of biliary distention is obstruction. In the absence of a mass in the pancreatic head, CT may not always show the nature of the obstructing process. The presence of biliary distention within the liver and a normal common bile duct in the pancreatic head gives fairly conclusive secondary evidence of obstruction, although the actual obstruction site may not be well shown. Lesions in the porta hepatis, particularly primary bile duct lesions such as cholangiocarcinoma, are extremely difficult to show on CT. MRI has not been shown to have any advantage to date in the evaluation of the biliary system.

Ultrasonography

The effectiveness of real-time ultrasonography in the evaluation of the biliary tree was established in the 1980s. In the hands of a skilled operator, this examination can be done quickly, effectively, inexpensively, and accurately. The presence of biliary distention can be detected easily, and the diameter of the common bile duct can be measured. The presence or absence of stones in the gallbladder is accurately evaluated. Stones are typically hyperechoic, resulting in acoustic shadowing. Stones within the common hepatic or common bile duct also are shown, but with a lesser degree of sensitivity (between 40% and 70%). In a patient in whom either gallbladder disease or biliary obstruction and distention is suspected, ultrasonography is often the initial examination.

Magnetic Resonance Cholangiography

It has become increasingly apparent that high-quality visualization of the biliary and pancreatic ducts during MRI can be achieved. Using imaging sequences that were first developed for vascular imaging, variations of these sequences now can show moderate anatomical detail of the ductal structures (Fig. 6-1); this is now referred to as MRCP. Advantages over other imaging modalities include the facts that MRCP is noninvasive and does not result in any radiation exposure. Also, it can be performed at the same time that MRI of the liver is being done so that the liver parenchyma and ductal structures can be evaluated during the same examination. Finally, the image can be projected in several planes, and coronal images can depict the entire biliary/pancreatic system, which is easily appreciated by clinicians. As further imaging advances are made, MRCP is expected to supplant other modalities.

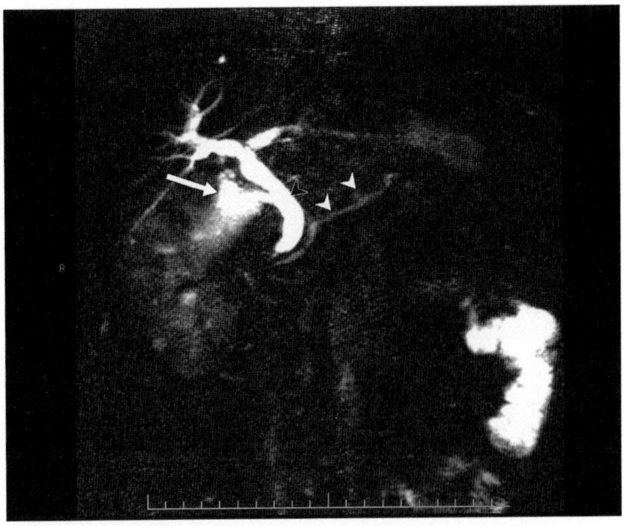

Figure 6-1 MRCP shows some bile leakage at the cystic duct stump *(arrow)*. Note common bile duct *(arrowheads)* and pancreatic duct.

Radioisotope Evaluation

Radioisotopes used for imaging the biliary system are cleared from the blood by the hepatocytes and excreted with bile into the biliary system. Scanning the right upper quadrant shows the biliary ducts and gallbladder. These agents are useful in evaluating patency of the cystic duct and the common hepatic and common bile duct and are effective in the evaluation of acute cholecystitis. Before the mid-1970s, rose bengal iodine-131 was the radiopharmaceutical used to show the biliary system. In the mid-1970s, a new series of technetium-labeled radiopharmaceuticals was developed with the advantages of a short half-life (6 hours) and a relatively low patient radiation dose. These agents are derivatives of iminodiacetic acid (IDA), and a variety of these derivatives have been developed, resulting in the well-known technetium-99m lidofenin (HIDA) and technetium-99m disofenin (DISIDA) scans that allow excellent visualization of the biliary system, even in the presence of mild to moderate jaundice.

Filling Defects

Calculi

Calculi are the most common cause of filling defects within the biliary system. For the most part, they originate within the gallbladder and traverse the cystic duct. Choledocholithiasis is common and may be seen in 6% to 10% of patients during cholecystectomy. Ductal stones also can migrate down the common bile duct and affect pancreatic secretion, resulting in gallstone pancreatitis (Fig. 6-2).

Filling defects in the common bile duct resulting from intraluminal stones are shown with relative ease on ERCP. If the stones are sufficiently large, they also can be

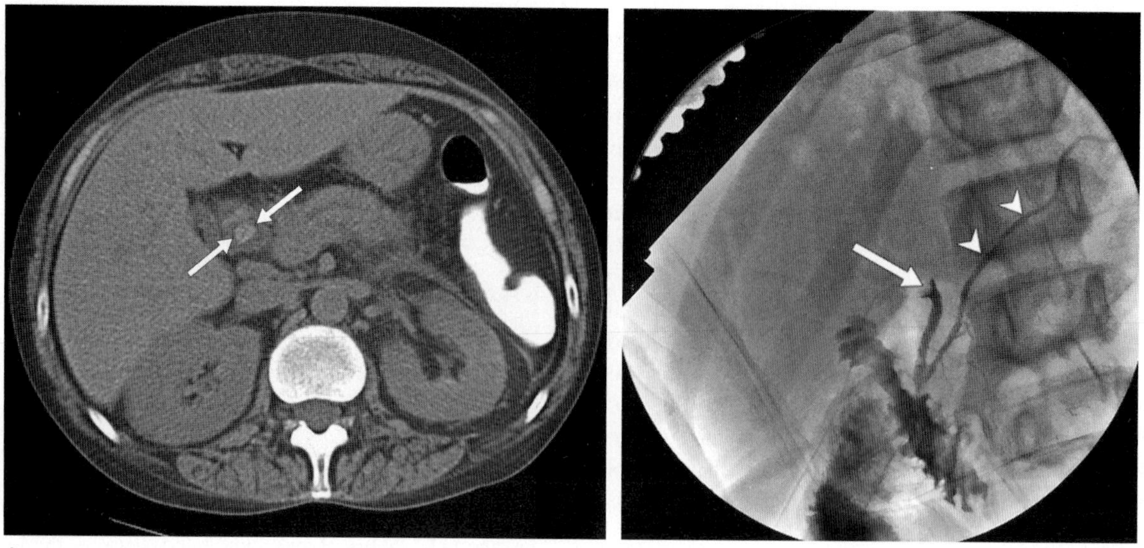

A B

Figure 6-2 **A,** A gallstone has become impacted in the distal common bile duct *(arrows),* causing a mild inflammatory change in the pancreas. **B,** ERCP with stone impaction higher in the common bile duct *(arrow)*. Note normal appearance of pancreatic duct *(arrowheads)*.

seen on CT. Stones within the cystic duct and the common bile duct can be missed easily on CT, however, especially when oral contrast material is used and the stone is obscured by opacified bowel. Ultrasonography may be helpful in showing common bile duct stones (Fig. 6-3). The reliability of the ultrasound examination in this region is much less than in the gallbladder (Fig. 6-4).

Primary stone formation in the common bile duct may occur, usually proximal to an area of narrowing in the duct. The origin of a prestenotic stone still may be the gallbladder, and as a result of obstruction and stasis, these stones accumulate within the common bile duct and increase in size. In the postcholecystectomy patient with a documented normal biliary system postoperatively,

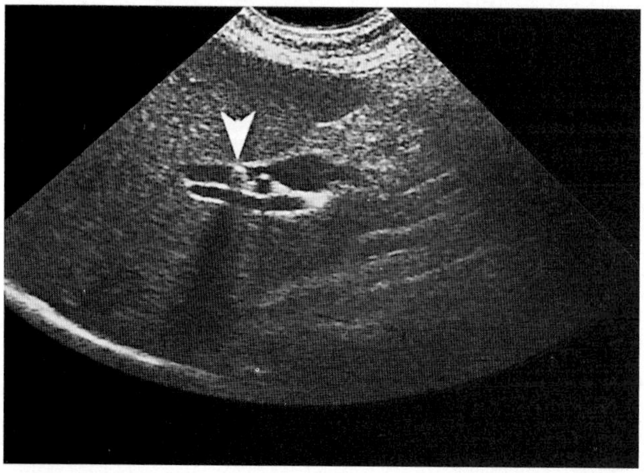

Figure 6-3 Ultrasound examination of the common bile duct shows a small stone within the duct *(arrowhead)* casting an acoustic shadow.

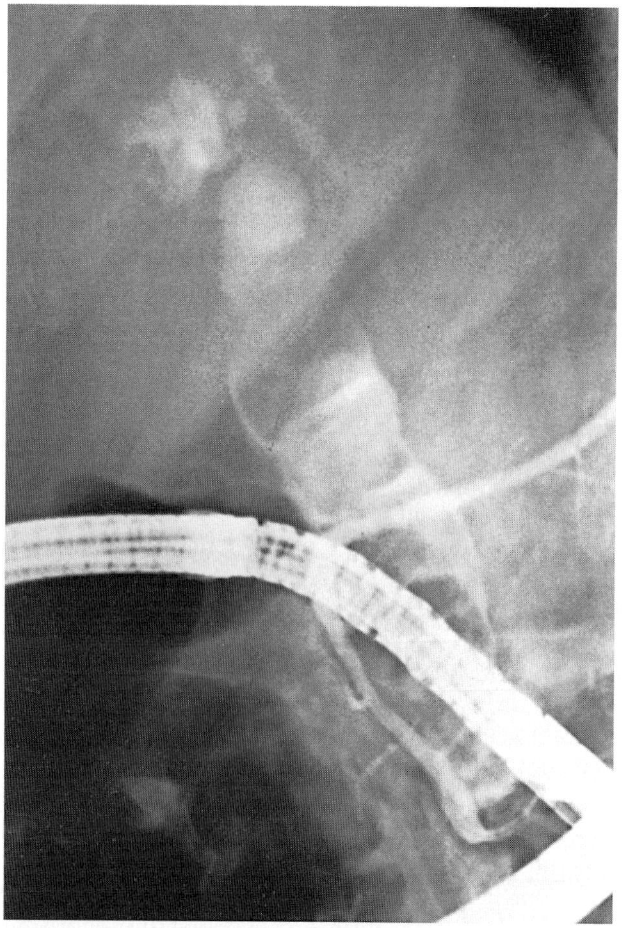

Figure 6-4 ERCP shows a markedly dilated common bile duct filled with multiple, large stones. An ultrasound scan of this region had failed to reveal the presence of the common bile duct stones. The presence of a gas-filled hepatic flexure of the colon seen at the margin of the liver would degrade the ultrasound evaluation of this region.

primary stone formation in the common duct or cystic duct remnant can be seen.

Differentiation of primary from secondary common bile duct stones may be impossible. Occasionally, the configuration of the stone is helpful. Ovoid stones or stone formations that seem to be developing a luminal configuration may suggest the presence of primary stones (Figs. 6-5 and 6-6).

Pseudocalculus

Although a solitary air bubble may mimic a calculus within the common bile duct, the term *pseudocalculus* is reserved for a convex filling defect in the distal common bile duct that has the appearance of the top of a stone (Fig. 6-7). No contrast material passes lateral or inferior to the convexity, however. This appearance is secondary to spasm of the sphincter of Oddi and can be confirmed by simply waiting a few minutes for relaxation to occur. If the spasm seems prolonged or the examiner is impatient, a 1-mg intravenous injection of glucagon usually results in the relaxation of the sphincter and resumption of a normal-appearing distal common bile duct (Fig. 6-8).

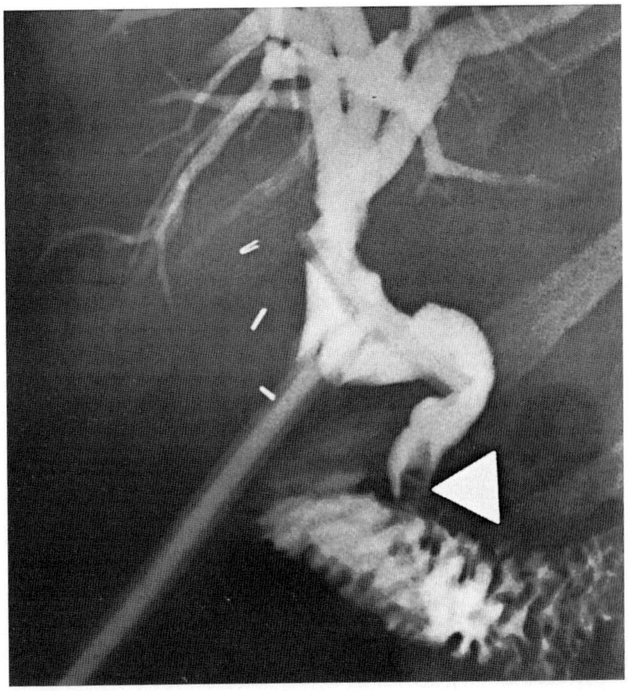

Figure 6-6 Postoperative T tube cholangiography shows a small, oval residual stone in the distal common bile duct *(arrowhead)*.

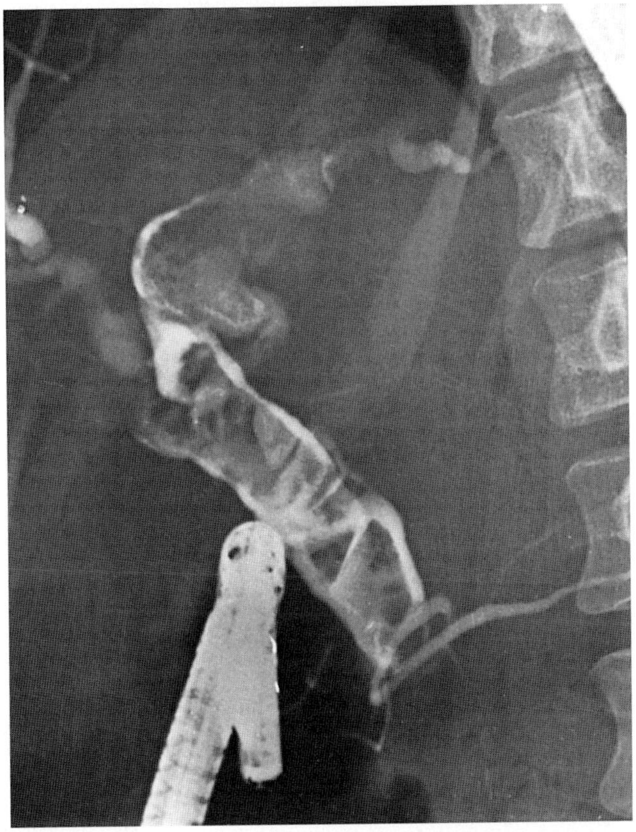

Figure 6-5 ERCP in a patient 13 years after cholecystectomy shows stones forming an intraluminal cast along the entire length of the common bile duct and common hepatic duct.

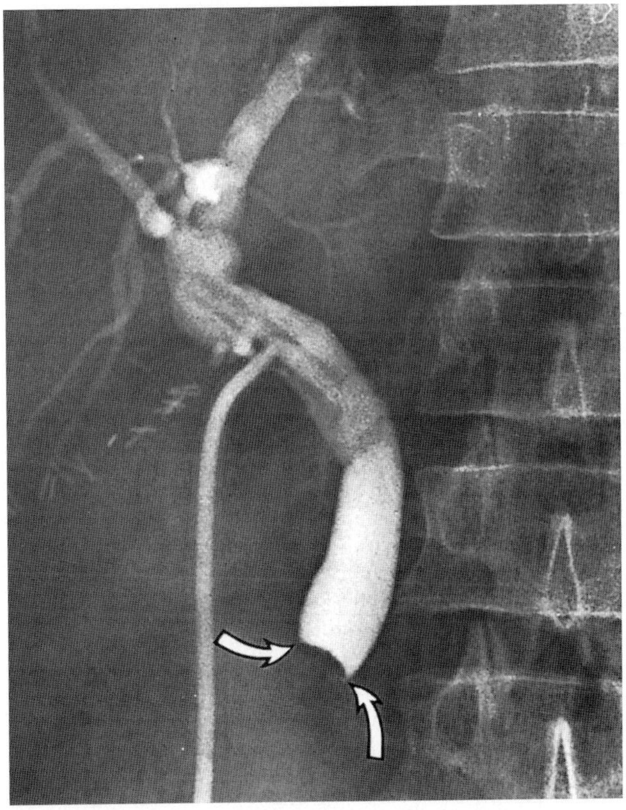

Figure 6-7 T tube cholangiogram shows a rounded filling defect in the distal common bile duct *(arrows)*, raising the possibility of an impacted stone.

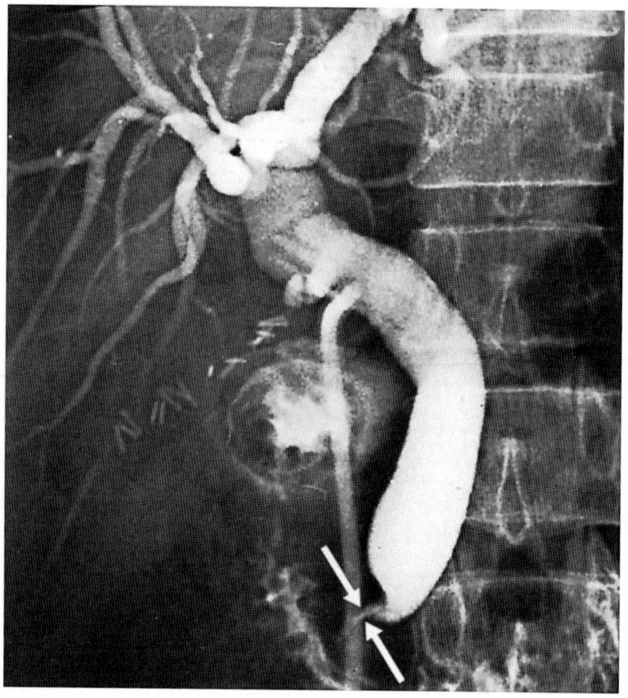

Figure 6-8 The same patient as in Figure 6-7 after the administration of intravenous glucagon. The apparent filling defect in the distal common bile duct has disappeared; it represented spasm of the sphincter of Oddi *(arrows)*.

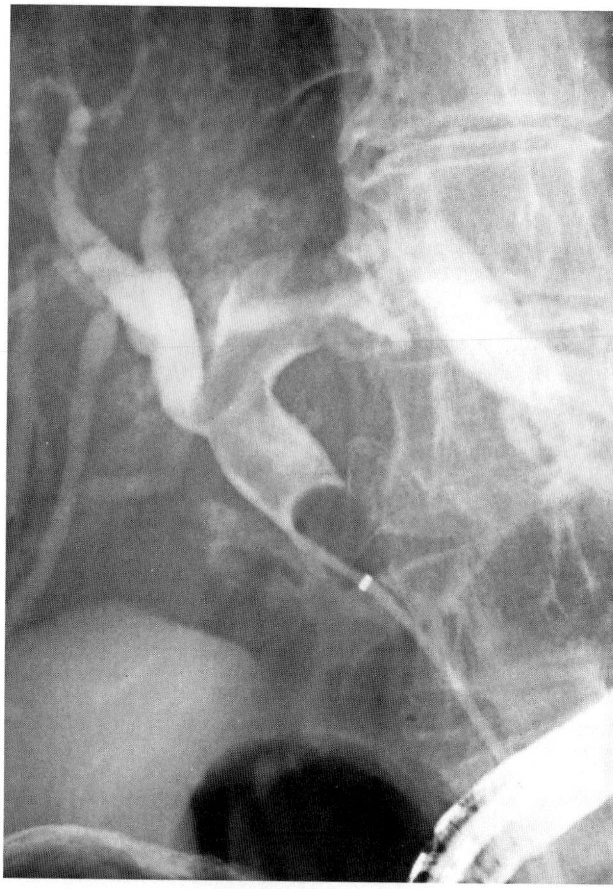

Figure 6-9 Injection of the bile ducts during ERCP shows a cast conforming to the bile ducts from a blood clot within the ductal system. The material is soft and pliable and conforms to the ductal system without significant obstructive changes.

Blood Clot

Hemorrhage into the biliary tract can result in a variety of appearances, from an isolated filling defect to several filling defects to a total cast of the lumen. The extent and rate of bleeding determine the appearance. Bleeding into the biliary tree, hemobilia, does not always result in the formation of a blood clot. This finding is becoming more common with the increasing availability of ERCP. The most common causes include trauma, instrumentation, tumor, and vascular abnormalities within the biliary tract. The presence of stones within the common bile duct also occasionally can result in bleeding. The cause is unclear, although stones passing through the cystic duct or the distal common bile duct may result in injured mucosa. The filling defects caused by clot formation are often different from the appearance of stones. They tend to be less defined and more ovoid (Fig. 6-9). There may be some changing of configuration as the filling defect moves. Blood clots almost never result in obstruction.

Benign Polypoid Lesions

Benign bile duct tumors are uncommon, but when present, they most frequently appear as small, rounded filling defects on the margin of the duct. These include such benign lesions as adenomas and papillomas and fibromas, neurofibromas, lipomas, hamartomas, and carcinoids (Fig. 6-10). These lesions are usually solitary, although multiple filling defects are present in biliary papillomatosis, a rare condition in which multiple papillomas are seen. This condition reputedly carries an increased risk of cholangiocarcinoma.

Parasites

Numerous parasitic infestations can affect the biliary system and result in typical filling defects within the common bile duct. The most common is the roundworm, *Ascaris lumbricoides*. The problem is worldwide, with the greatest prevalence in developing nations and rural areas, where overcrowding and unsanitary environments are common. The ingested ova hatch in the small bowel and usually make that site their habitation. The worm is capable of ascending the small bowel and reaching the duodenum. This proximal migration can result in some of the worms passing into the common bile duct, leading to degrees of biliary obstruction and possible secondary infection. Often this obstruction is

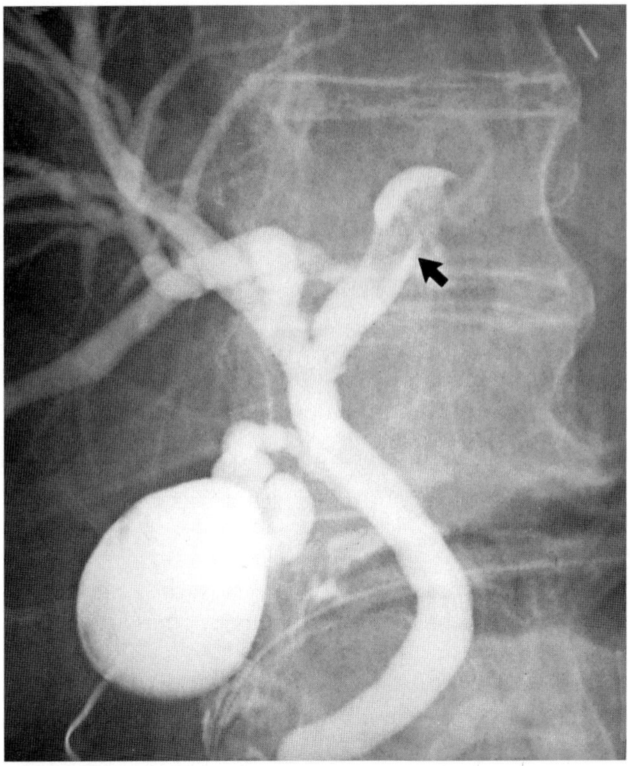

Figure 6-10 Filling defect *(arrow)* in the left hepatic duct is secondary to an adenoma of the bile ducts.

accompanied by pancreatitis, either as a secondary effect or as a result of worm migration into the pancreatic duct. Linear intraluminal filling defects are shown on contrast studies of the common bile duct. The intestine is much more commonly affected with this parasite than the biliary system. Intestinal ascariasis is often asymptomatic, but can be the basis of intestinal obstruction or intussusception. The worm, being quite mobile, can migrate into the biliary tree via the ampullary papilla of Vater.

Liver flukes, most commonly seen in the Far East, are occasionally seen in North America and Western Europe with the increase in worldwide travel and migration. The cysts are ingested, usually with raw fish. The larvae hatch in the duodenum and migrate to the liver and biliary system, where they can produce biliary obstruction and recurrent cholangitis. There is an increased incidence of cholangiocarcinoma in chronic infestation.

Hydatid echinococcal cysts of the liver also occasionally can communicate with the biliary tree and discharge daughter cysts into the biliary system, resulting in filling defects.

Inspissated Bile and Sludge

When conditions exist that produce stasis in the biliary system, the bile may congeal and produce a sludgelike deposit, mostly in the gallbladder, but sometimes in the bile ducts. This deposit appears as an intraluminal cast within the ducts that conforms to the internal lumen of the duct. Its appearance is similar to that of a blood clot. Although it is a rare filling defect, it is sometimes seen in patients who have had extensive biliary surgery, cholangitis, or liver transplantation. These individuals seem to be more susceptible to biliary stasis and resultant formation of biliary sludge. Treatment of this defect is usually accomplished at ERCP, when the endoscopist often can remove the cast by use of an inflatable balloon. Diagnosis is often made at that time because the bile cast is a soft, greenish black material.

Air

Small air bubbles, resulting in filling defects within the biliary system, are a common and troublesome finding during ERCP, PTC, and operative cholangiography. Generally, the defects are small, round, and mobile and can be distinguished from stones when patients are positioned in dependent and nondependent positions. In examinations in which patient positioning is a problem, such as operative cholangiography and occasionally ERCP, a small, rounded filling defect caused by an air bubble inadvertently injected with contrast material cannot be distinguished from a stone. Reinjection is often necessary to clear up the issue. The problem may be avoided entirely, however, if adequate precautions are observed during the contrast filling phase to exclude the possibility of injecting air.

Ductal Narrowing

Postinflammation

Chronic pancreatitis is one of the most frequent causes of common bile duct narrowing. This narrowing occurs as a result of changes in the pancreatic head, consisting of edema, chronic inflammation, and eventually fibrosis resulting in a mass effect. The combination of mass and cicatrization about the intrapancreatic portion of the common bile duct results in a smooth, tapered narrowing. Approximately 25% of these patients have sufficient narrowing to induce obstructive jaundice. When the stricture is the result of mass effect secondary to inflammation and edema and less due to cicatrization, the severity of the stricture may not be permanent, and some degree of relief may be observed as the pancreatic inflammatory process subsides. Prolonged strictures, resulting mostly from fibrotic changes about the common bile duct in the intrapancreatic portion, can result in permanent liver damage if unrelieved. These patients eventually go on to develop cirrhosis. This type of stricture is not amenable to dilatation, and the definitive treatment is choledochoduodenostomy or choledochojejunostomy.

The configuration of smooth, narrow tapering over a 2- to 4-cm segment of the distal common bile duct in its intrapancreatic portion is benign in most cases. Occasionally, malignancy manifests in such a manner, however. In a patient with no clinical or radiological evidence of pancreatitis or gallstone disease, the physician should be suspicious.

Other causes of stricture resulting from inflammation and fibrosis include trauma caused by difficult stone passage, ischemic and inflammatory damage that can occur as a result of hepatic artery chemotherapy infusion, and external penetrating and blunt trauma. Recurrent biliary infections also may result in stricture formation. Sclerosing cholangitis is discussed separately.

Postsurgery

Another important cause of benign strictures is accidental injury to the bile duct during cholecystectomy or other biliary surgery. Most of these strictures are amenable to surgery. The inadvertent placement of a ligature or a hemostat around the common bile duct or common hepatic duct is a common injury. Most frequently, the trauma involves the common hepatic duct, and depending on the degree of injury and the severity of the stricture, symptoms may occur weeks or years after the injury. Acutely, the patient may be jaundiced or experience intermittent attacks of cholangitis. Ductal stones develop above the stricture in about 25% of these patients. Long-term, unrelieved strictures eventually lead to obstructive biliary cirrhosis and liver failure. Careful fundal-to-ductal dissection by the surgeon to identify the common hepatic and common bile ducts clearly and routine use of intraoperative cholangiography reduce the incidence of these injuries.

Cholangitis

Several different conditions produce what can be termed a "cholangitis" appearance to the bile ducts (Box 6-1). This appearance consists of multiple areas of narrowing of the ductal structures, often involving intrahepatic and extrahepatic systems. The areas of narrowing can be of varying lengths and severity, even in the same patient or duct. The intervening portions of ducts can show a mild degree of dilatation, particularly as the disease becomes progressive. The development of cholangitis also can predispose patients to the later occurrence of cholangiocarcinoma. Cholangiocarcinoma is a well-known complication of sclerosing cholangitis from inflammatory bowel disease, but also can occur with parasitic cholangitides.

Sclerosing Cholangitis

Sclerosing cholangitis is a progressive inflammatory process involving all or parts of the bile duct system. Frequently, it involves the biliary system diffusely with extrahepatic and intrahepatic involvement. The inflammation results in diffuse thickening of the bile duct walls.

Box 6-1 Causes of Sclerosing Cholangitic Appearance of the Bile Ducts

- Ulcerative colitis
- Idiopathic causes
- Ascending (infectious) cholangitis
  - Postoperative
  - Immunosuppression (AIDS, transplants)
  - Parasitic
- Other
  - Retroperitoneal fibrosis
  - Crohn's disease
  - Riedel's thyroiditis
- Cholangiocarcinoma

The degree of severity commonly varies segmentally (Fig. 6-11). The disease occurs more commonly in men by a 2:1 ratio.

Several conditions are associated with sclerosing cholangitis, with ulcerative colitis being the most frequently observed. At least half of patients with sclerosing cholangitis have associated inflammatory bowel disease. Conversely, sclerosing cholangitis eventually develops in 3% to 10% of patients with ulcerative colitis and 0.5% to 1% of patients with Crohn's disease. The relationship is not understood. Some regression in the severity of the disease has been reported in patients with ulcerative colitis who have had total colectomies. Other conditions associated with sclerosing cholangitis

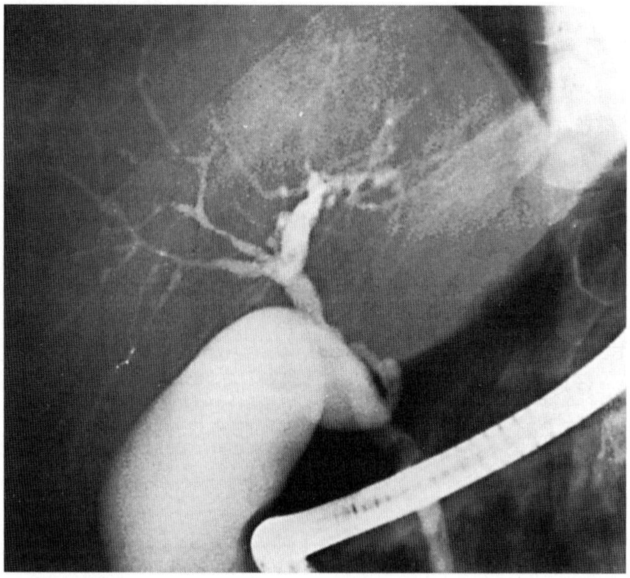

Figure 6-11 ERCP in a 32-year-old patient with ulcerative colitis and sclerosing cholangitis shows intrahepatic areas of segmental narrowing.

include Riedel's thyroiditis and retroperitoneal and mediastinal fibrosis. The incidence with these conditions is much less compared with that of ulcerative colitis or Crohn's disease.

The imaging diagnosis is best obtained by either ERCP or PTC. Although the small sclerosed ducts are difficult to aspirate with the percutaneous transhepatic approach, the use of the Chiba skinny needle in recent years has increased the success rate.

Diffuse or localized areas of alternating narrowing and relative dilatation are seen involving the intrahepatic and extrahepatic biliary system. The differential diagnostic considerations include a slow-growing scirrhous type of bile duct carcinoma and the possibility of congenital cystic disease when the strictures are segmental. In addition, cholangiocarcinoma may develop as a complication of sclerosing cholangitis, and the neoplasm's appearance is difficult to distinguish from the cholangitis. A secondary bile duct sclerosis can occur above chronic partial obstructions of benign causes. The appearance is similar to primary sclerosing cholangitis, and a clear limitation of the changes in the extrahepatic system should raise the suspicion of this possibility. These changes are postulated to result from the chronic recurrent cholangitis associated with partial obstruction.

Ascending Cholangitis

As previously discussed, chronic recurrent ascending cholangitis, proximal to a long-term partial obstruction of the common hepatic or common bile duct, results in proximal bile stasis, dilatation, and potential development of primary stone formation and bacterial cholangitis. Intrahepatic and extrahepatic ducts can be involved in a secondary sclerosing (ascending) cholangitis. The resultant changes in the biliary system can be indistinguishable from primary sclerosing cholangitis (Fig. 6-12). Patients are usually seriously ill with a biliary system that in the worst-case scenario is filled with pus at the height of the infectious process (Fig. 6-13). Numerous small pericholangitic abscesses may form and make the diagnosis easier. If untreated, the condition is usually fatal. Treatment and multiple recurrences of the infectious process are usually the scenario for the sclerosing ductal changes. Although the treatment of the septic process is primary, definitive treatment consists of relieving the distal obstructive process. Occasionally, tiny common bile duct diverticula are encountered that may indicate previous ascending cholangitis (Fig. 6-14).

Nonbacterial types of ascending cholangitis have been described in patients with acquired immunodeficiency syndrome (AIDS), with a radiological picture similar to primary sclerosing cholangitis. Biliary *Cryptosporidium,* although uncommon, is being encountered with more frequency with the increasing number of AIDS patients. Biliary cytomegalovirus and moniliasis, although rare, may produce similar pictures in immunocompromised patients.

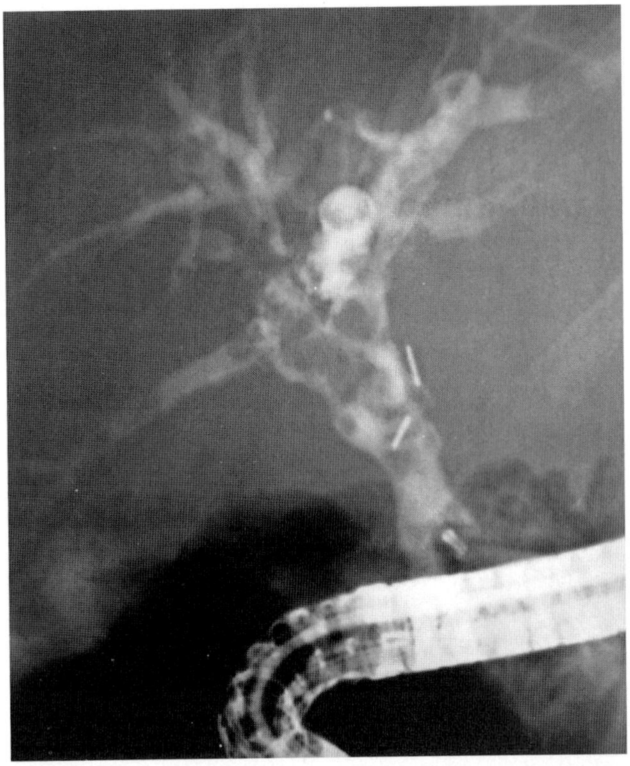

Figure 6-12 Areas of narrowing with filling defects in the ducts are secondary to ascending cholangitis with pus present within the ducts.

Parasitic Cholangitis

Although rare in developed countries, parasitic migration into the biliary system is one of the most common

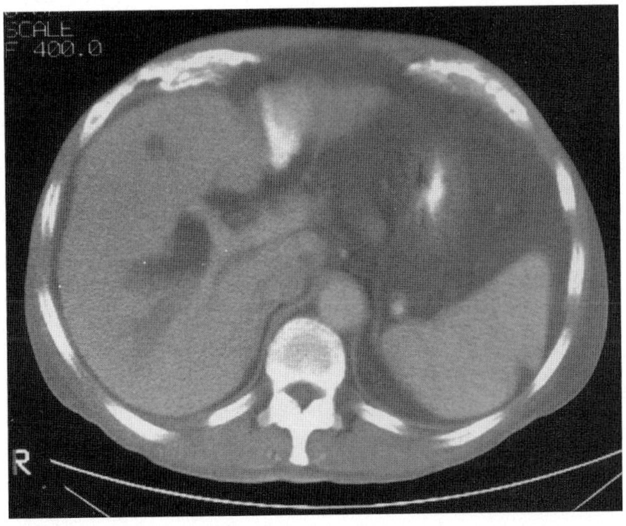

Figure 6-13 A case of ascending cholingitis. CT shows pus distending the intrahepatic biliary system.

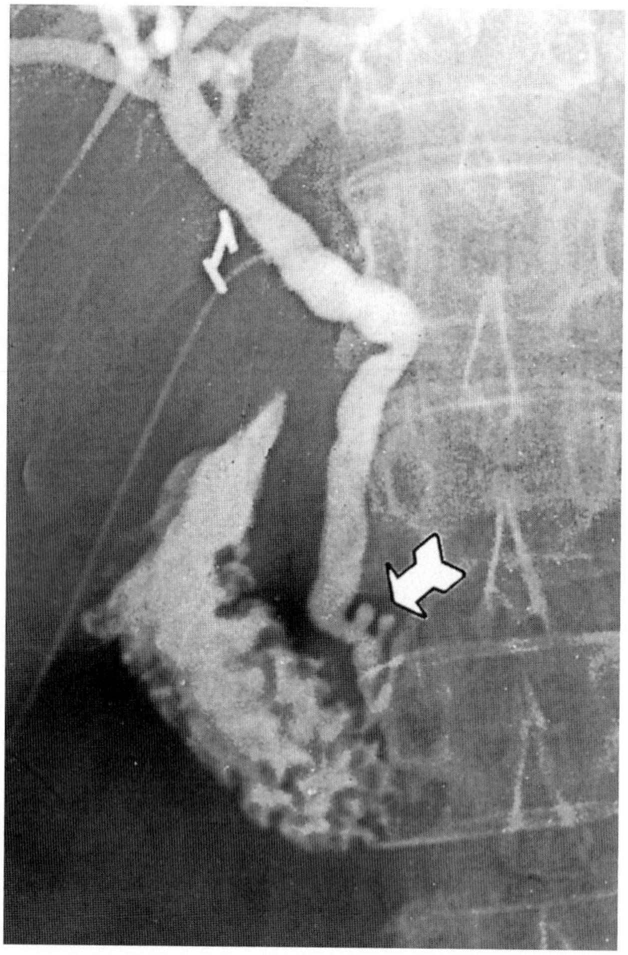

Figure 6-14 Cholangiogram shows several small diverticula *(arrow)* in the distal common bile duct associated with slight narrowing and irregularity, but no obstruction.

causes of cholangitis in the world. Intestinal parasites, such as *Ascaris lumbricoides* and *Clonorchis sinensis,* migrate from the intestinal tract into the biliary system. Echinococcal cysts have been known to rupture into the biliary system and produce cholangitis by a seeding process into the bile ducts.

A. lumbricoides is the most common cause of cholangitis in the world and infects a large proportion of the world's population. This large roundworm migrates up from the intestinal tract. It is easily recognizable as a long, tubular filling defect within the extrahepatic ducts. *C. sinensis* is a flatworm 1 to 2 cm in length. This parasite is most common in Southeast Asia. When it migrates into the biliary system, it tends to settle into the intrahepatic ducts. In contrast to ascariasis, the abnormalities in the intrahepatic ducts are more severely involved by *C. Sinensis*. Similar to sclerosing cholangitis with inflammatory bowel disease, the parasitic cholangitides are associated with an increased incidence of cholangiocarcinoma.

Box 6-2 Biliary Tract Abnormalities in Liver Transplantation

Leak
Stricture at anastomosis
Attenuated intrahepatic ducts (rejection)
Multifocal strictures (duct ischemia)

Liver Transplant Rejection

Several different conditions can affect the biliary system of the transplanted liver; this can occur from one third to one half of all transplanted patients and represents a major diagnostic challenge for the clinician and radiologist (Box 6-2). Some of these conditions, such as leakage, are not discussed here. Numerous conditions in the transplanted liver eventually produce some narrowing of the bile ducts.

During liver transplant rejection, edema and cellular infiltration of the liver parenchyma occur. These processes can be seen with acute and chronic rejection, although the biliary changes may be more pronounced with acute rejection. Imaging of the biliary radicles during rejection shows attenuation of the radicles and sometimes splaying (Fig. 6-15). The changes may become

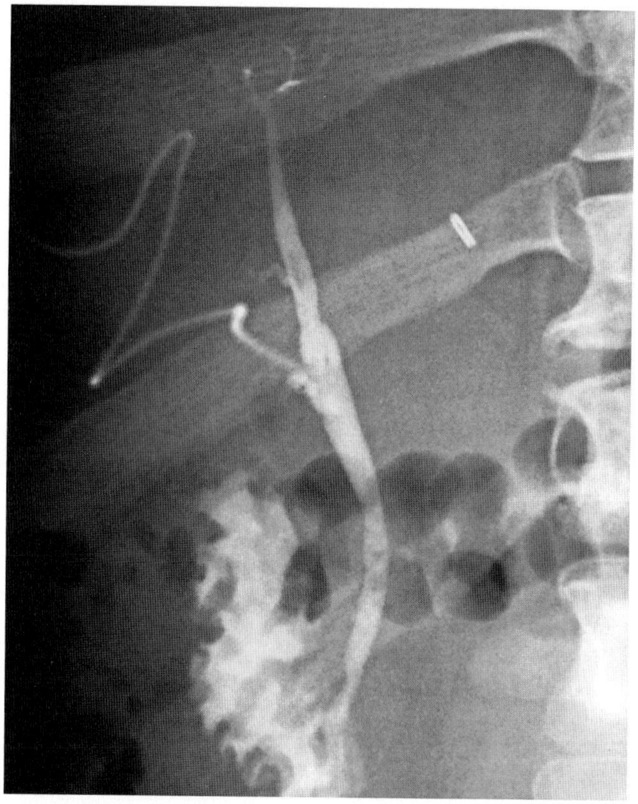

Figure 6-15 Markedly attenuated intrahepatic ducts are due to edema in this liver transplant patient with rejection.

pronounced, depending on the severity of the condition. Strictures of the extrahepatic biliary system also may be seen. The most common site of narrowing is the anastomosis site in the common bile duct. The cause for stenosis at the anastomosis may be scarring or sometimes focal ischemia. When strictures occur in a multifocal distribution after transplant, the most likely cause is ischemia. When liver transplantation is performed for sclerosing cholangitis, the potential exists for recurrence of the cholangitis. The appearance is similar to what is seen typically with sclerosing cholangitis.

Extrinsic Obstructive Processes

Stricture of the intrapancreatic portion of the common bile duct is a well-known result of acute (Fig. 6-16) and chronic pancreatitis and pancreatic carcinoma involving the pancreatic head; this has been discussed previously. Metastatic spread in the porta hepatis or the peripancreatic or periduodenal region also occasionally can produce sufficient extrinsic compression to cause bile duct narrowing and obstruction. Tumors from the gastrointestinal tract, lung, or breast are most commonly involved. Lymphomatous nodes, although large and bulky, seldom result in sufficient extrinsic pressure to narrow the common hepatic or common bile duct seriously except when accompanied by desmoplastic changes (Fig. 6-17).

Mirizzi syndrome and Mirizzi-like syndrome are unusual conditions that result in degrees of biliary obstruction. Mirizzi syndrome classically refers to a stone that becomes impacted in the neck of the gallbladder or the cystic duct, with the mass of the stone and accompanying inflammatory changes causing compression and narrowing of the adjacent common bile duct (Fig. 6-18). Malignant masses arising from the neck of the gallbladder or the cystic duct region can result in a Mirizzi-like picture as a result of contiguous spread, involvement of the common bile duct, and biliary narrowing and obstruction (Fig. 6-19).

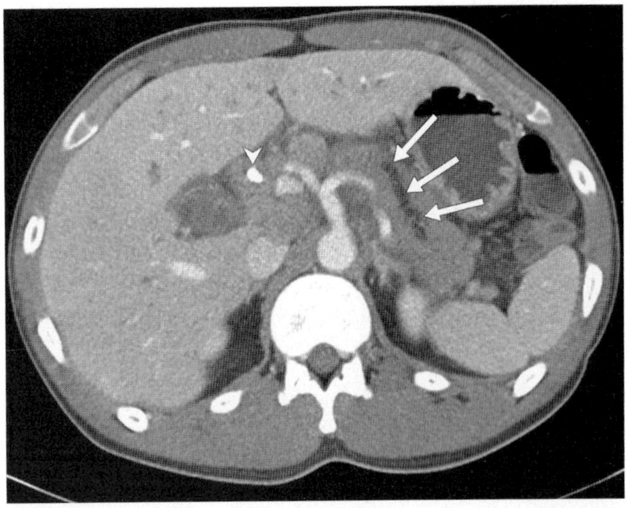

Figure 6-17 CT of upper abdomen shows severe lymphadenopathy with resulting obstruction of pancreatic duct *(arrows)* and common bile duct (*arrowhead* shows biliary stent). This is an unusual cause of ductal obstruction.

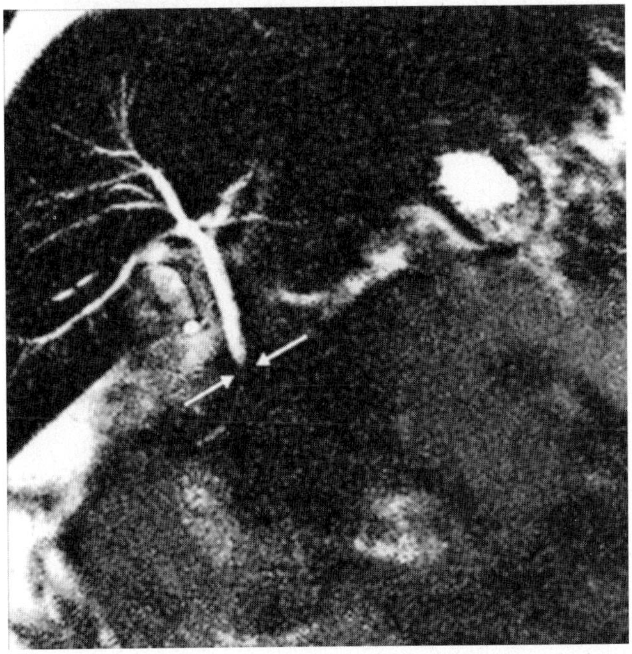

Figure 6-16 MRCP shows mild dilatation of the biliary system secondary to extrinsic impression and narrowing *(arrows)* of an acutely inflamed pancreatic head.

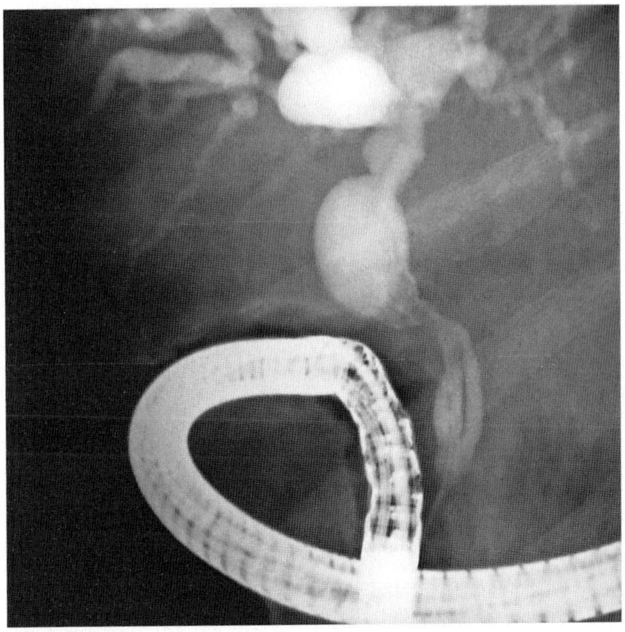

Figure 6-18 Narrowing of the midextrahepatic ducts is from a stone that has become impacted in the neck of the gallbladder with inflammatory changes (Mirizzi syndrome).

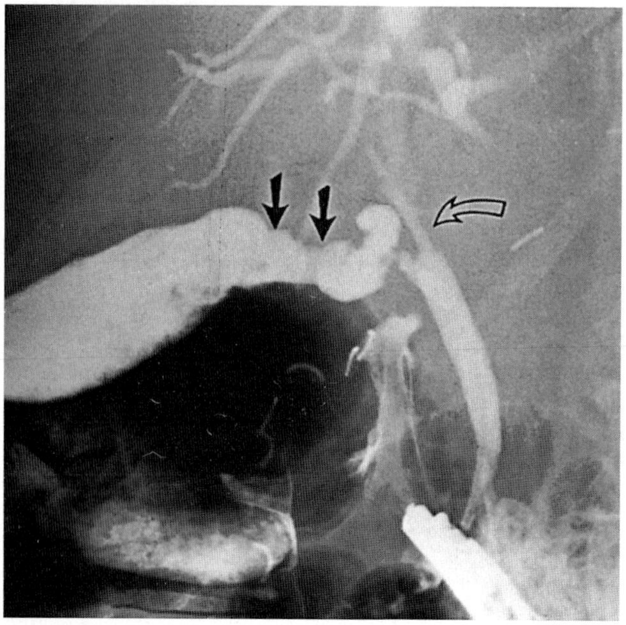

Figure 6-19 ERCP shows a lesion arising from the neck of the gallbladder *(arrows)* narrowing the gallbladder neck, cystic duct, and adjacent common hepatic duct *(curved arrow)*.

Cholangiocarcinoma

Cholangiocarcinoma is uncommon, but associated with high mortality. It occurs most often in adults 50 to 70 years old. Approximately 3500 new cases are seen in the United States annually. Ninety percent of cases are adenocarcinomas. The incidence of cholangiocarcinoma arising in patients with primary sclerosing cholangitis using imaging as the diagnostic tool has been reported to be 5% to 20%. The incidence is higher yet in patients receiving liver transplants and yet higher in postmortem studies. The risk of malignancy seems to increase with the presence of long-term sclerosing cholangitis (Box 6-3). There also is increased risk in any condition that results in chronic bile stasis, including Caroli's disease, choledochal cysts, widespread cystic disease of the liver, and certain parasitic infections. There is also an increased risk with chronic parasitic infections of the biliary system, with biliary papillomatosis, and in some environmental circumstances, such as are encountered in the chemical industry. Prognosis for this disease is poor, and there is no definitive treatment at present. Radiation therapy, chemotherapy, and ductal stenting offer some palliation. In a small select group of patients, some success has been reported with liver transplantation. In general, this option has had poor results, however, and cholangiocarcinoma is not generally considered an indication for transplantation. Survival after the diagnosis of this condition is 6 to 12 months. Few patients live beyond 1 year.

Although cholangiocarcinoma can present as a mass in the hepatic hilum (about 10% of cases), the most common presentation of cholangiocarcinoma is a short area of irregular biliary stenosis (Box 6-4). This stenosis is occasionally accompanied by marked desmoplastic changes and infiltration of the walls of the bile duct, and the lesion rarely can resemble sclerosing cholangitis. Approximately half of these tumors are located in the region of the bifurcation of the main biliary ducts (Klatskin's tumors) (Fig. 6-20). Morphologically, these

Box 6-3 Precursor Conditions for Cholangiocarcinoma

Sclerosing cholangitis
Choledochal cyst
Parasitic cholangitis
Biliary papillomatosis

Box 6-4 Radiographic Appearance of Cholangiocarcinoma

Focal stricture
Polypoid lesion
Diffuse narrowing (scirrhous)

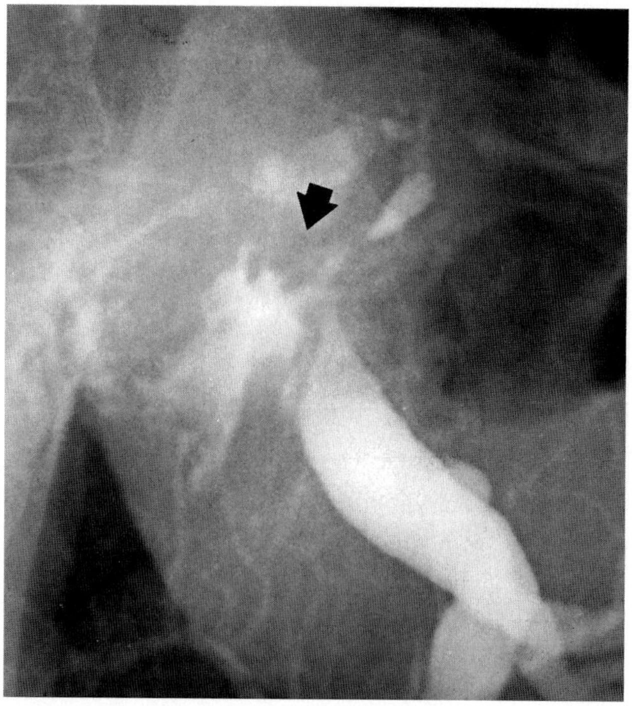

Figure 6-20 Cholangiography shows narrowing of the ducts at the bifurcation, representing a sclerosing cholangiocarcinoma *(arrow)*. This is called a Klatskin tumor.

lesions can be focally stenotic (most common) and polypoid or diffusely scirrhous in nature. CT and ultrasonography are often unable to show the tumor, although the secondary effects of biliary obstruction are readily identified using these modalities. ERCP is helpful, but in cases with high-grade obstructive lesions, PTC is superior in that it is able to show the proximal extent of the lesion. The value of MRI in this lesion is debatable. Some authorities suggest that the tumor may be more visible on certain MRI protocols. At this point, MRI does not occupy a primary role in the imaging workup, however.

The most common lesion pattern is a short, irregular stricture, although smooth margins are frequent. The polypoid form has the best prognosis, whereas the scirrhous form has the worst. Only a few patients are candidates for any form of surgical resection. For the remainder, when the diagnosis has been firmly established, biliary drainage is the goal. Drainage is accomplished by stenting the narrowed segment either from below (ERCP) or from above (PTC).

Adjacent Malignant Lesions

Malignant lesions arising in the tissues adjacent to the biliary system (Box 6-5), such as the liver in the case of hepatoma or occasionally hepatic metastatic lesions, can result in biliary stenosis caused by compression or invasion (Fig. 6-21). A similar pattern can be seen with cancer of the pancreatic head (Fig. 6-22). Cancer of the ampulla of Vater commonly constricts the distal common bile duct, leading to proximal distention. The bile ducts can be divided into pancreatic, suprapancreatic, and intrahepatic regions. If the pancreatic portion of the common duct is involved, the most likely process would be one arising from the pancreas, such as pancreatic carcinoma

Box 6-5 Bile Duct Stricture/Narrowing: Location versus Etiology

PANCREATIC

Pancreatic carcinoma
Pancreatitis
Cholangiocarcinoma

SUPRAPANCREATIC

Adenopathy (metastases)
Cholangiocarcinoma
Mirizzi syndrome (stone impacted in cystic duct)
Gallbladder neoplasm

INTRAHEPATIC

Cholangiocarcinoma
Liver metastases
Primary hepatic neoplasm

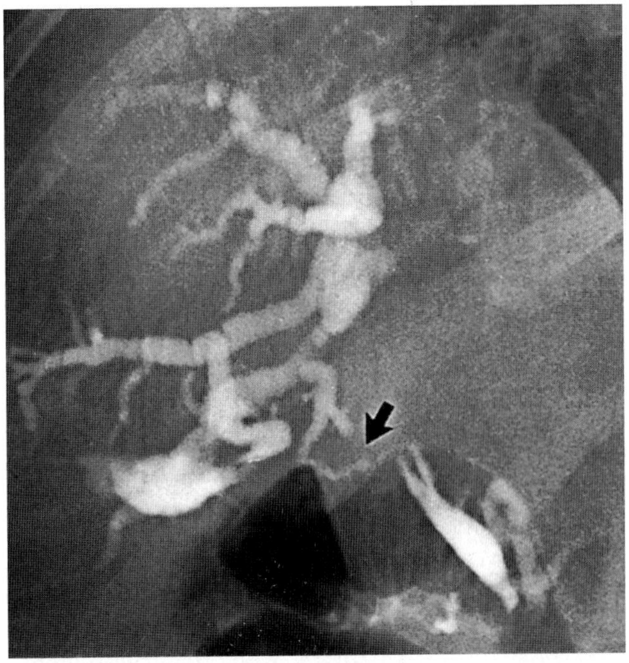

Figure 6-21 Cholangiogram in a patient with known breast cancer and disseminated metastatic disease shows obstruction of the biliary system at the level of the common hepatic duct *(arrow)* as a result of metastatic disease in the porta hepatis.

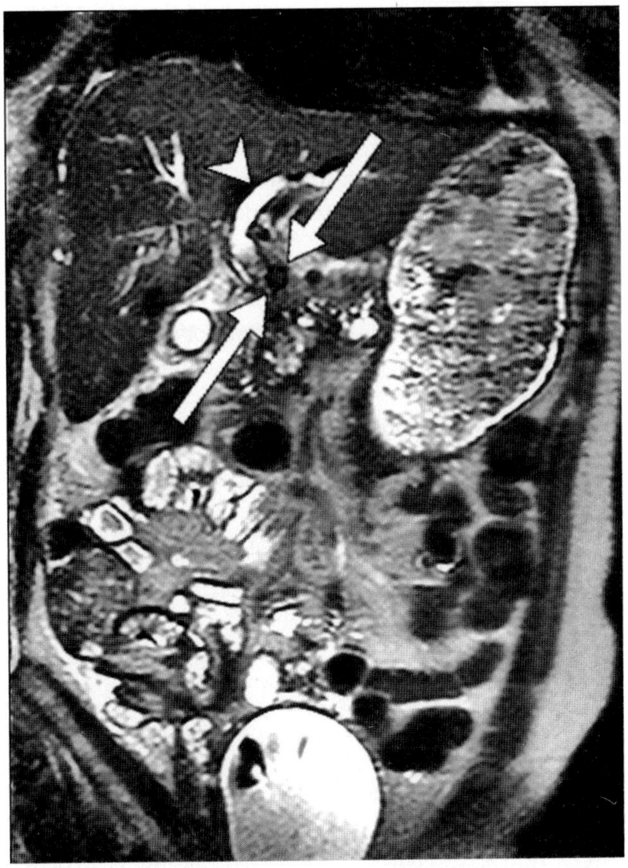

Figure 6-22 MRCP shows lesion in pancreatic head *(arrows)* and dilatation of left main bile duct *(arrowhead)*.

or pancreatitis. Above the pancreas, but still in the extrahepatic ducts, the most likely cause of narrowing is enlarged lymph nodes from either an abdominal or an extraabdominal tumor. Involvement by gallbladder disease, either malignant or inflammatory, also can produce narrowing. Intrahepatic involvement of the ducts is produced by hepatic neoplasms, usually metastatic.

Ampullary and Periampullary Processes

Carcinoma of the ampulla of Vater is often a nonspecific entity that includes lesions arising from the distal common bile duct, the pancreatic duct, and the adjacent duodenum. The appellation is more regional than histological, and in many instances it is impossible to differentiate these tumors histologically. True periampullary carcinomas are relatively rare. Carcinomas of the pancreatic head are three to four times more common (Fig. 6-23). Although the survival rate with pancreatic carcinoma is usually 1 year or less, true periampullary lesions can have a much better prognosis, with 5-year survival rates of 40% in patients with negative nodes. In this patient group, jaundice resulting from common bile duct obstruction is one of the most common presenting symptoms along with weight loss and anorexia. A palpable gallbladder (Courvoisier's gallbladder) is seen in at least 25% of patients.

Other assorted ampullary and periampullary processes that may result in biliary duct obstruction include polyps arising in the periampullary region. These are uncommon, but adenomas, particularly the villous type, are the most frequently encountered lesion (Fig. 6-24). Carcinoids of the periampullary region also have been described, along with most of the other benign tumors of the gastrointestinal tract.

Duodenal diverticula are a common and mostly innocuous finding on upper gastrointestinal (UGI) examinations. Most of the diverticula occur in the juxta-ampullary region, and the ampulla may empty into

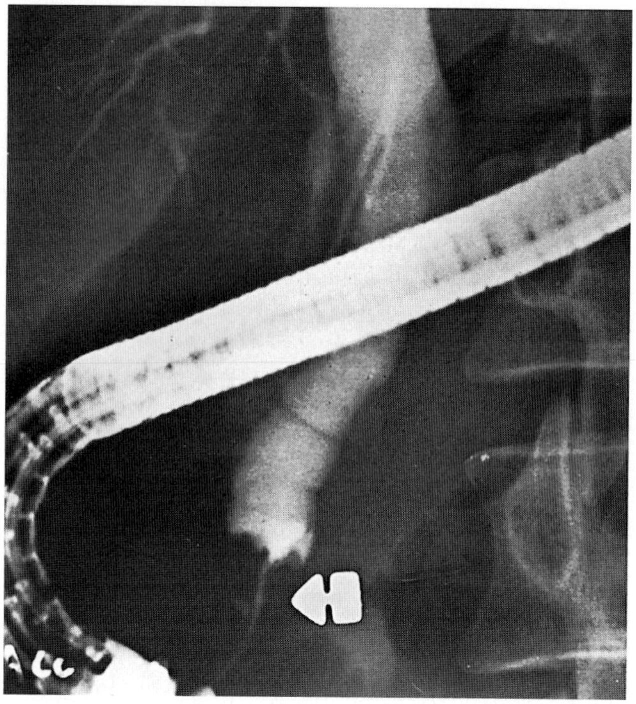

Figure 6-24 ERCP shows some dilatation of the common bile duct with narrowing distally *(arrow)*. The finding was persistent and proved to be a villous adenoma of the duodenum with extension into the distal common bile duct.

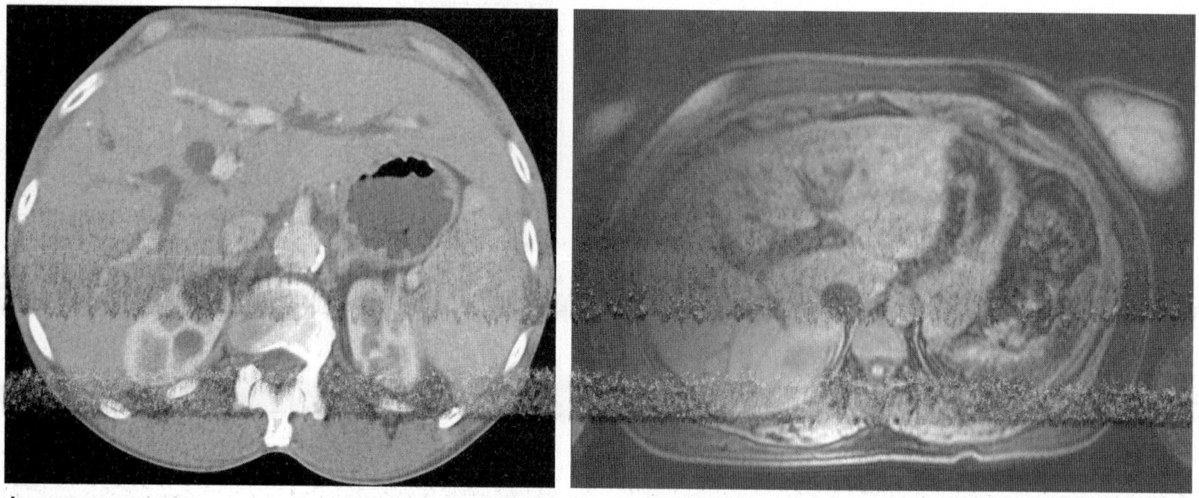

A B

Figure 6-23 **A,** A patient with pancreatic carcinoma presenting with biliary obstruction. A computed tomographic section through the liver shows a dilated intrahepatic system. **B,** MRI shows bile duct obstruction.

the diverticulum. In most instances, this condition provides little or no problem. Under certain circumstances, however, the anatomical arrangement becomes important. If the ampulla empties into the diverticulum, and there are duodenal inflammatory changes involving the diverticulum, the possibility of inflammatory and edematous changes resulting in some obstruction to the outflow of bile and pancreatic secretions is increased. This situation is uncommon. If the diverticulum is sufficiently large and bulky, it may present a mechanical difficulty by impressing the distal common bile duct. When the papilla is located within a diverticulum, the risk of papillary injury during cannulation is increased.

Biliary Atresia

Biliary atresia is defined as luminal obliteration of either the intrahepatic or the extrahepatic bile ducts during the neonatal period. It is the most common cause of jaundice and liver-related death in neonates. It may be congenital, although there is some suspicion that the lesions are caused by intrauterine, biliary, or hepatic infections and inflammation resulting in sclerosing changes within the ductal system. The symptoms usually develop shortly after birth, and without liver transplantation, life expectancy depends on the degree of biliary patency present. Life expectancy in general is approximately 2 years.

Trying to sort out the confusion surrounding the two neonatal conditions, biliary atresia and neonatal hepatitis, is an ongoing problem. Even with liver biopsies, a clear differentiation may not be possible. This observation has led some investigators to suggest that biliary cirrhosis and neonatal hepatitis may be manifestations of the same disease process.

Ductal Dilatation

Obstruction

The radiological problems of biliary stenosis and bile duct dilatation overlap, with one commonly leading to the other. The classification in this and the following section is at best arbitrary, choosing to emphasize the primary pathophysiological process. The most common cause of biliary duct distention is obstruction, many of the causes of which have been previously discussed (see Fig. 6-23). The problem of a dilated biliary ductal system is viewed in this section from the perspective of the dilated ducts as the primary problem instead of as the sequela of some other problem, such as stenosis. Bile duct obstruction can be obvious, even in unenhanced computed tomographic scans of the liver. Obstruction also can be subtle in its early stages, however, and the reader should be aware that the earliest change of bile duct obstruction is seen in the left lobe of the liver, whereas the right lobe may remain relatively normal (Fig. 6-25).

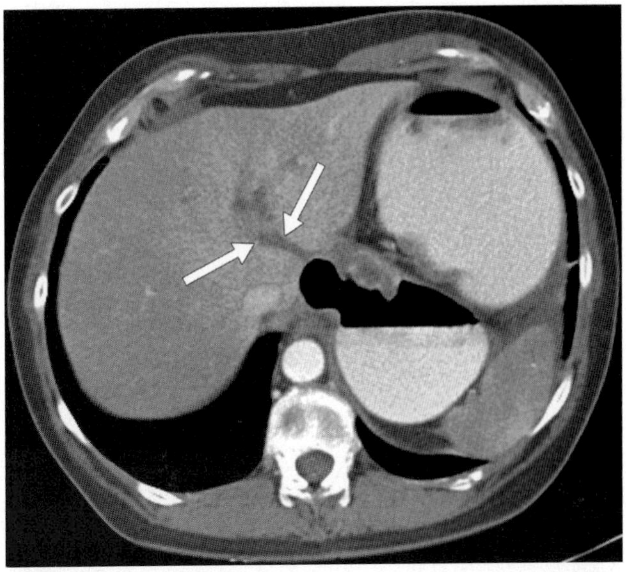

Figure 6-25 Early bile obstruction seen on CT of upper liver. Note that the left biliary system is more obviously dilated *(arrows)*.

Choledochal Cysts

Choledochal cysts are not true cysts, but rather cystic dilatations of the biliary tree. The condition is uncommon, although the Japanese report a higher incidence than the rest of the world. The changes in the biliary tree are thought to be congenital, but evidence suggests that some cases may be acquired as a result of an anomalous configuration of the pancreaticobiliary junction and subsequent reflux of pancreatic secretions into the bile duct. Whether the dilatation is congenital or acquired, it seems that it is a progressive process; choledochal cysts are only infrequently encountered in infancy.

The original classification of choledochal cysts divided them into three categories (Fig. 6-26). The first and most common presentation (80% to 90%) is manifested as a cystic dilatation of the entire common bile duct (type 1A). A subtype of this (type 1B) is focal dilatation of the common bile duct (Fig. 6-27). Another subtype (type 1C) is fusiform dilatation of the common bile duct (Fig. 6-28). In the type 1 form of choledochal cysts, the lesion is solitary and limited, and neither the cystic duct nor the intrahepatic system is involved. The cystic dilatation can be fusiform or saccular in configuration.

In type 2 (about 2% of all cases), a well-defined diverticulum with an ostium is seen arising from the common bile duct. The remainder of the biliary tree is usually normal. If the diverticulum becomes sufficiently large, it may begin to compress, narrow, and obstruct the common bile duct extrinsically. Type 3 choledochal cyst is a choledochocele, in which there is cystic dilatation of the intraduodenal portion of the common bile duct and protrusion into the duodenal lumen (2% to 5% of all cases).

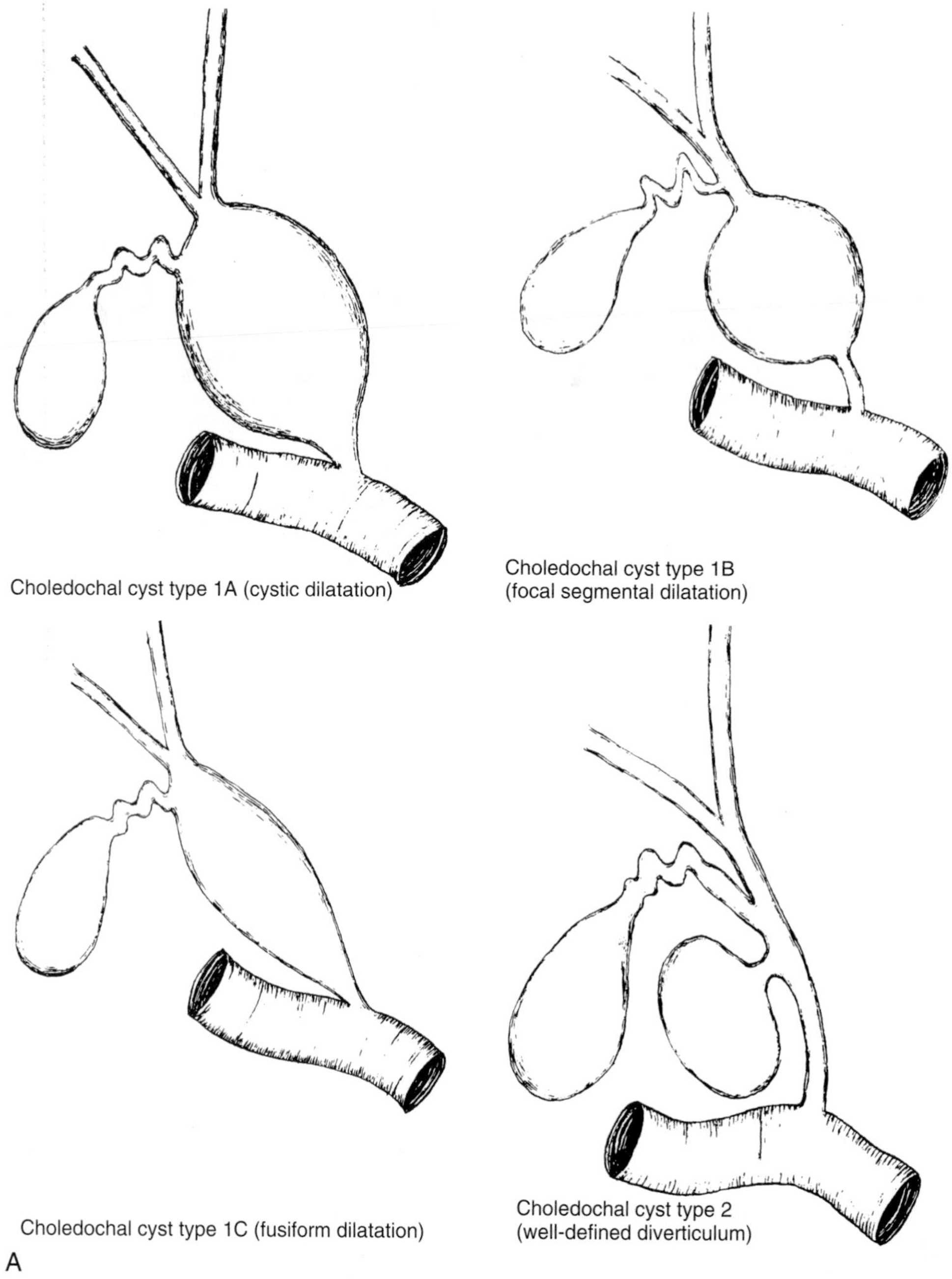

Figure 6-26 Classification of choledochal cysts.

In recent years, two categories have been added. Type 4A consists of multiple intrahepatic and extrahepatic segmental cystic dilatations (Fig. 6-29), and type 4B, an extremely uncommon type, is limited to extrahepatic segmental cystic dilatations. Type 5, which is a pattern of multiple intrahepatic cystic dilatations with sparing of the extrahepatic system (also known as Caroli's disease), is discussed separately.

Every medical student is familiar with the clinical triad of right upper quadrant pain, mass, and jaundice, which is said to represent the classic findings of choledochal cysts. As is frequently the case, the classic findings occur in only a few patients (22% to 40%). Right upper quadrant pain or discomfort is the most common symptom and is frequently attributed to the gallbladder, misdirecting the initial workup. Other clinical presentations include cholangitis and pancreatitis. Gallstones are found in a higher number of patients than expected who present as adults, and acute cholecystitis or gallstone-related pancreatitis occasionally can be the

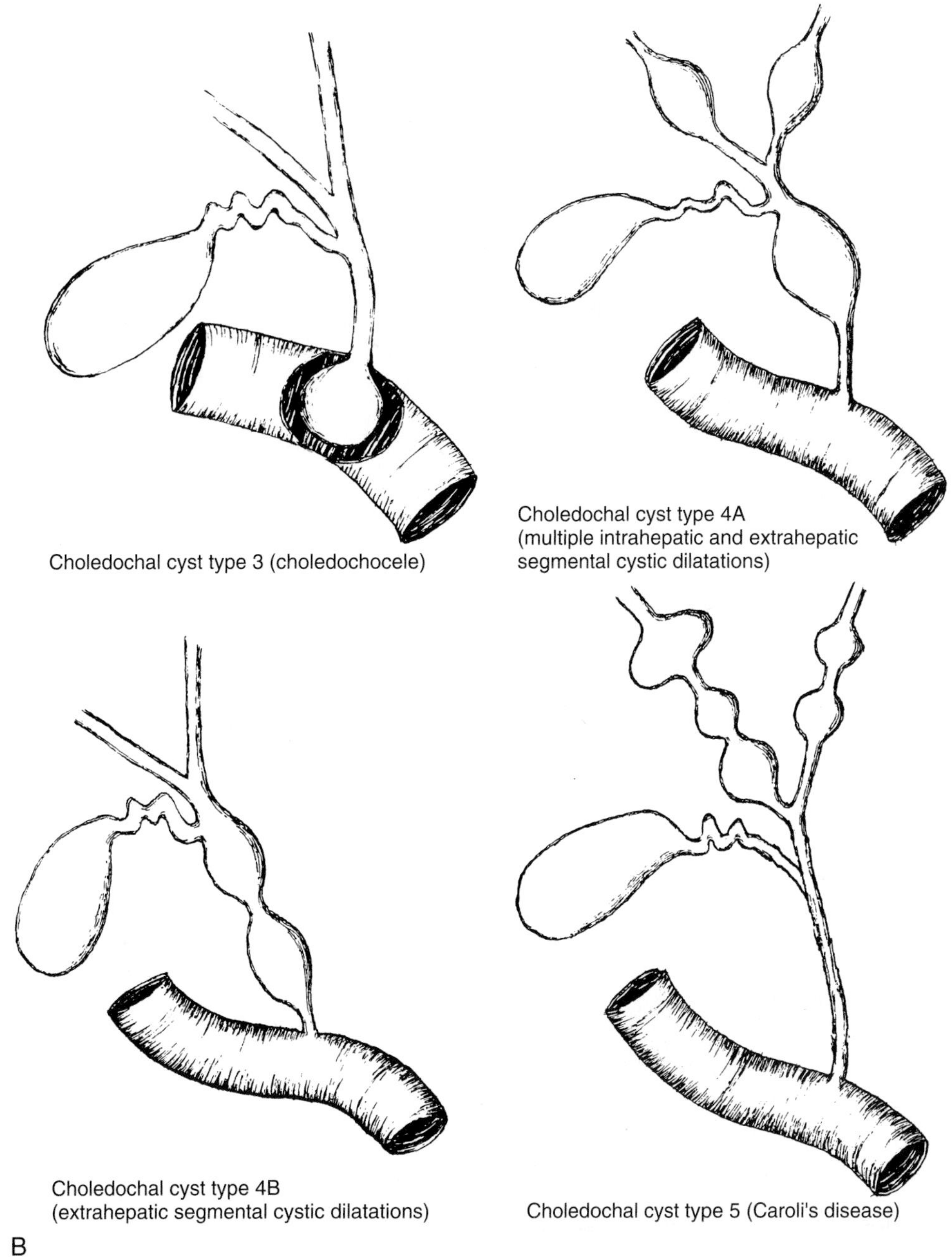

Figure 6-26 Cont'd

presenting problem. In many instances, the correct diagnosis is not made preoperatively.

Imaging methods of choice include ERCP and PTC, which permit the morphology of the ductal systems to be seen in detail. Ultrasonography, CT, and radionuclide scans also may be helpful, but in many cases it is impossible to rule out an obstructing process as the cause of ductal dilatation.

Caroli's Disease

Caroli's disease, also designated as type 5 choledochal cystic disease, is a condition usually limited to the intrahepatic ductal system and manifested as segmental saccular dilatations within a nonobstructed system. For some unknown reason, portions of the ductal system are spared in some patients. The process results in stasis and all the attendant complications associated with biliary stasis,

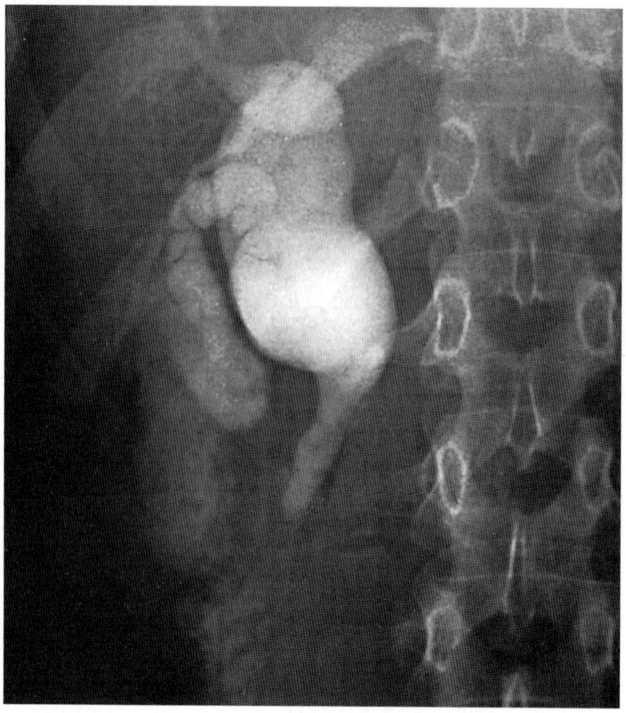

Figure 6-27 Choledochal cyst. Cholangiogram shows focal dilatation involving part of the common bile duct and common hepatic duct.

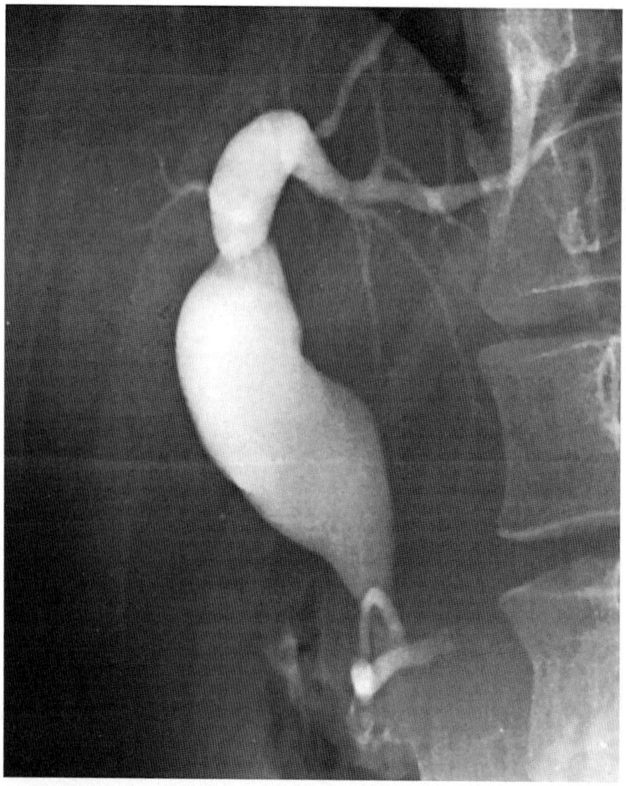

Figure 6-28 Choledochal cyst. Retrograde cholangiogram shows fusiform dilatation of the entire common bile duct.

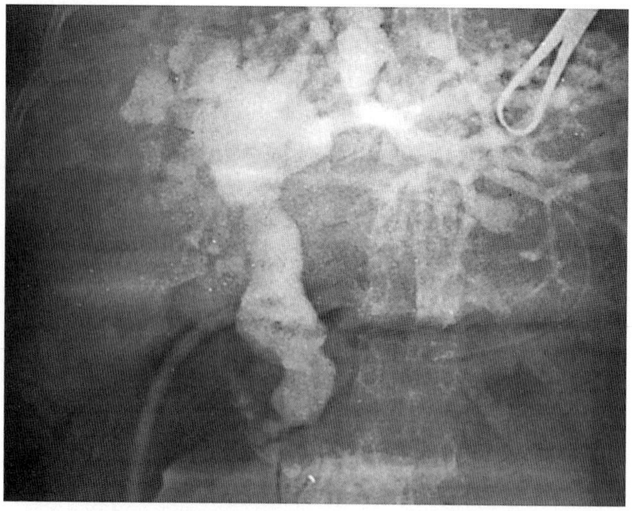

Figure 6-29 T tube cholangiogram shows multiple biliary cystic changes throughout the extrahepatic and intrahepatic system, consistent with Caroli's disease.

including infection and stone formation. These complications usually cause patients to seek medical attention. Liver function and portal blood flow are generally well preserved.

The disease is rare and probably is seen with considerably more frequency in written and oral board examinations than in actual practice. The course of the process is linked to the predisposition to develop bacterial cholangitis and a definite increased risk for cholangiocarcinoma. These patients have an approximately 100-fold increased risk for the development of this cancer.

Some controversy exists as to the cause of Caroli's disease. Some authorities believe that it is only one manifestation of a more generalized disease process that includes renal tubular ectasia (medullary sponge kidney), congenital hepatic fibrosis, and intrabiliary sacculations. Renal tubular ectasia and renal cystic disease are seen in almost 80% of reported cases. There is also an increased incidence of pancreatic cyst formation.

Ultrasonography and CT show multiple intrahepatic cysts (Figs. 6-30 and 6-31), but differentiation from polycystic disease may not be possible without luminal contrast studies, such as ERCP or PTC. These studies clearly show the ductal origin of the cystic structures and provide a better opportunity to evaluate potential complications.

Papillary Stenosis

Periampullary fibrosis or papillary stenosis can occur as a result of chronic inflammatory changes in the ampullary region. The difficult passage of a gallstone may account for some of the stenotic changes observed. It also may be possible that some of the stenosis could be iatrogenic as a result of previous failed sphincterotomies or repeated cannulations; this is one of the more common causes of mild diffuse dilatation of the bile

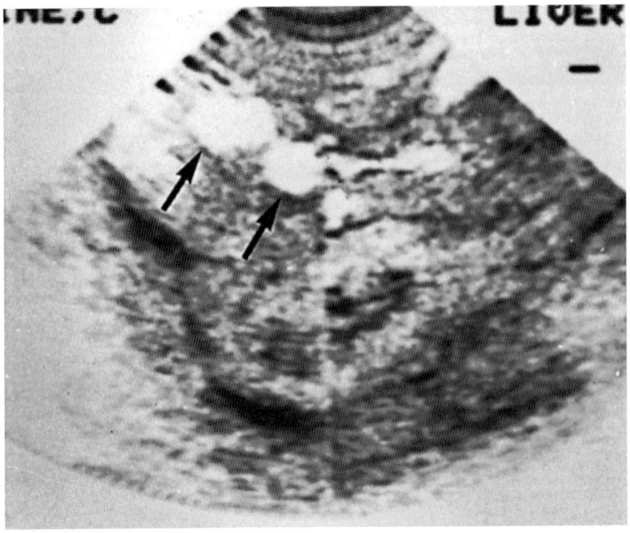

Figure 6-30 Ultrasound examination of the liver in a patient with Caroli's disease shows multiple cysts *(arrows)*.

ducts without any other underlying cause apparent. Often these patients have mild abnormalities in liver function tests, but the degree of jaundice is typically minimal. The diagnosis is made at ERCP and is one of exclusion, although some clinicians measure intraductal pressures. Treatment also can be done by the endoscopist, and sphincterotomy is usually all that is necessary for treatment.

Cholangitis

Recurrent bacterial cholangitis can result in changes in the intrahepatic ductal system that can produce dilatation in its initial stages. Numerous sacculations and strictures are the usual pattern in chronic disease, and the changes begin to resemble sclerosing cholangitis (Fig. 6-32).

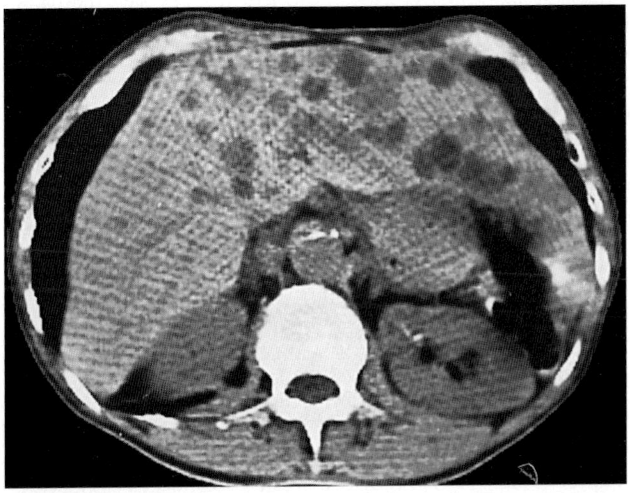

Figure 6-31 CT in a patient with Caroli's disease shows multiple cystic changes that are seen more prominently in the left lobe of the liver. Although most of the cysts seem discrete, some give the appearance of being part of the branching biliary system, suggesting this diagnostic possibility.

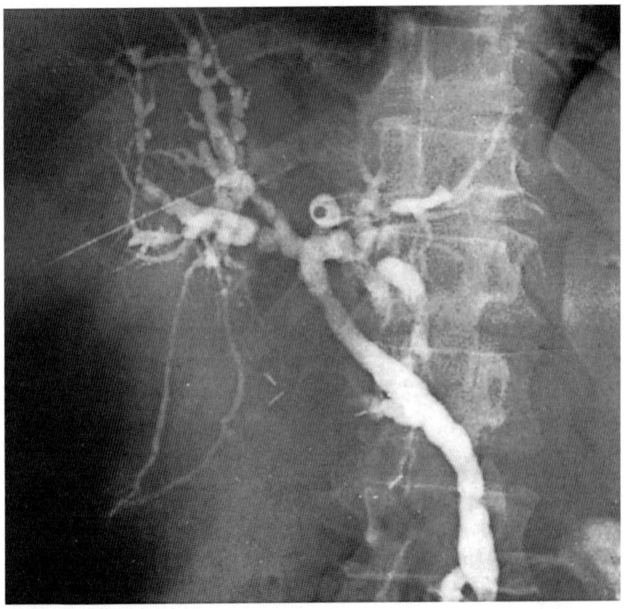

Figure 6-32 PTC in a patient with infectious cholangitis shows multiple strictures and sacculations of the intrahepatic system.

Chronic recurrent cholangitis is uncommon in North America and Europe. In the Far East, however, it is among the most common causes of abdominal emergencies leading to hospital admission. The extrahepatic ducts also can be involved. The most important causative factor is the antecedent presence of intrabiliary parasitic disease that results in an increased incidence of stone formation, obstruction, and subsequent infection.

Postcholecystectomy

It has been asserted that the common bile duct can become mildly dilated after cholecystectomy. The issue is controversial, and postsurgical common bile duct dilatation is not accepted by everyone. The literature reports the results of studies supporting both perspectives. Episodic right upper quadrant pain is seen in 5% to 40% of postcholecystectomy patients. In such symptomatic patients, there is an increased incidence of mild common bile duct dilatation.

Miscellaneous Conditions

Pneumobilia

The most common cause of pneumobilia is previous diverting surgery for biliary obstruction, such as choledochojejunostomy or choledochoduodenostomy (Box 6-6). In patients who have had previous sphincterotomies during ERCP, air may reflux from the duodenum into the biliary system. Any condition that undermines the competence of the sphincter of Oddi, whether it be traumatic, inflammatory, neoplastic, or iatrogenic, can result in air in the biliary system. On plain abdominal films, the

Box 6-6 Causes of Air in the Biliary System

Prior surgery or sphincterotomy
Fistula, biliary-enteric
- Ulcer
- Gallstone erosion
- Crohn's disease
- Carcinoma

Emphysematous cholecystitis/cholangitis

air is seen as linear branching lucencies (Fig. 6-33), and during UGI studies barium also may be seen within the biliary system. The air collections within the biliary system are generally centralized as a result of the centripetal flow of bile (Fig. 6-34). This observation helps distinguish air in the biliary system from air in the portal venous system, which is carried peripherally.

One cause of air in the biliary system is biliary-enteric fistula. This condition is discussed in more depth in the gallbladder section because the fistulous connection is almost always between the gallbladder and the adjacent bowel. Most cases involve the duodenum, although fistulous connection from the gallbladder to the colon can occur (Fig. 6-35). Even less common is a fistulous connection to the stomach. These conditions most commonly result from chronic cholecystic inflammation combined with erosion of a stone through the gallbladder wall and communication with the adjacent bowel lumen. In about half of cases, a permanently open fistulous tract remains, and air can be seen within the biliary tree. The next most common cause is peptic ulcer disease, usually from the duodenal bulb. The common bile duct is in close apposition to the proximal duodenum, and ulcers in that location may perforate into the duct. Other unusual causes of biliary fistula include Crohn's disease and neoplasms and rarely biliary-pancreatic fistula (Fig. 6-36).

In most inflammatory conditions of the duodenum, even the more severe peptic processes, the biliary system is unaffected. Reflux of air into the biliary tree has been seen rarely, however, in patients with severe involvement of the duodenum with Crohn's disease. Whether this reflux is due to distortion, deformity, and subsequent incompetence of the sphincter of Oddi or is a result of fistulous connections between the duodenum and common

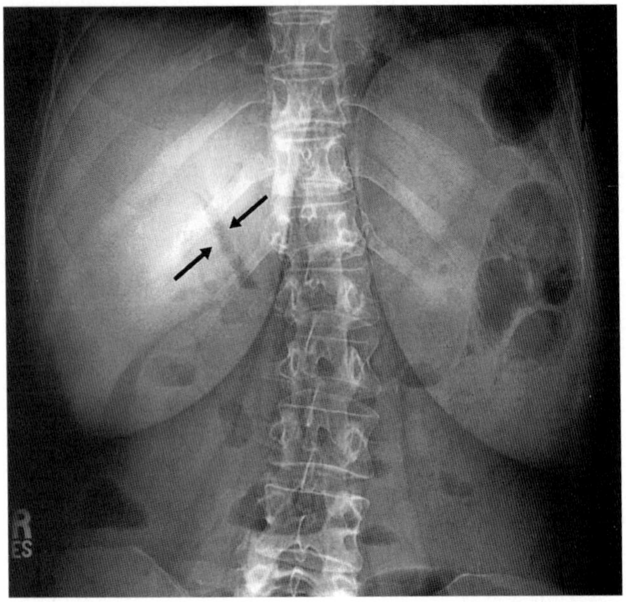

Figure 6-33 Plain film of abdomen shows air in branching structures of the biliary tree *(arrows)*.

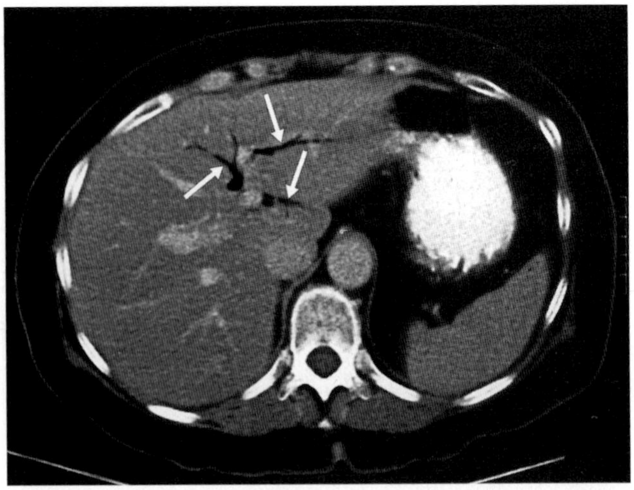

Figure 6-34 CT shows air in the central biliary system *(arrows)*.

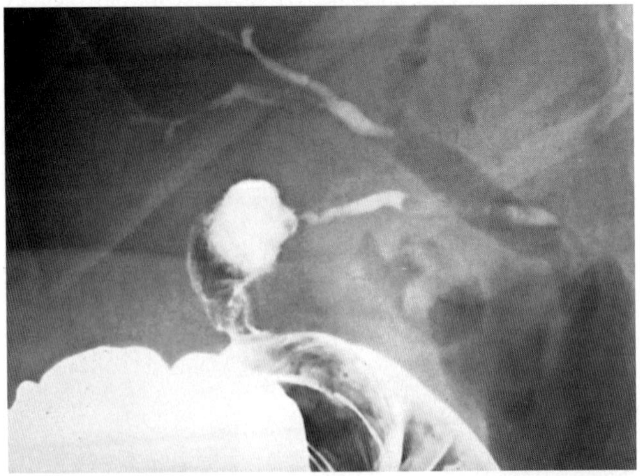

Figure 6-35 Film from a barium enema shows barium filling a small, tubular structure adjacent to the colon and just superior to the hepatic flexure that proved to be a small, contracted gallbladder continuous with the colon as a result of a fistulous connection.

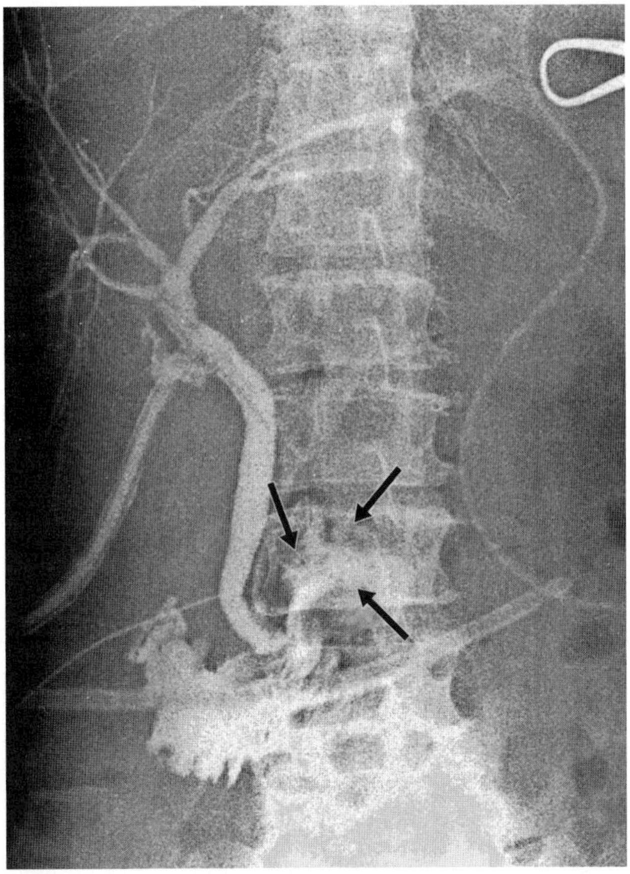

Figure 6-36 Intraoperative cholangiogram shows contrast material in the head of the pancreas *(arrows)*.

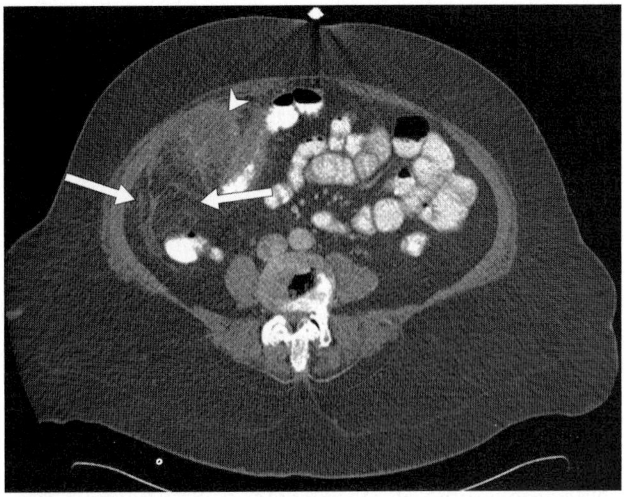

Figure 6-37 This is a computed tomographic section through the lower portion of the gallbladder in a patient with severe inflammation and gangrene of the gallbladder *(arrowhead)* wall and a pericholecystic stranding *(arrows)*.

bile duct is unclear. Occasionally, a periampullary neoplastic process sufficiently affects the sphincter of Oddi to induce incompetence and reflux of air.

Rarely, biliary air may be seen in asymptomatic patients with no evidence of current disease or history of previous disease or surgery. This finding may be related to anomalous pancreaticobiliary duct relationships.

Bile Peritonitis and Biloma

Leakage of bile from either the gallbladder or the biliary ductal system can result from several conditions. Focal bile leakage after biliary surgery or after PTC is common, although serious consequences associated with these leaks are much less common. Abdominal trauma, particularly penetrating trauma, is another important cause of bile leakage. Serious free spillage of bile into the peritoneal cavity can result in bile peritonitis with the clinical picture of an acute surgical abdomen. If the bile leakage is sequestered and loculated, usually in the right upper quadrant of the abdomen, a biloma develops. Bilomas that mature for a few weeks usually are round and have a thin capsule. Patients present with abdominal tenderness and a mass in the right upper quadrant in most cases. The biloma can occur in the midabdomen or left upper quadrant, however, in about one third of the cases. If the biloma ruptures, the clinical presentation is more dramatic, similar to that of frank bile peritonitis. Additionally, a biloma can decompress itself by eroding into an adjacent hollow viscus and possibly setting up a fistulous connection between the bowel and biliary system.

Gallbladder perforation is also a known complication of acute cholecystitis in approximately 10% of cases (Fig. 6-37). The spillage of infected bile (which is almost always the case in this complication of acute cholecystitis) into the peritoneal cavity results in a fulminating peritonitis that requires immediate surgical intervention. Approximately half of patients with acute cholecystitis and perforation of the gallbladder form a biloma that usually becomes infected as well. This condition may manifest several days to weeks after the perforation as a pericholecystic abscess.

GALLBLADDER

Examination Techniques

Oral Cholecystogram

In February 1924, a method for opacifying the gallbladder was reported by Graham and Cole in the *Journal of the American Medical Association*. The original contrast agent used was the sodium salt of tetrabromophenolphthalein. In the ensuing decades, more efficient and safer cholecystographic agents were developed. Iopanoic acid (Telepaque), a triiodobenzene ring compound, was introduced in the 1950s and along with variations has been the standard oral cholecystographic agent.

Having been displaced by the ultrasound scan, the OCG is now viewed as a secondary imaging study of the gallbladder. It is reserved for some patients for whom chemical dissolution or lithotripsy is being considered. As these therapeutic techniques are becoming less common, the OCG is becoming an even more obscure imaging examination. Because the OCG is the only imaging modality that is an actual reflection of hepatocellular physiology, however, it is a worthwhile exercise for the training radiologist to have a basic understanding of the examination and the significance of its results.

Being mostly lipid soluble, orally administered iopanoic acid is readily absorbed from the gut into the portal bloodstream, where it is bound to serum albumin and transported to the liver. In the hepatocyte, the bound cholecystographic agent undergoes conjugation in a manner similar to bilirubin. It is excreted into the biliary ductal system, where it ultimately collects in the gallbladder. In a fasting, fat-restricted patient, gallbladder contractility is diminished, and the contrast agent remains within the gallbladder, where concentration can occur as a result of water absorption. In most patients, the gallbladder is sufficiently opacified for imaging 18 to 24 hours after the ingestion of the contrast agent (Fig. 6-38).

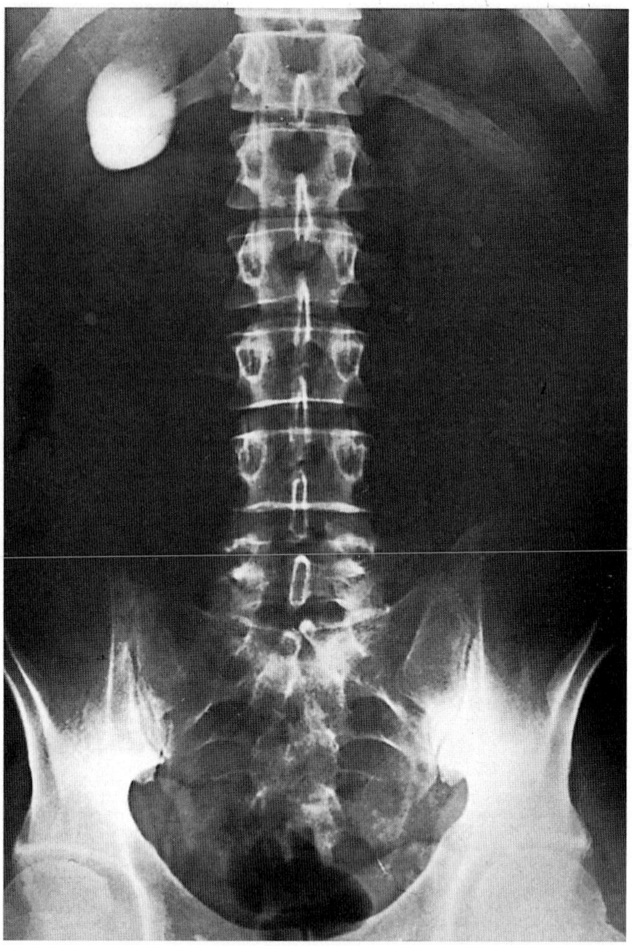

Figure 6-38 Normal opacification of the gallbladder is seen after the ingestion of oral cholecystographic contrast material.

Not all of the ingested contrast agent is absorbed. Some passes through the small bowel into the colon and appears as dense flecks of contrast sprinkled throughout the lower bowel. Not all conjugated contrast material is retained in the gallbladder. In the bowel, the conjugated excreted contrast agent is seen as a homogeneous, hazy, luminal opacity. It also has been estimated that a sizable amount (one third) of conjugated agent is excreted through the kidneys. As a result, renal toxicity is a known but rare complication of oral cholecystography.

For years, the usual dosage has consisted of 3 g (six tablets) of the oral contrast agent. Approximately 30% of patients have faint or no opacification of the gallbladder after this dosage. Two thirds of these patients have gallbladder visualization after the administration of a second 3-g dose. This two-dose schedule is incorrectly referred to as a double-dose examination in many radiology departments and occasionally results in a patient's receiving 6 g (12 tablets) of oral contrast agent at the same time. This dosage may reduce the chances of opacification because of the significant diarrhea it often causes. The correct application of this regimen, which is now routinely used by many institutions, is to administer 6 g of the contrast agent to the patient divided into 3-g doses over a 2-day period. A fat-restrictive diet is maintained.

In a diseased or obstructed gallbladder, little or no opacification occurs. In a diseased nonobstructed gallbladder, the reason for nonopacification may relate to the inability of the sick gallbladder to concentrate the bile and the contrast agent. Inflammatory changes involving the wall of the gallbladder, in particular the mucosal surface, resulting in edema and hyperemia, may impair the integrity of the gallbladder mucosa. This impairment increases its permeability to the contrast agent, and some of the contrast agent may escape the gallbladder via absorption through the mucosal surface with vicarious excretion through the kidneys.

Although the failure to opacify the gallbladder after a repeat-dose examination is presumptive evidence of gallbladder disease, there may be other causes of nonopacification not directly related to gallbladder pathology, and these causes must be excluded (Box 6-7). Some causes include the following:

- *Problems with patient compliance.* Most commonly, the problem of patient compliance is a result of the patient's failure to understand the instructions for the ingestion of the tablets and dietary restrictions. These problems are best avoided by a careful explanation to the patient accompanied by a simple set of written instructions and the phone number of a person within the department who may be reached if the patient has questions or concerns.

Box 6-7 Causes of Nonvisualization of the Gallbladder During Oral Cholecystogram

Patient noncompliance
Failure to absorb contrast material
Liver dysfunction
Gallbladder disease
Normal (<10%)

- *Failure to reach the absorbing surface.* Unless the contrast material reaches the absorbing surfaces of the small bowel in adequate amounts, insufficient absorption occurs, and poor opacification is the result. This situation can occur for many reasons. Diverticula anywhere in the gut proximal to these absorbing surfaces can sequester contrast material, greatly diminishing flow distally. These diverticula can be located in the esophagus, the gastric fundus, the duodenum, or the jejunum. Patients with or without diverticula who are sick, immobile, and limited to the supine position also may sequester the contrast material in the fundus of the stomach. Gastric outlet obstruction, of any cause, whether inflammatory or neoplastic, can result in lack of presentation of the contrast material to the small bowel. A patient with constant vomiting may lose much of the contrast material before it reaches the small bowel. Patients with gastric atony or gastrocolic fistulas also can be expected to present some difficulty in achieving opacification of the gallbladder.
- *Absorbing surface abnormalities.* Absorbing surface abnormalities are a relatively uncommon cause of nonopacification, even among patients with known inflammatory bowel disease and malabsorption syndromes that affect the absorbing surface of the small bowel. Occasionally, a patient with Crohn's disease or extensive small bowel resection who has a normal gallbladder can show nonopacification at OCG because of inadequate absorption. Patients with severe acute pancreatitis and accompanying malabsorption may fall into the same category.
- *Hepatocellular abnormalities.* Because the contrast agent must undergo conjugation within the hepatocyte before being excreted into the biliary system, the presence of normal hepatic function is necessary for the OCG. Patients with elevated bilirubin levels (>2 mg/dL), whether from primary hepatocellular disease or from biliary ductal obstructing processes, are not candidates for the OCG. Diminished opacification or nonopacification occurs in these patients not only because of the impairment of the intrahepatic capacity to transport the contrast agent, but also because the contrast agent molecule competes with bilirubin for the hepatobiliary-excretion mechanisms.

The use of the OCG declined dramatically during the 1980s with the widespread use of ultrasonography in the evaluation of the gallbladder. As previously mentioned, in recent years use of the OCG increased modestly for a period concomitant with the use of biliary lithotripsy to evaluate for stone size, number, and calcification.

Despite the decrease in the number of OCGs being performed in the United States, this is a simple, safe, inexpensive, and accurate method for examining the gallbladder. Its sensitivity in detecting gallstones approaches that of ultrasonography, whereas the cost of an ultrasound scan ranges from $1\frac{1}{2}$ to 2 times that of an OCG. The sensitivity for detection of gallstones with the OCG is said to be around 94% compared with 98% for ultrasound scan.

A significant limitation of the OCG is that diagnostic information is limited to the gallbladder. In a patient with a clinical history and symptoms that are most consistent with gallstone disease, an OCG, under certain circumstances, still may be considered a reasonable inexpensive first step in the evaluation of the patient. Filming procedure for the OCG includes upright, oblique, and compression views of the gallbladder.

Ultrasonography

Ultrasonography has the advantage of being noninvasive and not using ionizing radiation. It is highly accurate in detecting gallstones. It can provide additional valuable information regarding gallbladder wall thickness and pericholecystic abnormalities and an evaluation of the liver and pancreas (Fig. 6-39).

With the widespread use of real-time ultrasonography, this method of imaging has become the primary

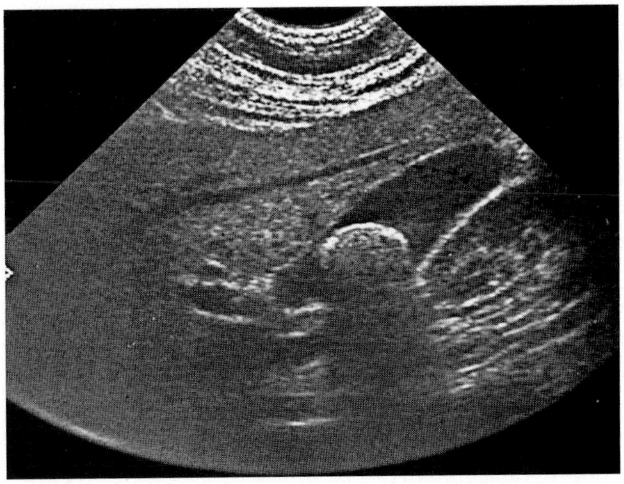

Figure 6-39 Ultrasound examination of patient shows a large, solitary gallstone casting a prominent acoustic shadow.

diagnostic modality for gallbladder and biliary pathology. When the OCG is contraindicated, an ultrasound scan is an effective alternative; this applies in jaundiced patients with abnormal bilirubin levels and in patients with known allergies to iodinated contrast material. Any patient with known structural abnormalities, such as high small bowel obstruction or gastric outlet obstruction, predictably would have an unsuccessful OCG examination. In these instances, ultrasonography always should be considered the first choice. In any instance in which the OCG is not conclusive or there is nonopacification of the gallbladder, ultrasonography is indicated.

Radioisotope Studies

Direct radionuclide imaging of the biliary system and gallbladder may be obtained using technetium-99m-labeled derivatives of IDA (HIDA, DISIDA, mebrofenin), which are excreted directly into the biliary tract and can show patency with a high degree of sensitivity. The most obvious use of radionuclide imaging is in the evaluation of cystic duct patency in patients with signs and symptoms of acute cholecystitis.

After the administration of the radionuclide, concentration can be detected in the liver within 5 to 10 minutes. Usually by 40 to 60 minutes, the biliary system, including the gallbladder, common bile duct, and possibly the cystic duct, may be seen, with some activity already present within the adjacent small bowel loops. Cholecystokinin or an analogue may be given before the examination to contract and empty the gallbladder and possibly promote filling during the study. This maneuver should be considered in patients in whom normal dietary stimulation of the gallbladder is ineffective.

In some instances, the efficiency of gallbladder contraction and emptying can be determined using the same agent by measuring uptake over the gallbladder before and after intravenous injection of cholecystokinin. It is assumed that some patients who have no evidence of stones or inflammation but have symptoms similar to those seen in gallstone disease have biliary dyskinesia, which can have identical symptoms. This diagnosis is controversial.

Nonvisualization of the gallbladder after 1 hour usually indicates cystic duct obstruction. Delayed gallbladder visualization beyond 1 hour after the common bile duct and the adjacent bowel already have been identified does not rule out the possibility of acute cholecystitis, although such a finding would be unusual. More commonly, delayed visualization of the gallbladder is associated with chronic cholecystitis. Generally, the longer the delay, the greater the likelihood of chronic cholecystitis.

Computed Tomography and Magnetic Resonance Imaging

CT cannot be considered a primary examination technique for simple gallbladder evaluation at this time. If gallstones are calcified, they may be detected on CT depending on the location of the stones and the thickness of the slices. Most stones, being composed of cholesterol, tend to blend into the bile environment within the gallbladder and often are not seen. Pericholecystic fluid or masses can be well shown on CT, however. MRI has not played a significant role to date in the evaluation of gallbladder disease.

Dilated Gallbladder

Physiological Causes

Patients undergoing prolonged fasting or starvation accumulate increased amounts of bile within the gallbladder, with resultant distention of the organ. These individuals also have an increased risk of stone formation. A similar picture is encountered in patients receiving prolonged hyperalimentation. After bone marrow transplantation, patients commonly show some distention of the gallbladder on ultrasound scan and computed tomographic scan of the abdomen. Often this distention is accompanied by sludge or stone formation. The exact cause of these findings is unclear.

Courvoisier's Gallbladder

Progressive, painless enlargement of the gallbladder with late development of jaundice has long been recognized as a high-probability sign for pancreatic cancer with secondary involvement and narrowing of the distal common bile duct (Fig. 6-40). Other lesions, such as carcinoma of the ampulla of Vater or the peripapillary duodenum, can result in a similar clinical presentation. Additionally, benign processes, such as villous adenomas or carcinoids involving the region of the papilla, have

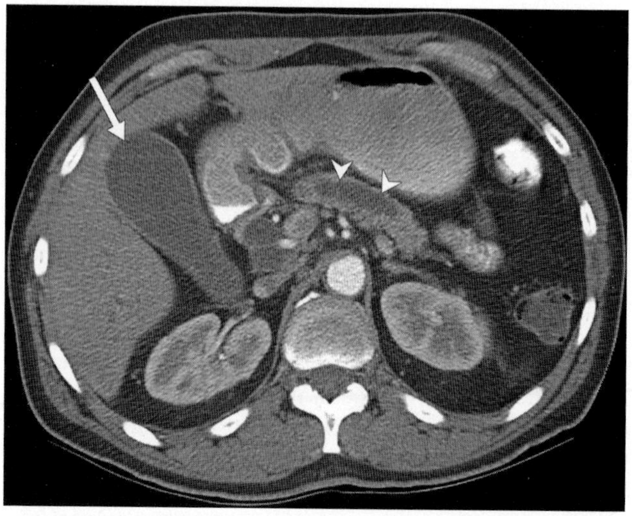

Figure 6-40 CT in a patient with known carcinoma of the pancreas and passive dilatation of the biliary system and gallbladder *(arrow)*. Note dilatation of the pancreatic duct *(arrowheads)*.

been noted to result in Courvoisier's sign. The general clinical significance of Courvoisier's gallbladder is that a palpable, nontender gallbladder in a jaundiced patient is more likely to be related to a neoplastic process than to an inflammatory process or a stone. Progressive, slow obstruction of a normal gallbladder results in a considerable amount of painless distention. Conversely, distention in chronic disease is less likely, even with significant obstruction, because of gallbladder wall thickening and fibrosis. Distention secondary to stones is commonly intermittent, incomplete, and painful. Inexplicably, some patients with complete cystic duct obstruction who do not present in the acute stage go on to manifest one of several conditions associated with chronic aseptic cystic duct obstruction. These conditions include porcelain gallbladder, milk of calcium bile, cholesterol impregnation of the gallbladder wall and mucosal surface (strawberry gallbladder), and hydrops of the gallbladder.

Hydrops

In most instances, patients with gallstone obstruction of the gallbladder neck or cystic duct present with acute cholecystitis. These patients frequently have a distended, painful gallbladder. The treatment of acute cholecystitis varies, depending on the condition of the patient and operative risks. Most commonly, early surgery is favored. In a few individuals who have chronic obstruction of the cystic duct, the gallbladder can become distended and surprisingly large, containing a clear or mucoid, milky aseptic bile. This is the condition known as hydrops of the gallbladder. Some patients have little or no history of gallbladder disease, and the finding can be incidental. Most patients have degrees of right upper quadrant discomfort and possibly biliary colic, however. These patients are almost never jaundiced, unless some intervening process results in common bile duct obstruction. Complications of hydrops of the gallbladder include gallbladder empyema (when the gallbladder content becomes infected), perforation, or, rarely, infarction. Although radionuclide imaging is the examination of choice in suspected acute cholecystitis, ultrasonography has been found to be a superior method of evaluation in the chronic situation, with remarkably easy and quick identification of the dilated, distended gallbladder. If the obstructing stone can be shown in the gallbladder neck or cystic duct, the diagnosis is complete.

Neuromuscular Abnormalities

Gallbladder atony and enlargement are common among patients with diabetes mellitus, occurring in half of patients with insulin-dependent diabetes. The incidence may be higher in patients with peripheral vascular disease or diabetic neuropathy. Additionally, patients with diabetes have a decreased ability to empty the gallbladder, with resultant increased bile stasis and increased risk of stone formation. The increased size of the gallbladder relates to contractile abnormalities of the muscular wall of the gallbladder secondary to neuromuscular changes associated with the disease.

Postvagotomy patients may have increased gallbladder size. An increased incidence of gallstone formation in these patients also has been observed. Truncal vagotomies are more frequently associated with increased gallbladder volume and selective vagotomies less so.

Small, Shrunken Gallbladder

Chronic Cholecystitis

The term *chronic cholecystitis* has meant different things to different clinicians in various specialties. In a few patients, obstruction of the cystic duct results in hydrops of the gallbladder with intermittent or persistent symptoms. These patients may be said to have chronic cholecystitis. More frequently, chronic cholecystitis refers to the presence of chronic inflammatory changes in the gallbladder wall with associated thickening of the wall. The gallbladder is small and often contracted and in 95% of the cases contains numerous stones. This pattern is probably the most commonly encountered form of gallbladder inflammation seen at surgery. These patients frequently have intermittent biliary colic resulting from intermittent cystic duct obstruction. Typically, the pain is severe, in the right upper abdomen, possibly radiating to the back or shoulder. The pain has a tendency to escalate shortly after the onset of symptoms and diminish slowly over the next few hours, as opposed to acute cholecystitis, in which the pain continues to increase and is prolonged beyond 5 or 6 hours.

The diagnosis of chronic cholecystitis may be suggested on computed tomographic or ultrasound studies in which a small, contracted gallbladder is shown with a thickened wall and gallstones (Fig. 6-41). Small amounts of pericholecystic fluid may be seen, although this is more common in acute cholecystitis. The diagnosis also can be suggested by biliary scintigraphy when the gallbladder is seen to fill in a delayed fashion either spontaneously or with pharmacological assistance, such as the administration of 2 mg of intravenous morphine sulfate to induce spasm of the sphincter of Oddi.

Cystic Fibrosis

Gallbladder changes are seen in approximately one third of patients with cystic fibrosis. A small, hypoplastic gallbladder is common in these patients. In addition, the bile is thicker than normal, and it is assumed that some impairment of bile flow is present, accounting for the increased incidence of gallstones. These changes are unusual in infancy and are usually seen during the teen years.

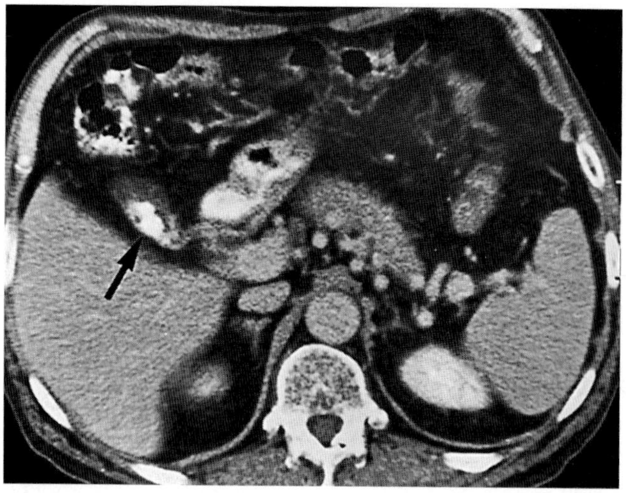

Figure 6-41 CT through the inferior aspect of the liver shows a small, contracted gallbladder containing several calcified stones *(arrow)*.

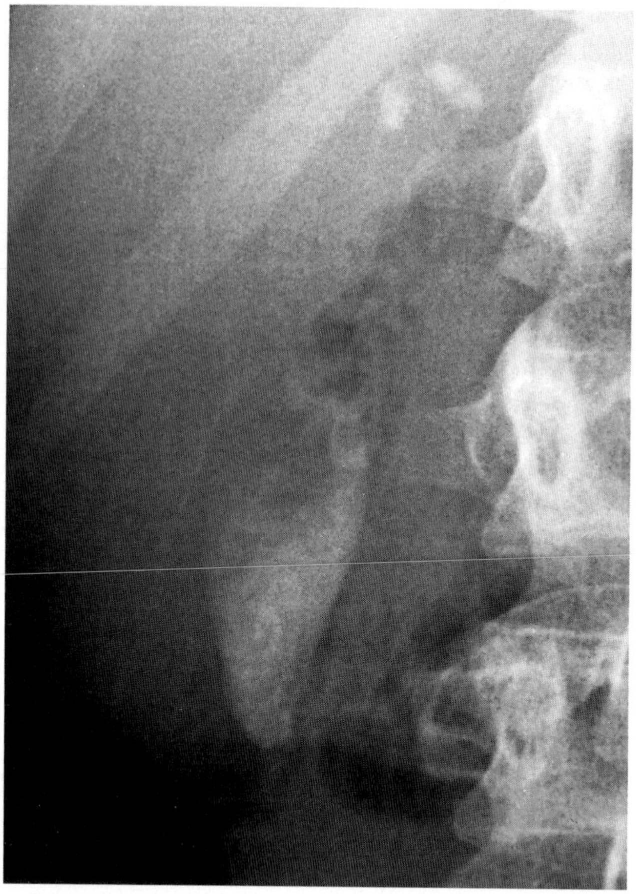

Figure 6-42 A small, poorly functioning gallbladder as seen in cholesterolosis is seen.

Hyperplastic Cholecystoses

The term *hyperplastic cholecystoses* refers to two conditions that lead to thickening of the gallbladder wall and, in advanced conditions, to diminished size or lack of distensibility of the gallbladder (Fig. 6-42). The two diseases are adenomyomatosis and cholesterolosis. These conditions are discussed in further detail in a later section. Both conditions limit the size and distensibility of the gallbladder when they begin to involve the gallbladder diffusely.

Filling Defects

Artifacts and Spurious Filling Defects

A significant problem encountered with the OCG was that of spurious lucencies projected over the gallbladder and mimicking gallstones. These are usually air bubbles in the adjacent hepatic flexure of the colon or the duodenal bulb. If multiple positional views are routinely obtained, this is usually not a serious problem. Routine compression views also diminish the potential of mistaking overlying air bubbles for gallstones. Occasionally, a tiny, persistent filling defect in the neck of the gallbladder can be seen, representing a slight invagination of the cystic duct into the neck of the gallbladder lumen.

Calcification in the anterior ribs, liver, right kidney, lymph nodes in the right upper quadrant, pancreatic head, and abdominal wall projecting over the gallbladder occasionally can be mistaken for calcified stones. Supine, upright, and compression views as a routine part of the examination should deal with the problem. In some instances, fluoroscopy may be required to sort out some of these calcifications.

Gallstones

It is estimated that approximately 20 million individuals in the United States have gallstones. Of these, an estimated 500,000 annually undergo cholecystectomy. The estimates of the prevalence of gallbladder disease depend to a large extent on the method by which information is gathered and the type of imaging techniques used. Many of the epidemiological studies have produced incidences based on interviews or questionnaires regarding a history of gallbladder surgery or reported findings of gallstones on previous imaging studies. The figures obtained are, at best, loose estimates of the prevalence of the disease. Realistically, we probably do not know with certainty what the incidence is and probably have underestimated it. We do know, however, that most removed gallstones (80%) are composed of cholesterol, whereas the remainder contain a variety of calcium salts. Approximately 15% of gallstones are sufficiently calcified to be seen on plain films of the abdomen (Fig. 6-43); this is increased with the use of CT (Fig. 6-44). Stones that are predominantly pigmented tend to occur in patients with hemolytic types of anemias, such as sickle cell disease. Cholesterol stone formation is more common in women than men, slightly more common in whites, and much more common in Native Americans. There is a relationship between obesity and the incidence of gallstone formation, particularly in young women.

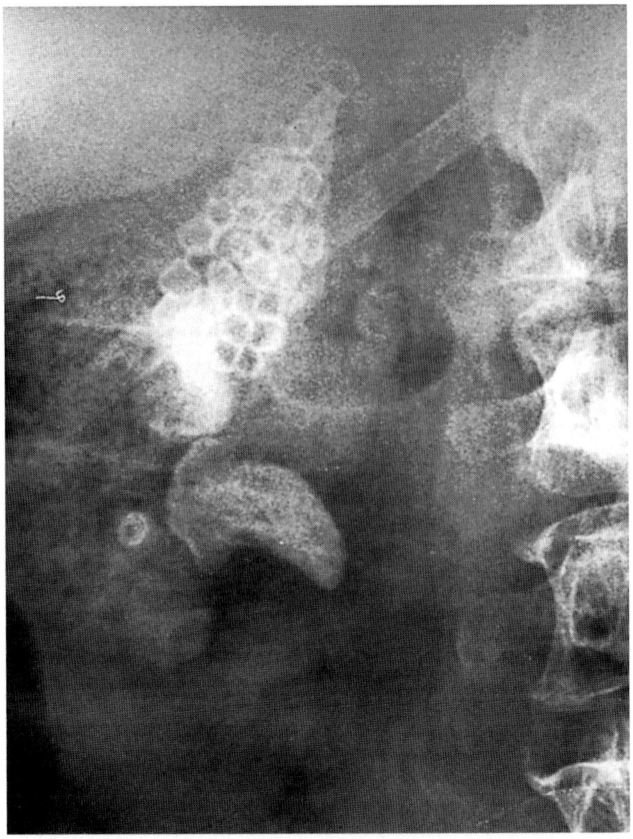

Figure 6-43 This is a right upper quadrant, coned-down view of supine abdomen in a patient with numerous faceted gallstones filling the entire gallbladder. Prominent renal calcifications can be seen adjacent to this.

Other causative factors include chronic liver disease, the use of certain types of antilipidemic agents, and hyperalimentation. In recent years, MRI has been used successfully to determine the composition based on the differences in signal intensity of the component materials that make up a gallstone.

Most gallbladder stones are never diagnosed. Many patients with stones are asymptomatic, whereas others

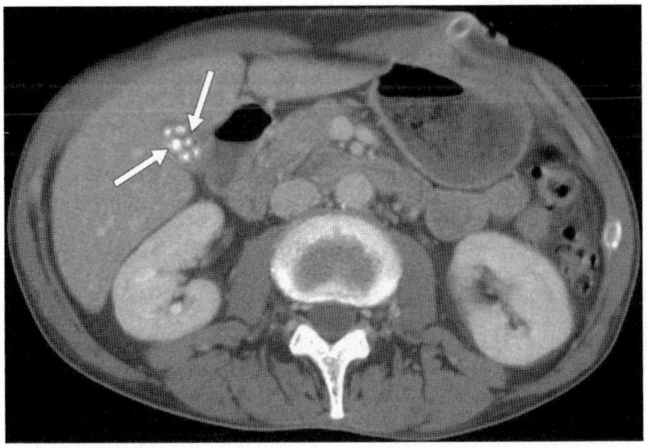

Figure 6-44 Gallstones are seen on CT *(arrows)*.

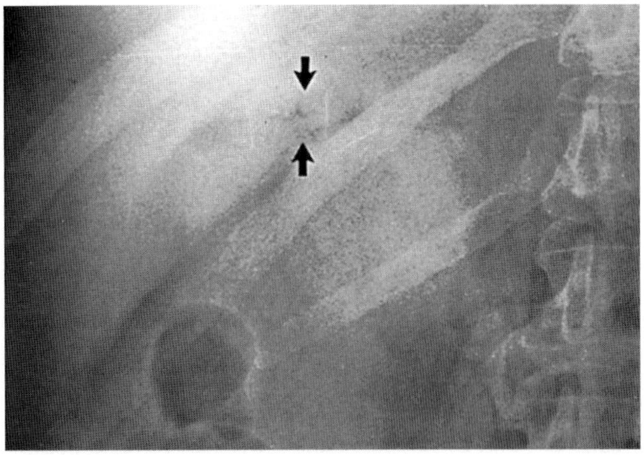

Figure 6-45 A coned-down view of the right upper quadrant shows a subtle stellate lucency *(arrows)*, representing gas within a large, fissured gallstone (Mercedes-Benz sign).

have vague nonspecific symptoms. Only a fraction of patients come to cholecystectomy. The heightened attention to alternative therapies for the treatment of cholelithiasis has brought about a renewed interest in the composition and the pathophysiological processes that lead to the formation of gallstones. Gallstone pharmacological dissolution and biliary lithotripsy or combinations of both therapies have been used in the treatment of gallstones over the past 2 decades.

As previously mentioned, 15% of gallstones can be diagnosed on the basis of plain films of the abdomen. Plain film diagnosis of cholesterol stones with fissured interiors containing gas is a rare occurrence and a curious phenomenon of gallstone formation (Fig. 6-45). When present, this phenomenon is usually manifested by cross-shaped or stellate thin lucencies in the right upper quadrant; this has been referred to as the "Mercedes-Benz sign" and is pathognomonic of gallstones (Fig. 6-46).

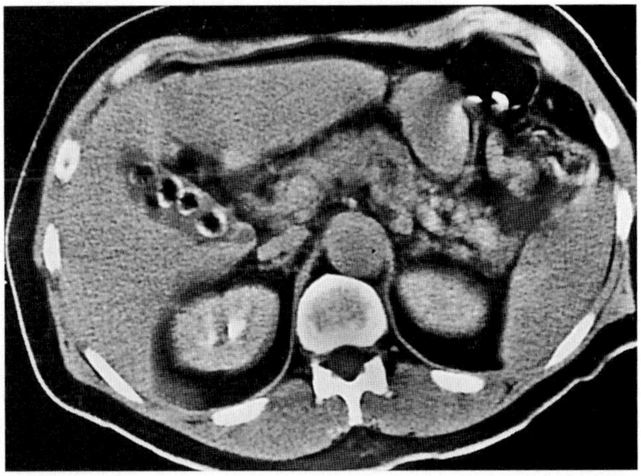

Figure 6-46 CT through the liver shows numerous gallstones, calcified in their rim with internal fissures and gas collections, resulting in the Mercedes-Benz sign seen on plain film.

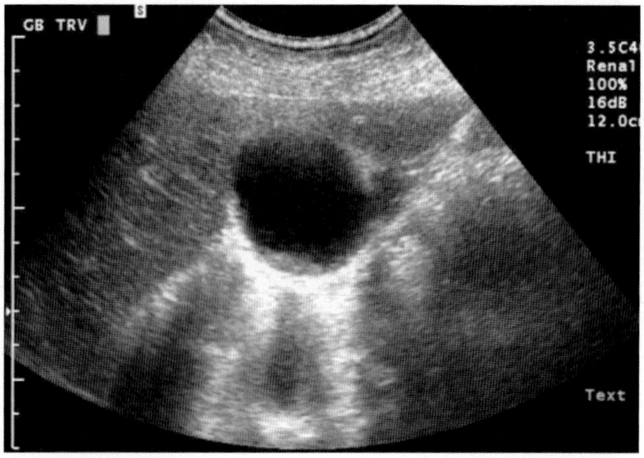

Figure 6-47 Small gallstones and sludge throw a prominent acoustic shadow on this ultrasonogram.

The principal method of imaging gallstones is ultrasonography (Fig. 6-47). The sensitivity for the detection of stones is quite high. Although the OCG is used infrequently today, it has some advantages and some limitations. The OCG requires some patient preparation and the use of ionizing radiation. It shows not only gallbladder morphology, but also gallbladder and liver function. Ultrasonography does not show function, but is highly sensitive in the detection of stones and can give additional information regarding the surrounding organs. Little or no patient preparation is necessary for ultrasound examination.

On the OCG, with opacification of the gallbladder, noncalcified stones show as filling defects of varying number and size (Fig. 6-48). A single stone may be present, or the gallbladder may be distended with numerous stones. Stones may be sandlike, rounded, or faceted. On ultrasound examination, the presence of acoustic shadowing in the dependent portion of the gallbladder is typical of gallstones. The composition of the gallstone does not seem to be a factor in the degree of acoustic shadowing present. Occasionally, gallstones float, particularly pure cholesterol gallstones. The layering out process can be observed in ultrasound scans and OCGs. A striking finding on the OCG occurs when multiple small stones layer out and form a radiolucent band across the gallbladder lumen (Fig. 6-49).

New approaches to gallstone therapy have led to a mild resurgence in use of the OCG. Methods for chemical stone dissolution and biliary lithotripsy have been major topics for discussion in the medical literature and in the lay media. Initially, oral bile salts were used in an attempt to dissolve gallstones. Success was limited and not always reproducible, and recurrence was common. Newer, direct-dissolving agents have been developed, the most noteworthy of which is methyl *tert*-butyl ether (MTBE). Dissolution of gallstones using MTBE requires the direct application of the chemical to the gallstones,

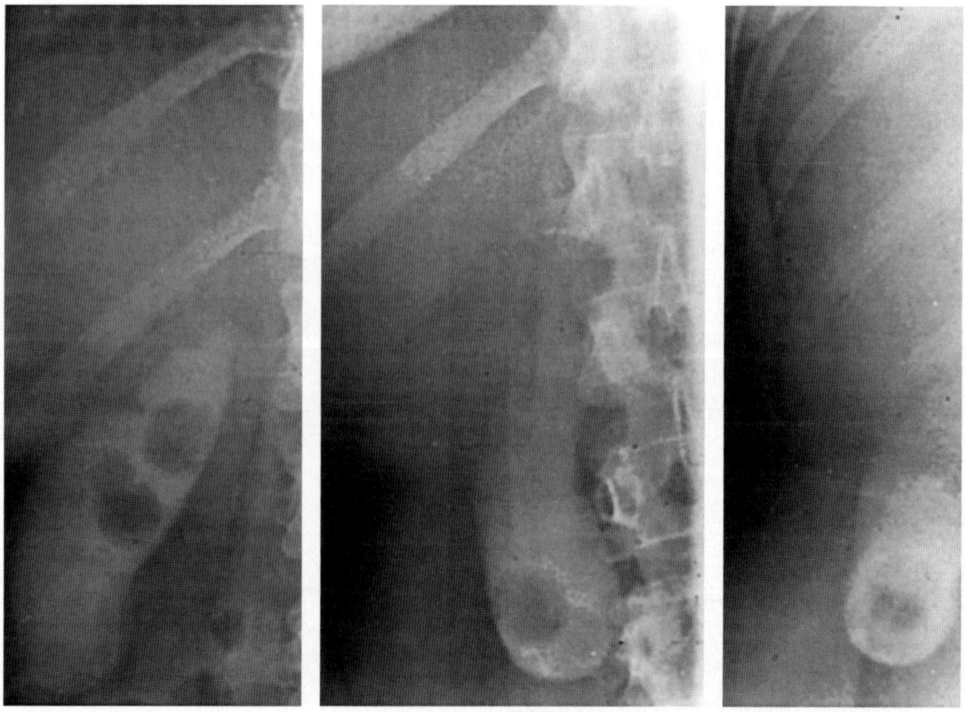

Figure 6-48 Gallstones. OCG shows good opacification of the gallbladder that has at least two rounded mobile lucencies within it.

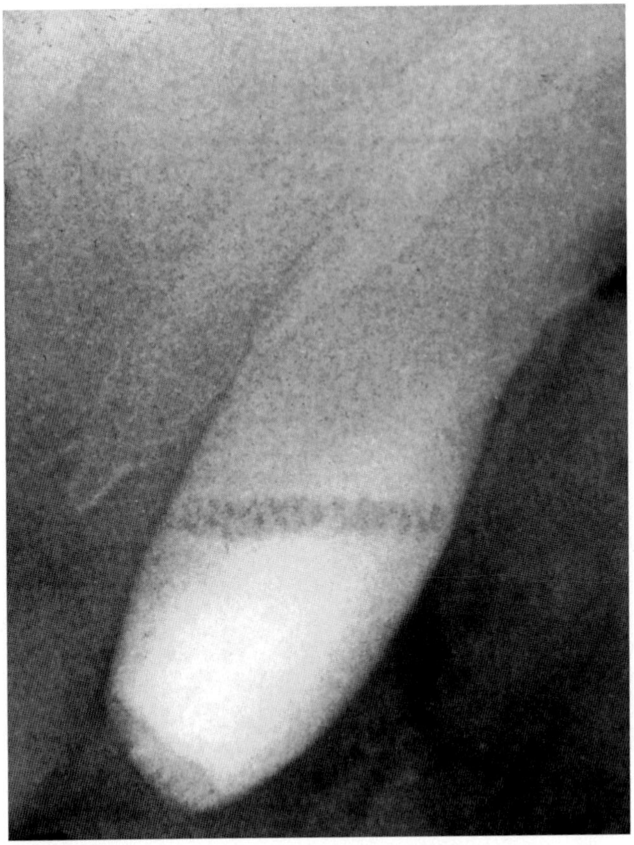

Figure 6-49 OCG in a patient in the upright position shows numerous tiny cholesterol stones layering out, forming a linear radiolucent band across the lumen of the gallbladder.

which requires a percutaneous transhepatic route or endoscopic cannulation of the cystic duct. Infusion and aspiration of MTBE follow, resulting in complete dissolution of the stones in 30% to 60% of patients. Stone recurrence is a problem after MTBE treatment, more so in patients with multiple stones.

Length of hospital stay is often greater for MTBE treatment than for laparoscopic cholecystectomy, particularly if the transhepatic percutaneous route is used. A few patients (5% to 10%) experience complications related to transhepatic puncture or cystic duct perforation.

The first extracorporeal shock-wave lithotripsy (ESWL) treatments were undertaken in the mid-1980s after success in renal stone therapy. The goal of ESWL is to shock gallstones into tiny fragments that can pass through the biliary system into the gut or be dissolved more easily by MTBE. Focused shock waves, generated by either electromagnetic or piezo-ceramic techniques, are used to produce a high-pressure shock effect over an area of several centimeters. The tissue damage to the gallbladder and adjacent organs is minimal and, with the exception of an occasional case of mild pancreatitis, seems to be of little consequence. The amount of fragmentation seems to depend on the number, size, and composition of the stones. Best results are obtained in patients with a few small, noncalcified stones. The recurrence rate of gallstones after complete clearance is significant, ranging from 10% to 15%. Combining ESWL with powerful dissolving agents such as MTBE seems to produce a slightly higher rate of success. The unresolved question is the relative cost of different therapies with the advent of laparoscopic surgery. In general, the enthusiasm for ESWL seen during the 1980s has waned significantly. In symptomatic patients for whom surgery is contraindicated, however, ESWL represents an encouraging alternative.

Nonadenomatous Polyps

The most common cause of polypoid (nonmobile) filling defects within the gallbladder is cholesterol polyps (Fig. 6-50). These polyps arise from a condition of the gallbladder known as cholesterolosis, in which deposits of cholesterol and cholesterol precursors are found

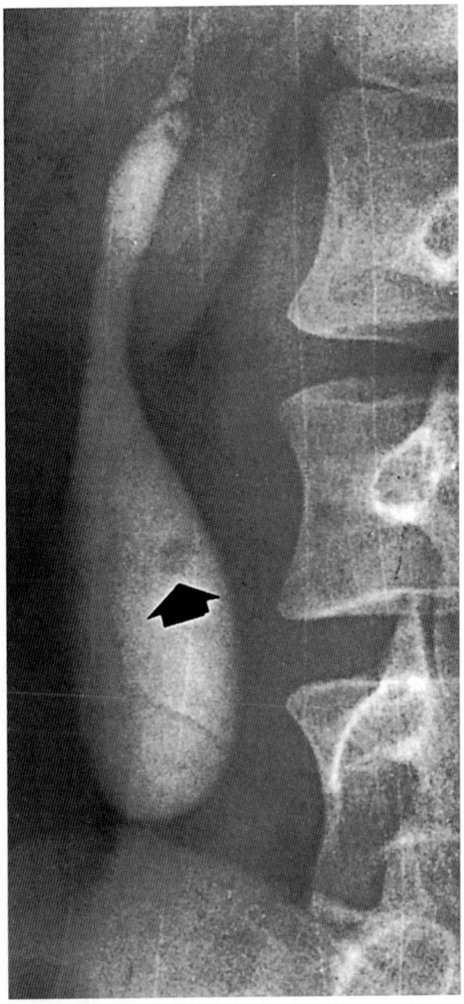

Figure 6-50 OCG in a patient with a single, nonmobile filling defect within the gallbladder *(arrow)*, which was found to represent a solitary cholesterol polyp.

within the gallbladder wall. The typical OCG and ultrasound findings are similar to those of a gallstone, with the exceptions that the lesion is fixed on the gallbladder wall, and there is no acoustic shadowing on ultrasound. The morphological changes can be either a focal buildup forming a discrete cholesterol polyp or diffuse surface deposition over the gallbladder mucosa, giving rise to an unusual surface texture and pattern, sometimes referred to as "strawberry gallbladder."

Cholesterolosis and its manifestations are part of a larger group of conditions often referred to as the hyperplastic cholecystoses, first described by Jutras in 1960. Under the same heading, he also included adenomyomatosis and several rare and unusual conditions. The validity and significance of the latter conditions have been questioned, and for the most part cholesterolosis and adenomyomatosis are considered the only two important conditions under the hyperplastic cholecystoses classification. Jutras used the term *hyperplastic cholecystoses* to describe a group of gallbladder disorders that had common functional abnormalities, such as hyperconcentration, hyperexcretion, and hypercontractibility. Adenomyomatosis is discussed in more detail in subsequent sections.

Other nonadenomatous polypoid lesions of the gallbladder are rare and include lipomas, leiomyomas, fibromas, hemangiomas, and neurofibromas. Carcinoid tumors of the gallbladder have been reported. Rarely, granular cell myoblastomas (also a rare finding in the esophagus) also have been described in the gallbladder. Papillomas of the gallbladder and of the biliary tree have been reported and produce multiple filling defects (Fig. 6-51). In addition to the aforementioned conditions, an unusual but troublesome filling defect in the gallbladder is seen rarely as a result of a gallstone adherent to the gallbladder mucosa.

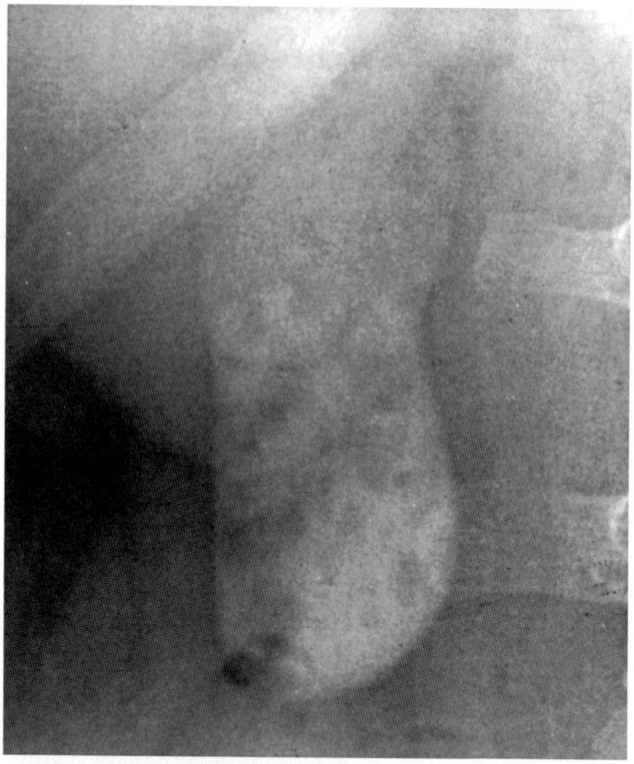

Figure 6-51 Multiple filling defects are seen within the gallbladder resulting from papillomatosis.

Adenomatous Polyps

True epithelial adenomas are uncommon. When present, they can occur as either sessile or pedunculated filling defects. They can occur in any portion of the gallbladder, and multiplicity is a frequent finding. The possibility that gallbladder adenomas represent a definite precursor to carcinoma, such as in the colon, lacks convincing scientific support. The presence of carcinoma in situ in some reported cases of gallbladder adenomas makes it a real possibility, however.

Carcinoma

An estimated 6000 individuals in the United States each year die as a result of gallbladder carcinoma. The incidence is higher in women and Native Americans and Hispanics. Gallbladder carcinoma has a 5-year survival rate between 2% and 4%. If the patient is symptomatic, the prognosis is always grave. Patients who are asymptomatic and whose lesions are discovered fortuitously have a higher 5-year survival rate. The cause of gallbladder cancer is poorly understood. It must include the possibility of malignant degeneration of gallbladder adenomas. The development of gallbladder cancer in patients with calcified gallbladder walls (porcelain gallbladders) is thought to be extremely high, ranging from 20% to 30%.

The relationship between gallstones and the development of gallbladder cancer is controversial. Similar to gallstone disease, gallbladder cancer is more common among women, and 80% of patients with gallbladder cancer have gallstones (Fig. 6-52). The size of the stones also has been suggested as a factor because patients with larger stones have an increased association with gallbladder cancer. The most common presentation of this cancer is a large mass in or around the gallbladder. This mass is easily shown with CT (Fig. 6-53) or ultrasonography. The effect of the tumor as it involves adjacent bowel, such as the duodenum or the hepatic flexure of the colon, can be seen with barium studies. The presence of calcium within the gallbladder wall, in cases of porcelain gallbladder, is nicely shown on CT. Intraluminal masses arising from the wall also may be seen on ultrasound examination of the gallbladder (Fig. 6-54). The correct diagnosis, particularly in advanced disease, is often difficult to make because of the marked contiguous spread

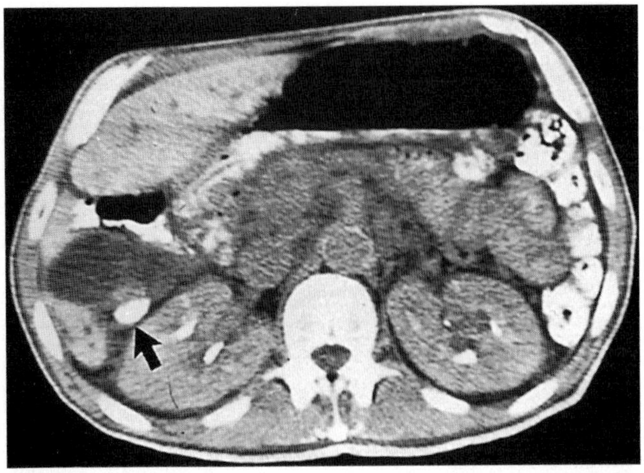

Figure 6-52 Computed tomographic section through the region of the gallbladder in a patient with carcinoma of the gallbladder shows perforation of the gallbladder with pericholecystic fluid and gallstones *(arrow)* seen outside the confines of the gallbladder.

of disease to the adjacent structures such that the actual site of origin cannot be determined.

Metastatic Disease

Metastatic disease is an uncommon cause of filling defects within the gallbladder. The most common metastatic lesion is melanoma. The known predisposition of melanoma to metastasize to the gastrointestinal tract is also known to include the gallbladder in approximately 15% of cases with gastrointestinal metastatic disease (Fig. 6-55). These metastatic lesions may be solitary

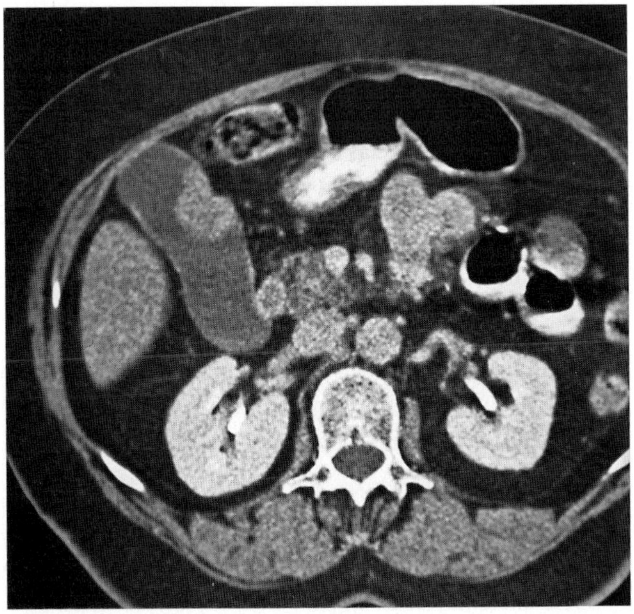

Figure 6-53 CT shows a soft tissue mass in the wall of the gallbladder in this patient with gallbladder carcinoma.

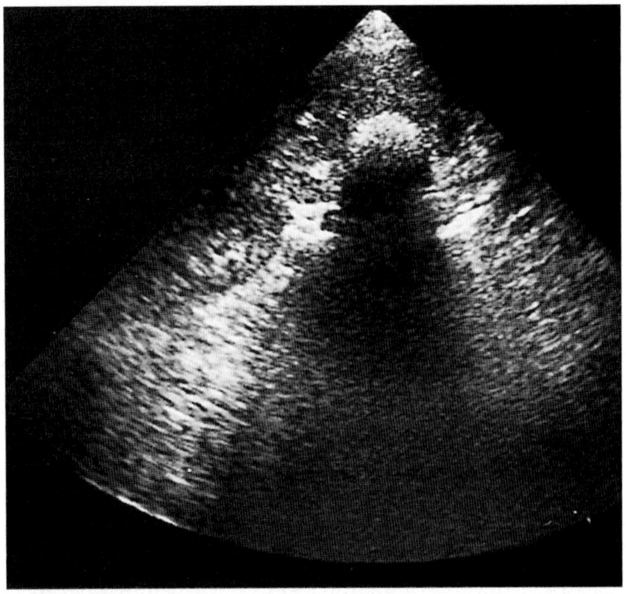

Figure 6-54 Ultrasonographic scan of a patient with porcelain gallbladder shows marked acoustic shadowing. There was also a mass associated with the gallbladder, which was found to be gallbladder carcinoma.

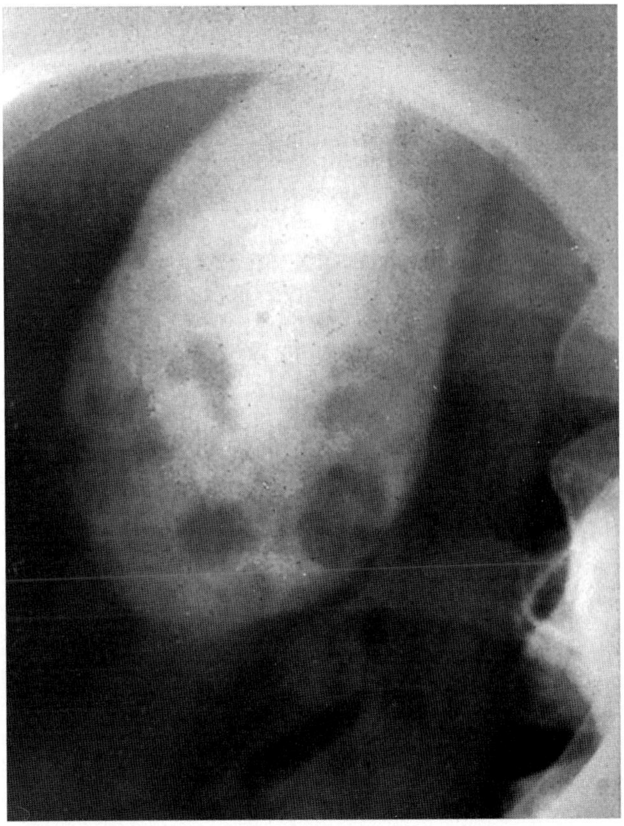

Figure 6-55 OCG in a patient with known malignant melanoma shows multiple, irregular nonmobile filling defects that proved to be metastatic lesions to the gallbladder.

or multiple. They are usually identified on ultrasound scan or the OCG as irregular polypoid lesions. In most cases, there is accompanying metastatic disease in the liver.

Thickened Wall

Thickening of the gallbladder wall is an imaging abnormality that can be identified by either ultrasonography or CT. It may represent either an actual or an apparent thickening and is related to the underlying condition. The actual thickness of the gallbladder wall is a nonspecific finding, and it is difficult to relate a specific measurement of the wall to the underlying disease entity (Box 6-8).

Cholecystitis

Thickening of the gallbladder wall can be identified in either acute or chronic cholecystitis. The cholecystitis can be related to inflammation of the gallbladder wall with infiltration by inflammatory cells and edema. Adjacent edema or fluid can accentuate the appearance of the wall thickening. The presence of stones with gallbladder wall thickening and enhanced on contrast CT is pathognomonic of cholecystitis. The condition becomes more difficult to diagnose without the presence of gallstones (Fig. 6-56).

Cholecystitis in the absence of gallstones is thought to occur in approximately 5% of cases, although the incidence seems to be higher in children. The signs and symptoms are identical to acute cholecystitis caused by gallstones. The lack of stones tends to make the diagnosis difficult, however, because the demonstration of the gallstones on imaging is often the central diagnostic feature. The difficulty in correctly diagnosing acalculous cholecystitis is not limited to any one imaging method. There may be faint or no opacification on the OCG. Ultrasonography also has proved to have less than an ideal sensitivity in detecting this condition, with a reported range of 60% to 70%. The diagnostic criterion in the absence of gallstones is often the thickness of the gallbladder wall, which has proved to be more nonspecific than previously realized (Box 6-9). The cause of acalculous cholecystitis is unclear. It has been suggested

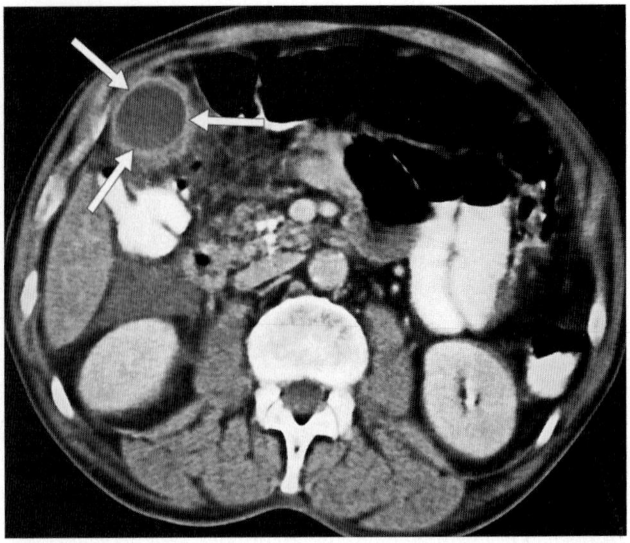

Figure 6-56 CT at the level of the gallbladder shows marked thickening of the wall with some enhancement *(arrows)* in a patient with acute cholecystitis.

that patients in the recovery phase from previous trauma, surgery, or severe systemic diseases may be more susceptible to acalculous cholecystitis. It has been suggested that radionuclide imaging may be more useful in the diagnosis of acalculous cholecystitis because the diagnosis does not hinge on the presence of stones (Box 6-10); however, this has not proved to be the case, and the diagnostic sensitivity is similar to that of ultrasonography.

Acute acalculous cholecystitis is considered a more dangerous process than acute calculous cholecystitis with respect to morbidity and mortality (Fig. 6-57). This most likely relates to difficulties in making an early diagnosis.

Adenomyomatosis and Cholesterolosis

Adenomyomatosis and cholesterolosis are hyperplastic cholecystoses that can result in some thickening of the gallbladder wall. Adenomyomatosis is the most interesting part of Jutras' classification of hyperplastic cholecystoses. It occurs as a result of poorly understood hyperplastic changes involving the mucosa and muscular wall of the gallbladder and the formation of intramural sinuses, known as the Rokitansky-Aschoff sinuses,

Box 6-8 Gallbladder Wall Thickening Identifiable by Ultrasonography or CT

Cholecystitis (acute or chronic)
Hyperplastic cholecystoses
Ascites
Edema (congestive heart failure, chronic renal failure, liver failure)
Carcinoma

Box 6-9 Sonographic Findings of Acute Cholecystitis

Cholelithiasis
Gallbladder wall thickening
Pain over gallbladder (Murphy's sign)
Intramural sonolucency
Pericholecystic fluid/abscess
Gas in lumen

Box 6-10 Causes of False-Positive Biliary Scintigraphy for Acute Cholecystitis

Prolonged fasting
Failure to obtain delayed views
Chronic cholecystitis
Pancreatitis
Systemic illnesses
Gallbladder neoplasm

which are characteristic of this disease. Involvement of the gallbladder may be diffuse or segmental. There seems to be an increased association with gallstones. The focal fundal type of adenomyomatosis shows characteristic changes involving the gallbladder fundus with round, smooth polypoid filling defects frequently accompanied by filling of Rokitansky-Aschoff sinuses with contrast material (Fig. 6-58). Involvement of the gallbladder also may be segmental, with a well-defined narrowed waist within the body of the gallbladder in which marked wall thickening, including sinus formation, may be shown (Fig. 6-59). Diffuse involvement is also well known, with narrowing and irregularity of the gallbladder lumen, possible focal filling defects, and filling of multiple, intramural sinuses.

The diagnosis of segmental or diffuse adenomyomatosis is relatively easy using the OCG or ultrasonography. Focal adenomyomatosis is more difficult to diagnose and can be missed; this is supported by the pathological examination of gallbladders in which focal changes are seen more frequently than shown on imaging studies.

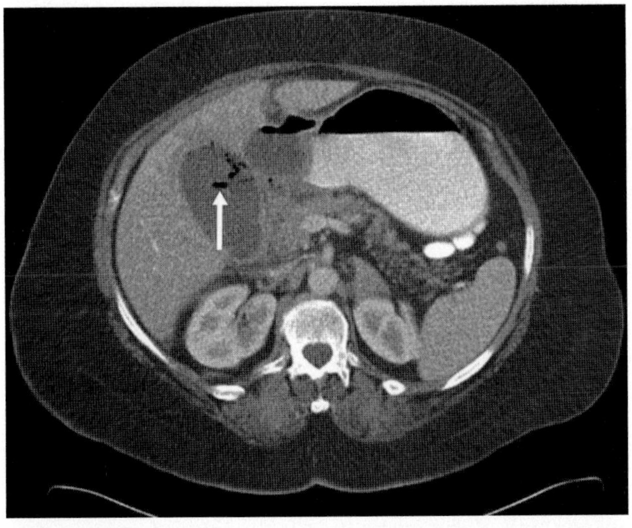

Figure 6-57 CT shows a thickened gallbladder wall in a patient with perforated gallbladder *(arrow)*. Note air bubbles within the gallbladder.

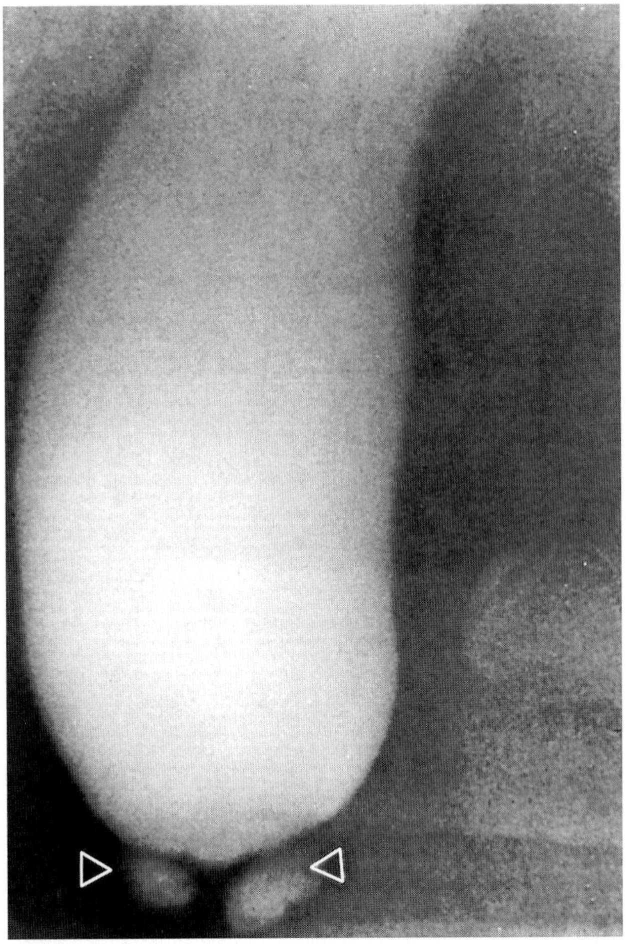

Figure 6-58 OCG in a patient with adenomyomatosis shows filling of prominent intramural sinuses *(arrowheads)* at the tip of the gallbladder fundus.

Ultrasound scan shows gallbladder wall thickening and occasionally may show sinus formation. Segmental involvement of the gallbladder is easily shown on ultrasound scan. OCG findings in this condition generally include good function and opacification of the gallbladder. There may be filling of the intramural sinuses with contrast material. Often this filling is incomplete, and the addition of a fatty meal or the use of cholecystokinin enhances the demonstration of the Rokitansky-Aschoff sinuses (Fig. 6-60).

Adenomyomatosis represents a benign proliferation of normal tissues and cannot be considered a neoplastic process. There is no evidence that it is premalignant. Many patients are asymptomatic. Treatment of symptomatic patients is controversial. There is evidence to suggest, however, that symptomatic patients who receive cholecystectomy frequently experience abatement of symptoms.

Cholesterolosis has been described in the previous section. In this condition, cholesterol deposits form in the wall of the gallbladder. Often they manifest as small

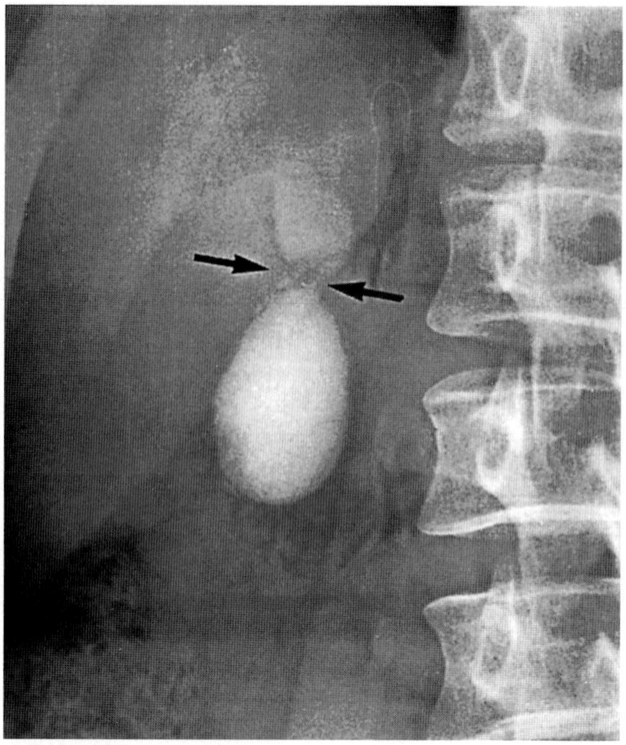

Figure 6-59 OCG in a patient with segmental adenomyomatosis of the gallbladder shows focal narrowing *(arrows)* of the body of the gallbladder.

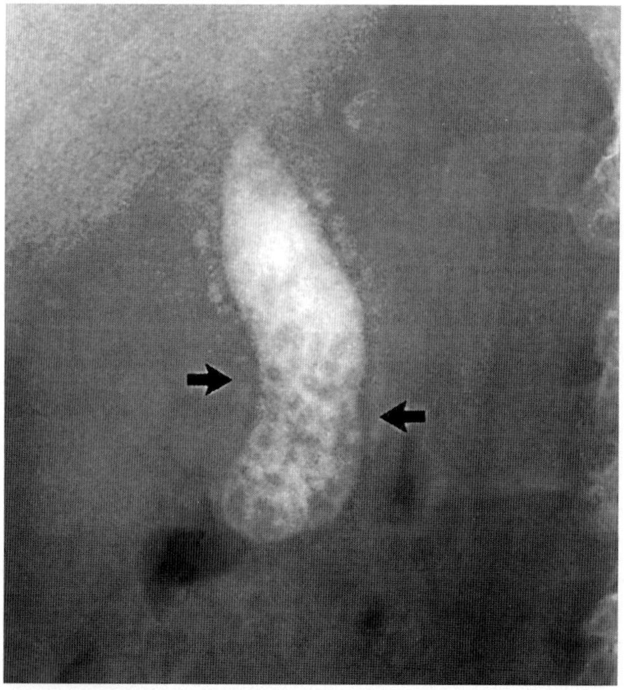

Figure 6-60 After ingestion of a fatty meal, the intramural sinuses of Rokitansky-Aschoff, faintly seen in Figure 6-59, are well shown *(arrows)*.

polyps and are seen as filling defects. Sometimes the deposition is in a diffuse fashion, with an irregular thickened gallbladder mucosa developing, which can be seen with cross-sectional imaging as a thickened wall.

Miscellaneous Causes

Occasionally, the presence of neoplastic infiltration of the gallbladder wall causes the appearance of wall thickening. This is not a common presentation, however. When ascites or pericholecystic fluid is present, the gallbladder wall may have the appearance of thickening on ultrasonography or CT. Sometimes this is just a spurious finding. Any medical conditions that result in edema can cause gallbladder wall thickening because edema develops in the wall of the gallbladder; this is apparent in hypoalbuminemia or other causes of low protein, including liver failure. Patients in chronic or acute renal failure also may develop wall thickening, and it can also be seen in congestive heart failure.

Calcifications

Stones

As previously mentioned, approximately 15% of gallstones contain sufficient calcium to be radiopaque on plain films. CT, being more sensitive to smaller amounts of calcium, yields a higher percentage. Radiopaque gallstones commonly have calcium in their outer rim. Calcification can vary in its pattern, however. Some stones have an irregular, mottled calcification, whereas others have a laminated appearance. Some stones have a small, central calcified nidus around which radiolucent cholesterol layers accumulate.

Porcelain Gallbladder

Porcelain gallbladder refers to a gallbladder that has undergone chronic inflammation and subsequent calcification in its wall (Figs. 6-61 and 6-62). The wall is usually thickened, and the gallbladder is often small and contracted. The cystic duct is always obstructed. The relationship between porcelain gallbladder and gallbladder carcinoma is striking, with gallbladder carcinoma developing in 20% to 30% of patients with porcelain gallbladder. Conversely, most patients with gallbladder carcinoma do not have antecedent porcelain gallbladder. A small, contracted calcified gallbladder, seen as a rounded, ringlike density in the right upper quadrant, can be easily mistaken for a large gallstone on a plain film of the abdomen (Fig. 6-63).

Milk of Calcium Bile

Another manifestation of chronic cholecystitis and obstruction of the cystic duct is the condition known as milk of calcium bile. This condition represents a situation in which the bile contained within the obstructed gallbladder becomes radiopaque because of the high

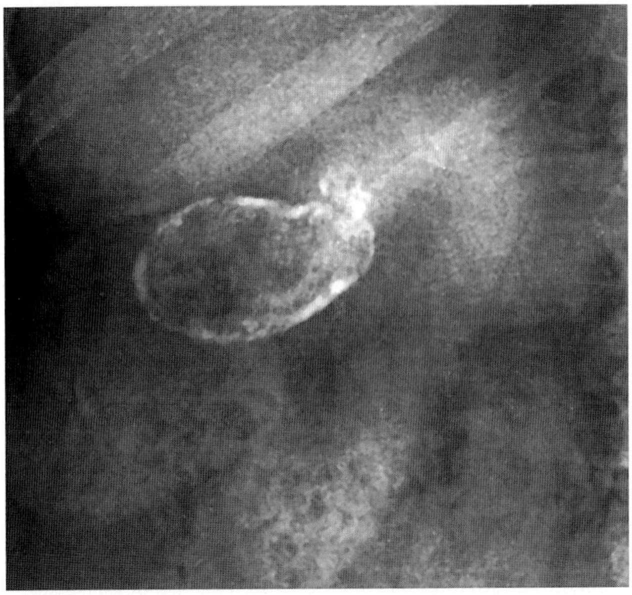

Figure 6-61 Porcelain gallbladder with segmental calcification throughout the wall is seen.

concentration of calcium carbonate and its resultant precipitation. Milk of calcium bile can be shown easily by obtaining upright, supine, and decubitus views of the gallbladder in which the fluid character of the radiopacity is visible (Fig. 6-64). Although the gallbladder is commonly small and contracted, occasionally the appearance can simulate a contrast-filled gallbladder seen during CT or ERCP.

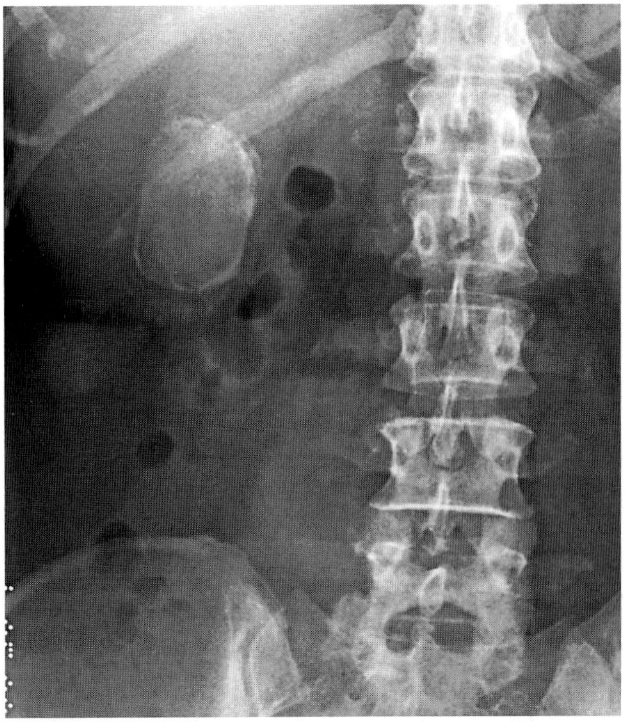

Figure 6-63 An oblong calcification in the right upper quadrant initially was thought to represent a large calcified gallstone, but proved to be a porcelain gallbladder.

Miscellaneous Conditions

Emphysematous Cholecystitis

Emphysematous cholecystitis is a rare condition in which bubbles and streaks of gas appear within the wall and possibly the lumen of the gallbladder (Fig. 6-65). There may be collections of gas in the pericholecystic region as well. The cause of the gas is almost always related to the presence of gas-forming organisms involved in the infectious and inflammatory processes occurring in or around the gallbladder. The condition is seen most commonly in patients with diabetes mellitus

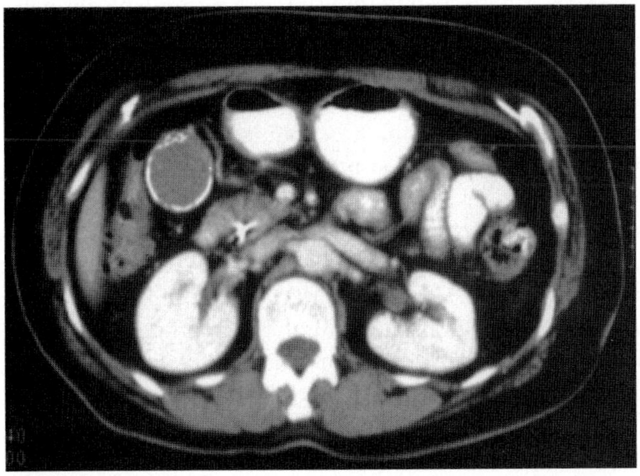

Figure 6-62 CT of calcified gallbladder wall, representing porcelain gallbladder.

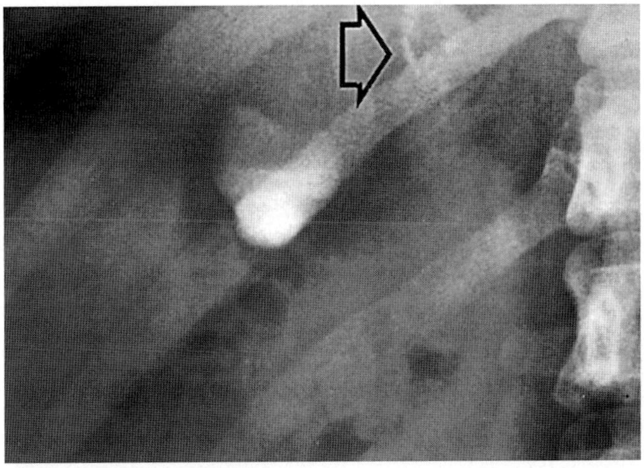

Figure 6-64 A patient with chronic cystic duct obstruction and milk of calcium bile. Note the layering of the milk of calcium bile in the fundus of the gallbladder on this upright view. Also seen is the calcified stone *(arrow)* obstructing the gallbladder neck and cystic duct.

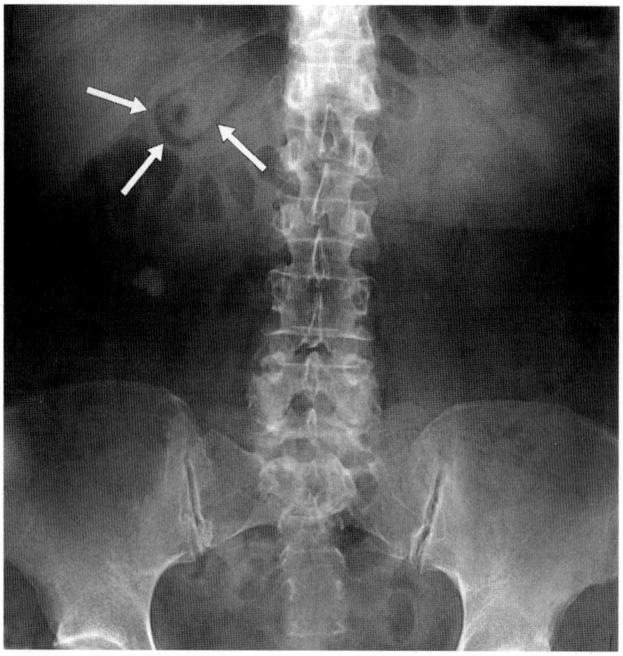

Figure 6-65 This patient has emphysematous cholecystitis; air is seen within the gallbladder and the gallbladder wall *(arrows)*.

and, in contrast to most gallbladder inflammatory processes, is more commonly seen in men (Box 6-11).

On plain films of the abdomen, the most important diagnostic criterion is intramural gas in the gallbladder wall. Occasionally, mottled collections of gas can be seen around the gallbladder fossa. The radiological finding of gas confined to the gallbladder lumen or the biliary tree without intramural or pericholecystic gas should lead one away from the diagnosis of infection and toward consideration of benign causes of pneumobilia. Those patients are seldom ill, in contrast to the severe toxic state of patients with emphysematous cholecystitis. Clinically, patients with emphysematous cholecystitis present with sudden and rapidly progressive right upper quadrant pain accompanied by fever and elevated white blood cell counts. Treatment and diagnosis must be prompt because the mortality rate is significantly higher than that of the usual acute cholecystitis. The ongoing inflammatory and infectious processes can lead quickly to gangrenous changes within the gallbladder wall, perforation, and catastrophe. Treatment is prompt cholecystectomy.

Box 6-11 Characteristics of Emphysematous Cholecystitis

Elderly patients, usually men
Diabetes in approximately half of cases
High incidence of perforation
Clostridium welchii a common organism

Box 6-12 Three Features of Gallstone Ileus

Air in biliary system
Bowel obstruction, typically small bowel
Calcified gallstone visible in the bowel

Gallstone Ileus

Gallstone ileus (Box 6-12) is a misleading name of a condition in which the most striking finding is intestinal obstruction. The obstruction results from the erosion of a gallstone (usually >2.5 cm) into the adjacent duodenum, forming a cholecystoduodenal fistula. The stone passes distally until it reaches the narrowest portion of the small bowel in the distal ileum, where it becomes lodged, resulting in intestinal obstruction. The condition is much more common in women and generally seen in older individuals.

If the stone is smaller, it may pass through the gut without resulting in obstruction. The patient may not be left with a cholecystoduodenal fistula because many of these seal off. Deformity in the gallbladder and duodenum may be seen, however, on UGI examinations and CT. Approximately 10% of cholecystoenteric fistulas are between the gallbladder and the adjacent hepatic flexure of the colon. In this instance, most stones pass through the colon without causing obstruction. Rarely there may be erosion of a gallstone into the adjacent stomach, possibly leading to pyloric obstruction (Bouveret's syndrome).

In more than half of the cases of patients presenting with small bowel obstruction as a result of gallstone ileus, air can be seen within the biliary tree. The absence of air in the biliary tree does not exclude the diagnosis. The presence of a calcified stone in the right lower quadrant may be helpful. Lacking this, diagnosis may be extremely elusive, which accounts for the higher mortality rate seen in this condition than is normally associated with other causes of small bowel obstruction. The erosion of a gallstone into the colon is unlikely to lead to obstruction and may be the preferable site for fistulous communication. Residual cholecystocolonic fistula is not a happy proposition to contemplate, with gram-negative coliform organisms ascending the biliary system. Abdominal CT performed for evaluation of possible gallstone ileus should be done without oral contrast material so as to increase the possibility of detecting the obstructing stone (Fig. 6-66).

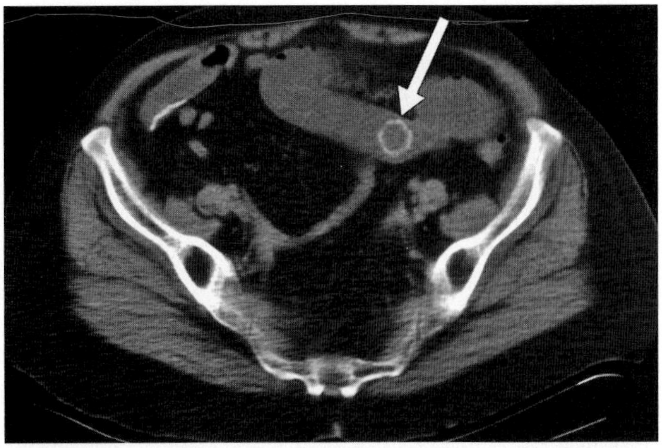

Figure 6-66 CT of lower abdomen shows calcified gallstone *(arrow)* that has become impacted in the distal ileum, causing the so-called gallstone ileus.

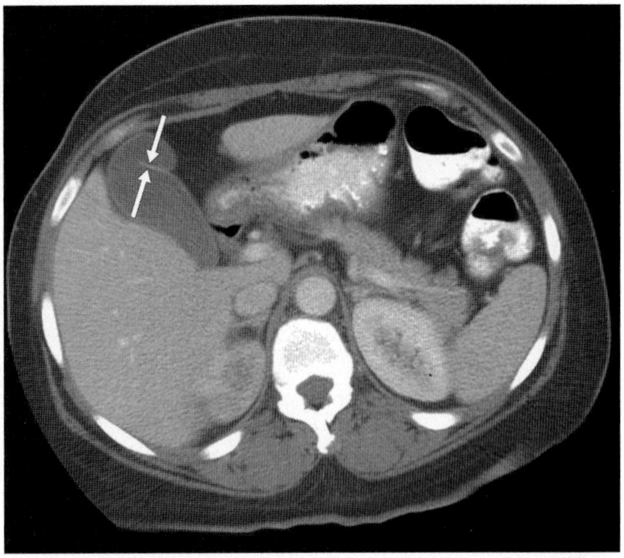

Figure 6-67 Bandlike narrowing *(arrows)* across the fundus of the gallbladder is a phrygian cap deformity and is of no clinical significance.

Postcholecystectomy Syndrome

Although most patients with symptoms relating to gallstones are cured after cholecystectomy, approximately 5% to 40% have persistence of symptoms or recurrent symptoms. These patients fall within a confusing category known as the postcholecystectomy syndrome.

Residual common bile duct stones may account for symptoms in a small percentage of patients. The routine use of operative cholangiography during cholecystectomy has reduced significantly the incidence of residual stones, however.

Additionally, intraoperative trauma and resultant injury to either the ductal system or the sphincter of Oddi may be implicated in a few patients. In most instances, a clear anatomical cause for the symptoms is not found. Nonbiliary causes, such as duodenal or gastric ulcer or pancreatitis, also should be considered as potential sources of the symptoms.

There is an increasing tendency to implicate changes in the papilla of Vater in postcholecystectomy syndrome. It is postulated that patients with underlying, unrecognized papillitis or papillary stricture most likely undergo cholecystectomy as a result of their symptoms. Frequently, the pathological changes at the sphincter are not anatomical, but physiological, and manometry of this segment and a careful ERCP examination of the biliary tree with delayed images to evaluate for biliary emptying can be helpful. The common bile duct in symptomatic postcholecystectomy patients tends to be mildly dilated.

VARIATIONS AND ANOMALIES

Phrygian Cap

Normal anatomical variations within the gallbladder, representing either folding of the gallbladder on itself or intraluminal septations, occur and should not be confused with disease. A fold or septation near the gallbladder fundus is a relatively common finding and represents the well-known "Phrygian cap" (Fig. 6-67), referring to the hats worn by slaves in the ancient Greek province of Phrygia in Asia Minor. This finding is of no clinical consequence.

The size and configuration of the gallbladder can vary considerably from patient to patient. There also may be a variation in the position of the gallbladder. In most patients, the gallbladder is located in the subhepatic fossa. In a few particularly tall, slender individuals, the gallbladder is vertically oriented with its fundus in the lower abdomen. In such individuals, the gallbladder is frequently on a long mesentery and may be found in ectopic locations (Fig. 6-68). In addition, herniations into the lesser sac through the foramen of Winslow have been reported. Conversely, a few individuals have the gallbladder in an intrahepatic position (Fig. 6-69). Patients with small left lobes of the liver frequently have a malpositioned gallbladder (Fig. 6-70).

Ectopic Gallbladder

Rarely, the gallbladder is congenitally absent. When this occurs, there is a high incidence of common bile duct stones. This congenital anomaly also is associated with other malformations seen within the cardiovascular system and the gastrointestinal system. Agenesis of the gallbladder is difficult to distinguish radiologically from any condition in which the gallbladder fails to function or in which there is obstruction of the cystic duct.

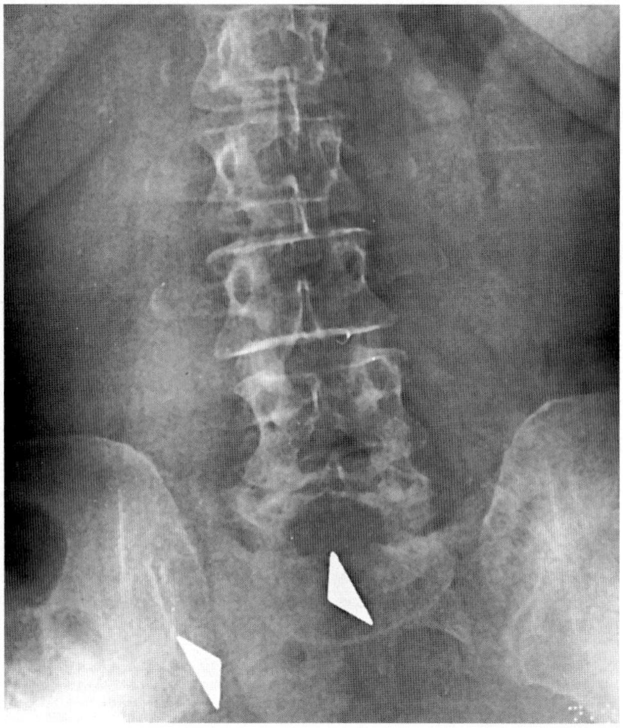

Figure 6-68 OCG shows relatively faint opacification of a gallbladder that is located at the pelvic inlet *(arrowheads)*.

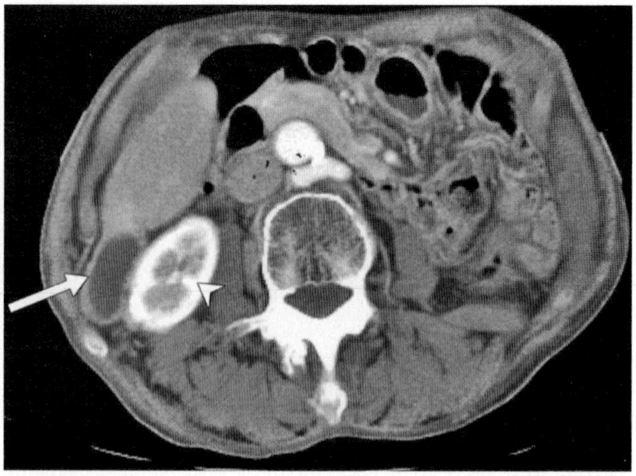

Figure 6-70 CT shows unusual position of gallbladder *(arrow)* adjacent to and touching the right kidney *(arrowhead)*.

Duplications and Septations

Duplication of the gallbladder and cystic duct has been reported, but is extremely rare. Occasionally, an apparent double gallbladder can be seen on the OCG when a long, slender gallbladder is found to have turned on itself, giving the appearance of two well-opacified gallbladders. Often these are just septations that may be occurring within the gallbladder because of abnormalities in recanalization of the lumen (Fig. 6-71).

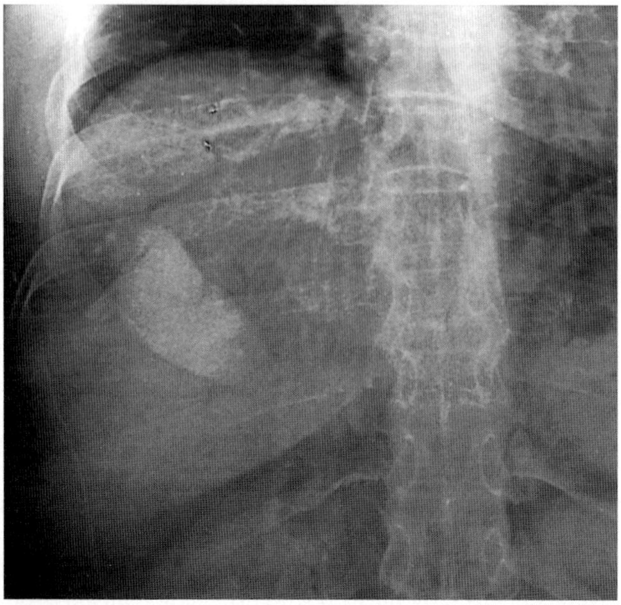

Figure 6-69 OCG shows good opacification in a patient with an intrahepatic gallbladder.

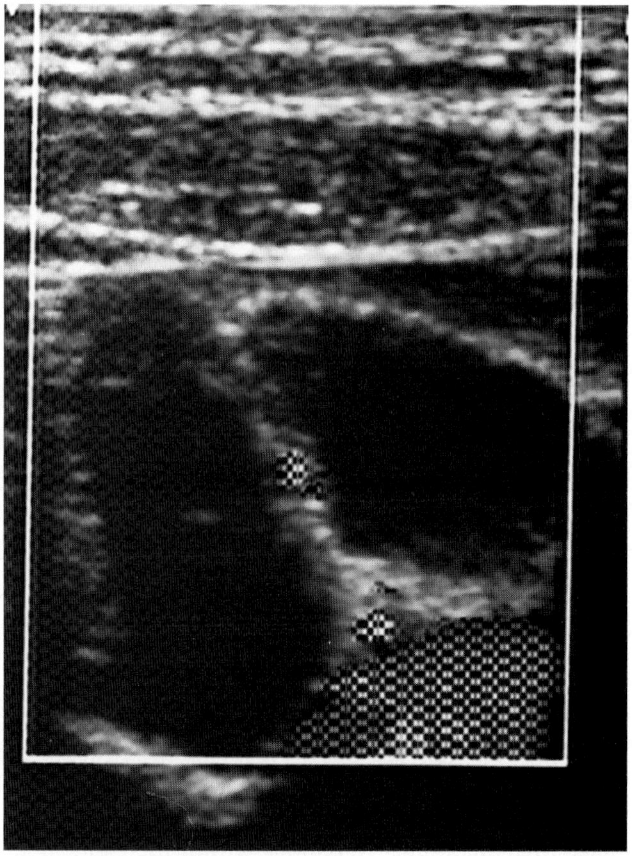

Figure 6-71 Ultrasonographic scan shows two distinct gallbladder lumens because of a duplication.

With a long, tortuous gallbladder that may be on a mesentery, the potential for torsion of the gallbladder increases. This is unusual, but is almost always associated with the aforementioned condition. Clinically, the presentation is that of severe acute cholecystitis. The potential for gangrenous changes and perforation is greatly increased. Other uncommon causes of gallbladder deformity are pericholecystic adhesions and adhesive bands. These are thought to be congenital in nature and probably of little clinical significance.

Anomalous Ductal Insertions

Of great clinical concern is the presence of anomalous position of some of the ducts because the potential for injury during surgery or interventional procedures is greatly increased. As noted previously, the bile ducts form as a bud from the ventral pancreas and gradually arborize as they branch into the liver. Unusual branching patterns of the ducts commonly are seen. Sometimes the major left or right branches are seen to insert quite low into the extrahepatic ducts (Fig. 6-72). In these situations, the likelihood of injury during surgery is greatly increased. Some ducts have been known to drain into the gallbladder or cystic duct.

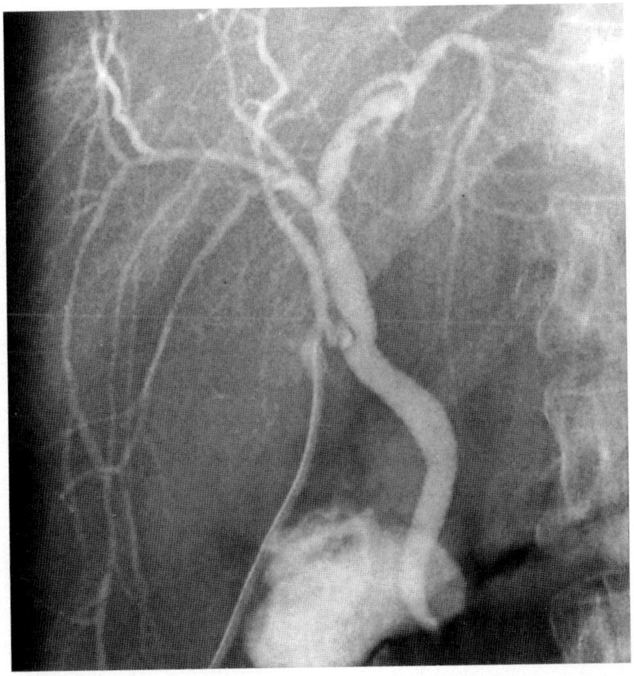

Figure 6-72 Aberrant right hepatic duct inserts into the side of the cystic duct. It was narrowly missed at surgery and was evident only during the cholangiogram.

SUGGESTED READINGS

Berk RN, Armbuster TG, Saltzstein SL: Carcinoma in the porcelain gallbladder. Radiology 106:29-31, 1973.

Bucceri AM, Brogna A, Ferrera R: Common bile duct caliber following cholecystectomy: two-year sonographic survey. Abdom Imaging 19:251-258, 1994.

Chan YL, Chan ACW, Lam WWM, et al: Choledocholithiasis: comparison of MR cholangiography and endoscopic retrograde cholangiography. Radiology 200:85-91, 1996.

Chen RC, Liu MH, Tu HY, et al: Value of ultrasound measurement of gallbladder wall thickness in predicting laparoscopic operability prior to cholecystectomy. Clin Radiol 50:570-578, 1995.

Crittenden SL, McKinley MJ: Choledochal cyst—clinical features and classification. Am J Gastroenterol 80:643-647, 1985.

Grand D, Horton KM, Fishman E: CT of the gallbladder: spectrum of disease. AJR 183:163-170, 2003.

Hall-Craggs MA, Allen CM, Owens CM: MR cholangiography: clinical evaluation in 40 cases. Radiology 189:423-427, 1993.

Haller JO: Sonography of the biliary tract in infants and children. AJR 157:1051-1058, 1991.

Huntington DK, Hill MC, Steinberg W: Biliary tract dilatation in chronic pancreatitis: CT and sonographic findings. Radiology 172:47-50, 1989.

Jutras JA: Hyperplastic cholecystoses. AJR 83:795-827, 1960.

Kim OH, Chung HJ, Choi BG: Imaging of the choledochal cyst. Radiographics 15:69-88, 1995.

Koehler RE, Melson GL, Lee JKT, et al: Common hepatic duct obstruction by cystic duct stone: Mirizzi syndrome. AJR 132:1007-1009, 1979.

Kumar A, Aggarwal S: Carcinoma of the gallbladder: CT findings in 50 patients. Abdom Imaging 19:304-310, 1994.

Larsen CR, Scholz FJ, Wise RE: Diseases of the biliary ducts. Semin Roentgenol 11:259-267, 1976.

LaRusso NF, Wiesner RH, Ludwig J, et al: Primary sclerosing cholangitis. N Engl J Med 310:899-903, 1984.

Lim JH: Cholangiocarcinoma:morphologic classification according to growth pattern and imaging findings. AJR 181:819-827, 2003.

Lim JH, Yoon KH, Kim SH, et al: Intraductal papillary mucinous tumors of the bile ducts. Radiographics 24:53-67, 2004.

Li-Yeng C, Goldberg HI: Sclerosing cholangitis: broad spectrum of radiographic features. Gastrointest Radiol 9:39-47, 1984.

Malet PF, Baker J, Kahn MJ, et al: Gallstone composition in relation to buoyancy at oral cholecystography. Radiology 177: 167-169, 1990.

Mall JC, Gharemani CG, Boyer JL: Caroli's disease associated with congenital hepatic fibrosis and renal tubular ectasia. Gastroenterology 66:1029-1035, 1974.

Miller FH, Hwang CM, Gabriel H, et al: Contrast-enhanced helical CT of choledocholithiasis. AJR 181:125-130, 2002.

Miller WJ, Sechtin AG, Campbell WL, et al: Imaging findings in Caroli's disease. AJR 165:333-340, 1995.

Moliver CL, Saltzstein EC: Common bile duct distensibility after cholecystectomy. South Med J 84:719-721, 1991.

Mujahed Z: Factors interfering with the opacification of a normal gallbladder. Gastrointest Radiol 1:183-185, 1976.

Reinhold C, Bret PM, Guibaud L, et al: MR cholangiopancreatography: potential clinical applications. Radiographics 16:309-331, 1996.

Rizzo RJ, Szucs RA, Turner MA: Congenital abnormalities of the pancreas and biliary tree in adults. Radiographics 15:49-68, 1995.

Rooholaminia SA, Tehrani NS, Razavi MK, et al: Imaging of gallbladder carcinoma., Radiographics 14:291-310, 1994.

Savader SJ, Benenati JF, Venbrux AC, et al: Choledochal cysts: classification and cholangiographic appearance. AJR 156: 327-331, 1991.

Schuster DM, Pedrosa MC, Robbins AH: Magnetic resonance cholangiography. Abdom Imaging 20:353-361, 1995.

Sheng R, Campbell WL, Zahko AB, et al: Cholangiographic features of biliary strictures after liver transplantation for primary sclerosing cholangitis: evidence of recurrent disease. AJR 166:1109-1116, 1996.

Silva AC, Friese JL, Hara AK, Lui PT: MR cholangiopancreatography: improved distention with intervenous morphine administration. Radiographics 24:677-687, 2004.

Taourel P, Bret PM, Reinhold C, et al: Anatomic variants of the biliary tree: diagnosis with MR cholangiopancreatography. Radiology 199:521-527, 1996.

Ward J, Sheridan MB, Guthrie JA, et al: Bile duct strictures after heptobiliary surgery: assessment with MR cholangiography. Radiology 231:101-108, 2004.

Wedmann B, Borsch G, Coenen C, et al: Effect of cholecystectomy on common bile duct diameters: a longitudinal prospective ultrasonographic study. J Clin Ultrasound 16:619-624, 1988.

Weltman DI, Zeman RK: Acute diseases of the gallbladder and biliary ducts. Radiol Clin North Am 32:933-954, 1994.

Wiot JF, Felson B: Gas in the portal venous system. AJR 86: 920-929, 1961.

CHAPTER 7 Colon and Rectum

The colon and rectum are two common sites for disease in the gut, with a wide spectrum of disease processes encountered on a daily basis in medical practice. The steady increase in the incidence and mortality resulting from colorectal cancer (CRC) has focused the medical and lay communities' attention on early detection and potentially effective screening strategies for this disease. With the great impact of colonoscopy and the refinement of air-contrast barium enemas (ACBE), there has been some improvement in overall survival and mortality rates in the past 4 decades. Until more recently, there has been relatively little detailed analysis, however, of the screening strategies put forth by various groups. In recent years, more careful scrutiny has shown most screening strategies to be either not efficient or not cost-effective. The addition of computed tomography (CT) colonoscopy is exciting, but as yet this modality has not been shown to be at least as nearly accurate as conventional colonoscopy and ACBE. More important, the cost-effectiveness of the technique is an important issue at this time of increasing heath care costs.

The question of efficiency and cost-effectiveness of any technique or combination of techniques of various screening strategies may be considered, to some extent, to be not entirely answered at this time. The barium enema, whose demise was forecast by our clinical colleagues in the late 1970s and early 1980s, still seems to be quite useful and, although much less prevalent than in the 1980s, is still widely used. The barium enema could be a better and more cost-effective method of examining the colon than previously realized and, along with CT colonoscopy, may play a role in future screening strategies. Before we see that, however, many questions regarding screening for CRC remain to be answered. With CT colonoscopy added to the choices, among the choices or combination of choices for screening, what is the most cost-effective method? Even more fundamental, does any form of widespread screening for CRC significantly reduce mortality in the population, such as has been shown with mammography for breast cancer or the Papanicolaou test for cervical cancer? At this point, accumulating data suggest that this may be the case. The U.S. Preventive Services Task Force recommended that screening for CRC be performed for all persons older than 50 years of age with annual fecal occult blood tests; the American Cancer Society and the World Health Organization recommend yearly fecal occult blood tests and flexible sigmoidoscopy every 3 to 5 years. Although the intent is commendable, screening that does not examine the entire colon is a curious proposition, given that at least 50% of lesions are proximal and detected by the area of examination. The American College of Physicians, considering the evaluation of the entire colon as a necessity for appropriate screening, has proposed screening strategies to include flexible sigmoidoscopy, colonoscopy, and ACBE at 10-year intervals. Considerable evidence is mounting in the literature regarding the role of CT colonoscopy (virtual colonoscopy) in the screening process, however, and with the continued refinement of this process and the apparent increased patient acceptance of the CT colonoscopy, this examination is expected to play a large role in colonic diagnosis and screening in the future.

EXAMINATION TECHNIQUES

Computed Tomography Colonoscopy

With the arrival of 16, 64, and eventually 128 multidetector CT scanning, the world of colonic screening and diagnosis will undoubtedly be greatly impacted. Patients tend to report the CT colonoscopy examination to be more acceptable than either the ACBE or conventional colonoscopy. The actual imaging phase consists of a few minutes or less. Generally, no sedation is necessary, and patients are free to drive and return to the workplace almost immediately.

After carbon dioxide or air insufflation has taken place, the patient is imaged in both the supine and prone positions. More recent reports in the literature suggest that CT colonoscopy is effective at detecting cancerous lesions and most polyps measuring greater than 6 mm. The interpretative phase can be more time-consuming than the ACBE, however. Image reconstruction includes three-dimensional intraluminal images and sagittal and coronal reconstructions of the colon. Two-dimensional cross-sectional axial images may number in the thousands. If this technology is to become a routine, radiologists will need to rethink the format of how they would interpret these studies (Fig. 7-1).

Double-Contrast Barium Enema

Although the number of barium enemas has declined significantly since the 1990s, there seems to be a renewed interest and increased use of the double-contrast barium enema (DCBE). The DCBE study remains one of the mainstays in the diagnostic evaluation of the colon. It is an effective and relatively inexpensive method for evaluation of the entire colon. Good double-contrast technique also is reliable for excellent evaluation of the rectum. The detection rate for CRC varies from study to study, but is probably about 94%. The ability to detect small polyps (<1 cm) is less than with colonoscopy, whereas ACBE has been shown to be the equal of colonoscopy in detecting larger polyps (>1 cm). The risk of perforation is considerably greater with colonoscopy (10 to 25 times) than with ACBE. The examination can be done quickly and requires no sedation, no extended time off work, and no accompanying person to drive the patient home.

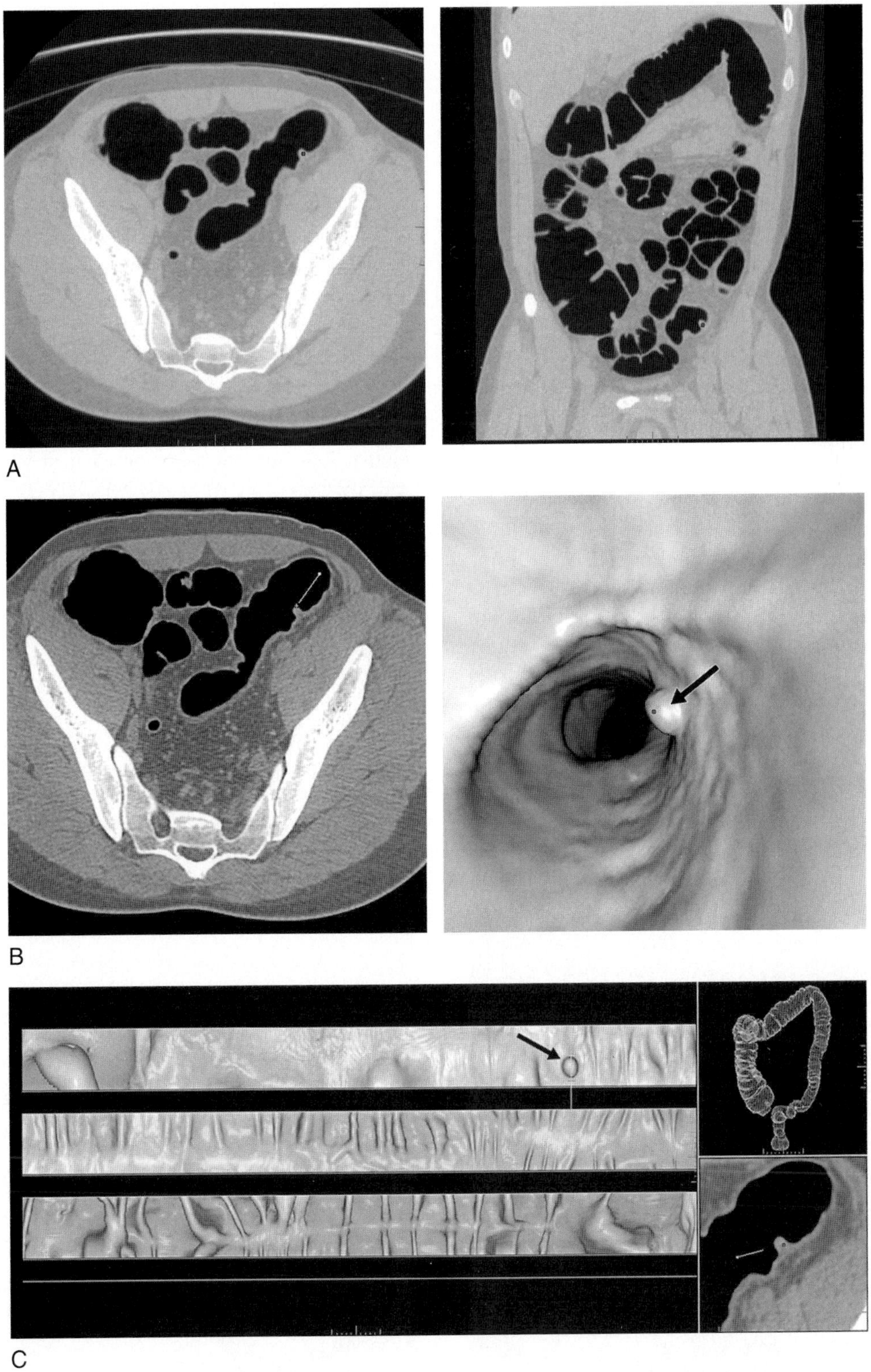

A

B

C

Figure 7-1 **A,** CT colonoscopy with insufflated carbon dioxide in the colon. Transaxial and coronal views are shown. **B,** Transaxial images with corresponding intraluminal image reconstruction show a small sessile polyp *(arrow)*. **C,** Newer software technology is able to lay the luminal view of the colon in striplike, open patterns so that the mucosal surface may be more readily evaluated. Note the small sessile polyp *(arrow)*. (**C** courtesy of GE Healthcare Systems.)

The three types of diagnostic contrast enemas used today are the DCBE, the single-contrast barium enema (SCBE), and the water-soluble contrast enema. It is beyond the scope of this book to instruct in the technique and mechanics of performing these examinations. It is important, however, to discuss certain general principles regarding how a radiologist decides which type of examination to use in a given clinical situation.

For all practical purposes, the DCBE is considered at this time the standard radiological examination of the colon (Fig. 7-2). There are still good indications, however, for the SCBE and the water-soluble contrast enema. The issue rests on preexamination diagnostic goals. In patients with bleeding, mild to moderate degrees of diarrhea, nonspecific abdominal pain, or a risk for polyp or cancer development, the DCBE study should be used. These patients require an efficient bowel preparation, for which a variety of commercially prepared products are available. The polyethylene glycol electrolyte solution for colonic lavage is becoming popular. It is the same preparation commonly used for colonoscopy. This type of bowel preparation tends to leave the colon clean, but with a wet ascending colon, which can be dealt with by the administration of bisacodyl suppositories at appropriate intervals before the examination (Figs. 7-3 and 7-4).

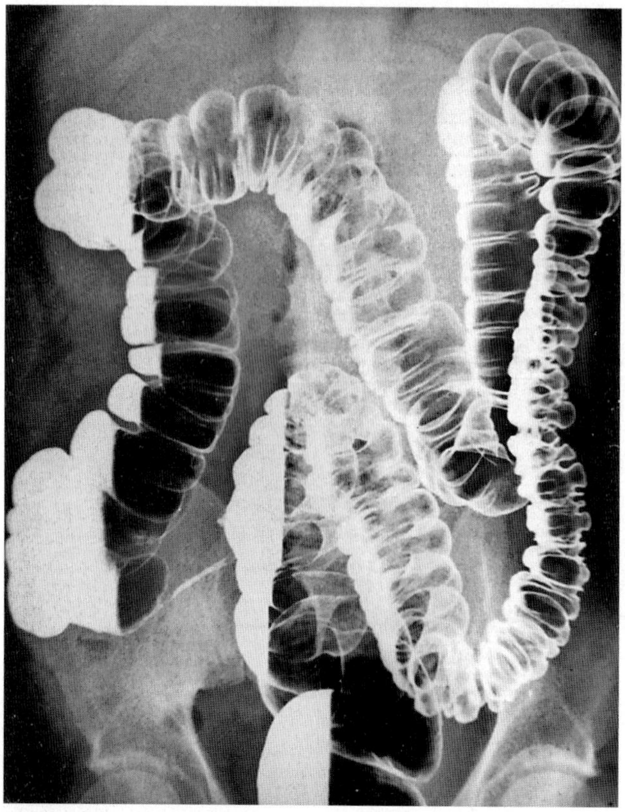

Figure 7-2 A right decubitus film from a DCBE. Decubitus films with compensation filtration are the most important overhead views in this examination.

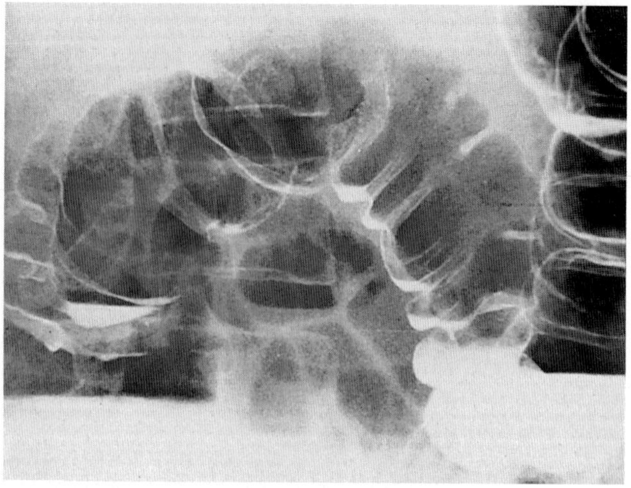

Figure 7-3 Air-contrast examination in which residual fluid makes coating of the ascending and transverse colon ineffectual. Lesions can be missed easily under these circumstances. Rotating the patient and washing the area with barium can result in additional coating.

All bowel preparations should be used with some knowledge of the patient's current clinical status and the diagnostic questions to be addressed. In some instances, particularly in inflammatory bowel disease (IBD) or bowel obstruction, colonic bowel preparation may require modification or, in some cases, be totally omitted.

Double-contrast technique consists of administering a high-density, low-viscosity barium into the colon followed by air insufflation and the demonstration of the entire mucosal surface of the rectum and colon.

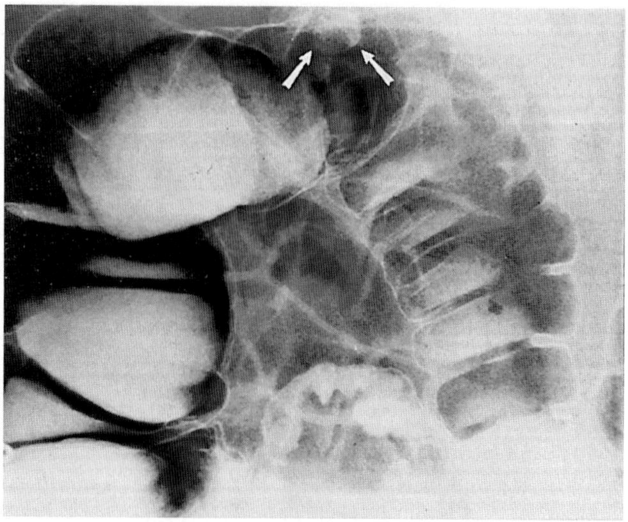

Figure 7-4 Same patient as shown in Figure 7-3. Because of the wetness and poor coating of the right colon, the patient was rotated, and additional barium was allowed to wash over the area, showing a rounded polyp on the superior margin of the hepatic flexure *(arrows)*.

In a well-prepared patient, this is a sensitive examination, detecting cancer in 94% of cases in sites when it is commonly performed by a radiologist well trained in the technique. The DCBE also is able to detect early mucosal inflammatory changes. The guiding principle in the performance of this procedure, similar to all radiological procedures, is to achieve a high-quality examination that results in maximum information about the state of the patient's colon. It also should be a high priority of the examining radiologist to attempt to achieve this goal with certain well-founded patient concerns in mind.

The technologist who prepares the patient for the examination explains the examination in detail and does much to allay most of the patient's concerns. Nevertheless, it is not advisable for the physician practicing radiology to meet the patient for the first time while that patient is on the fluoroscopic table with a rectal tube in place. Despite the acknowledgment that it is an efficient examination for the detection of disease, the barium enema over the decades has achieved a notorious reputation among lay individuals as a well-devised form of medical torture. The wise radiologist endeavors to use every psychological and physical advantage in attempting, to some extent, to debunk this reputation, while not sacrificing the efficiency of the examination.

The psychological state of the patient is often crucial to the successful completion of the study, and this is particularly the case in more difficult examinations. It is reasonable to greet the patient before the examination, elicit a brief history, explain the examination, and address whatever concerns the patient has regarding the study. It is also important that the radiologist not lose sight of patient anxiety, discomfort, and embarrassment that are commonly associated with this procedure. All of these issues can be addressed during the course of the examination. The number of films, fluoroscopic time, and overall radiation exposure should be kept to the minimum necessary to achieve an efficient examination. The radiologist should strive to ensure that the amount of time the patient spends on the fluoroscopic table is as short as possible. Concerns with patient dignity and modesty should be dealt with by ensuring the patient is properly draped at all times. Many radiologists have perfected the procedure to the point that they are able in many instances to remove the rectal tip relatively early in the examination; this results in a significant decrease in patient discomfort and an increased patient tolerance for the remainder of the study. There are also excellent diagnostic reasons for early removal of the rectal tip because low rectal lesions can be missed if the tip or balloon obscures the lesion (Figs. 7-5 to 7-7).

For similar reasons, some radiologists prefer the tableside fluoroscopic examination to remote control facilities. In some cases, the patient needs to be talked through the difficult parts of the examination, and being beside the patient with a hands-on directive approach sometimes can make the difference between success and failure. A spectral voice emanating from a loudspeaker somewhere in the room while the table moves and the overhead tower arcs above the patient does little to allay the anxieties of many patients. Controversy and disagreement exist on this issue while the number of remote units in use continues to grow. Nevertheless, whether tableside or remote fluoroscopic technique is used, the patient is the center of the radiological practice, and it is reasonable to expect that radiologists practice patient-centered, rather than machine-centered, radiology. There is perhaps no other area in radiology in which patient-centered technique can be practiced with such gratifying results as fluoroscopy.

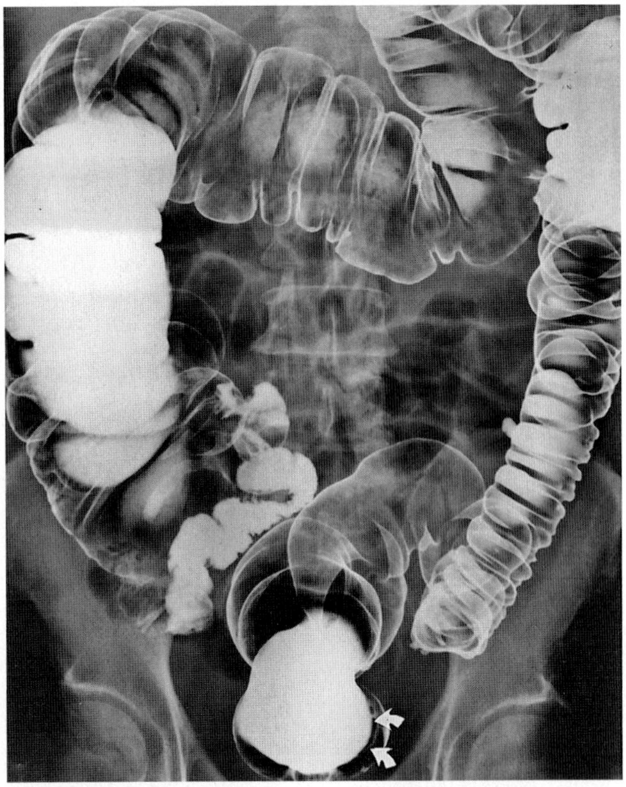

Figure 7-5 DCBE overhead film. A rectal carcinoma is obscured by the barium pool and the retained rectal tip and balloon. A subtle edge of the mass is all that is visible *(arrows)* on this study.

Single-Contrast Barium Enema

In most large medical centers, most barium enema studies are DCBE. Some patients have well-defined reasons for using the SCBE, however. Before the study, the radiologist should review the goals of the study carefully to establish the technique to be undertaken. In patients in whom colonic obstruction must be excluded, a single-contrast examination suffices to address the question.

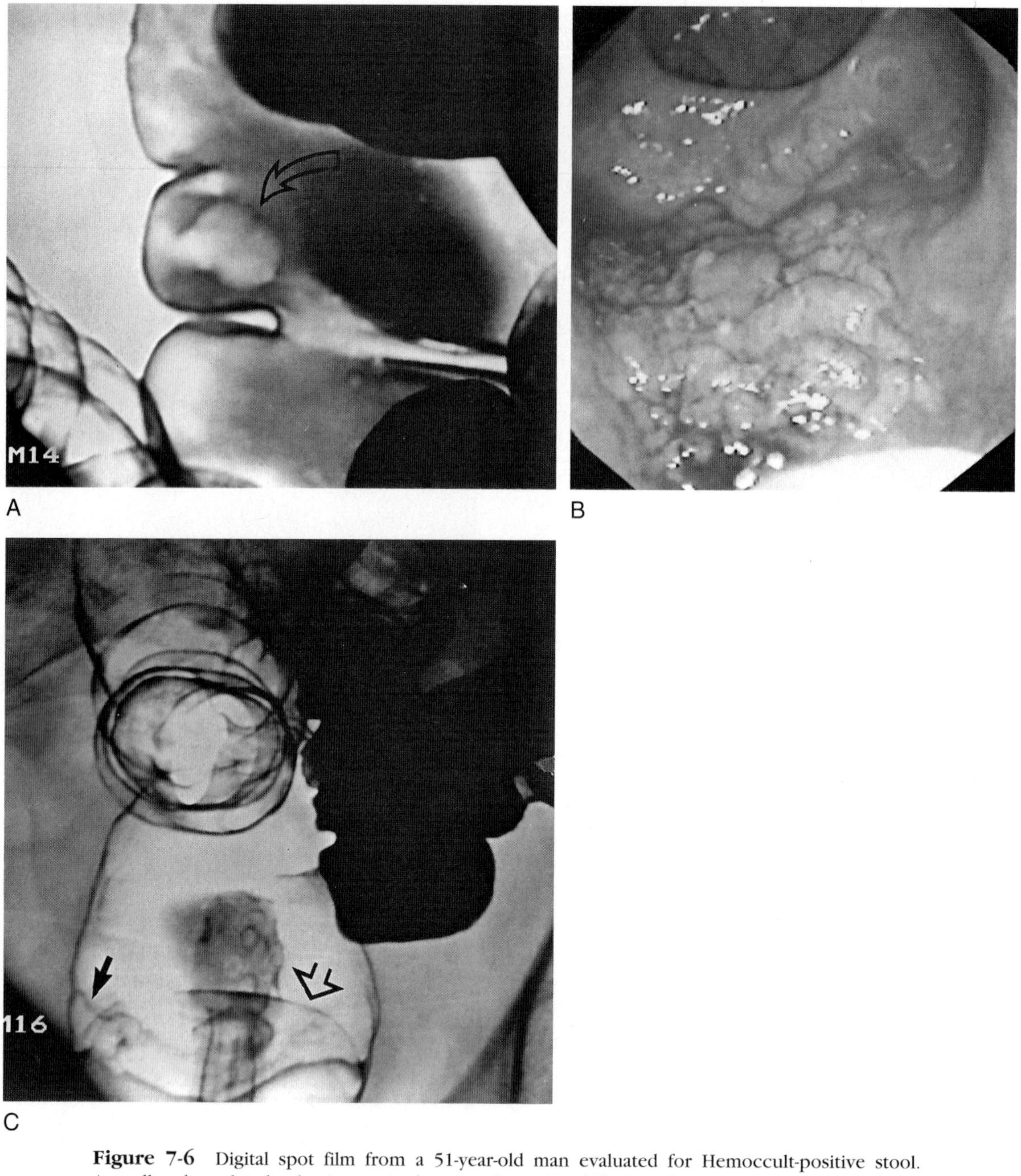

Figure 7-6 Digital spot film from a 51-year-old man evaluated for Hemoccult-positive stool. A small pedunculated polyp is seen in the ascending colon **(A)**. On colonoscopy, a rectal carcinoma is also discovered **(B)**. Review of films with image processing **(C)** shows the irregular margin of the rectal lesion *(solid arrow)* mostly obscured by the rectal balloon *(open arrow)*.

In many cases, these patients have undergone incomplete bowel preparation or none at all.

In questionable cases of diverticulitis, some radiologists prefer the SCBE, believing that the radiological findings of diverticulitis are better shown with a single-contrast study. This belief is based on the supposition that thinner, less viscous barium flows more readily into intramural or paraluminal tracts or abscesses than the more dense and viscous double-contrast barium.

In instances in which patients are impaired and cannot move or roll to the extent required for a successful DCBE study, the SCBE should be seriously considered. This is particularly the case in older, debilitated, severely mentally retarded, or extremely ill patients. Although a double-contrast examination has been shown to be more sensitive for the detection of inflammatory and polypoid processes, a bad double-contrast examination is worse than a bad single-contrast examination. This is a good

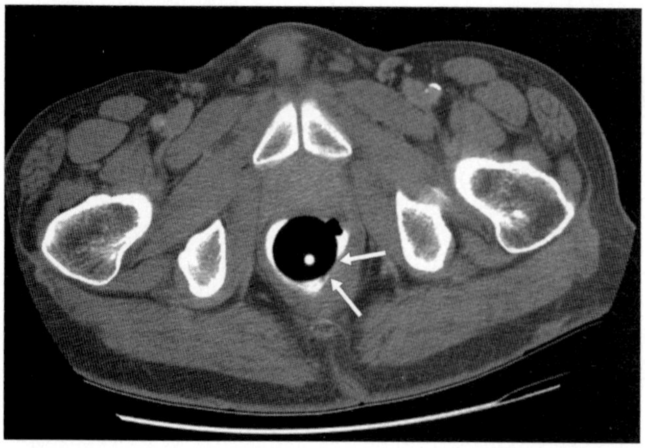

Figure 7-7 Inflated balloon in rectum obscures rectal wall lesion *(arrows)*.

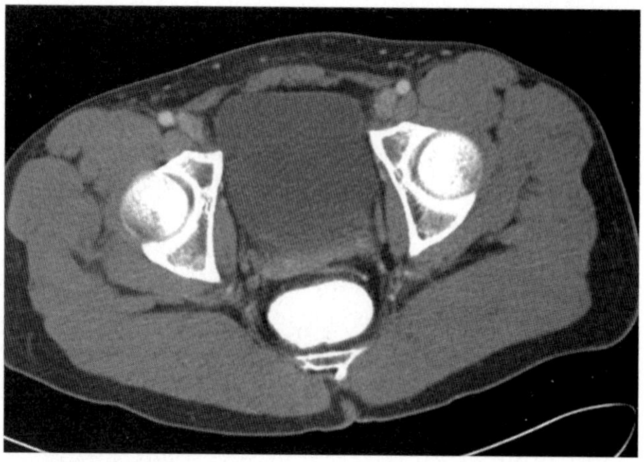

Figure 7-8 CT with barium administered by rectum.

rule of thumb to remember, and, given a choice in a situation in which a very limited or poor DCBE is possible, one should opt for the SCBE.

Water-Soluble Contrast Enema

There is an increasing but limited role for the water-soluble contrast enema. This technique is used almost entirely for the evaluation of a patient with suspected perforation. Frequently, these patients have experienced recent trauma, instrumentation, or surgery. The water-soluble contrast enema also may be used in the evaluation of a colon in which the potential for perforation may be high. This includes patients with colonic dilatation and particularly a cecum that may be acutely dilated to a preperforation state.

Additionally, a limited examination to rule out colonic obstruction can be performed with water-soluble contrast because many of these patients require CT of the abdomen within the next few hours or days. Retained colonic barium causes severe CT artifacts, making the examination useless and resulting in delays in the workup in such patients.

Computed Tomography and Magnetic Resonance Imaging

The role of routine CT of the abdomen and pelvis continues to become more important in colonic diagnosis. Many sites routinely use bowel contrast per rectum to delineate the colon better during CT (Fig. 7-8). The ability of CT to detect bowel wall thickening makes it more sensitive in the detection of diverticulitis than the barium enema. In addition, paraluminal abscesses are readily identified with CT. The ability to evaluate adjacent structures is an added dimension of the examination. Although the occasional dramatic demonstration of a colonic malignancy with CT is encountered (Fig. 7-9), there is no direct role for routine CT in the primary evaluation of colonic polyps and masses. This situation is likely to change, however, with the refinement of CT colonoscopy. Three-dimensional intraluminal images are generated using thin-section helical computed tomographic scans of the abdomen and pelvis after colonic insufflation of air or carbon dioxide. This examination must be preceded by a thorough bowel preparation. Types of limited bowel contrast material that adhere to stool and newer software that subtracts the tagged stool from the image may address one of the most perplexing problems in CT colonoscopy. Additionally, software permitting volume rendering imaging techniques are now used to achieve a progressive three-dimensional passage through the colonic lumen, evaluating the mucosal surface along the way. The introduction of multidetector CT means evaluation of CT colonoscopy using multiplanar images has finally been refined to the point that it is being routinely used. These techniques are relatively early in

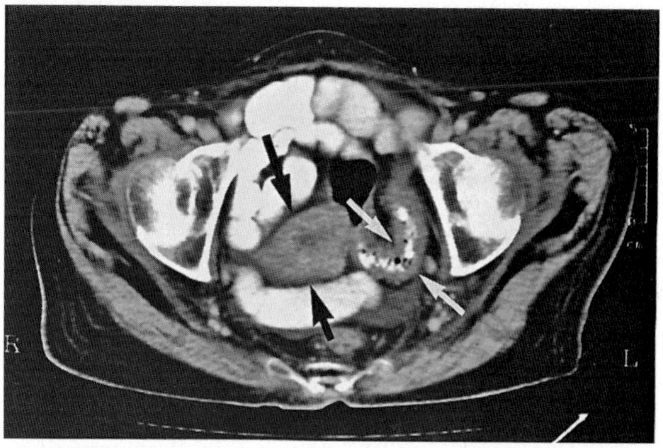

Figure 7-9 CT to look for metastatic disease in a 35-year-old woman with breast cancer. Thickening of the sigmoid colon *(white arrows)* is revealed, which proved to be primary carcinoma of the colon. The other mass in the pelvis *(black arrows)* is the uterus.

development with many technical difficulties to be overcome. The early work is startling and dramatic, however, holding exciting possibilities for the near future. In particular, it may revolutionize the way radiologists view CT images. The standard two-dimensional transaxial view may be replaced as the primary method of viewing the colon (and other organs) by three-dimensional volume rendering, with the radiologist resorting to two-dimensional images only if needed.

Although routine CT is able to show bowel wall thickening to advantage, the evaluation of superficial inflammatory disease within the colon or adjacent small bowel requires additional examinations, either colonoscopy or barium studies. At this point, CT colonscopy can detect bumps and masses in the colon, but cannot yet detect inflammatory changes in the mucosa.

The role of magnetic resonance imaging (MRI) in colorectal imaging is extremely limited at this time. MRI is being increasingly used, however, in evaluating rectal tumors for staging purposes. Although there is some evidence to suggest that MRI may be slightly superior to CT in evaluating the extent of tumor invasion of pelvic structures, it apparently is less reliable in the detection of abnormal nodes.

Ultrasonography

Except for abscess detection, conventional ultrasound imaging has a relatively small role in the evaluation of colonic abnormalities. Although some early success has been reported using conventional ultrasonography to examine water-filled colons, its potential as a routine method of colon evaluation is questionable. The use of endoscopic sonography in the evaluation of rectal disease has increased, however, in most medical centers, with clinical research indicating that it is as accurate as, if not more accurate than, CT in the detection of disease, evaluation of the extent of disease, and determination of the absence or presence of affected regional lymph nodes. Ultrasonography is a safe examination with no significant complications reported to date.

SOLITARY FILLING DEFECT

The radiological problems of the colon and rectum are discussed as they relate to standard intraluminal contrast examinations of the colon. Other imaging techniques are included as part of the relevant discussion of the radiological problem under consideration.

Filling defect is a term historically rooted in the development of the SCBE and suggests displacement of barium by a space-occupying entity. For a focal area, a thinner barium column is presented for the x-ray beam to penetrate, resulting in less attenuation and producing a focal lucency. The term is used frequently when describing polypoid lesions on double-contrast studies, although technically these are usually not filling defects in the strict definition.

Box 7-1 Alone and Surrounded by Barium: Solitary Filling Defects of Colon

Cancer
Lipoma
Leiomyoma
Carcinoid
Unusual diverticula (more frequent than realized)
Lymphoma
Inverted appendiceal stump
Foreign body

The radiological problem of an intraluminal filling defect presents a wide variety of diagnostic possibilities and can be divided into benign neoplastic, malignant neoplastic, and a wide assortment of miscellaneous causes (Box 7-1). Inflammatory causes of a solitary filling defect are rare.

Adenoma

Most adenomatous polyps are solitary. In the presence of carcinoma, the incidence of multiple adenomatous polyps increases. Approximately 25% of patients with CRC have one or more adenomatous polyps elsewhere in the large bowel. It also is suggested that the presence of multiple hyperplastic polyps may be associated with an increase in the number of adenomas. The chance for multiplicity increases with age.

Adenomatous polyps histologically fall within the classification of tubular (80%), tubulovillous (10%), and villous adenoma (10%). Villous adenoma tends to have the greatest malignant potential, whereas tubular adenoma has the least. Adenomatous polyps are primarily tubular adenomas and frequently are smooth surfaced or lobulated. They may be sessile or pedunculated, having a stalk of varying lengths (Figs. 7-10 and 7-11). The stalk usually is composed of normal mucosal tissue and often is associated with larger polyps. Progressive peristaltic activity results in stretching of the base of the polyp and, over a prolonged period, elongation into a well-defined stalk. The villous adenoma has the typical frondlike papillary surface, often described by pathologists as being "velvety." They are almost always sessile, and the amount of lobulation may be considerably more than is seen with the tubular adenoma. The superficial "carpet lesions" of the colon are almost always villous adenomas or superficial carcinomas (Fig. 7-12). These surface characteristics,

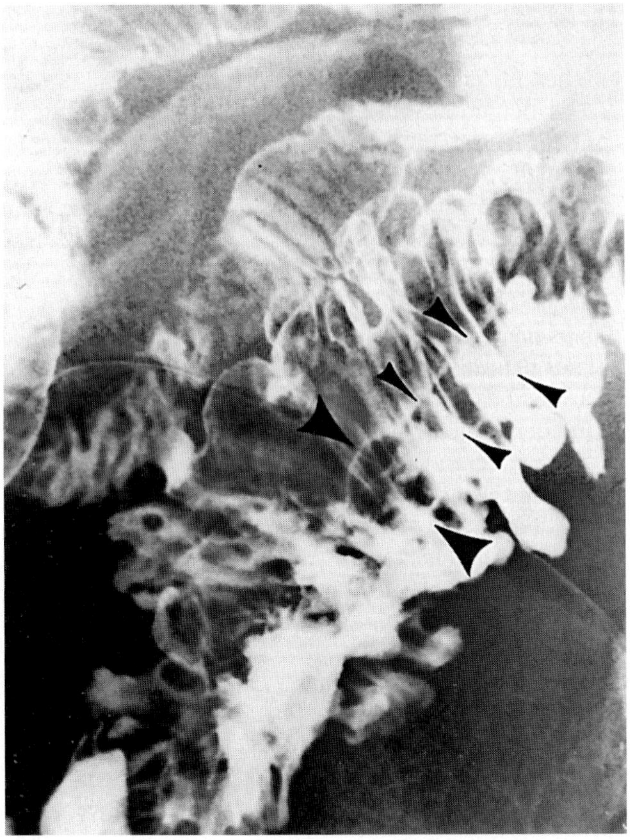

Figure 7-10 DCBE in a patient with severe diverticular disease of the sigmoid colon. A polyp on a long stalk is present *(arrowheads)* but is obscured by the multiple diverticula.

so familiar to radiologists, hold true for polyps greater than 1 cm but are less reliable for smaller lesions. The classic presentation of a villous adenoma is that of a patient presenting with watery diarrhea as a result of fluid and electrolyte loss from the large surface area of the lesion. This classic clinical presentation is, as with many "classic presentations," uncommon, but eventually is encountered by most radiologists (Fig. 7-13).

The frequency of adenomatous polyps in the general population has been found to vary markedly from study to study. Autopsy studies may provide the most consistent data, placing the incidence of adenomas larger than 1 cm

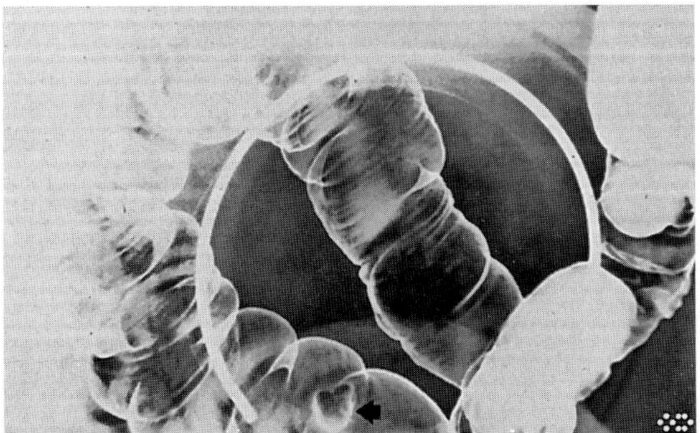

Figure 7-11 A sessile sigmoid polyp *(arrow)* is shown on DCBE.

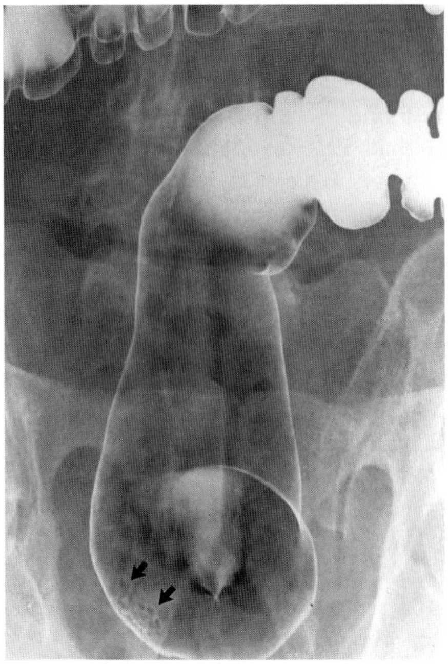

Figure 7-12 Focal nodularity (carpet lesion) of the rectum *(arrows)* proved to be villous adenoma.

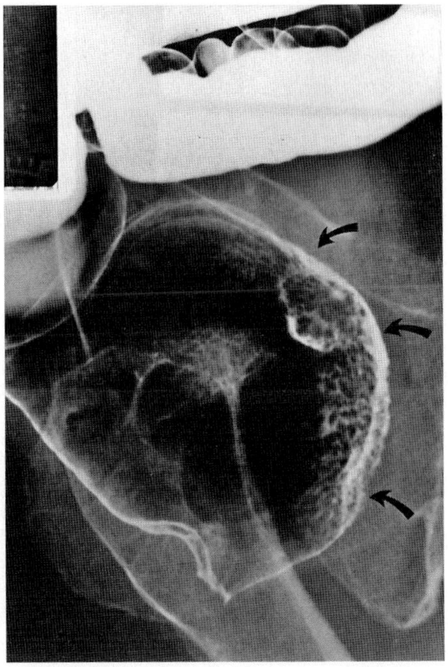

Figure 7-13 Large carpet lesion of the anterior rectum *(arrows)* in a patient presenting with diarrhea and incontinence. The lesion proved to be large villous adenoma.

between 10% and 15% of the population. The incidence increases significantly with age.

Various studies have indicated that most adenomatous polyps are found in the rectosigmoid region. It has been estimated that 50% of adenomas occur in this area, although in recent years some research has suggested a so-called proximal migration of colonic polyps. This migration may represent a combination of an increasingly aging population and improvements such as colonoscopy and DCBE in examining the colon.

It is now widely accepted that most CRCs result from malignant transformation of benign adenomatous polyps, the adenoma-carcinoma sequence. Estimations of the risk of malignant degeneration are imprecise; however, the well-differentiated tubular adenomas have a smaller risk than the more volatile villous adenomas. Only 0.01% of polyps less than 5 mm show dysplastic changes, whereas frank malignancy is virtually unknown among these "diminutive polyps." Malignant foci are seen in less than 1% of polyps measuring 5 to 10 mm. In polyps greater than 2 cm, the incidence increases dramatically to 30% to 40%. The time progression of adenoma to carcinoma evolution is estimated at 10 to 20 years, although startling exceptions are encountered from time to time (Fig. 7-14).

Most adenomas are asymptomatic. The most common presentation is rectal bleeding, either occult or overt. Additionally, polyps can act as the lead point for intussusception, although this is unusual in the colon. The classic association of large villous adenomas with loss of fluid and electrolytes (especially potassium) is infrequently encountered.

The detection rate of polyps is higher with double-contrast technique than with single-contrast technique. A high-kilovoltage, full-column technique, using fluoroscopic manipulation and compression, may have an equally high yield for polyps greater than 1 to 2 cm. Polyps less than 1 cm are detected with less frequency in both types of studies, although the ability to detect smaller polyps seems to be significantly higher in double-contrast studies than in single-contrast studies. As of yet, it is not clear that CT colonoscopy is an improvement over ACBE in the detection of small polyps (Figs. 7-15 and 7-16).

The radiographic appearance of polyps on full-column, single-contrast studies is often that of the traditional filling defect. The appearance on double-contrast studies is more complex because this technique provides the ability literally to see through the colon, observing both mucosal surfaces at the same time. As a result, the polyp can be seen profiled, en face, or tangentially, resulting in different well-known appearances, such as the "Mexican hat" sign (Fig. 7-17) or the "bowler hat" sign. Evaluation of the polyp should include size, the presence or absence of a stalk or pedicle, description of the surface features, and the presence or absence of ulceration. With respect to size, at least an approximate 25% magnification distortion should be figured into the final estimation of the polyp size.

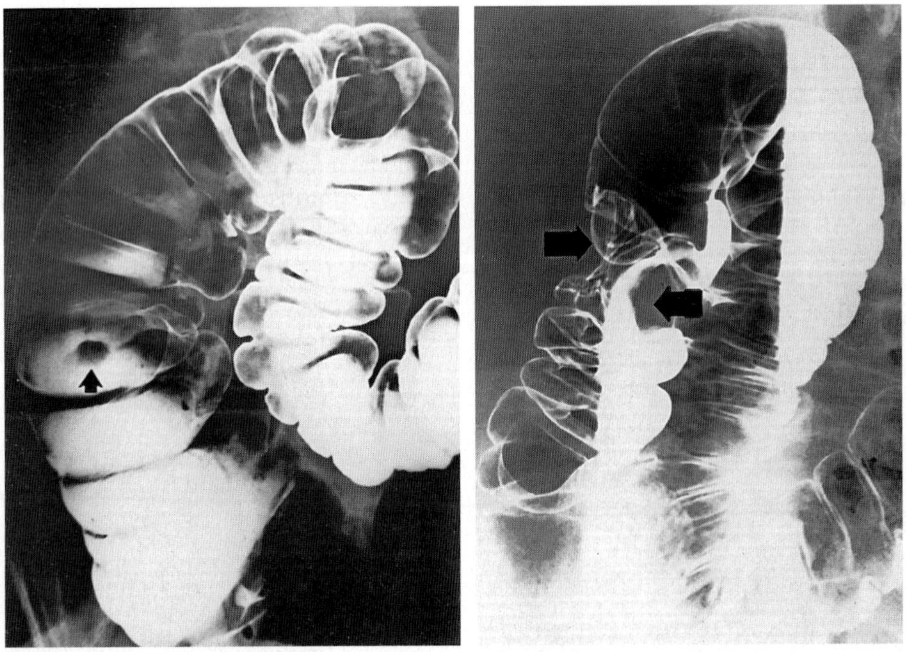

A B

Figure 7-14 **A,** Barium enema discloses a 1.5-cm pedunculated polyp in the ascending colon *(arrow)*. **B,** DCBE obtained less than 2 years later in the same patient reveals an annular carcinoma at the site of the polyp seen on the earlier examination.

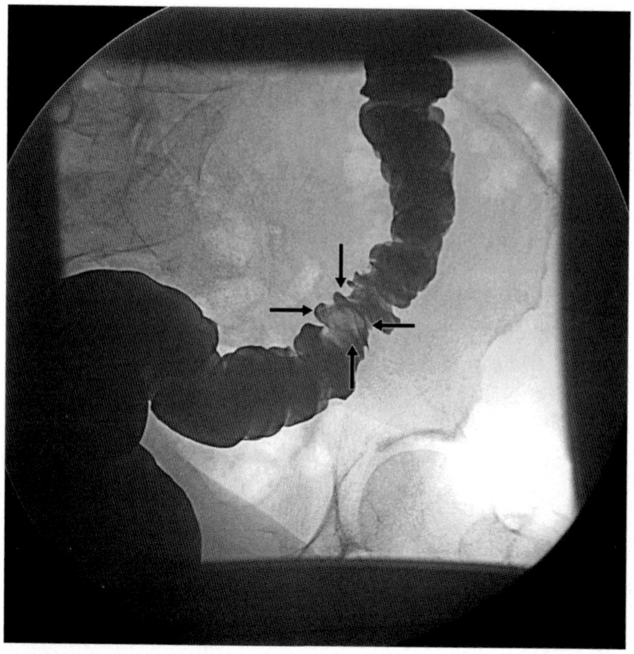

Figure 7-15 Barium shows filling defect caused by polyp in sigmoid colon *(arrows)*.

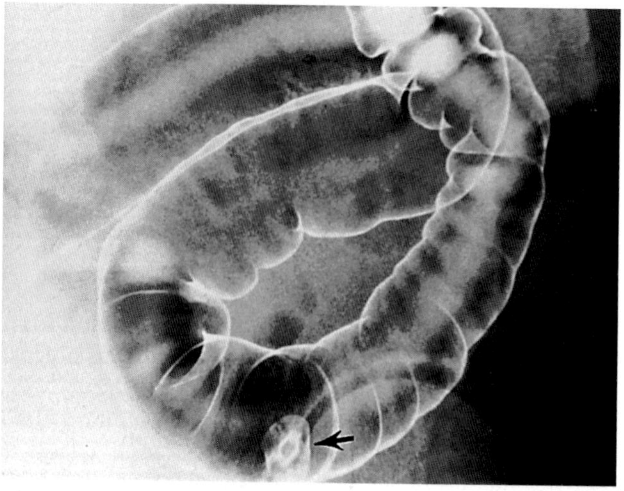

Figure 7-17 Sigmoid spot film shows a polyp *(arrow)* with a central "ring shadow" representing barium coating of the short stalk of the polyp. This configuration is sometimes known as the Mexican hat sign.

The polyp that often provides the most difficulty in radiological diagnosis during DCBE is the polyp on a long stalk (Fig. 7-18). Because it shifts position with the various views, it may be misinterpreted as residual stool. Occasionally, these polyps can be quite large, reminding us that the interpretation of double-contrast studies by necessity must include a meticulous evaluation of the various lines and contours of the colon. There is a dictum in gastrointestinal radiology that double-contrast radiology of the colon is an excellent examination, with the only difficulties being lesions that are extremely tiny or are extremely large. This dictum occasionally can become an embarrassing reality.

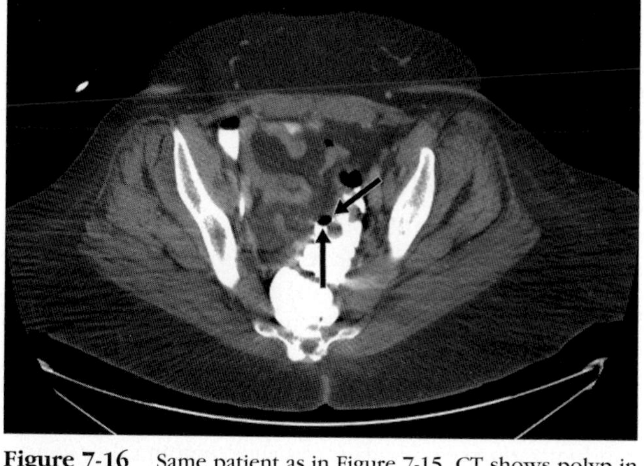

Figure 7-16 Same patient as in Figure 7-15. CT shows polyp in sigmoid *(arrows)*.

Carcinoma

In 2001, 135,000 new cases of CRC were diagnosed. Around 57,000 deaths were attributable to this disease in 2001. Cases of CRC are estimated to increase slightly over the next decade. In 1992, one estimate was that between 150,000 and 160,000 new cases would be seen by 1998. In fact, the rate has leveled off. Mortality rates also have declined in recent years, after several decades of relative stability. Even so, CRC still remains the most common newly diagnosed malignancy after cancer of the prostate, breast, and lung. The CRC rate among men and women is about equal. Only lung cancer exceeds CRC in terms of cancer deaths. For any given patient, survival depends on how early the lesion is diagnosed. Dukes' classification (first introduced in 1929 and modified many times over the years), on which the staging of CRC is based, reflects the extent of tumor involvement and the prognosis. Dukes' stage A represents lesions confined to the mucosa and has an 85% 5-year survival rate. Dukes' stage B1 represents lesions that have extended to, but not through, the muscularis propria. Stage B2 is representative of tumor penetrating the muscularis propria but with no lymph node involvement. These are associated with a 70% 5-year survival rate. With Dukes' stage C1 representing bowel wall involvement and C2 penetration of the bowel wall and both with spread to regional lymph nodes, the survival rate declines to 33%. Distant metastatic disease, Dukes' stage D, has a 5% 5-year survival rate. It has been estimated that 40% to 50% of patients have hepatic metastatic disease at the time of diagnosis.

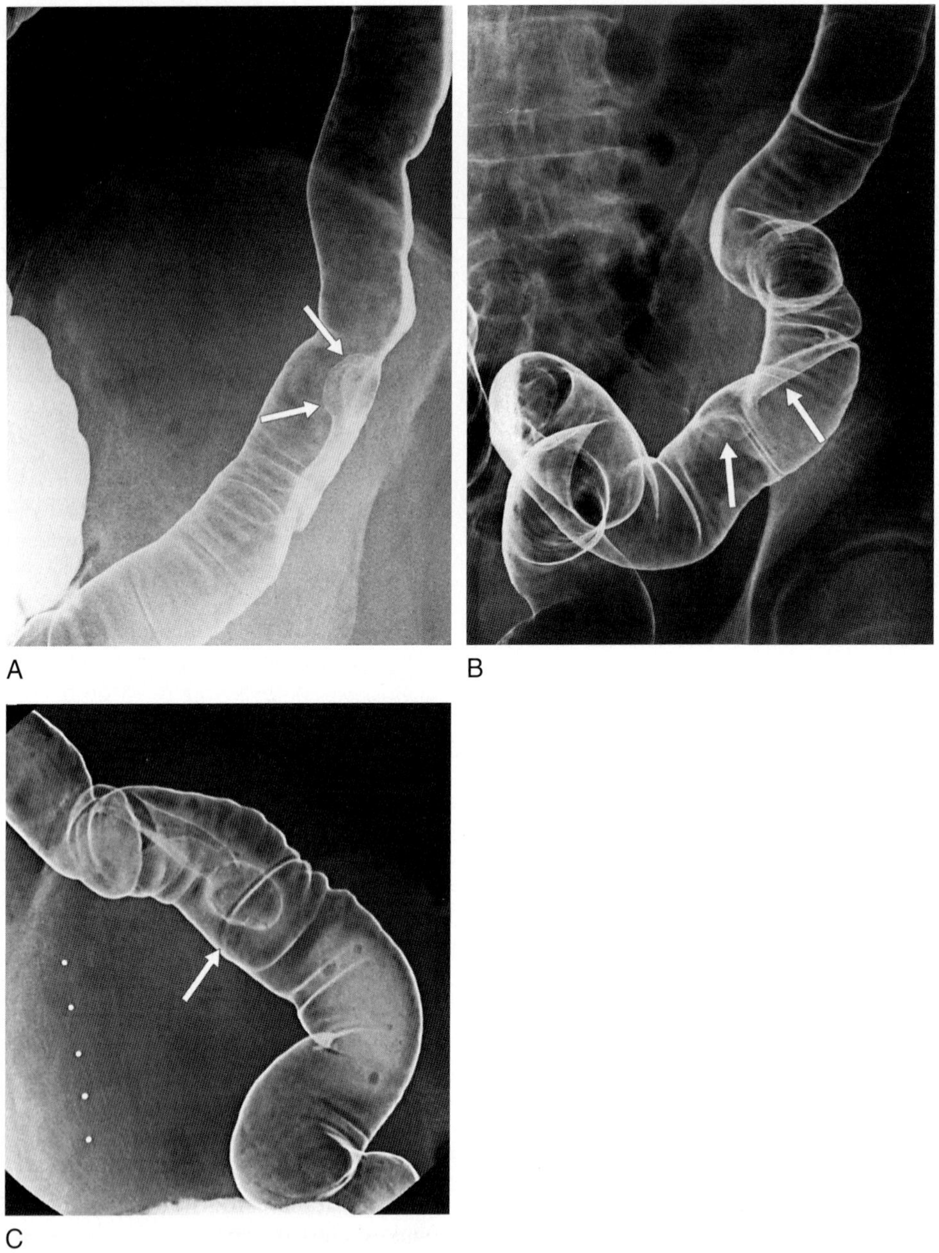

Figure 7-18 A 76-year-old man presented with blood in his stool. A polyp on a long stalk is seen in the distal descending colon. **A,** On left-side-down decubitus view, the polyp lays out along the lateral wall *(arrows)*. **B,** On right-side-down decubitus view, the polyp and stalk cross the lumen near the medial wall *(arrows)*. **C,** A digital spot view nicely shows the entire polyp *(arrow)*.

In an attempt to define a universally more applicable and orderly process across the world, the American Joint Committee on Cancer introduced the tumor-node-metastases (TNM) classification for colorectal malignancies (Box 7-2). In the randomization of patients in therapeutic trials, the TNM classification has largely replaced Dukes' classification. This classification divides the classification of tumor into five stages dependent on the extent of tumor (*T*), the status of regional lymph node involvement (*N*), and the presence or absence of distant metastatic disease (*M*). Individual cases are assigned according to the extent of disease based on TNM values and are grouped further into five stages, 0 to IV. The TNM classification is in common usage at institutional tumor boards or conferences all over the United States and most of the world and is crucial in the uniform randomization of patients for various ongoing therapeutic trials.

Box 7-2 American Joint Committee on Cancer Tumor-Node-Metastases Staging System

STAGE 0

Carcinoma in situ—T_{is}, N0, M0

STAGE I

Tumor invading submucosa—T1, N0, M0
Tumor invading muscularis propria—T2, N0, M0

STAGE II

Tumor penetrates beyond muscularis propria into subserosa but not peritoneum—T3, N0, M0
Tumor penetrates into peritoneum or directly invades other structures or organs—T4, N0, M0

STAGE III

Any degree of bowel wall penetration with regional lymph node spread
N1—one to three pericolic or perirectal lymph nodes involved
N2—four or more lymph nodes involved
N3—metastatic disease in any lymph node along a vascular trunk
Any T, N1 or N2 or N3, M0

STAGE IV

Tumor invasion of bowel wall with or without lymph node involvement, but distant metastatic disease
Any T, any N, M1

CRC continues to be mainly a disease of Western industrialized nations. It is a disease of older individuals, with the median patient age at diagnosis in the 60s. The etiological and epidemiological data associated with this disease are ponderous and cannot be addressed in detail. The issues and controversies surrounding the possible causes are becoming more openly discussed in the lay media as the United States becomes more conscious of nutrition and health and as notable individuals in the public eye have had this illness. The controversy surrounding suspected causes and associated risk factors includes dietary intake, with particular emphasis on increasing the ingestion of dietary fiber and decreasing the ingestion of animal fats. Observations have been put forth suggesting that intake of vitamin C, aspirin, or nonsteroidal anti-inflammatory drugs on a regular basis may confer some degree of protection. In 1997, there were reports that vitamin E bestowed some protection from the disease. Additionally, there has been further evidence that vitamin D and dietary calcium may confer some protection. These are interesting possibilities, but require considerable further investigation.

There are some things about which clinicians are more certain, and one is that most CRCs progress through the adenoma-to-cancer route. A few may arise de novo from dysplastic changes within the mucosal surface, although this is believed to be uncommon in patients without IBD. IBD, in particular, ulcerative colitis, carries a higher risk for the development of CRC. Certain familial polyposis syndromes carry an extremely high, if not absolute certain, risk of cancer. CRC can run in families with sporadic manifestation, and in approximately 25% of new cases there is a family history of CRC. It has been estimated that individuals who are first-generation relatives of patients with CRC have a 10% to 15% increased risk above that of the general population.

Hereditary nonpolyposis CRC has been recognized in recent years as a disease of autosomal dominant inheritance in which colon cancers arise via the recognized adenoma-to-cancer mechanism, but the marked colonic polyposis of familial polyposis (hundreds or thousands of polyps) does not occur. The definition of hereditary nonpolyposis CRC has been standardized. Families must have at least three relatives with CRC, one of whom must be a first-degree relative of the other two. CRC must involve at least two consecutive generations, and one case must occur before age 50. These families may be divided further as being at risk for only CRC (Lynch syndrome I) or other cancers (particularly of the female genital tract) in addition to CRC (Lynch syndrome II). It is estimated that hereditary nonpolyposis CRC may account for 5% to 6% of CRCs (Box 7-3).

The clinical presentation of CRC depends to a large extent on the site of the lesion. During early stages of growth, the patient may be asymptomatic or there may be undetected occult bleeding (Fig. 7-19). The most insidious lesions usually arise from the right side of the colon; this occurs because the wider luminal diameter, greater distensibility of the right colon, and more liquid nature of the colonic content on the right side delay the onset of obstructive symptoms and allow the lesion to become larger and more invasive before the diagnosis is finally made (Fig. 7-20). Patients with right-sided lesions often present with frank bleeding or positive fecal occult blood testing. They may experience crampy, nonspecific

Box 7-3 Risk Factors for CRC

Habitation in an industrialized region of the world
Diet
Familial polyposis
Family history of hereditary nonpolyposis CRC
Chronic ulcerative colitis
First-generation family member with CRC
Presence or history of colonic adenomatous polyps

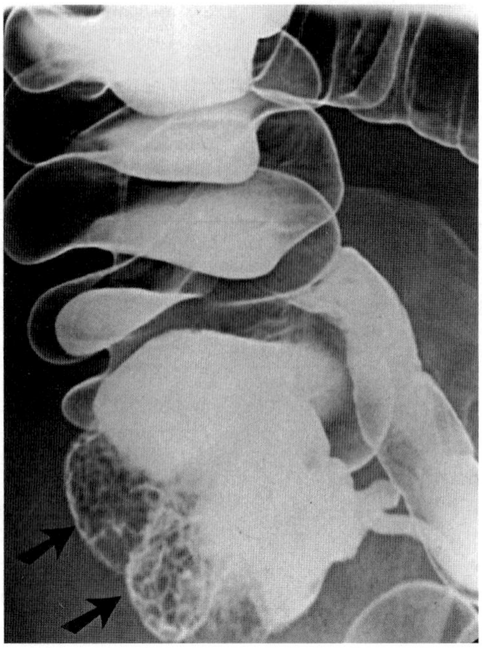

Figure 7-19 A 53-year-old patient presented with Hemoccult-positive stool. ACBE shows superficial spreading carcinoma of the cecum *(arrows)*.

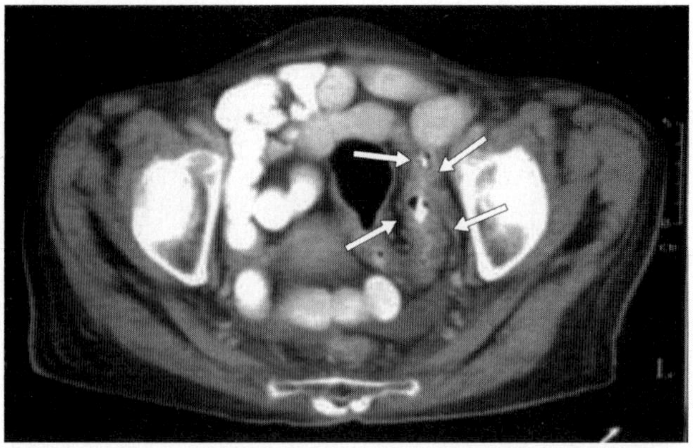

Figure 7-21 Thickened wall and narrowed lumen are a common presentation of a right-sided malignant lesion *(arrows)*. Note the length of the stricture, which could be confused with diverticulitis.

right-sided abdominal pain. The most common presenting problem is iron deficiency anemia as a result of chronic blood loss. Tumors on the left side, in the descending and sigmoid colon, tend to manifest earlier (Fig. 7-21); this is a result of the smaller luminal diameter of the colon in this region and the firmer colonic content. Changes in the luminal diameter, secondary to tumor growth, most commonly result in obstruction (Figs. 7-22 and 7-23). A common exception should be mentioned, however, regarding left-sided lesions. Some tumors in the sigmoid colon or descending colon that are slow growing can attain significant size without resulting in the expected obstruction. Because of the indolent nature of the lesion, its physical contours to some extent can be molded by the fecal stream, assuming a form of "flap valve" configuration. It is possible to find a distal lesion with complete retrograde obstruction on barium enema, with no physical or radiological evidence of antegrade obstruction (Fig. 7-24). Lesions in the rectum commonly present with bright red bleeding and changes in bowel habits. Generally, lesions in the distal colon are detected earlier, and survival is better. Approximately 50% of lesions are found distal to the mid-descending colon. Rarely, colonic adenocarcinoma can perforate, and the patient may present with a pericolic abscess.

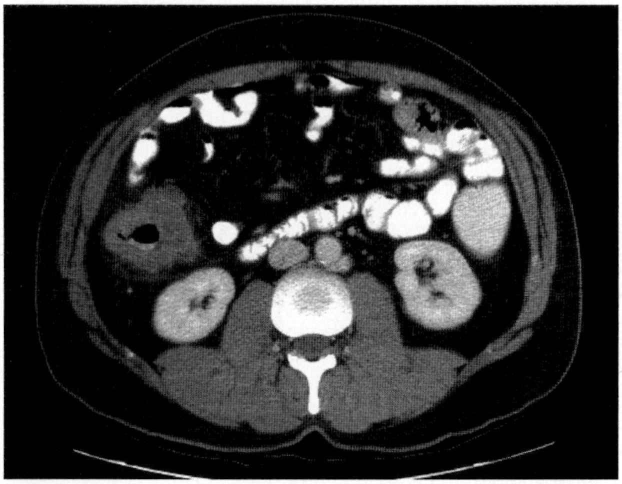

Figure 7-20 CT shows thickened irregular cecal wall with pericolic stranding caused by adenocarcinoma.

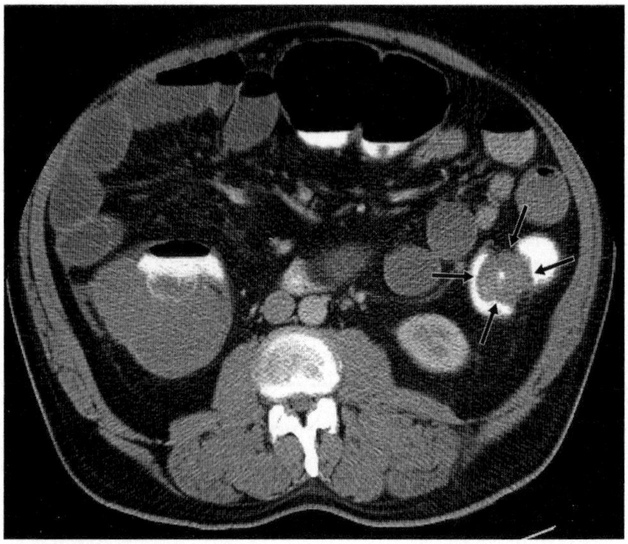

Figure 7-22 An apple core lesion is seen in the descending colon *(arrows)*, causing narrowing, obstruction, and proximal dilatation.

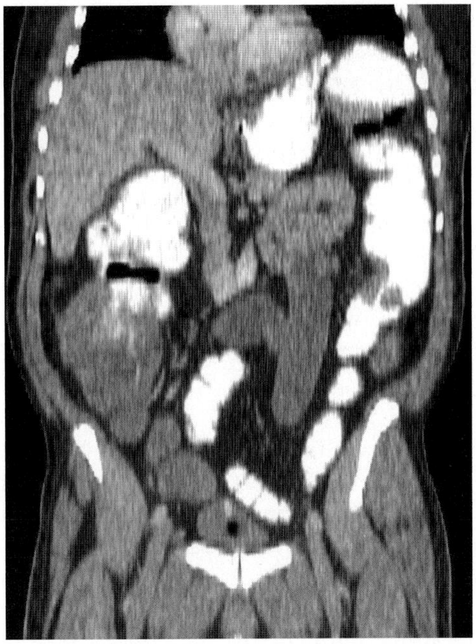

Figure 7-23 Coronal reconstruction of the same patient as in Figure 7-22 shows the obstructing lesion to advantage.

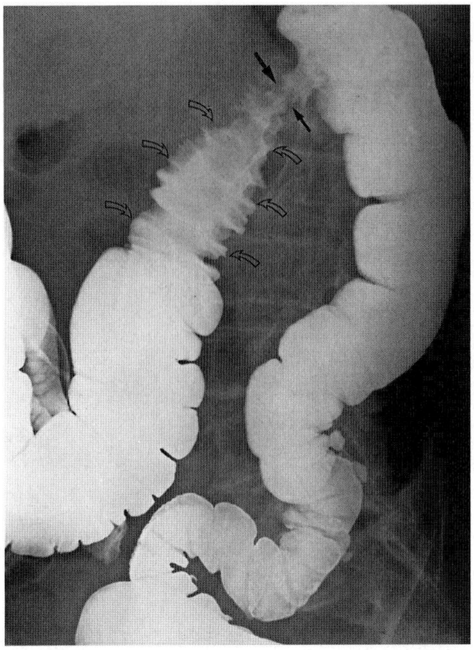

Figure 7-25 SCBE in patient with carcinoma of the distal transverse colon *(solid arrows)* and evidence of fold thickening proximal to the lesion *(open arrows)*, which proved to be ischemic changes.

Also seen infrequently are lesions with ischemic changes immediately proximal to the malignancy (Fig. 7-25).

Given the impact of CRC in terms of morbidity and mortality, a complete examination of the colon is required. Although flexible sigmoidoscopy can examine 50 cm, this still results in approximately half of the lesions being undetected. Colonoscopy permits direct examination of the mucosal surface of the entire length of the colon and is without doubt the most effective tool available for the complete and most efficient examination of the colon. It can be of considerable value because it permits removal of polyps and the retrieval of tissue specimens for pathological diagnosis. The examination is incomplete, however, in at least 10% of attempts (Fig. 7-26). Colonoscopy is a relatively expensive undertaking, and its use as a screening agent would be a prohibitive burden on the strained health care resources in the United States.

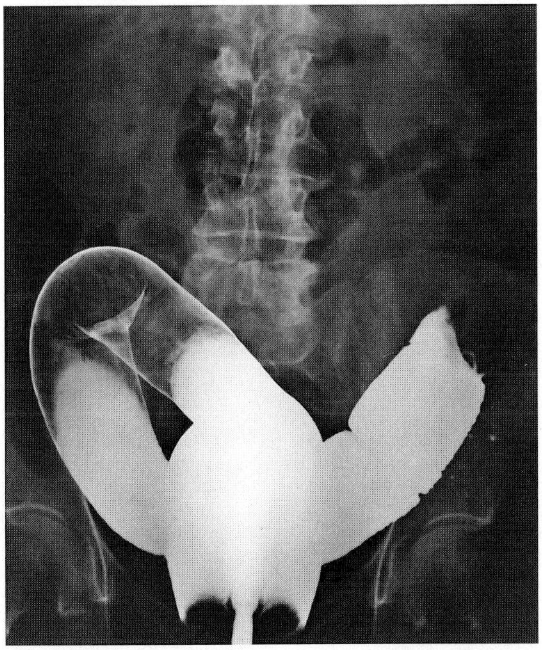

Figure 7-24 A 68-year-old woman presented with gastrointestinal bleeding, but no evidence of bowel obstruction. ACBE shows obstructing lesion at junction of sigmoid colon and descending colon. The retrograde obstruction is complete. Note the radiological evidence of complete lack of antegrade obstruction.

The DCBE is a relatively low-cost examination with a relatively high rate of detection for CRCs (94%) and an extremely low rate of incomplete examinations. This examination is considerably safer than instrumentation, having one tenth to one hundredth the incidence of bowel perforation associated with colonoscopy.

Problems associated with DCBE relate to bowel preparation and coexistent diverticular disease. Both of these factors can render the examination less sensitive. The presence of extensive diverticular disease in the sigmoid region results in such significant bowel distortion that it may be impossible to identify a polypoid lesion. Single-contrast compression views of this area would be much more useful in detecting polypoid lesions in this situation. Additionally, residual stool can be troublesome. Double-contrast examinations ought to include decubitus

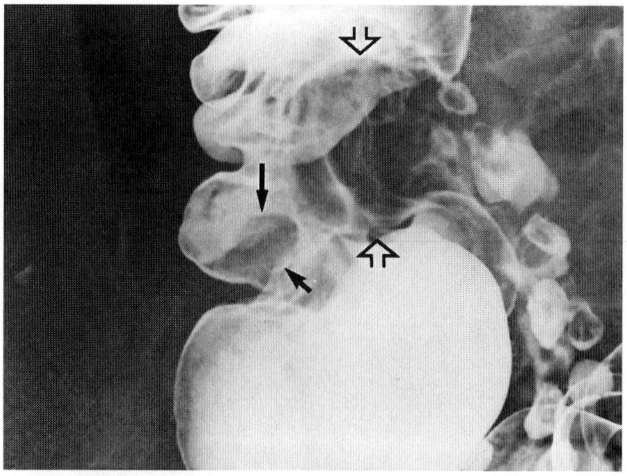

Figure 7-26 A 65-year-old woman presented with Hemoccult-positive stool. Colonoscopy is incomplete, and the right colon is unexamined. ACBE shows a lesion arising in *(open arrows)* and around *(solid arrows)* the ileocecal valve.

views, which often can sort out these problems. Other areas of difficulty include the ileocecal region and the wall of the ascending colon, where subtle or occult lesions can hide (Fig. 7-27). Most missed CRCs on double-contrast examination have been shown to be errors of perception. The importance of meticulous and careful analysis of double-contrast views of the colon cannot be overstated. Interpretation of these studies is an exercise in self-discipline and concentration.

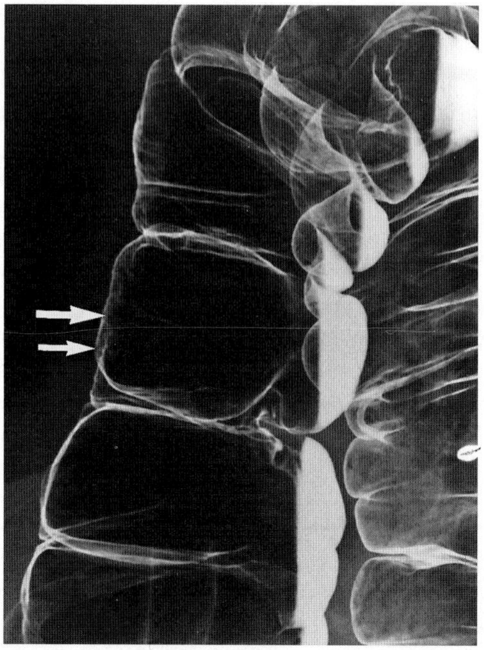

Figure 7-27 A 70-year-old woman with a family history of carcinoma of the colon. ACBE shows a focal area of marginal irregularity in the ascending colon *(arrows)*. Biopsy showed it to be superficial spreading carcinoma.

Box 7-4 Radiological Presentations of CRC

COMMON

Annular lesions
Polypoid lesions

LESS COMMON

Infiltrative lesions with little mass effect
Superficial surface (carpet) lesions

The radiological findings of CRC can include numerous configurations (Box 7-4), from round polypoid filling defects to encircling, constricting lesions. They also can be seen as raised, ulcerated masses or as irregular, villous-appearing lesions (Fig. 7-28). More subtle lesions may be manifested as distortions in the normal haustral pattern or bowel wall contours (Figs. 7-29 to 7-31).

Frequently, CT of the abdomen reveals a soft tissue mass adjacent to or within the colonic lumen (Fig. 7-32). One should take care not to misinterpret a prolapsed ileocecal valve or stool as a cecal mass (Figs. 7-33 and 7-34). There may be evidence of extension of the tumor beyond the wall or involvement of adjacent organs, such as lymph nodes or the liver. Ultrasonography may show a large hypoechoic mass with some central echoes representing thickened bowel wall and the central lumen. This finding is nonspecific and can be seen in other conditions, such as lymphoma, Crohn's disease, or intussusception. Transrectal endosonography has been shown to be a potentially useful technique in the evaluation of the spread of rectal carcinoma into the perirectal soft tissues.

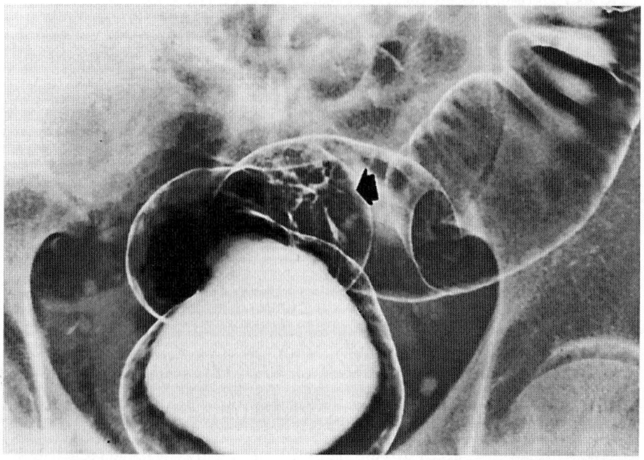

Figure 7-28 Spot film from DCBE reveals a focal area of raised, irregular mucosa with radiation toward a small, central mound *(arrow)*. Biopsy specimen showed villous adenoma with malignant degeneration.

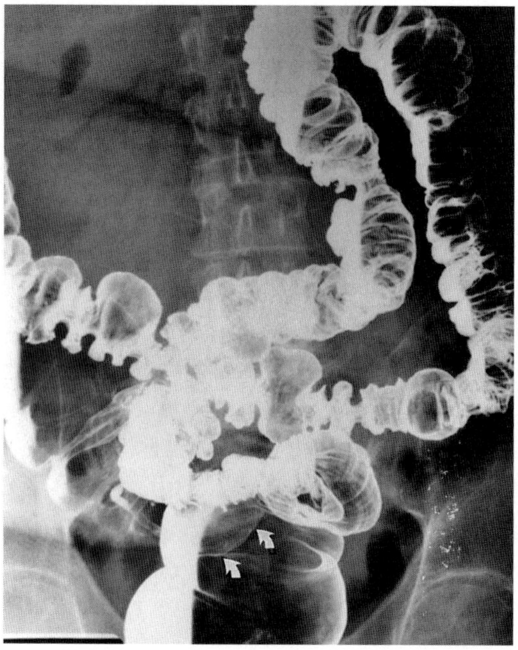

Figure 7-29 A polypoid lesion of the rectum *(arrows)* seen clearly only on the left decubitus film.

Early reports suggest that it is more accurate than conventional CT in evaluating the extent of invasion.

Metastatic spread of CRC can be seen in a variety of presentations. Large bulky masses may be seen in the mesentery or retroperitoneum (Fig. 7-35). Widespread disease can occur throughout the liver (Fig. 7-36). Metastatic lesions may be seen in the adrenals (Fig. 7-37). Bony metastases are common in CRC (Fig. 7-38).

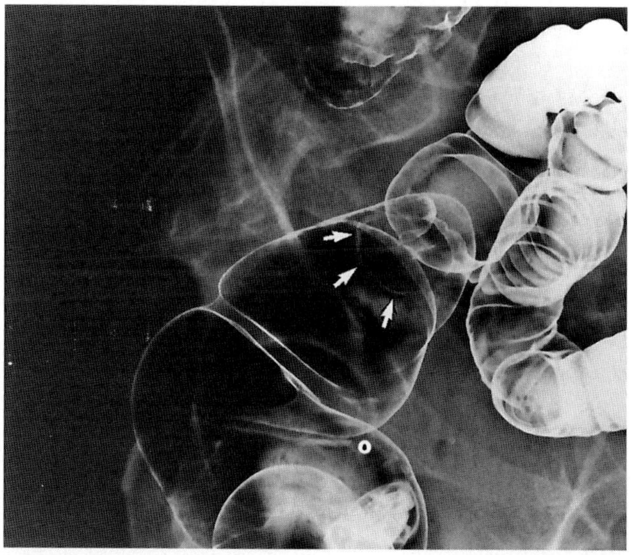

Figure 7-30 A 58-year-old man presented with Hemoccult-positive stool. A subtle polypoid carcinoma is seen in the sigmoid as an abnormal margin *(arrows)*.

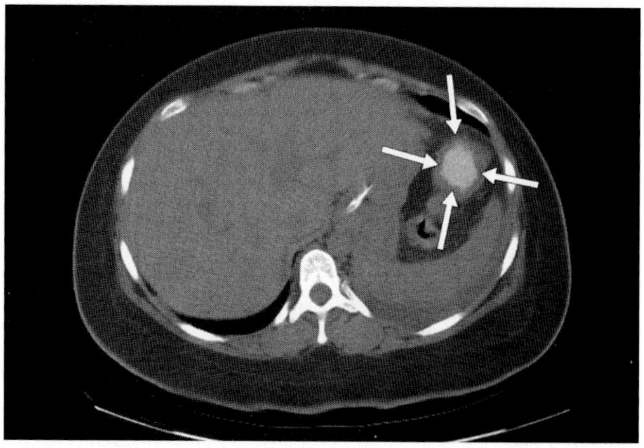

Figure 7-31 Colonic carcinoma of the splenic flexure is seen as bowel thickening and irregularity on CT *(arrows)*.

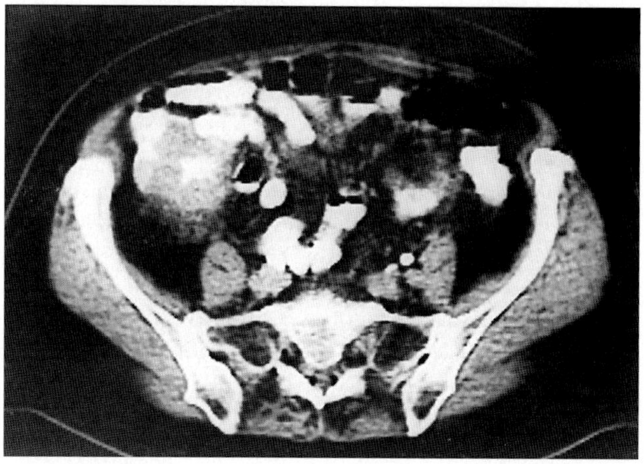

Figure 7-32 CT of the pelvis in an anemic patient reveals a mass within the cecum with extension beyond the cecal wall posteriorly. There is no evidence of obstruction, and the lesion proved to be an adenocarcinoma.

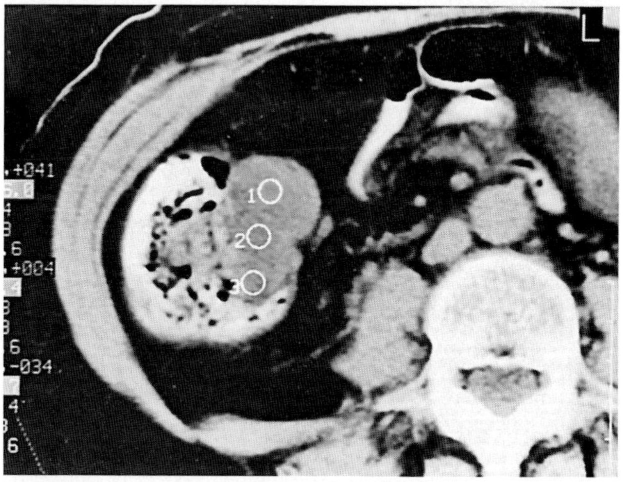

Figure 7-33 CT in a patient with vague abdominal complaints. A cecal mass was diagnosed *(circles)*, and a barium enema examination was performed for further evaluation (see Fig. 7-34).

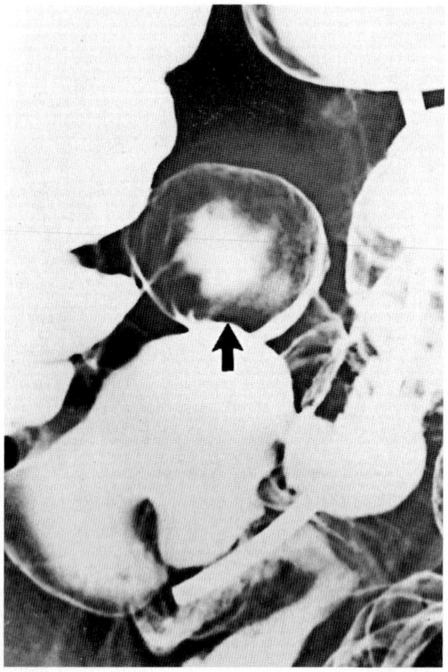

Figure 7-34 DCBE obtained in a patient with diagnosis of a cecal mass (see Fig. 7-33) on CT shows a normal cecum. Reflux into the terminal ileum shows some focal dilatation without evidence of obstruction or disease *(arrow)*. This fluid-filled terminal ileum, partially prolapsed through the ileocecal valve, accounts for the CT findings.

It is not unusual to encounter a relatively small, apparently contained lesion on the ACBE only to find widespread distribution on CT (Fig. 7-39). Other common sites of metastasis include lungs and brain. Intraperitoneal spread of colorectal lesions often is accompanied by malignant ascites (Fig. 7-40).

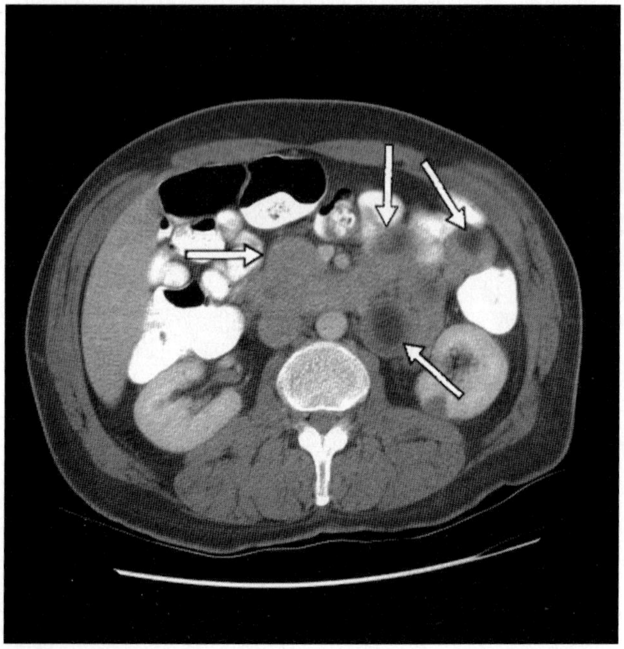

Figure 7-35 Metastatic CRC is seen as large mesenteric and retroperitoneal masses *(arrows)*.

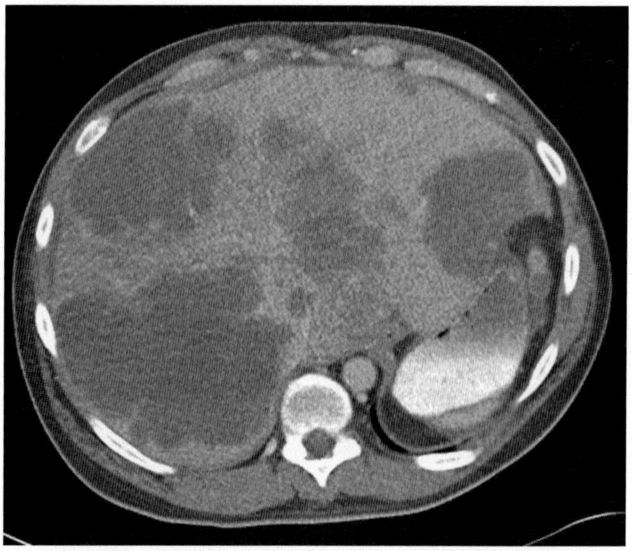

Figure 7-36 Widespread involvement of the liver with metastatic colon carcinoma is seen.

Rectal malignancies can manifest as large, bulky lesions or as intramural infiltrative lesions or both (Fig. 7-41). An unusual lesion under the category of rectal carcinomas is the cloacogenic carcinoma (Fig. 7-42). This is a rare tumor seen at the anorectal junction and arising from remnants of the cloacal membrane. The lesion is aggressive, and in more than half of the patients lymphatic spread will have occurred at the time of diagnosis. The tumor varies in its radiological presentation. It is seen most commonly on the anterior rectal wall and has all the appearances of a typical bulky rectal adenocarcinoma. Additionally, well-defined submucosal masses or mucosal plaques may be seen.

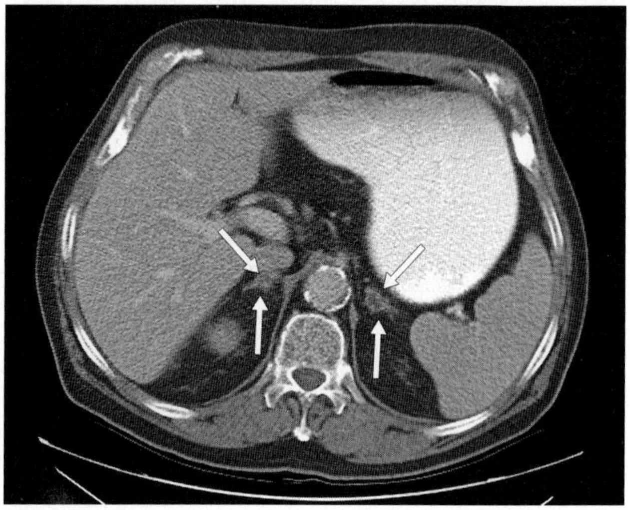

Figure 7-37 Small colorectal metastases are seen in both adrenal glands *(arrows)*.

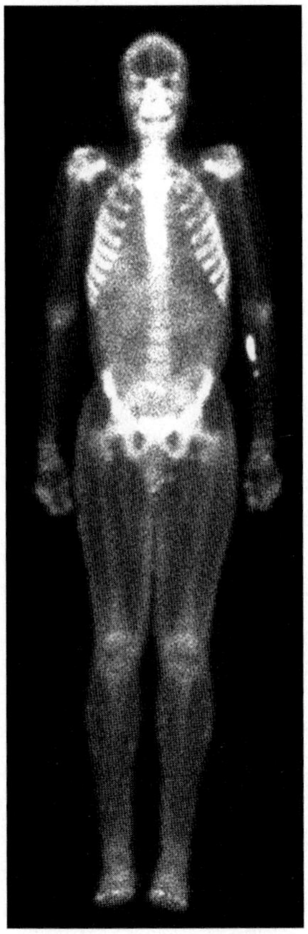

Figure 7-38 A bone scan of a patient with colon carcinoma shows extensive involvement of the bony structures in the upper body.

Synchronous CRC lesions (two or more lesions discovered at the same time) are uncommon, occurring in only 1% to 2% of cases (Fig. 7-43). Metachronous lesions (a second lesion discovered subsequently and unrelated to the previous lesion) can occur in approximately 5% of patients.

Lipoma

Lipomas of the colon are uncommon, but represent the next most common benign tumor of the large bowel after adenomas. These lesions are not included in the spectrum of mesenchymal tumors now called "stromal cell tumors" of the gastrointestinal tract. They are mostly solitary lesions and can occur anywhere within the colon, although the right side seems to be the most frequent site.

The lesion is usually asymptomatic, but erosions or ulcers on the mucosal surface overlying the lipoma can result in bleeding. The lipoma generally is 1 to 3 cm in size and rarely exceeds 4 cm. It shows the typical radiological findings of a submucosal lesion with a smooth surface and a right or obtuse angle formed with the adjacent mucosal surface. Occasionally, there can be some pedunculation of the lipoma. Because of the softness of the tumor, these lesions, particularly the larger ones, can change shape with compression, and this can be a helpful method of differentiating them from other neoplasms. The old diagnostic trick of performing a water enema to show the lipoma (which is less than water density) is virtually useless. CT of a sufficiently large lesion (>2 cm) can show the lipoma definitively as a fatty tumor. Lipomatous infiltration of the ileocecal valve is not considered a neoplastic process.

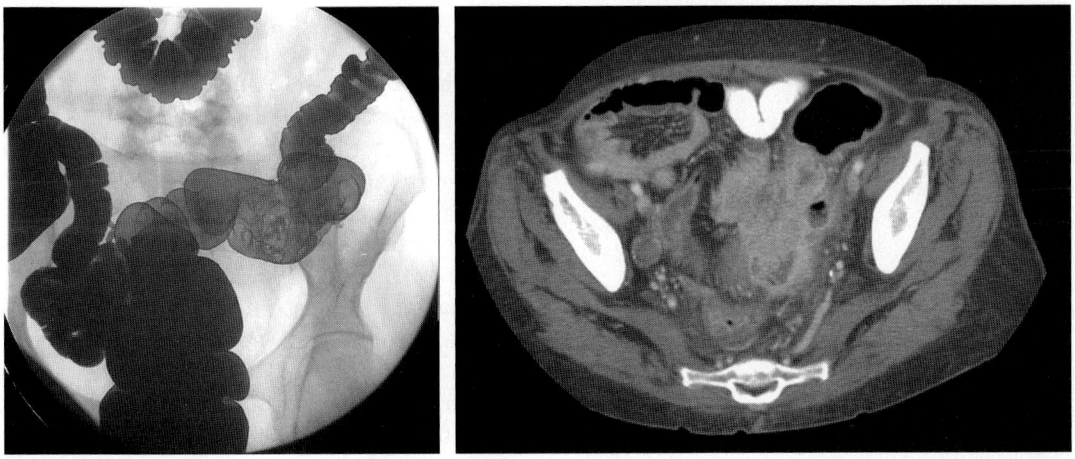

A B

Figure 7-39 **A,** ACBE shows marked nodularity and irregularity in the sigmoid colon. There is no obstruction or unusually large masses. This was seen to be adenocarcinoma on biopsy. **B,** CT through the pelvis in the same patient shows widespread invasion of adjacent structures, lymph nodes, and mesentery.

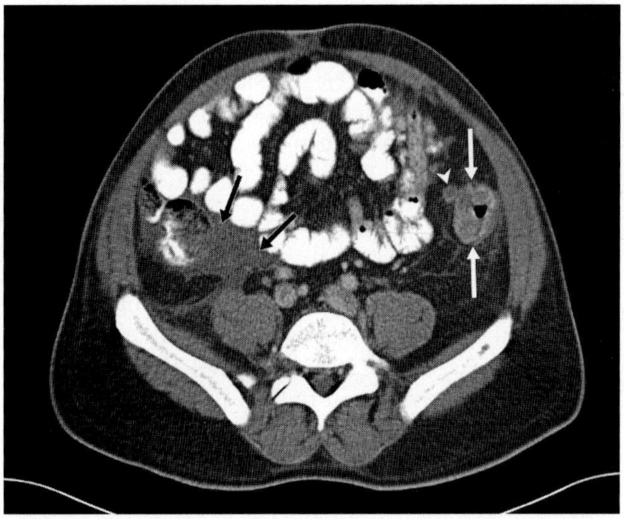

Figure 7-40 Intraperitoneal spread of colorectal lesion *(black arrows)* is accompanied by ascites *(white arrows)* and nodules *(arrowhead)*.

Stromal Cell Tumor (Leiomyoma)

Although common in the more proximal gastrointestinal tract, stromal cell tumors, which are benign mesenchymal (spindle or epitheloid) tumors, are relatively uncommon in the colon; they constitute less than 5% of these lesions seen in the gut (Fig. 7-44). In the anorectal area, they are extremely rare. Stromal cell tumors usually manifest as a submucosal colonic mass with the usual radiological findings (Fig. 7-45). They also may manifest as an exophytic lesion. Patients are mostly asymptomatic. Bleeding from ulceration on the stretched mucosal surface over the stromal cell tumor may result in the patient presenting with rectal bleeding or anemia. Rarely, the stromal cell tumor may act as a lead point for an intussusception. Intussusception in adults should be viewed with some alarm, however, because most of these are the result of malignant lesions.

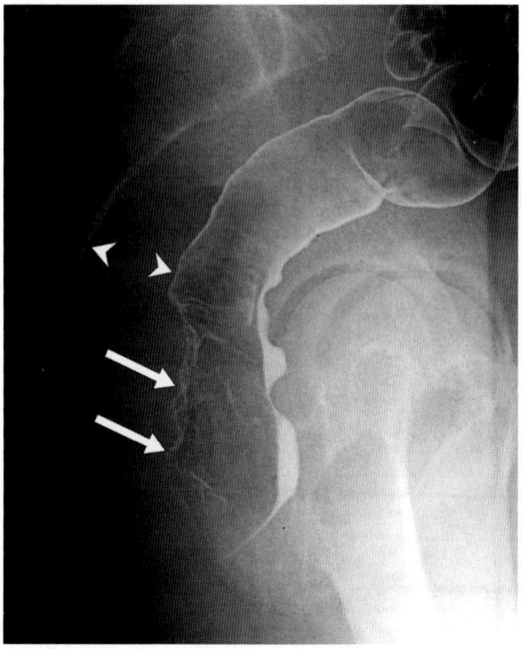

Figure 7-41 A large, primarily infiltrating lesion involving the rectum *(arrows)*. Note the widening of the presacral space *(arrowheads)*.

Another rare mesenchymal tumor that has been described in the colon is the hemangioma. These tumors are often located distally in the colon and are almost always multiple. Calcified phleboliths are occasionally seen on plain films. These patients most commonly present with bleeding.

Carcinoid Tumor

Approximately 85% to 90% of all carcinoid tumors of the gastrointestinal tract occur in the appendix and are benign. Although previously thought to be tumors arising from the neural crest, there is now evidence to suggest the origin of carcinoid tumors may be primary differentiation from within the intestine itself. Being neuroendocrine lesions, they may be seen in multiple endocrine neoplasia type I. Approximately 10% of patients with multiple endocrine neoplasia type I have a carcinoid tumor. Carcinoids also have been linked loosely to the APUD grouping of tumors (tumor of amine precursor uptake and decarboxylation). The ileum is the next most common site. Colorectal carcinoids compose about 20% of all carcinoids, with the more common sites being the rectum and, to a lesser degree, the cecum and ascending colon. The incidence of rectal carcinoids has been increasing over the past few decades. The tumors are often quite small, measuring 1 cm on average. They also may be of considerable size, however, particularly in the right side of the colon. Smaller lesions may have a typical mucosal polypoid appearance on barium enema. Larger lesions may be indistinguishable from an adenocarcinoma. Overall, survival seems to be greater with the rectal lesions. In general, survival with malignant carcinoids is related to the size of the tumor at the time of diagnosis.

Imaging diagnosis in the colon can be difficult, and the inclusion of a suggestive history by referring physicians (as would be expected in any physical or imaging examination of the body) and the knowledge of elevated 5-hydroxyindoleacetic acid significantly improves diagnostic accuracy. Multidector CT, ACBE, positron emission tomography, and nuclear medicine all have a role to play in the diagnostic workup of these patients.

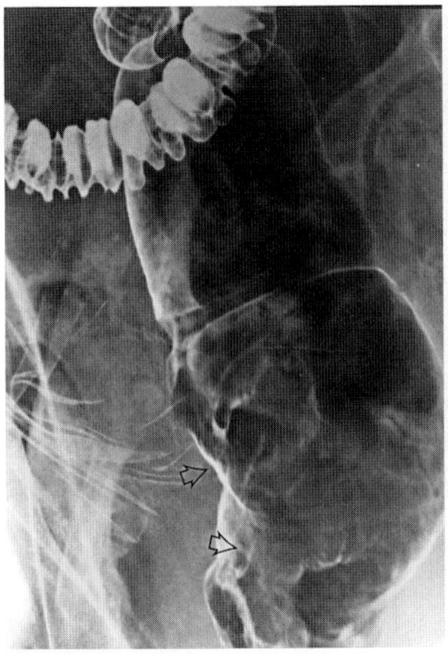
A

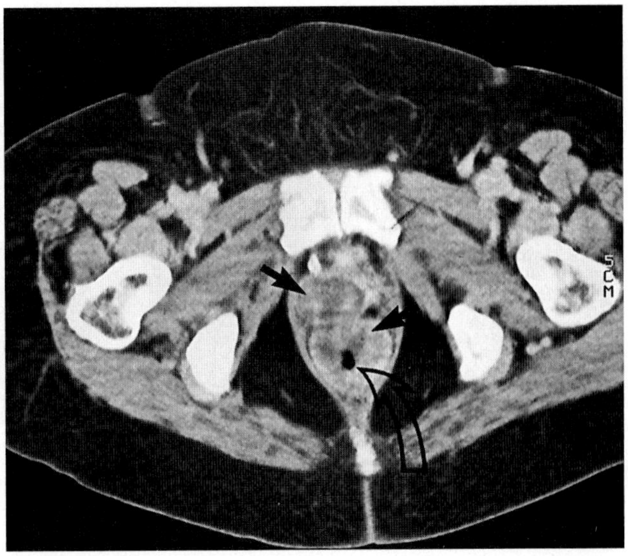

B

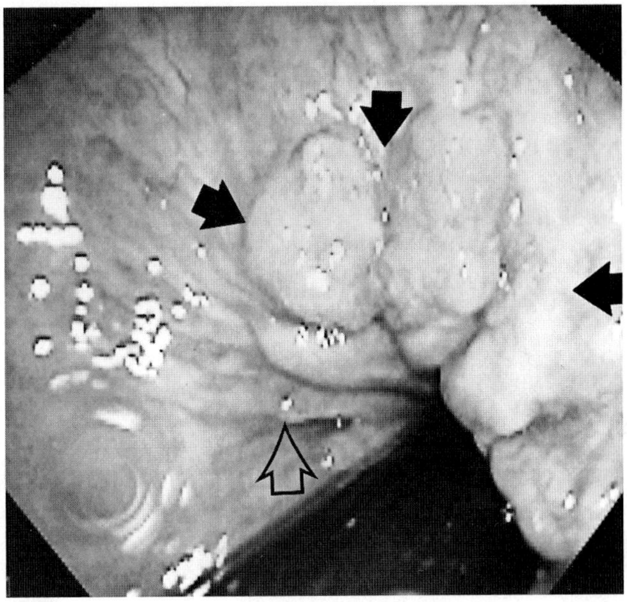
C

Figure 7-42 A 71-year-old woman presents with low rectal mass with extension into the vagina. **A,** ACBE shows anterior wall nodular rectal mass *(arrows)*. **B,** CT shows rectal mass with anterior extension *(black arrows)*. A rectal lumen also is shown *(open arrow)*. **C,** Retroflexed sigmoidoscope view shows nodular mass *(arrows)* on low anterior rectal wall. Biopsy and resection confirmed a cloacogenic carcinoma. The anterior *(black arrows)* and posterior *(open arrow)* margins are shown.

Lymphoma

Lymphoma is a relatively uncommon tumor of the colon and probably represents less than 1% of all malignant neoplasms of the large bowel. The most commonly involved area tends to be the right side of the colon, particularly the cecum. The clinical presentation includes weight loss, weakness, diarrhea, and bleeding. A palpable mass may be discovered if the lesion is sufficiently large. Obstruction is unusual.

The most common radiological presentation is a large, bulky lesion identical in appearance to an adenocarcinoma. Less commonly, it may present as a diffuse nodular or polypoid process. An occasional case of Burkitt's lymphoma of the colon is seen in the small bowel and right colon of children and young adults in

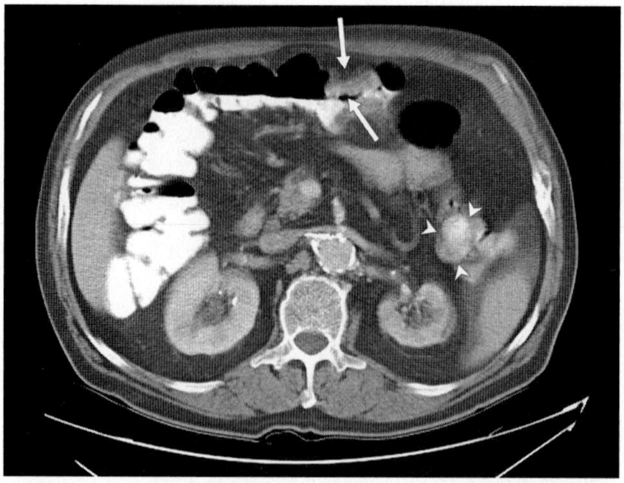

Figure 7-43 A single slice on CT shows synchronous lesions in the transverse colon *(arrows)* and the descending colon *(arrowheads)*.

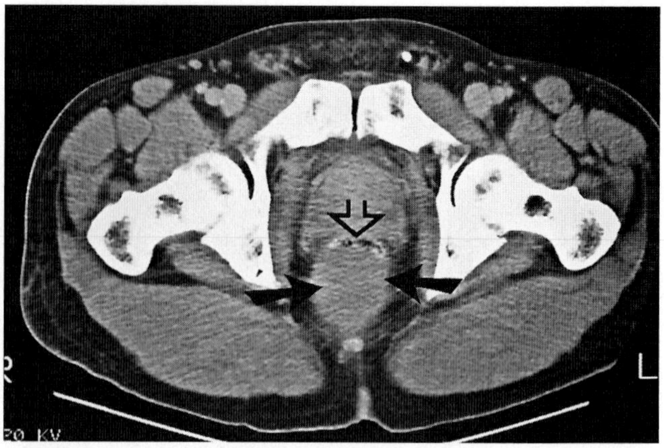

Figure 7-45 A 54-year-old man presents with a rectal mass. CT shows a mass in the posterior rectal wall *(solid arrows)* with some anterior displacement of the rectal lumen *(open arrow)*. Surgical resection revealed a stromal cell tumor.

North America. This disease is histologically identical to that described by Burkitt in Uganda during the 1950s that almost exclusively involved children, with the primary site being the mandible. In some parts of Africa, Burkitt's lymphoma is the most common malignant neoplasm of childhood. The lesion has been linked to Epstein-Barr virus. The North American variety of Burkitt's lymphoma more commonly occurs intra-abdominally. When colonic involvement is present, it is usually in the ascending region (Fig. 7-46).

Colonic Duplication

Colonic duplication is thought to result from intrauterine vascular insults. Duplications can occur virtually anywhere, from cecum to rectum. The duplication may or may not communicate with the main colonic or rectal lumen. The symptoms depend on the amount of luminal narrowing associated with the mass effect of the duplication. This condition is rare.

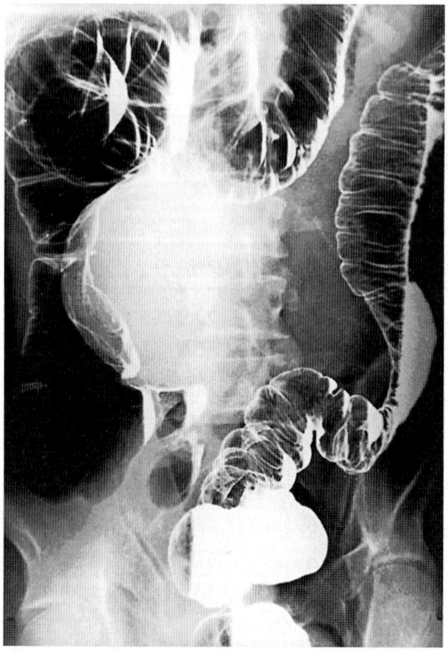

Figure 7-44 A large leiomyoma is seen arising from the medial wall of the ascending colon. The lesion is largely exophytic in nature.

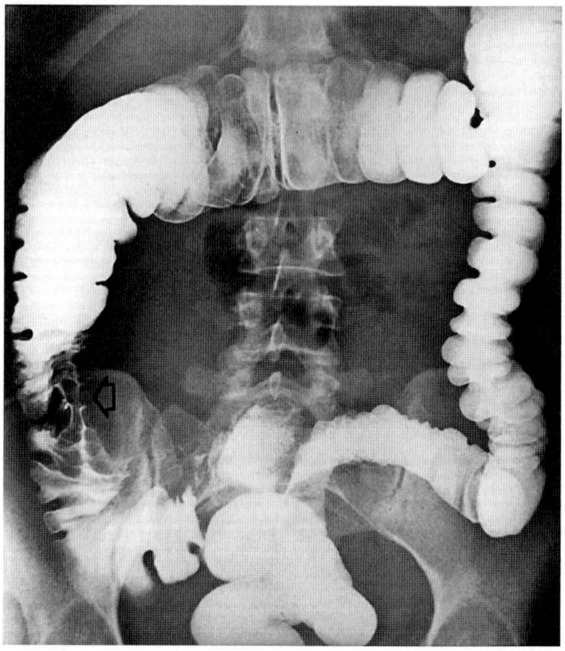

Figure 7-46 Burkitt's lymphoma involving the ascending colon *(arrow)* is seen.

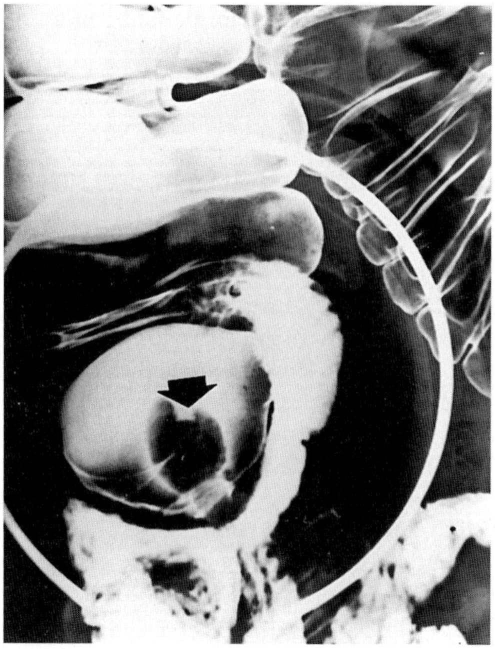

Figure 7-47 Prominent and slightly irregular polypoid filling defect *(arrow)* is seen at the expected site of the inverted appendiceal stump. This finding represents a variant of a normal inverted appendiceal stump and is most likely a result of suture granuloma.

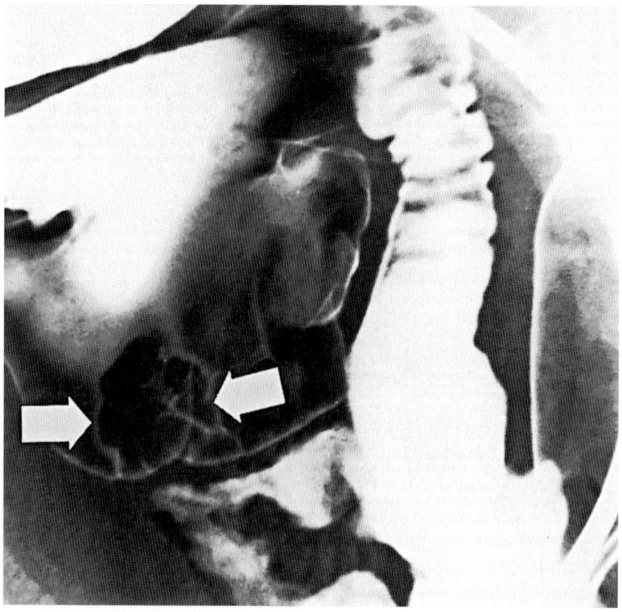

Figure 7-48 A lobulated filling defect at the cecal tip *(arrows)*. Endoscopic follow-up showed adenocarcinoma arising from the appendiceal stump.

Inverted Appendiceal Stump

In a patient with a history of appendectomy, a round, smooth mucosal defect in the cecal tip at the expected orifice of the appendix is almost invariably an inverted appendiceal stump. Some irregularity can be associated with the stump, however, usually as a result of suture granuloma, which may give a suspicious appearance radiologically and result in the necessity of direct visualization (Fig. 7-47). Adenocarcinoma of the appendiceal stump is seen rarely (Fig. 7-48).

Unusual Diverticulum

Under normal circumstances, there is no difficulty in differentiating diverticula from intraluminal filling defects. The so-called unusual diverticulum does occur and can manifest as a filling defect. This can happen for a couple of reasons. The diverticulum may invert into the lumen, producing a smooth, rounded filling defect (Fig. 7-49). Additionally, the diverticulum may become distended and impacted with stool, some of which may project into the lumen, resulting in a filling defect. During fluoroscopic evaluation, this problem often can be sorted out by the use of compression technique or by rotating the patient in an attempt to profile the diverticulum. Additionally, postevacuation films commonly show some barium within the diverticulum that occurred during evacuation (Fig. 7-50).

Foreign Bodies

Occasionally, medication or vitamin tablets that have traversed the entire small bowel and arrive intact and undissolved in the colon are seen. These are mobile and usually present little difficulty in diagnosis. Metallic foreign bodies in the colon or rectum are not a diagnostic problem. Plastic, glass, latex, and rubber are less obvious but usually apparent.

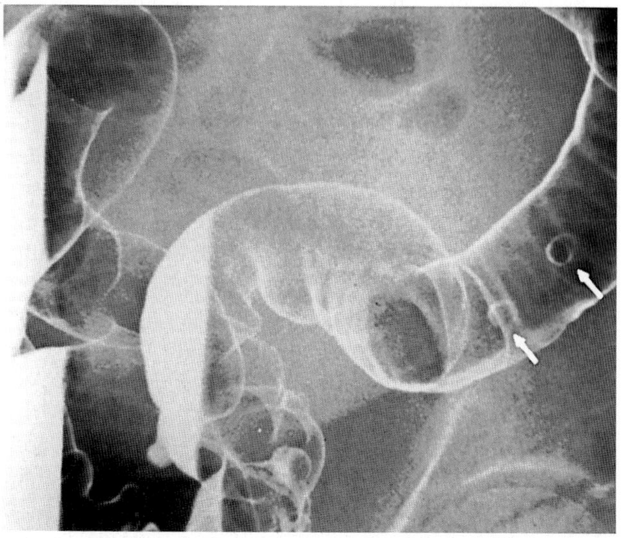

Figure 7-49 Two small, circular lesions *(arrows)* seen in the proximal sigmoid colon. Both proved to be diverticula. Note how the barium margin fades toward the center of the more distal lesion, an expected finding with a diverticulum.

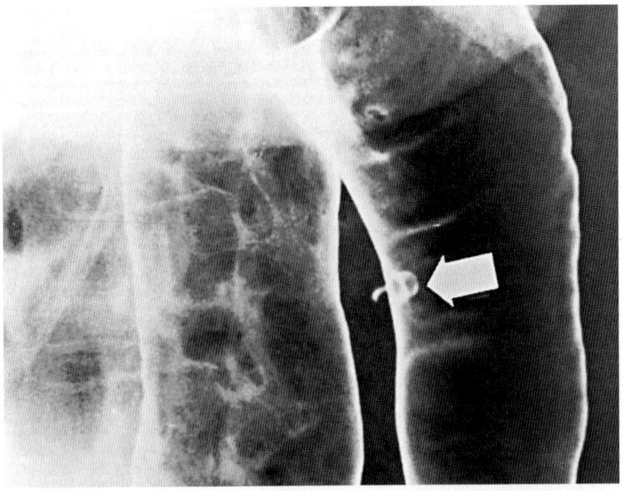

Figure 7-50 A rounded, smooth filling defect in the splenic flexure *(arrow)* seems to represent a typical polyp. A small amount of barium has seeped into the diverticulum, however, and is projected outside the lumen, revealing this polypoid lesion to be a diverticulum.

MULTIPLE FILLING DEFECTS

Hyperplastic Polyps

Hyperplastic polyps of the colon represent the most common type of colonic polyp. The incidence and number of polyps tend to increase with age. Histologically, one finds evidence of epithelial hyperplasia with accompanying elongation and cystic dilatation of the glandular structures. These polyps also are referred to as "metaplastic polyps." They are thought to present no increased risk of malignancy.

Radiologically, the polyps are usually small, measuring from a couple of millimeters to 1 cm, and are almost always sessile. Although in themselves the hyperplastic polyps are associated with no particular clinical symptoms, they do present some difficulty during barium enema because of the inability of the radiologist to distinguish between small adenomatous polyps and hyperplastic polyps. There is also considerable difficulty during colonoscopy in making the differentiation. This difficulty and more recent observations that suggest that the number of diminutive polyps (<5 mm) that are adenomatous is greater than previously thought has led to the assertion that all colorectal polyps should be removed, regardless of size. This position is controversial in the light of widely accepted data that the incidence of carcinoma in adenomatous polyps less than 1 cm is less than 1% and is considerably less in polyps less than 5 mm. Although there is little or no evidence to indicate any malignant potential in hyperplastic polyps, some concern has been expressed regarding the company they keep. There have been reports of increased incidence of adenomas and carcinomas in patients with multiple hyperplastic polyps of the colon.

Polyposis Syndromes

The colonic polyposis syndromes are compared in Table 7-1.

Familial Polyposis

Familial polyposis represents the most well-known and important of the colonic polyposis syndromes. It is inherited as an autosomal dominant trait with equal distribution among males and females. The frequency of individuals with the gene for this disease ranges from 1:7000 to 1:8000 in the general population. The first appearance of colonic adenomatous polyps is usually manifested during the teen years. Polyps, although predominantly concentrated within the colon, also may be seen within the stomach, small bowel, and rectum (Fig. 7-51). The large bowel is usually carpeted with several hundred to several thousand small adenomatous polyps.

The disease may be relatively asymptomatic (Fig. 7-52) until rectal bleeding occurs. Patients may present in their 20s or 30s with vague abdominal pain or diarrhea and occult or frank rectal bleeding. Because the potential for malignant transformation is so great, frank rectal bleeding may indicate the presence of a malignant lesion. In two thirds of patients, malignant degeneration already has occurred at the time of diagnosis. If untreated, patients with familial polyposis eventually develop colon cancer, usually in their 30s or 40s.

Radiological examination discloses a colon carpeted with multiple, small polypoid lesions. Distribution may be uniform throughout the large bowel, or it may be more concentrated on the left side. Examination of the stomach and small bowel also should be included as part of the patient's workup to evaluate for the presence of polyps in these sites. Gastric and duodenal polyps can be detected in approximately half of the patients.

Gardner's Syndrome

Gardner's syndrome, representing a form of colonic familial adenomatous polyposis, has been a recognized syndrome since the 1950s and is characterized by extracolonic manifestations such as epidermoid cysts, fibromas, and osteomas of the skull. It also is inherited by autosomal dominant transmission. The potential for malignant transformation, as in familial polyposis, is 100% if untreated. Radiological evaluation of the colon discloses numerous colonic polyps. Frequently, the number of polyps is less than is seen in typical familial polyposis. Additionally, some of the polyps may be large and pedunculated. Many of these patients also present with symptoms that result from malignant transformation (Fig. 7-53).

Table 7-1 Colonic Polyposis Syndromes

Syndrome	Type	Inheritance	Other Gastrointestinal Sites	Extragastrointestinal Sites	Cancer Risk
Familial polyposis	Adenomatous	Autosomal dominant	Stomach, duodenum, small bowel	Uncommon	High (100%)
Gardner's syndrome*	Adenomatous	Autosomal dominant	Polyps mostly limited to colon	Epidermoids, cysts, fibromas, osteomas	High (100%)
Turcot's syndrome	Adenomatous	Autosomal recessive	None	CNS tumors, mostly glioblastomas	High; malignant CNS tumors
Peutz-Jeghers syndrome	Hamartomatous	Autosomal dominant	Small bowel most common, but also stomach, rectum	Perioral pigmentations, GU abnormalities in women	Low (2-3%); increased risk of breast cancer
Juvenile polyposis	Hamartomatous	Possibly autosomal dominant	Mostly limited to colon, rarely generalized in gut	Increased incidence of congenital malformations, retroperitoneal fibrosis	Low (10%)
Cronkhite-Canada syndrome	Mixed inflammatory/ hamartomatous	Unknown	Stomach, small bowel, rectum	Alopecia, skin pigmentations, onychodystrophy	Low (10%)
Cowden's syndrome (multiple hamartoma syndrome)	Mixed hamartomatous/ fibrosis	Autosomal dominant	Esophagus to rectum	Skin keratoses, oral papillomas, faciotrichilemmomas, thyroid abnormalities	Low; increased risk of breast cancer

*May be a variant of familial polyposis.
CNS, central nervous system; GU, genitourinary.

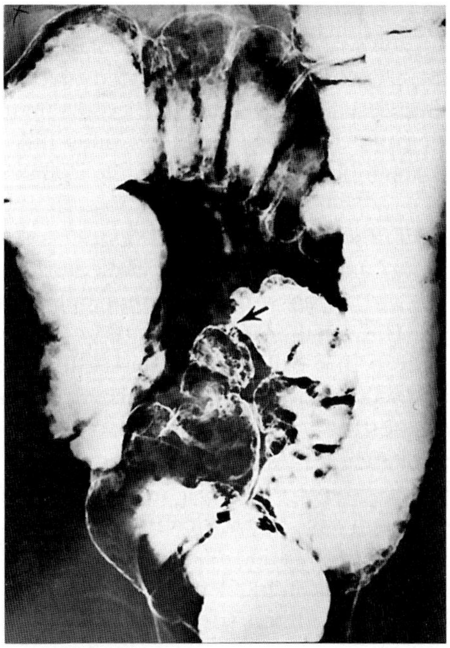

Figure 7-51 Overhead film from DCBE reveals numerous polyps throughout the entire length of the colon. An area of stricturing *(arrow)* representing malignant degeneration is shown in the midsigmoid colon in this patient with familial polyposis.

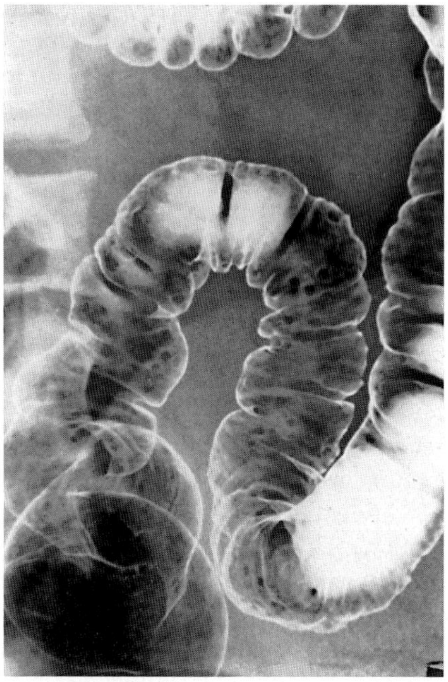

Figure 7-52 Spot film of the sigmoid colon in a patient with a family history of familial polyposis. The patient is asymptomatic, and the examination was done because of the family history. Numerous, small sessile polyps are seen throughout the sigmoid and the remainder of the colon.

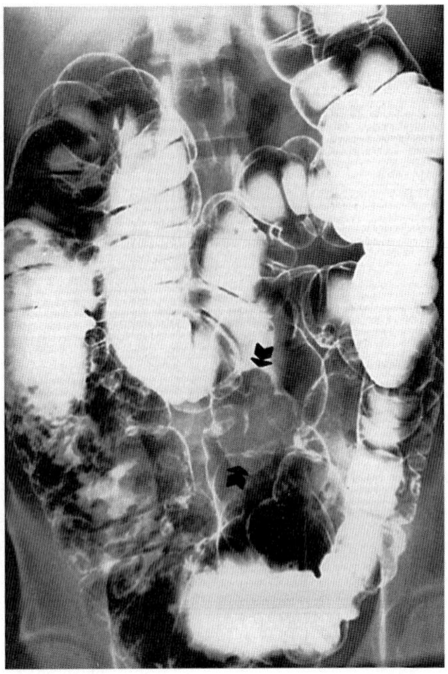

Figure 7-53 DCBE in a patient presenting with rectal bleeding and a family history of Gardner's syndrome. Multiple polyps of varying sizes are seen throughout the colon. A large, lobulated distal sigmoid mass *(arrows)* is seen and was found to be a polypoid carcinoma.

Turcot's Syndrome

Turcot's syndrome is a rare colonic polyposis condition characterized by adenomatous polyps of the colon, usually larger and in fewer numbers than are seen in Gardner's syndrome or familial polyposis. The syndrome also includes central nervous system tumors, most commonly glioblastoma multiforme and astrocytomas. Despite the high risk of colon cancer, most patients die early as a result of central nervous system lesions. The syndrome is thought to be inherited as an autosomal recessive process.

Peutz-Jeghers Syndrome

Peutz-Jeghers syndrome is an unusual autosomal dominant inherited disorder consisting of gastrointestinal polyps, usually of hamartomatous origin, accompanied by mucocutaneous pigment changes of the face and perioral region. The polyps may be asymptomatic or associated with hemorrhage or intermittent small bowel intussusception. The patient may present with iron deficiency anemia or intermittent cramping and abdominal pain.

The small bowel is the most common site for polyps in the Peutz-Jeghers syndrome, although polyps are seen in the colon and stomach. Polyp size varies from a few millimeters to 2 to 3 cm. The number of polyps also varies. Radiologically, the polyps of this syndrome are indistinguishable from adenomas. The main clinical factor, which increases suspicion, must be the pigmented mucocutaneous lesions that often precede the appearance of the gastrointestinal symptoms.

Peutz-Jeghers syndrome seems to be associated with a slightly increased risk of gastrointestinal cancer. It is unknown, however, whether the carcinoma arises as part of the hamartomatous process or spontaneously and coincidentally. At this time, the latter perspective seems to be favored. Women with this syndrome seem to have an increased risk for developing breast carcinoma. There also may be a slight increase in ovarian cancer in these patients.

Juvenile Polyposis

Juvenile polyposis is a disorder thought to be inherited as an autosomal dominant trait. These polyps are hamartomas and may be solitary or multiple, occurring in the colon and rectum of children or young adults, called infantile or juvenile. Polyps can result in gastrointestinal bleeding, intussusception, and obstruction. In recent years, increased attention has been directed at the relationship between this condition and a possible increased risk of carcinoma. The polyps are not neoplastic, however, and no actual malignant degeneration of a polyp composed of hamartomatous elements is known. There may be an increased incidence of adenomatous polyps in these patients.

Associated extracolonic manifestations may include congenital abnormalities and malformations and an increased incidence of retroperitoneal fibrosis. Radiologically, the polyps can attain surprisingly large proportions. Often they are pedunculated. Occasionally, the larger polyps break free of their stalk, resulting in significant rectal bleeding. An isolated juvenile polyp, and in some cases multiple juvenile polyps, can be seen with a negative family history and does not seem to represent the inherited form of juvenile polyposis.

Cronkhite-Canada Syndrome

Cronkhite-Canada syndrome was first described in the mid-1950s and is an apparent nonfamilial polyposis syndrome. The condition is characterized by gastrointestinal polyps that can be distributed throughout the gut from stomach to rectum. Associated extragastrointestinal manifestations include alopecia, onychodystrophy, and hyperpigmented lesions of the skin.

The polyps tend to be most numerous in the small bowel, although colonic polyps are common. Patients are often middle-aged and present with diarrhea relating to an associated protein-losing enteropathy. Although initial reports considered the polyps to be adenomas, subsequent studies consistently showed a lesion resembling a juvenile polyp with hamartomatous and inflammatory elements. Occasional reports of colon cancer in patients with this condition have raised the question of whether there may be a slightly increased risk. From a clinical perspective, the chronic diarrhea seems to present more of a threat to the patient's health than the presence of gastrointestinal polyps does.

Cowden's Syndrome

Cowden's syndrome is uncommon and is characterized by multiple hamartomatous polyps of the esophagus, stomach, small bowel, and colon. The polyps themselves are not known to be associated with any clinical symptoms. The significant aspect of the syndrome is the extragastrointestinal manifestations, which include skin changes, perioral papillomas, faciotrichilemmomas, thyroid abnormalities (including goiter and cancer), and an increased risk of breast cancer.

Neurofibromatosis

Neurofibromatosis (von Recklinghausen's disease) is a condition in which the most well-known manifestations are multiple subcutaneous neurofibromas. Involvement of the gut with disseminated neurofibromatosis is unusual but does occur (Fig. 7-54). Although involvement of the gut usually is associated with the cutaneous manifestations, the disease also may be confined to the gastrointestinal tract. Most reports of colonic involvement are in children. Children usually present with intussusception or rectal bleeding. There is a slightly increased risk of malignant degeneration.

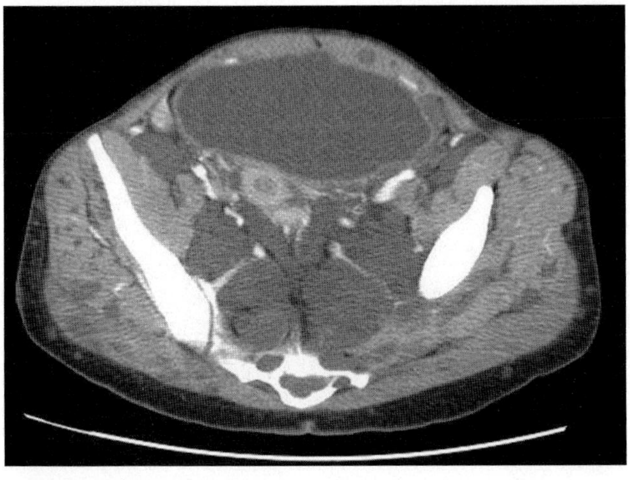

Figure 7-54 Large intraabdominal tumors of neurofibromatosis compress segments of small bowel and colon.

Pseudopolyps

Pseudopolyps are polypoid protrusions into the lumen of a colon exhibiting the changes of severe IBD and are truly named, in that they are not polyps in the typical sense. The pseudopolyp is actually residual edematous mucosa sitting, like an island, on a sea of surrounding ulceration. The denuding of the adjacent mucosa and the swelling of the remaining island of mucosa result in the classic polypoid appearance of the pseudopolyp. Pseudopolyps may be seen in virtually any IBD involving the colon, although the most common is ulcerative colitis. Pseudopolyps are a particularly prominent feature of toxic megacolon.

Postinflammatory Polyps

The appearance of colonic postinflammatory polyps (Box 7-5) is a direct effect of IBD, in particular, ulcerative colitis. Postinflammatory polyps may be seen less commonly in Crohn's disease and other inflammatory conditions of the colon.

These polyps are composed of normal mucosa. They are often filiform or comma-shaped and tend to be found mostly in the distal colon. These projections of normal mucosa into the lumen occur as a result of mucosal healing after severe IBD. They represent what were, during the height of the inflammatory process, pseudopolyps. When the healing process begins, reepithelialization of the surrounding ulcerated areas occurs. This reepithelialization process extends into the undermined base of the pseudopolyp. As a result, when healing is complete, a projection of normal mucosa, usually in a filiform shape and often readily identifiable, is seen (Fig. 7-55). This projection may be seen on a background of normal colonic mucosa or recurrent disease. Residual fecal debris sometimes closely mimics postinflammatory polyposis, and a careful and detailed examination of the configuration of the "polyps" along with the absence of any evidence of new or old inflammation usually sorts out the problem (Fig. 7-56). Unusual presentations of postinflammatory polyposis include mucosal bridges, which are occasionally seen and represent reepithelialization of a thin strip of viable mucosa that has been

Box 7-5 Postinflammatory Polyps: How They Come to Be

1. Starts as inflammatory colonic disease (usually ulcerative colitis)
2. Inflammation results in severe ulceration and near-denuding of mucosal surface
3. Residual "islands" of edematous mucosa (pseudopolyps) are spared
4. Healing occurs with reepithelialization of ulcerated surfaces
5. Reepithelialization process surrounds and involves the undermined edges of the pseudopolyps, giving classic appearance of postinflammatory or filiform polyps

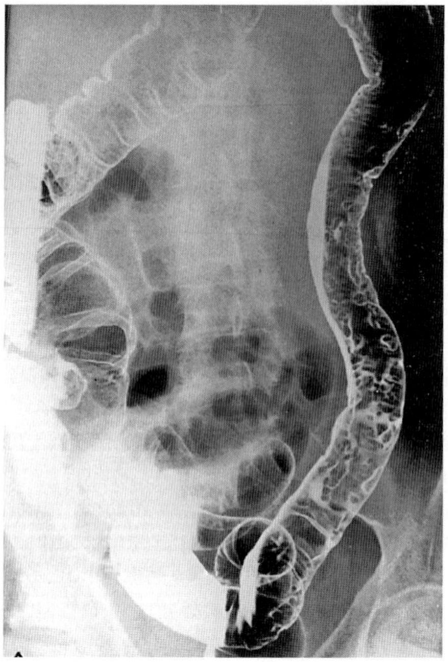

Figure 7-55 DCBE in a patient with a previous history of ulcerative colitis reveals a tubular-appearing left colon with numerous filiform filling defects representing postinflammatory polyposis.

totally undermined by ulceration. Additionally, large masses of postinflammatory polyps have been reported, having, in some instances, the appearance of a large villous tumor. These have been called giant postinflammatory polyps.

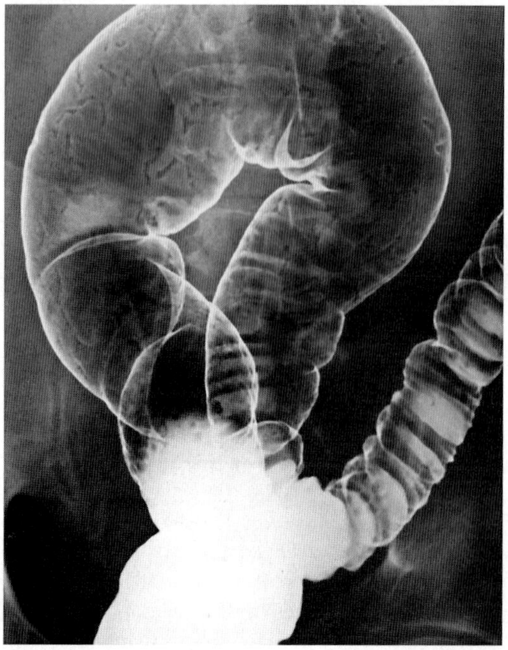

Figure 7-56 Mucus stranding in the rectum was initially called *filiform polyposis* on ACBE. Sigmoidoscopy was normal.

Lymphoid Hyperplasia/Lymphoid Follicular Prominence

The diagnosis of nodular lymphoid hyperplasia presents a dilemma. This diagnostic title suggests a disease, whereas the presence of prominent lymphoid follicles throughout the colon is usually a normal finding in children and is seen with much more frequency than previously thought in adults. In most instances, these small lymphoid nodules of the colon are considered a normal variant. They usually measure 1 to 3 mm and are rounded elevations of the mucosa with poor definition of the borders (Fig. 7-57). They tend to occur in areas where lymphoid follicles are most numerous, such as the ileocecal area and rectum. They also can be seen distributed throughout the entire colon. When these nodules are larger than 3 mm, the condition is commonly referred to as lymphoid hyperplasia and characterized radiologically by a tiny, central, barium-filled dimple seen on ACBE. This is not a disease, but more likely the reaction of the lymphoid follicles to an adjacent inflammatory or infectious process, although the process may not always be apparent. The presence of nodular lymphoid hyperplasia in the small bowel and possibly the colon of patients with hypogammaglobulinemia and associated giardiasis also has been noted. It has been suggested that lymphoid hyperplasia may represent the earliest changes of IBD or lymphatic disease, although this is speculative and has never been proved.

Pneumatosis Cystoides Coli

Pneumatosis coli manifests two distinctive patterns. The condition is characterized by air in the bowel wall. The most common form is subserosal cystic blebs (Fig. 7-58). The actual cause is unknown. Speculation

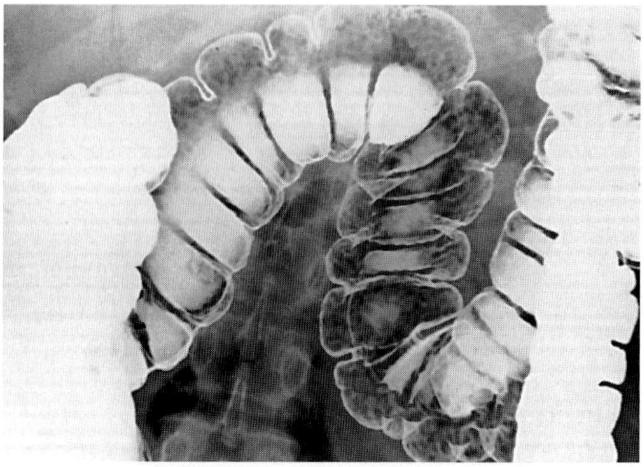

Figure 7-57 Numerous, tiny filling defects are seen throughout the colon in this adult patient, representing a prominent lymphoid follicular pattern.

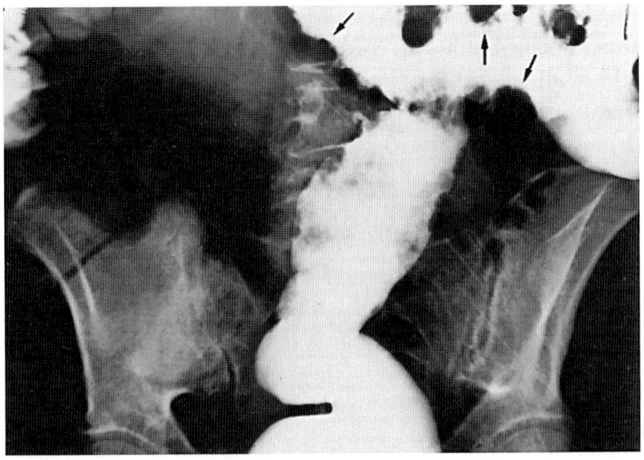

Figure 7-58 Barium enema reveals numerous marginal nodular filling defects, some of which have the appearance of thumbprinting *(arrows)*. The filling defects are air-filled, however, and represent pneumatosis coli.

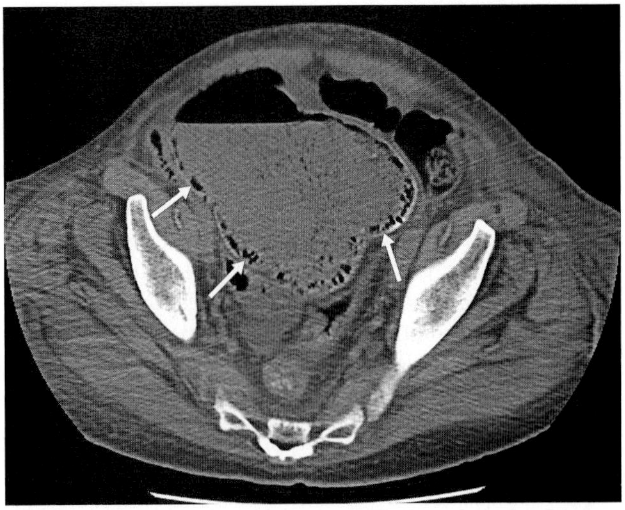

Figure 7-59 CT in patient with transverse colon volvulus shows distended colon and air in the wall of the affected bowel *(arrows)*.

has largely centered on coexistent chronic obstructive pulmonary disease in which microruptures of the alveoli occur, and air dissects through the vascular-bronchial interstitial pathways to the mediastinum, down the mediastinum into the retroperitoneum, and into the root of the mesentery. Upward migration of air into the neck probably also occurs, but is in such small amounts as not to be noticed. Further dissection of air occurs along the leaves of the mesentery until it reaches the peritoneal surface of the bowel. Most of the subserosal cystic air collections are seen in the distal colon, with abrupt termination at the peritoneal reflection off the rectum. The oxygen is largely absorbed, and the remaining gas is primarily nitrogen. Another condition that has been associated with this is scleroderma. These patients are almost always asymptomatic, and the findings are usually incidental. Rarely, if a subserosal cyst is sufficiently large, there can be stretching of the overlying mucosa and potential ulceration and bleeding. Additionally, the subserosal blebs occasionally can rupture, and the patient can have a benign pneumoperitoneum. Such a finding often can cause confusion in the emergency department.

Another, more ominous form of pneumatosis coli is the presence of linear intramural collections of air. These are not subserosal in location, but usually submucosal intramural. This finding is most frequently associated with underlying acute vascular insults to the bowel, ischemia, and infarction (Figs. 7-59 and 7-60). Air that has percolated into the submucosa as the result of a loss of mucosal integrity is, similar to food nutrients, taken up in the portal venous system and transported through the mesenteric veins to the portal vein. From there, it can be carried into the intrahepatic portal venous system; this can be identified on plain radiographs as tiny, branching, tubular collections of air in the periphery (as opposed to larger air-filled branching structures centrally seen in the biliary tree) of the liver. In most instances, at the time of radiological evaluation, these patients are sufficiently toxic to allow the radiologist to make the diagnosis confidently. The findings of air in the bowel wall may precede by several hours the onset of catastrophic decline in the patient's physical status, however. Some patients undergoing major bowel infarction may have little more than complaints of abdominal pain

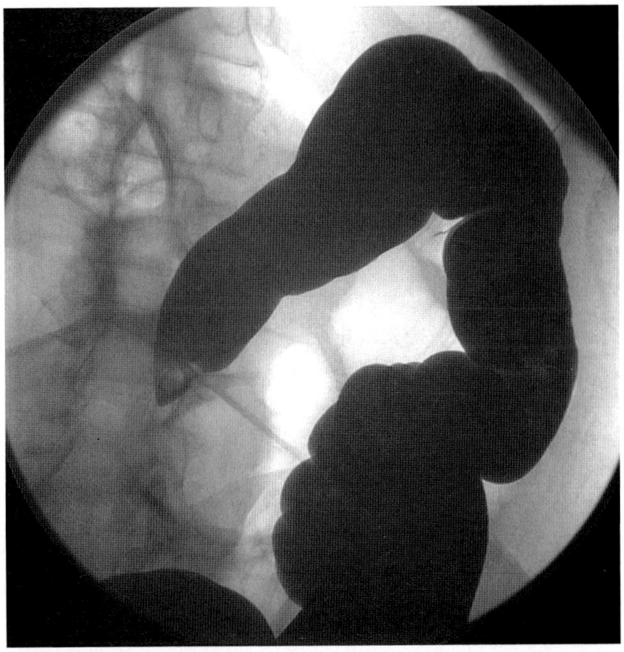

Figure 7-60 Barium enema in same patient as Figure 7-59 shows typical "beaklike" configuration at the point of torsion obstruction in the transverse colon.

and will not survive 24 hours. This may be especially true in older individuals.

A major problem for the radiologist is the occasional discovery of extensive linear submucosal air collections or air within the portal venous system in a relatively asymptomatic patient. This condition can occur as a benign finding unrelated to bowel wall ischemia or necrosis. Such conditions include gastrointestinal surgery, pyloric obstruction, peptic ulceration, instrumentation, and mucosal trauma. In these situations, the cause of the condition is related to mechanical and surgical factors rather than bowel necrosis. Linear pneumatosis on plain film or abdominal CT should always lead to an immediate consultation with the referring clinician.

Metastatic Disease

Metastatic spread of tumor to the colon and rectum can produce a variety of radiological findings and clinical symptoms. The spread to the colon may occur as a result of seeding through the intraperitoneal pathways, local contiguous spread, or hematogenous dissemination. Tumors that can spread in such a manner and produce multiple and, rarely, solitary filling defects include breast cancer, malignant melanoma, and bronchogenic carcinoma. Radiographic appearances vary and may include well-defined intramural polypoid masses or large, bulky, irregular masses with superficial ulceration. Lesions originating in the ovary and stomach most commonly spread through the intraperitoneal pathways and result in narrowing and stricture. Lesions from the stomach via the gastrocolic mesentery and retroperitoneal lesions affecting the transverse colon via the transverse mesocolon occasionally may be seen. Involvement of the rectum by cervical cancer or prostatic cancer usually results from contiguous invasion.

Colitis Cystica Profunda

Colitis cystica profunda is an unusual nonneoplastic condition characterized by the presence of mucus-filled cysts in the submucosa and is usually confined to the rectum or distal sigmoid colon. The radiographic appearance varies, with a classic description of numerous, smooth polypoid lesions that may be indistinguishable from adenomatous polyps. Occasionally, the polyps are clustered and irregular, even assuming a masslike configuration that requires differentiation from malignant neoplasm. Clinically, these patients present with rectal bleeding and passage of excessive mucus per rectum.

The etiological basis of the condition is confusing. It is believed by some authorities to originate as a primary focal glandular abnormality of the distal large bowel and rectum. Conversely, there is also a fairly convincing argument that this is a variant of the solitary rectal ulcer syndrome. Solitary rectal ulcer syndrome is probably a result of chronic internal rectal prolapse, resulting in superficial ulceration, interval episodes of inflammation and healing, and invagination of the glandular structures that become cystic over time.

Kaposi's Sarcoma

For decades, Kaposi's sarcoma had been known as an indolent cutaneous neoplastic disease of older men and was considered uncommon. With the advent of acquired immunodeficiency syndrome (AIDS), however, it has come to the forefront of diagnostic considerations. Of patients with AIDS, 30% to 40% have Kaposi's sarcoma somewhere in the gastrointestinal tract. Virtually all cases of Kaposi's sarcoma of the gut are associated with AIDS. The lesions can affect the esophagus, stomach, small bowel, or colon. They may predate the cutaneous lesions. Barium enema commonly shows multiple nodular lesions, usually in the distal colon. Infiltrative or irregular masses also can be seen.

Patients may present with gastrointestinal bleeding as a result of ulceration of the larger nodules. In some instances, this bleeding may be the presenting complaint before the diagnosis of AIDS is known. The presence of Kaposi's sarcoma within the bowel indicates a poor prognosis, and few patients survive beyond 12 to 18 months after diagnosis.

Colonic Lymphoma

In most instances, lymphoma is indistinguishable from primary adenocarcinoma. Occasionally, this lesion may present as multiple nodular polypoid lesions within the colon, usually on the right side (Fig. 7-61). Rarely, the multinodular appearance is indistinguishable from the more well-known polyposis syndromes (Fig. 7-62).

Colonic Schistosomiasis

Colonic schistosomiasis is a condition rarely encountered in North America, but is occasionally seen in travelers who have visited areas of endemic disease. It presents in the colon as ulcerations associated with polypoid filling defects (Fig. 7-63).

Colonic Varices

Varices are encountered in patients with portal hypertension, most frequently associated with liver cirrhosis. The collateral pathways are usually via the gastroesophageal veins, the mesenteric veins, and occasionally the umbilical veins. Colonic varices are rare. They are usually associated with pathways that develop as a result of the anastomosis of veins on the visceral surface of the bowel with systemic venous channels in the abdominal wall. This occurs, in almost all cases, in patients with

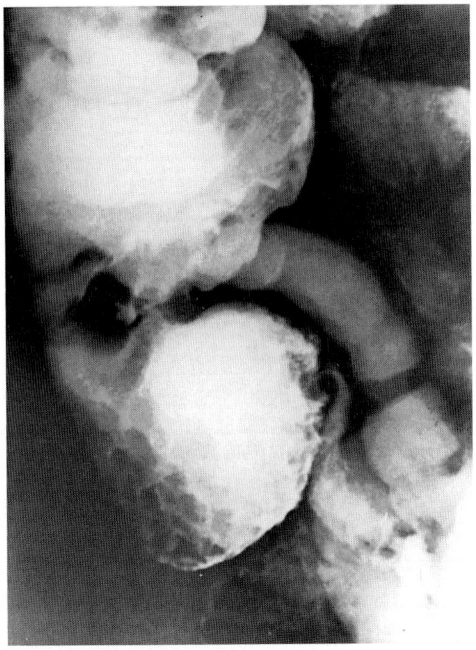

Figure 7-61 Spot film of the cecum shows multiple mucosal nodules in the cecal tip, giving a mosaic pattern and representing lymphoma. Other conditions that can give a similar appearance include ischemic changes, Crohn's disease, and *Yersinia* colitis.

portal hypertension and a history of prior abdominal surgery and resection who develop adhesions between bowel loops, setting the stage for possible abnormal venous collateralizations on the surface of the bowel (Fig. 7-64).

EXTRINSIC DEFECTS

Extrinsic defects affecting the colon may fall within the normal or abnormal category (Box 7-6). In the normal category, one can expect to see impressions from the right lobe of the liver, particularly Riedel's lobe, in which the inferior aspect of the right lobe is elongated and impresses the ascending colon. A patulous or prominent gallbladder may be seen impressing the superior margin of the proximal transverse colon. Splenic impressions are common, but their presence does not indicate splenomegaly. Occasionally, individuals with a prominent sacral promontory have some posterior impression at the rectosigmoid junction.

Virtually any intraabdominal mass can result in colonic displacement or compression. This ranges from abscesses, the most common of which are due to diverticular, periappendiceal, and pelvic inflammatory disease, to cystic lesions, most commonly of the ovary. Significant cystic disease of the kidney also can impress the colon. Intraabdominal tumor masses can compress, displace, or invade the colon.

ULCERATION

Ulcerative Colitis

Of the group of diseases generally known as IBD, ulcerative colitis and Crohn's disease represent the

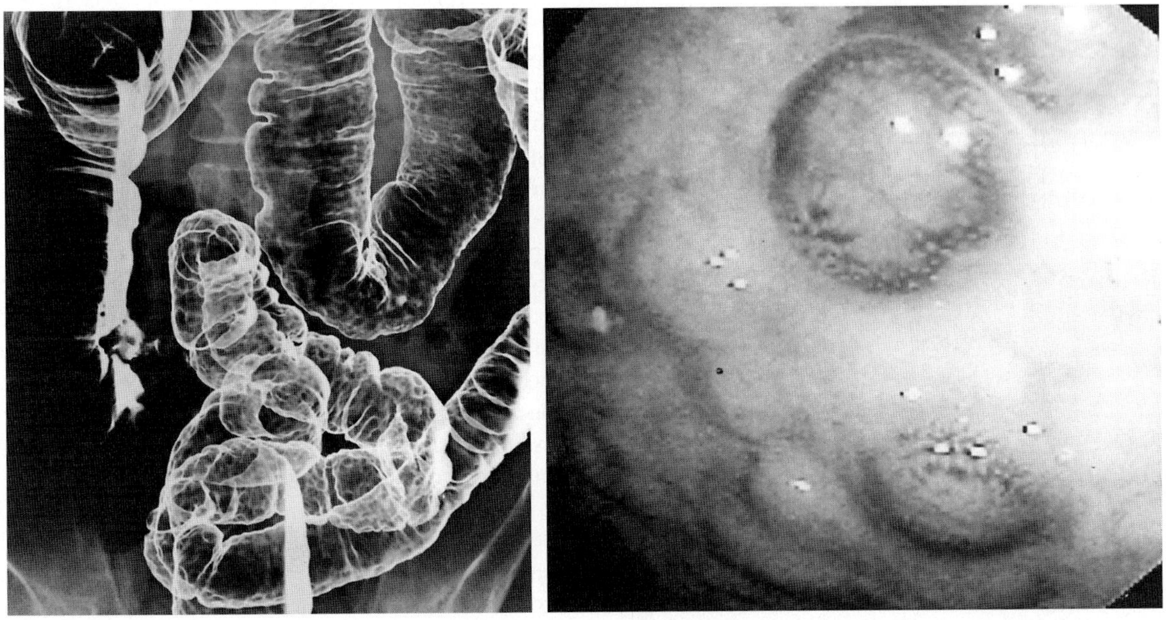

A B

Figure 7-62 A 53-year-old man presented with Hemoccult-positive stool, but was otherwise well. **A,** ACBE reveals multiple colonic polyps. **B,** Colonoscopy reveals multiple atypical-appearing polypoid lesions. Biopsy specimen showed lymphomatous polyposis of the colon, a presentation of colonic lymphoma.

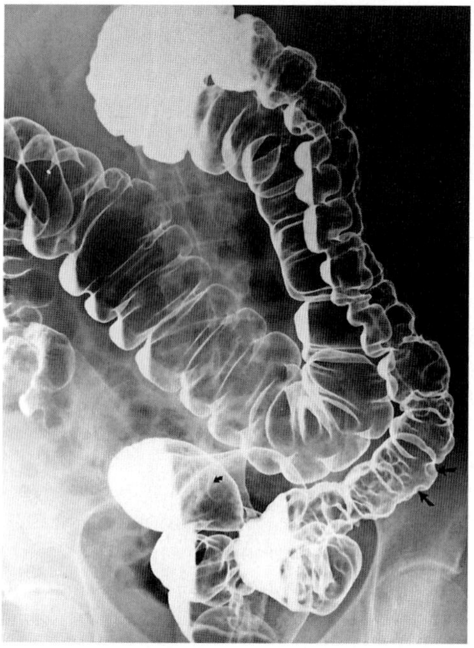

Figure 7-63 A 46-year-old woman presented with abdominal pain and diarrhea after a trip to the Middle East. ACBE shows multiple polypoid lesions in the distal colon *(arrows)*, which is one form of presentation of colonic schistosomiasis.

two most important conditions (Table 7-2). Ulcerative colitis is a mucosal disease that involves the colon distally and may progress to affect the proximal colon. If limited to the rectum at the time of diagnosis, the disease is referred to as ulcerative proctitis.

The cardinal clinical features are diarrhea and rectal bleeding. The severity of the clinical presentation often depends on the amount of large bowel involved.

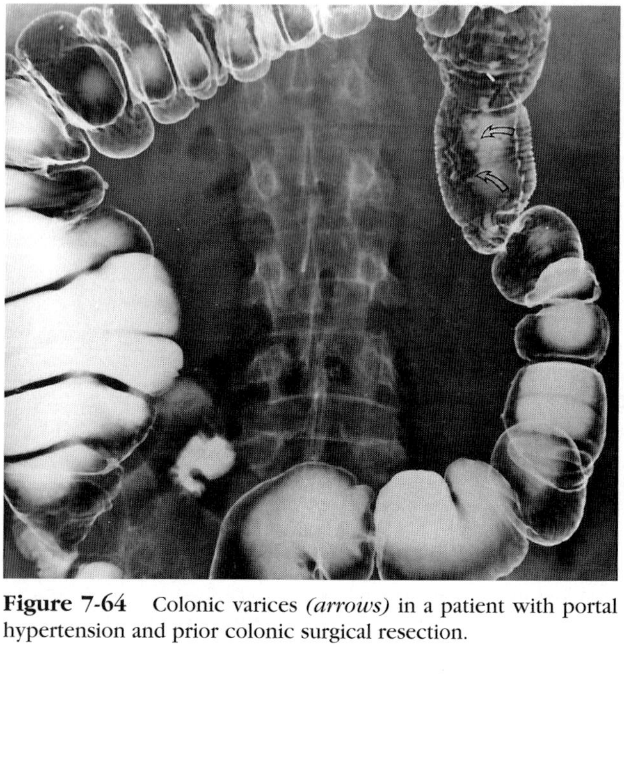

Figure 7-64 Colonic varices *(arrows)* in a patient with portal hypertension and prior colonic surgical resection.

Box 7-6 Pushing the Colon Around: Extrinsic Sources of Normal and Abnormal Impressions on the Colon

- Liver
- Gallbladder
- Spleen
- Pelvic masses, especially ovarian
- Renal disease
- Abscesses, especially diverticular or periappendiceal
- Mesenteric masses
- Small bowel disease

Approximately one third of patients have pancolonic involvement at initial presentation. The disease can present as an acute process, a recurrent process, or a chronic ongoing condition. It is mostly a disease of young individuals, although it can be seen in any age group. The pathological characteristic of the disease is continuous and concentric superficial involvement of the bowel wall with inflammatory changes, mostly limited to the mucosa. In severe fulminating disease, the extent and depth of disease can increase significantly and become transmural, as in the case of toxic megacolon.

When early active disease is present, the mucosal surface becomes hyperemic, granular, and edematous. Tiny punctate ulcers also may be seen in the acute phase on ACBE. Uniform wall thickening of the distal colon, without small bowel involvement or adenopathy, is the typical finding on CT. The haustral pattern is usually diminished, but not absent. Progression of disease results in increased ulceration and friability of the mucosal surface. Severe ulceration and denuding of the mucosal surface can occur. As previously mentioned, islands of residual edematous mucosa on this background of ulceration are known as pseudopolyps. Healing can occur with complete restoration of the normal colonic appearance if the initial insult was not sufficiently severe to cause chronic fibrotic changes.

With more severe disease, there may be distortion of the haustral pattern after healing. Mucosal tags, or postinflammatory polyposis, may be present. With chronic disease, the bowel loses its haustral pattern entirely, assuming a "tubular" appearance. In addition, there is marked foreshortening of the colon. The terminal ileum is usually normal. The condition known as backwash ileitis has been described, resulting from chronic fibrotic changes involving the ileocecal valve and an uninterrupted continuum of the distal ileum and cecum. The terminal ileum appears dilated, but is usually not involved in the inflammatory process.

Microscopic changes in the mucosal surface during the initial inflammatory phase reveal not only vascular

Table 7-2 Inflammatory Bowel Disease

	Ulcerative Colitis	Crohn's Disease
Etiology	Unknown	Unknown
Pathology	Superficial mucosal inflammation	Transmural, granulomatous inflammation
Peak age of onset	20-40 years	Bimodal, mostly 20-30 years, very small secondary peak 60-70 years
Male/female ratio	Equal	Equal
Colorectal involvement	100%	65%-70%
Fistula and abscess formation	Rare	Common
Malignant potential	Related to extent and duration of disease, 10%-15%	Rare in colon, 2%-5% in small bowel with associated small bowel disease
Rectal involvement	Always, may be limited to rectum initially	Approximately 50% with colonic disease
Disease pattern	Continuous, diffuse ulceration, symmetrical involvement of the bowel	Discontinuous, asymmetric skip lesions, asymmetric punctate, linear or branching (cobblestoning) ulceration
Perianal disease	Unusual, can be associated with diarrhea	Common (approximately 50%) with colonic disease
Gastroduodenal disease	No	10%-30%
Major clinical symptoms	Rectal bleeding/diarrhea	Diarrhea, abdominal pain, bleeding less common
Colonic strictures	Yes	Yes (more common)
Pseudopolyp formation	Common	Less common
Toxic megacolon	2%-10%	1%-3%
Extracolonic manifestations		
Arthritis	20%	10%
Skin lesions	Yes	Yes
Liver/biliary	Sclerosing cholangitis 1%-5%	Increased incidence of gallstones
Renal disease	No	Increased incidence of kidney stones
Ophthalmologic disease	4%-5%	Unknown

congestion and leukocytic infiltrates, but also inflammatory changes that occur within the crypts of Lieberkühn and resultant microabscesses. Most patients present with mild to moderate disease. A few patients (<10%) can present initially with a severe fulminant form of the condition.

Various extracolonic manifestations of ulcerative colitis have been described. Among the most severe is primary sclerosing cholangitis. Although almost half of patients with ulcerative colitis may have degrees of abnormality of liver function, only a few have significant hepatobiliary disease, representing approximately 1% to 5% of patients. This includes patients with severe hepatocellular disease and cirrhosis and patients with sclerosing cholangitis.

In about 20% of patients, significant periarticular disease is present. Most commonly, this is a monarticular arthritis involving the lower limbs, usually the ankles or knees. There is also an increased incidence of sacroiliitis and ankylosing spondylitis in patients with ulcerative colitis.

Skin changes also are seen in ulcerative colitis. The most common of these is erythema nodosum, seen in approximately 10% to 15% of patients. Less commonly, pyoderma gangrenosum is seen in patients with severe colonic disease. Other important complications include ocular lesions, such as conjunctivitis, iritis, and episcleritis.

Other recognized, but relatively uncommon complications include an increased incidence of thromboembolic disease, growth retardation, and secondary amyloidosis. The potential for the development of colon carcinoma in patients with ulcerative colitis is well known. The risk seems to increase with the extent and duration of disease. A patient with pancolitis and disease more than 10 years in duration has a 10% to 15% risk of developing a malignant lesion, with the risk increasing over time.

The use of the DCBE over the past few decades has greatly enhanced the ability of the radiologist to identify mild early mucosal changes of ulcerative colitis. These findings include mucosal granularity, diminished colonic folds and loss of rectal valves, and the presence of mucosal erosions (Fig. 7-65). In general, the single-contrast study is not sensitive for the detection of these early changes. Unless there is frank ulceration, these changes are often missed with single-contrast technique. With more pronounced disease, both techniques can show the diagnostic findings easily. Frank ulcerations, including the classic "collar button" ulcers, are easily shown on the margins of the bowel using either technique (Fig. 7-66).

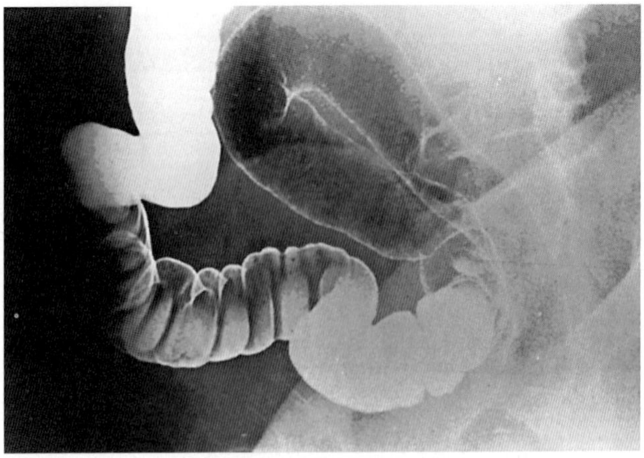

Figure 7-65 Spot film of the rectosigmoid colon in a patient with acute ulcerative colitis reveals loss of haustral folds through the affected area, with granularity and tiny, superficial punctate ulcers involving the rectum and distal sigmoid colon.

The collar button type of ulceration indicates penetration into the submucosa and the undermining of mucosa leading to this classic configuration.

In the chronic phases of ulcerative colitis, colonic foreshortening and narrowing of the lumen can occur. The flexures may virtually disappear. Fistula formation is extremely uncommon; if present, it should prompt the clinician to reconsider the diagnosis. After healing or in chronic recurrent disease, postinflammatory polyps may be present.

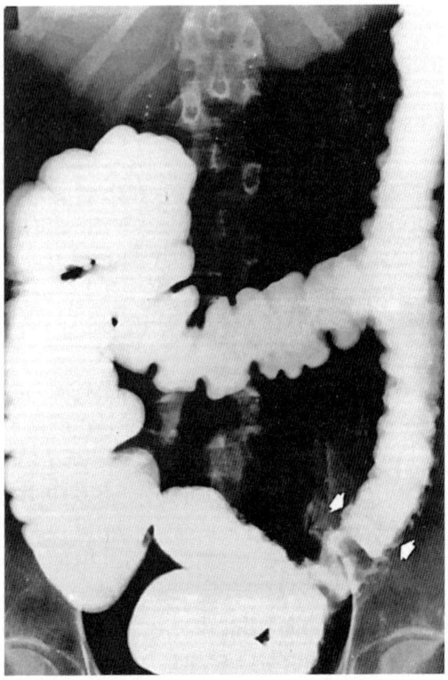

Figure 7-66 Single-contrast examination of the colon in a patient with bloody diarrhea reveals numerous marginal ulcers *(arrows)*, with undermining of mucosa and a collar button appearance.

Crohn's Disease

Crohn's disease is a chronic inflammatory process that, in contrast to ulcerative colitis, is transmural in nature (see Table 7-2). The cause of the disease remains a mystery. It is largely a disease of young persons, 20 to 30 years old, although a smaller subset of patients with onset of symptoms after age 50 is now being identified.

Three primary clinical and anatomical presentations are recognized: small bowel involvement only (30%), distal small bowel and colonic involvement (45%), and colonic involvement only (25%). The pattern of involvement often dictates the clinical presentation. Although diarrhea and abdominal pain tend to be common to all presentations, bowel obstruction and fistula formation are seen most frequently in patients with small bowel involvement. Conversely, rectal bleeding and perianal disease tend to indicate colorectal disease.

The transmural granulomatous type of inflammatory changes is discontinuous within the colon, resulting in the well-known skip lesions recognized by pathologists and radiologists. In addition, the pattern of involvement tends to be asymmetric (e.g., one wall of the colon at any given point may be more or less involved than the opposite wall). This is an important observation, and it contrasts with ulcerative colitis, in which involvement is continuous and concentric.

The full-thickness inflammatory disease eventually results in a thickened rigid segment of bowel, with progressive increase in mesenteric fat over the inflamed serosal surface (creeping fat) first described by pathologists and now appreciated by radiologists with CT (Fig. 7-67). Initially, the mucosal changes may be little more than aphthoid types of erosions on the mucosal surface. Care should be taken regarding the diagnosis of

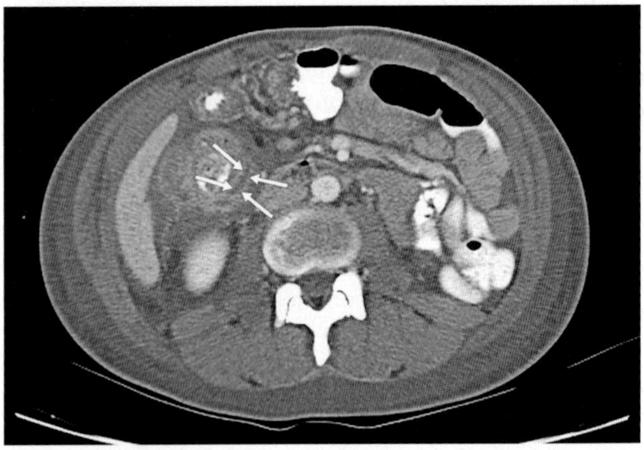

Figure 7-67 Crohn's disease involving the ascending colon with marked wall thickening, haziness of the pericolic fat, and some low-density, concentric, ringlike structures, which might be fluid or fat *(arrows)*.

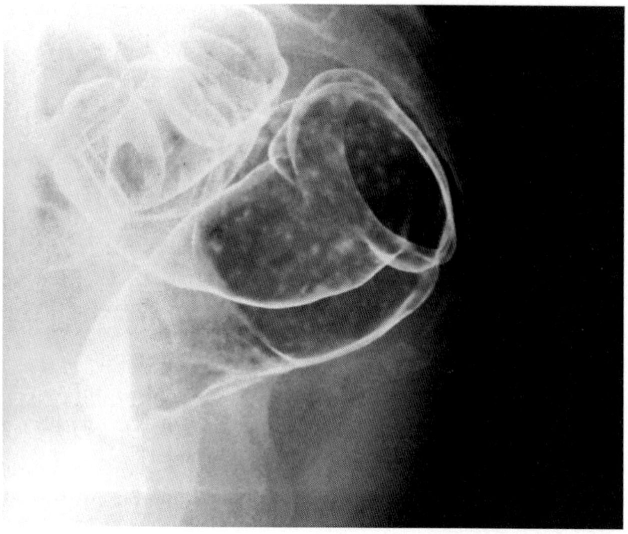

Figure 7-68 A 35-year-old patient with abdominal pain and bloating. Aphthous ulcers of the rectum were diagnosed on ACBE. Sigmoidoscopy was normal. Appearance of rectal mucosa is a normal variant.

aphthous ulcers in the colon and rectum because a prominent lymphoid pattern and variations of the normal rectal pattern can simulate the appearance (Fig. 7-68). Aphthous ulcers can enlarge, deepen, and extend into long linear ulcerations (Fig. 7-69). Extensive branching linear ulcerations can result in the classic "cobblestone" effect described in the early radiological literature. Penetration of the inflammatory process to the external serosal surface of adjacent bowel or adjacent structures accounts for the high incidence of bowel-to-bowel or bowel-to-bladder fistulas and perforation with abscess formation. These represent the most common complications of Crohn's disease and are rarely seen in ulcerative colitis (Figs. 7-70 and 7-71). Free perforation in Crohn's disease is unusual. There is a slightly increased risk of malignancy as a complication of Crohn's disease. These neoplasms almost always occur in the small bowel in patients with small bowel involvement. Adenocarcinoma and lymphoma may occur. Colonic malignancy is rare.

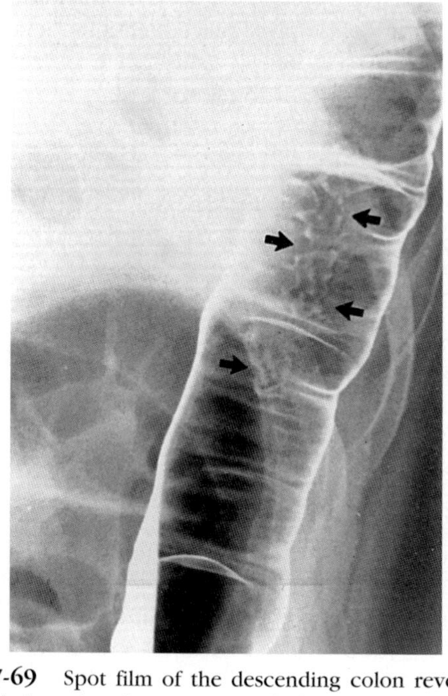

Figure 7-69 Spot film of the descending colon reveals linear superficial ulceration *(arrows)* typical of early Crohn's disease.

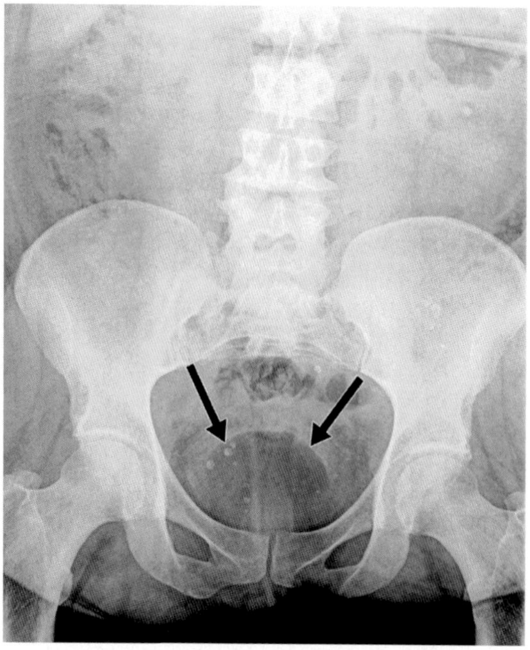

Figure 7-70 Patient with Crohn's disease was shown to have air in the bladder on plain abdominal image *(arrows)*.

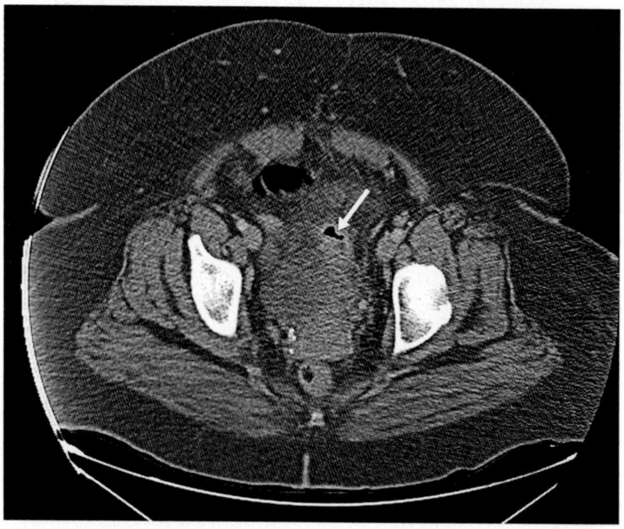

Figure 7-71 Same patient as in Figure 7-70. CT through the pelvis shows fistulous connection of diseased bowel to adjacent bladder. Air is seen in the fistulous tract *(arrow)*.

Other important complications include toxic megacolon (less common than in ulcerative colitis) and enterovaginal, enterovesical, and enteroureteric fistula formation. In addition, as in ulcerative colitis, there are extragastrointestinal manifestations of the disease. Approximately 10% of patients have peripheral arthritis. Dermatological manifestations include erythema nodosum and pyoderma gangrenosum.

The radiological evaluation of Crohn's disease begins with the plain film of the abdomen in most patients. Typically, changes include a bowel gas pattern showing thickened irregular folds (Fig. 7-72). The plain film is also of particular benefit in the evaluation for toxic megacolon. Additionally, unusual gas collections may suggest abscess formation.

The radiological evaluation of a patient with nonfulminant disease and no evidence of toxic megacolon or free air should be with double-contrast technique. The early superficial aphthous-type erosions are missed on a single-contrast study. These tiny erosions are surrounded by apparently normal mucosa.

More severe disease is manifested by deeper and more extensive ulceration, including long linear ulcers (Fig. 7-73). The rectum is histologically involved in more than 50% of cases of colonic Crohn's disease, but may appear grossly normal on radiological examination. Skip lesions and eccentric involvement of the colon should be identified if present (Fig. 7-74). Fistulas, sinus tracts, and periluminal abscesses may be seen in more advanced disease. The involvement tends to be greater in the proximal portions of the colon. If the disease involves the ileocecal valve, the valve may be seen as enlarged and rigid. Generally, if the ileocecal valve is involved, this indicates terminal ileum involvement (Fig. 7-75).

CT of the involved segments shows the expected thickened, rigid bowel wall. CT is especially valuable, however, in the documentation of intraabdominal complications, such as abscess formation (Fig. 7-76). It is extremely useful in evaluating right lower quadrant masses, which may be matted, inflamed loops of bowel, but must be differentiated from abscess. CT also is valuable in performing diagnostic aspiration and therapeutic drainage of intraabdominal pus collections. Small clusters of slightly enlarged lymph nodes may be seen in the mesentery and retroperitoneum.

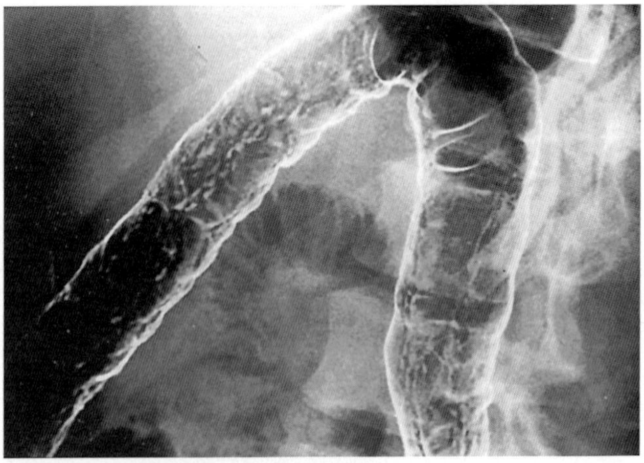

Figure 7-73 Spot film of the splenic flexure shows eccentric involvement of the flexure with focal areas of more severe involvement (skip lesions). Numerous superficial linear and branching ulcers are seen, particularly in the proximal limb.

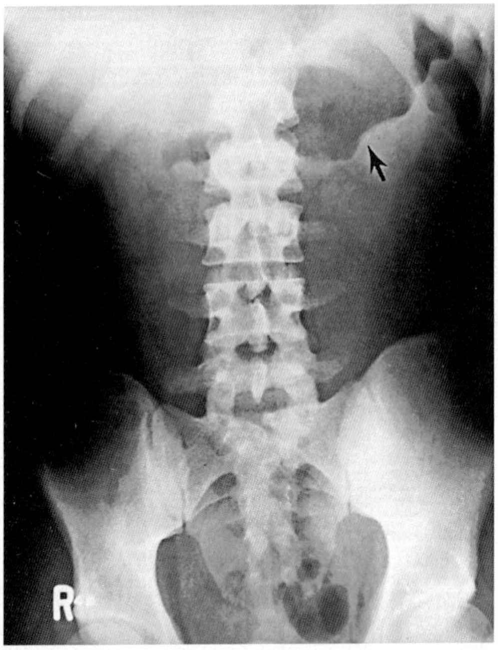

Figure 7-72 Plain film of the abdomen shows abnormal contours *(arrow)* of the air-filled distal transverse colon in a patient with colonic Crohn's disease. The normal haustral pattern is absent, and narrowing of the mid-transverse colon is seen.

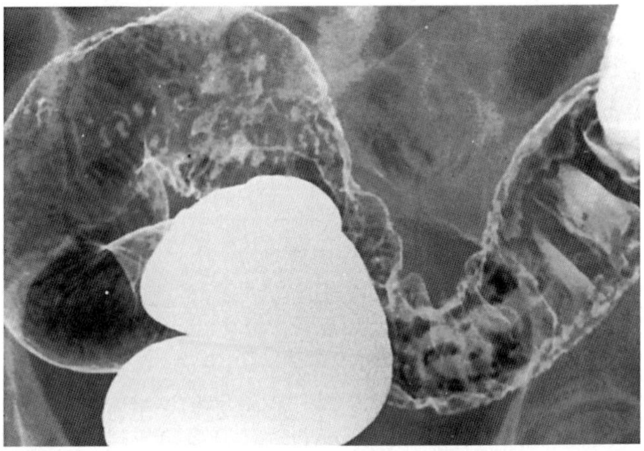

Figure 7-74 In a patient with severe Crohn's disease, DCBE shows marked involvement of the midsigmoid colon and relative sparing of the distal sigmoid colon and rectum.

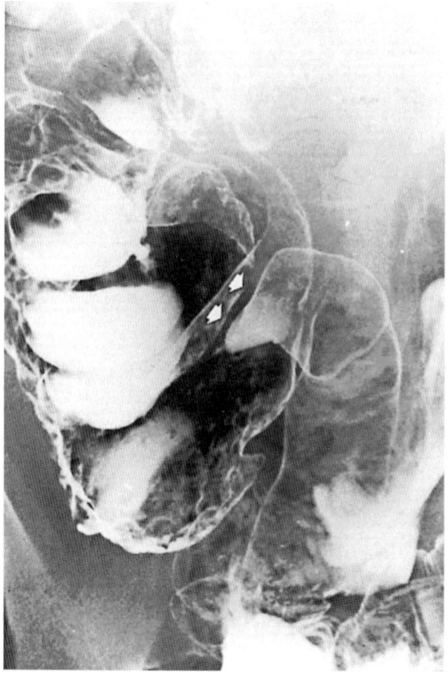

Figure 7-75 This patient had marked involvement of the colon, particularly the cecal region, with Crohn's disease. Note the sparing of the ileocecal valve *(arrows)* and the normal appearance of the terminal ileum.

Ultrasonography can show bowel wall thickening and is useful in the evaluation of possible abscess formation. Typically, abscesses are seen as sonolucent masses with internal echoes. Radionuclide scintigraphy using indium-labeled leukocytes also has been used in the evaluation of possible Crohn's disease in difficult cases. This modality tends to be more useful in small bowel than colonic disease.

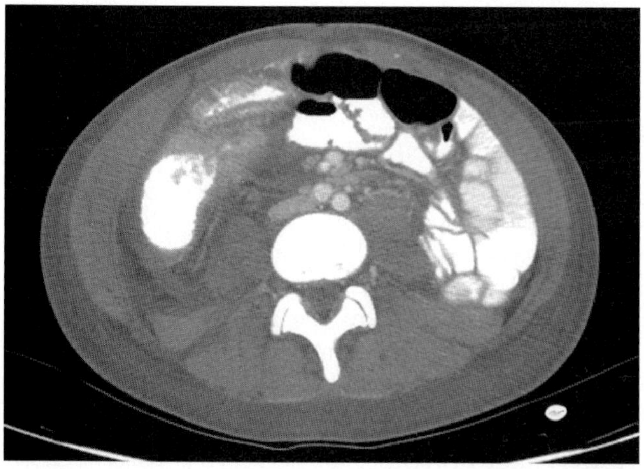

Figure 7-76 CT in a patient with Crohn's disease. Note the marked thickening of the ascending colon and hepatic flexure.

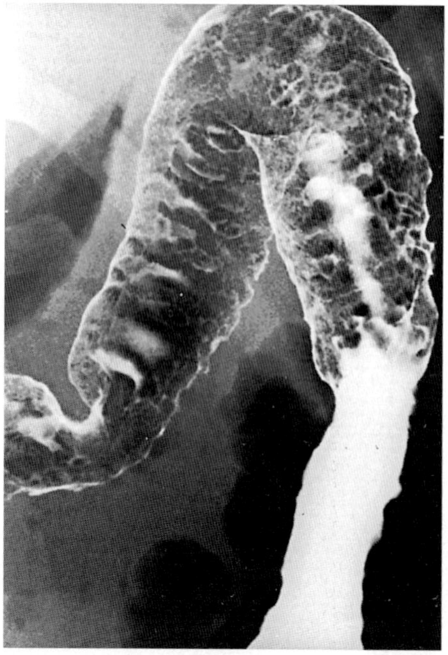

Figure 7-77 Spot film of the splenic flexure in a patient with AIDS who has severe CMV colitis. Note the marked ulceration and nodularity of the mucosal surface of the splenic flexure similar to Crohn's disease.

Viral Colitis

Cytomegalovirus (CMV) colitis is commonly seen in patients with AIDS and patients with other conditions that compromise the immunological system, such as posttransplant immunosuppression. CMV colitis can have a variety of presentations, from diffuse to focal deep ulcerations. Patients often present with bloody diarrhea (Figs. 7-77 and 7-78). Barium enema findings vary from nonspecific, mild, superficial inflammatory changes to dramatic, deep ulcerations. The presence of large, deep ulcers may suggest the possibility of CMV colitis, although biopsy is required for diagnosis.

Bacterial Colitis

Many bacterial infections of the colon, such as *Shigella, Salmonella, Clostridium,* and *Campylobacter* infections, can result in colonic ulcerations. Most of these are infrequently seen, and few barium enemas are performed for these conditions. The findings tend to be nonspecific. The findings seen in *Campylobacter* colitis have been reported to be identical to the findings seen in acute ulcerative colitis. *Yersinia* infections of the bowel are generally limited to the distal ileum, although the cecum can be involved. The radiological findings seem to be quite variable, with edema and ulceration the most common findings. Infectious processes that tend to be limited to the rectum include rectal gonorrhea

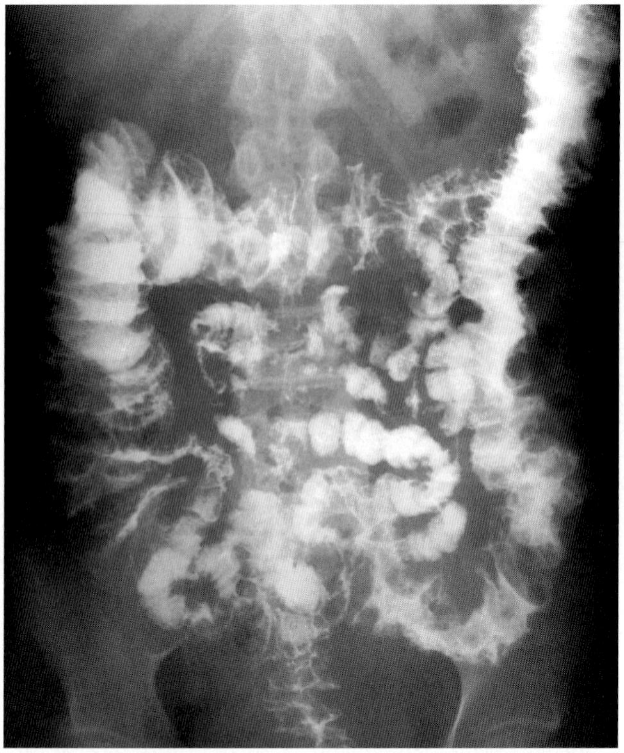

Figure 7-78 CMV colitis involving the entire colon in addition to the distal small bowel.

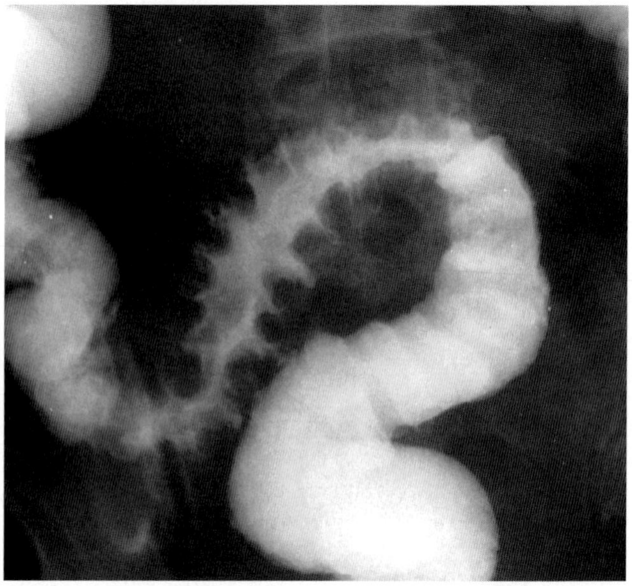

Figure 7-79 Ischemic colitis with marked fold thickening and thumbprinting.

and herpes and *Campylobacter* infections. All of these conditions can manifest with fold thickening and superficial ulceration.

Ischemic Colitis

Ischemic colitis is a condition resulting from the deprivation of adequate blood flow to the bowel, usually from the inferior mesenteric artery distribution. Often the condition is more related to hypoperfusion than to occlusive phenomena. Patients almost uniformly present with bloody diarrhea, occasionally accompanied by lower abdominal pain. The mucosa and submucosa, being most sensitive to the hypoperfusion state, tend to become quickly edematous, hyperemic, and susceptible to ulceration.

The condition is encountered most frequently in elderly patients, with the disease limited to the colon. Progression of the process to gangrene or to more extensive involvement of the colon, or even the distal small bowel, also can be seen and carries a higher mortality rate. Most episodes of ischemic colitis have a benign course, however, with more than half of patients recovering with no evident residual problems. Infection of disrupted mucosa can occur in a few patients, and perforation is uncommon.

The most common finding on either plain film or contrast examination of the colon is marked segmental wall thickening, resulting in the well-known "thumbprinting" sign. Ulceration of the mucosal surface is relatively common (Fig. 7-79). Intramural air can be seen on plain films, barium enema, and CT. The barium enema findings can be easily confused with inflammatory disease of the colon. The most common sites are in the distal colon. The overlapping of the distal middle and distal colic artery circulation around the splenic flexure has long been the basis of discussion as to whether the splenic flexure is more likely to be at risk, being the end of both circulations and most likely to be affected by episodes of hypotension, or whether the area of the splenic flexure is at less risk because of the overlapping circulation at the splenic flexure (Griffith's point). The fact that most ischemic episodes affect the lower descending colon and sigmoid colon seems to favor the latter argument.

Amebiasis

Amebic colitis is the result of colonic parasitic infection by the protozoan *Entamoeba histolytica*. Infection is limited to the colon in most cases, although widespread amebiasis can occur. The protozoan is ingested as a cyst in food or water and eventually passes into the small bowel and colon, where the cyst dissolves, and the uninuclear trophozoite form is released. These motile organisms invade the colonic mucosa, causing hyperemia and edema. Progression of the infectious process results in mucosal ulcers. The cecum and ascending colon are the areas most commonly affected within the colon. Involvement of the adjacent distal ileum is unusual.

In addition to widespread mucosal inflammation and ulceration, a more localized, masslike form of the process, an ameboma, is occasionally identified. An ameboma is a marked, localized reaction involving an extensive granulomatous type of inflammation, thickening of the bowel wall, and narrowing of the lumen. The configuration of an ameboma may look like carcinoma on endoscopic or radiological examination. Amebomas are uncommon and are seen in less than 0.5% of cases.

If the barium enema is used (and it is seldom used when the diagnosis is known), it often shows severely inflamed spastic bowel with widespread ulceration. In the early stages, superficial discrete ulcers may be identified on ACBE. The disease tends to be more prevalent in the proximal portions of the colon. In severe disease, there can be marked edema of the bowel wall, thumbprinting, and toxic dilatation (Fig. 7-80). The radiological findings on ACBE and CT are nonspecific, and any stage of the examination can resemble Crohn's disease or ulcerative colitis. Distinction between amebiasis and IBD is crucial because patients with amebiasis who are inadvertently treated with steroids may decline rapidly. The definitive diagnosis is made by detecting the organisms in the stool or endoscopic aspirate.

A helpful but nonspecific radiological finding is the "conical" cecum resulting from diffuse inflammation and spasm of the cecal tip. Other conditions, such as Crohn's disease, tuberculosis, actinomycosis, and even adjacent appendiceal disease, also can result in a conical cecum.

Radiation Colitis

Inflammatory changes secondary to radiation are seen most commonly in the rectum and sigmoid colon, usually as a result of radiation therapy for pelvic neoplastic disease. Radiation colitis seems to be associated most commonly with treatment of carcinoma of the cervix. Acute changes are nonspecific and mostly consist of edema and erythema. In more severe radiation damage or chronic radiation damage, the colon tends to lose its haustral pattern and become tubular (Fig. 7-81). Rectal folds may disappear completely. Frequently, there is widening of the presacral space. Ulceration may be present to varying degrees in the acute and chronic phases.

Tuberculosis

Tuberculosis involving the gastrointestinal tract can be either primary or secondary. Primary involvement, usually associated with the ingestion of nonpasteurized milk, is rarely seen in Western countries today. *Mycobacterium tuberculosis* primarily involving the lungs can infect the gastrointestinal tract secondarily as a result of swallowed organisms in the sputum. The disease tends to occur around the ileocecal region, possibly because of the abundant lymphoid tissue in that area. Clinical presentation tends to be nonspecific, with the most common presenting complaints being abdominal pain, weight loss, fever, and diarrhea. The radiological evaluation may be helpful in identifying an inflammatory

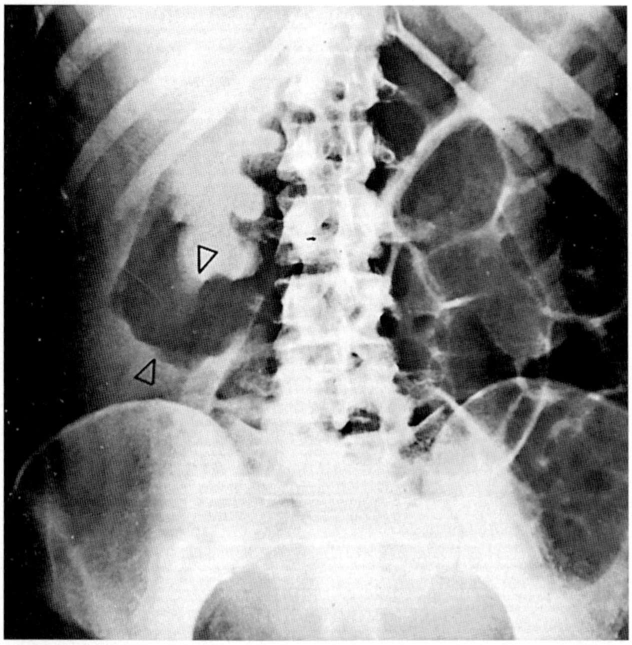

Figure 7-80 Plain film of the abdomen in a patient with fulminant amebic colitis. Note the narrowing of the proximal transverse colon and the prominent nodularity (thumbprinting) in this region *(arrowheads)*.

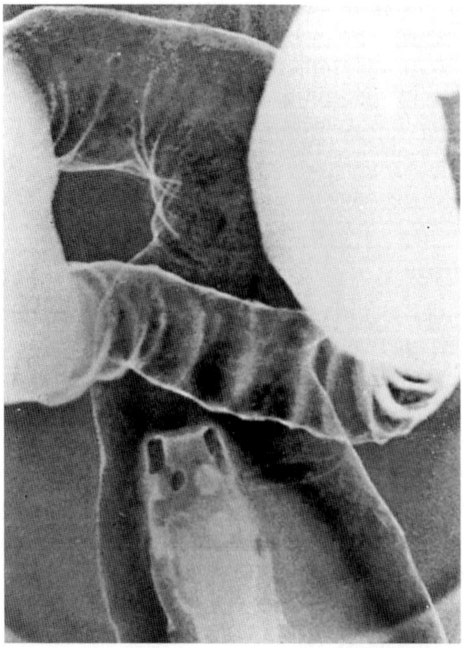

Figure 7-81 Rectosigmoid spot film in a patient with chronic radiation proctitis and sigmoiditis. There is a general loss of the haustral pattern with a tubular appearance of the bowel.

mucosal process, but is not diagnostic. The radiological appearance can mimic Crohn's disease, including mucosal ulceration, fold thickening, and occasionally stricture. The terminal ileum is commonly involved. In patients with known primary pulmonary tuberculosis, these findings raise the diagnostic possibility of gastrointestinal tuberculosis. The definitive diagnosis is made by identification of the organism.

The incidence of gastrointestinal tuberculosis has increased with an increasingly large AIDS population in the community. In addition to *M. tuberculosis,* another form of tuberculosis that has been seen with increasing frequency in these patients is *Mycobacterium avium-intracellulare,* now designated as *M. avium* complex. This organism is generally nonpathological. In immunocompromised patients, such as patients with AIDS, *M. avium* complex infections primarily involving the respiratory tract are seen with increasing frequency, however. In such patients, this organism occasionally may be found to be the basis of gastrointestinal infection as well.

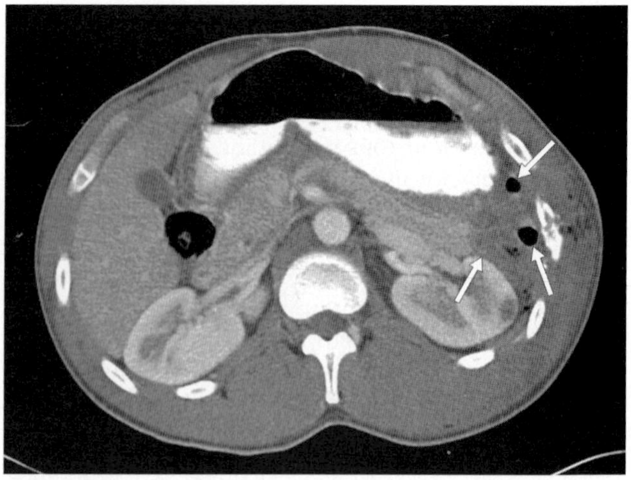

Figure 7-82 Gunshot injury to left colon. Note blood and air in left paracolic area *(arrows).*

Solitary Rectal Ulcer Syndrome

Solitary rectal ulcer syndrome, an unusual and confusing disorder, was first described in the early 1800s. It is most commonly seen in young or middle-aged adults, and the presenting findings are rectal bleeding and mucous discharge. Many patients also report difficulty passing stool. Ulcers frequently can be identified, although commonly there is more than a solitary ulcer present. Multiple etiological theories have been suggested. Perhaps the most important is the association of internal rectal prolapse and difficult rectal evacuation. The disease may be associated with or identical to colitis cystica profunda.

Radiologically, inflammatory changes including ulceration can be identified along the anterior rectal wall. The rectal valves often appear thickened. A polypoid inflammatory mass also may be identified and may mimic neoplastic disease.

Trauma

Although colorectal trauma may result from a variety of causes, such as gunshot wounds (Figs. 7-82 and 7-83), stabbing, or blunt trauma, most cases are probably iatrogenic. These can occur as a result of the traumatic effect of a barium enema tip on the rectal mucosa or intracolonic instrumentation, such as results from sigmoidoscopy or colonoscopy. Frequently, these instruments may cause mucosal lacerations, but infrequently result in serious complications, such as perforation.

Behçet's Disease

Behçet's disease is a condition sometimes referred to as the "silk route" disease because of its historical prevalence in the Mediterranean basin, where it was thought to have been brought back by Marco Polo, along with silk, from his overland journeys to the Far East. The disease is of unknown origin and is characterized by four main clinical findings: aphthous ulcers of the mouth, eyes, skin, and genitalia. It tends to be more common in men between ages 40 and 50. Gastrointestinal involvement occurs in less than half of patients and tends to be a minor manifestation of the condition. In a few patients, colonic involvement can be severe, and significant ulceration may be seen (Fig. 7-84).

The radiological evaluation may be confusing because Behçet's disease can simulate either Crohn's disease or, in some cases, ulcerative colitis. Additionally, because both of these idiopathic IBDs are known to have extracolonic manifestations that involve the eyes and skin, patients with Behçet's disease may carry the diagnosis of IBD for some time.

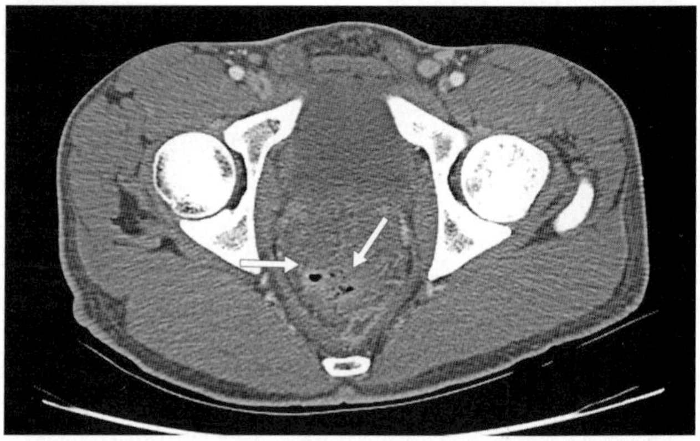

Figure 7-83 Gunshot wound in the rectum. There is blood as well as tiny air bubbles in the pararectal space *(arrows).*

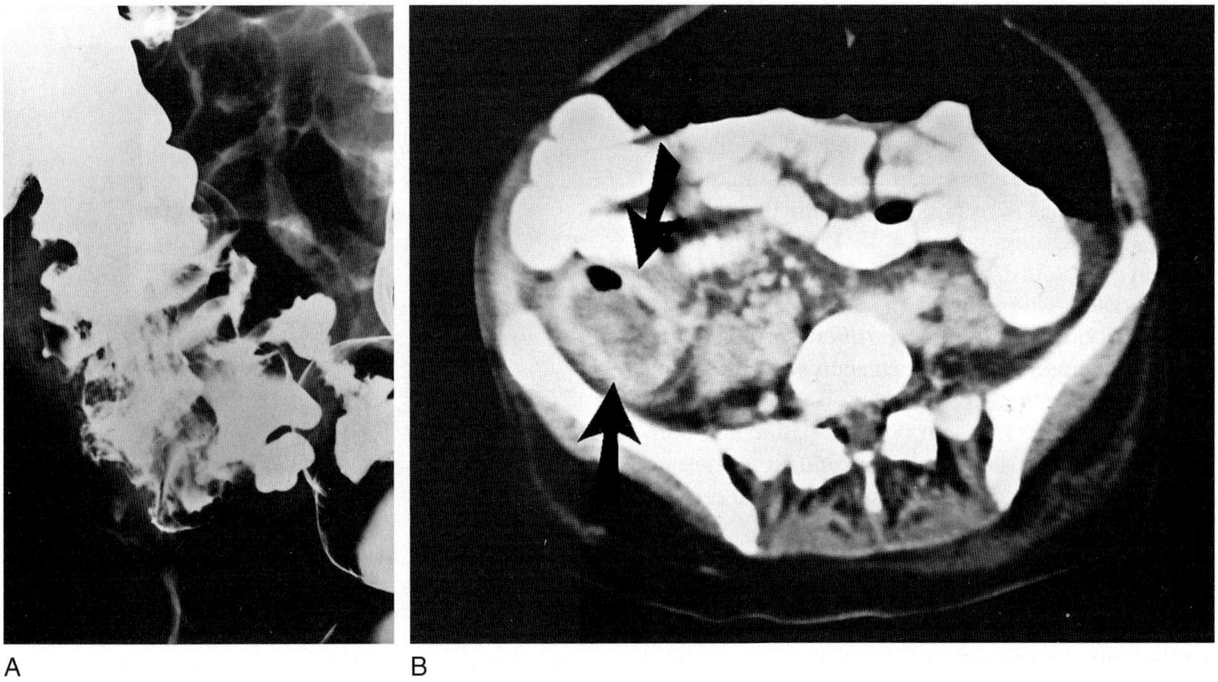

Figure 7-84 Patient with Behçet's disease with involvement of the right colon. **A,** ACBE shows thickened irregular folds with some areas of ulceration in the cecum. **B,** CT shows inflammatory changes in cecal wall *(arrows)*.

Diversion Colitis

In patients who have had their fecal stream diverted as the result of a proximal colostomy or ileostomy, a nonspecific inflammation involving the diverted portion of the colon may be seen, representing what has been termed *diversion colitis*. The radiological evaluation of the excluded colonic segment shows acute inflammatory changes similar to mild acute ulcerative colitis. This curious condition usually spontaneously regresses when the ostomy has been taken down and the fecal stream reestablished.

Gonorrheal Proctitis

Gonorrhea is a relatively common sexually transmitted infectious disease that involves the mucous membranes of the urethra, vagina, and cervix. Rectal involvement can occur in women as a result of infected vaginal discharge and secondary rectal infection or primarily as a result of anal intercourse. In men, it always results from direct sexual contact and is seen in homosexuals. The radiological findings are superficial inflammatory changes involving the mucosa of the rectum with fold thickening and areas of punctate ulceration (Fig. 7-85). The appearance may be identical to ulcerative proctitis seen early in the development of ulcerative colitis. Other infectious processes, such as *Campylobacter* and viral proctitis, can give a similar picture.

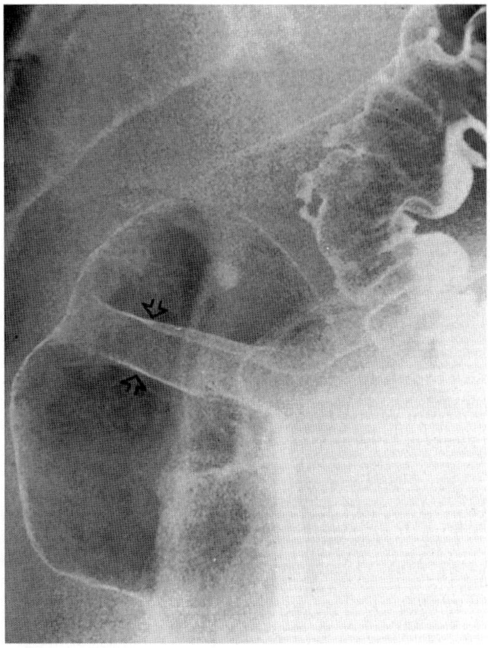

Figure 7-85 Spot film of the rectum in a patient with known gonorrheal proctitis. Note the thickening of the rectal folds *(arrows)* and the granular appearance of the mucosa.

COLONIC NARROWING

Adenocarcinoma

Although the physical manifestations of colonic adenocarcinoma are numerous, one common manifestation is focal irregular narrowing, classically described as the "apple core" configuration or the British equivalent, the "napkin ring" (Fig. 7-86). This lesion involves a short segment of colon, frequently with some degree of proximal dilatation or obstruction, especially in the sigmoid colon. Annular lesions tend to be relatively uncommon in the rectum, where large bulky polypoid lesions are considerably more frequent (Fig. 7-87). Rectal lesions also occur in a slightly older age group and are associated with a more aggressive course and slightly decreased survival time.

Diverticulitis

Diverticulitis represents one of the two common complications of diverticulosis of the colon (the other being bleeding), and as such, the underlying condition of diverticulosis requires some understanding before this complication can be fully understood. Diverticular disease of the colon is a condition of 20th century industrialized nations and was relatively uncommon before. Diverticula can occur anywhere in the colon, but are most common in the sigmoid region (Fig. 7-88). These diverticula develop at the site of penetrating blood vessels entering the bowel wall. The mucosa and submucosa of the bowel wall tend to protrude through these natural areas of wall weakness. This anatomical relationship of diverticula to penetrating blood vessels accounts for the high incidence of hemorrhage associated with diverticulum formation.

The etiological origins of diverticulum formation seem to be related to abnormally high intraluminal

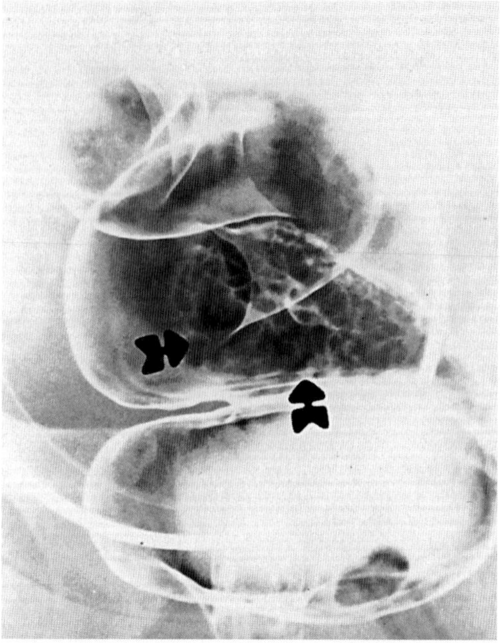

Figure 7-87 An air-contrast view of rectal carcinoma *(arrows)* shows a large, bulky polypoid lesion with a villous appearance.

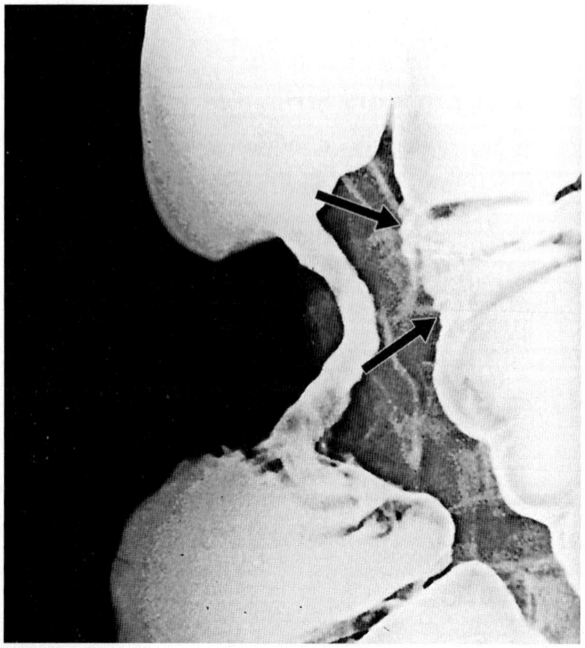

Figure 7-86 Typical apple core or napkin ring configuration of an annular carcinoma of the colon. Note the contiguous invasion of the adjacent colon *(arrows)*.

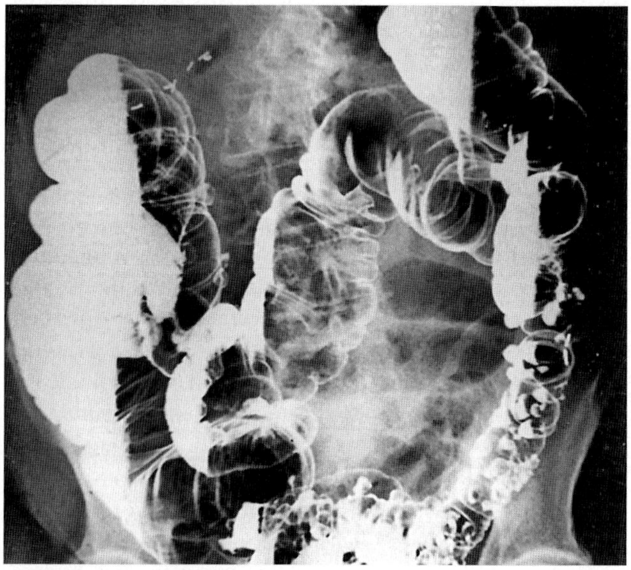

Figure 7-88 Decubitus view from DCBE shows marked diverticular changes concentrated in the sigmoid region, resulting in considerable distortion of the bowel and difficulty in evaluating the area.

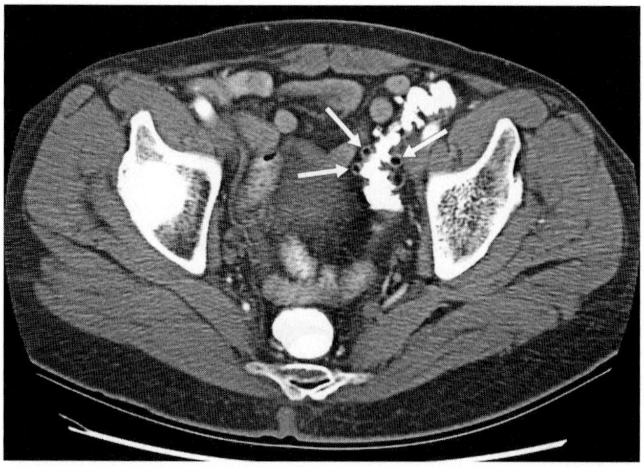

Figure 7-89 Diverticular changes *(arrows)* are seen in the sigmoid colon without evidence of diverticulosis.

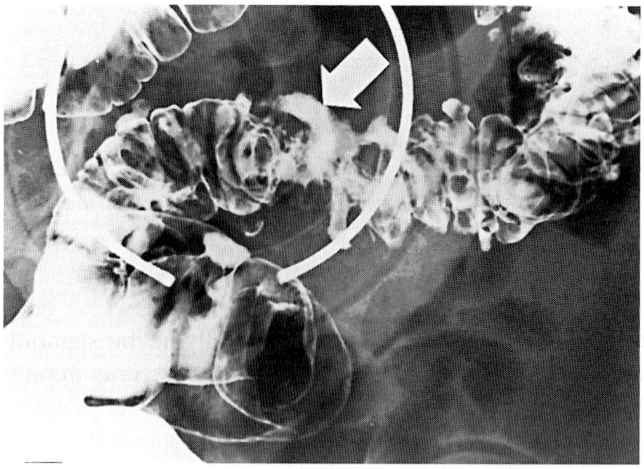

Figure 7-90 Spot film from DCBE reveals multiple diverticula in the sigmoid region with narrowing and irregularity. A lenticular collection of barium *(arrow)* represents a pericolic abscess secondary to diverticulitis.

colonic pressures and abnormally prolonged colonic transit times. Chronic disease results in muscular thickening, and when severe diverticulosis is present, there can be diffuse narrowing even without the presence of diverticulitis.

The incidence is thought to be slightly more common in women than in men and definitely increases with age. At age 60, 60% to 70% of patients examined by barium enema have some degree of diverticulum formation (Fig. 7-89). It is also suggested that the disease may be occurring in increasingly younger individuals.

As previously mentioned, this condition seems to be seen most commonly in Western industrialized nations and is almost unheard of in Africa and the Far East; this is thought to relate to differences in the fiber content of the diet and to significant differences in colonic transit times. It also has been observed that long-time vegetarians seem to have a decreased incidence of diverticular disease.

Most patients with uncomplicated diverticulosis are likely to be asymptomatic. There is a poorly defined group of patients who experience lower abdominal pain, exacerbated by dietary intake, who are given the diagnostic label of "irritable bowel syndrome." Whether the so-called irritable bowel syndrome is a manifestation of colonic intraluminal pressure abnormalities leading to diverticulum formation, or whether it is a coexisting condition is unclear, and there is difficulty in defining the irritable bowel syndrome. There have been assertions that a correlation exists between the two conditions, although this idea is controversial.

Patients who develop complications associated with diverticulosis most frequently develop rectal bleeding. The most common cause of massive lower gastrointestinal bleeding is diverticulosis.

Much the same way that appendicitis develops, diverticulitis can occur when a diverticulum becomes occluded by stool, and peridiverticular inflammatory changes associated with microperforations can occur. These can go on to frank pericolic abscess formation (Fig. 7-90). Areas of narrowing may occur as a result of spasm associated with the inflammation, even in the early changes of diverticulitis without abscess formation. With the presence of abscess formation, the narrowing results from a combination of spasm and mass effect. CT is useful in the evaluation of diverticulitis, showing thickened edematous bowel wall (Fig. 7-91) and pericolic abscesses (Fig. 7-92). The three classic barium enema findings are narrowing and spasm, mass effect, and barium in intramural tracts or pericolic abscess.

Postinflammatory Strictures

Many inflammatory conditions can cause focal stricturing and narrowing of the colon. They may occur

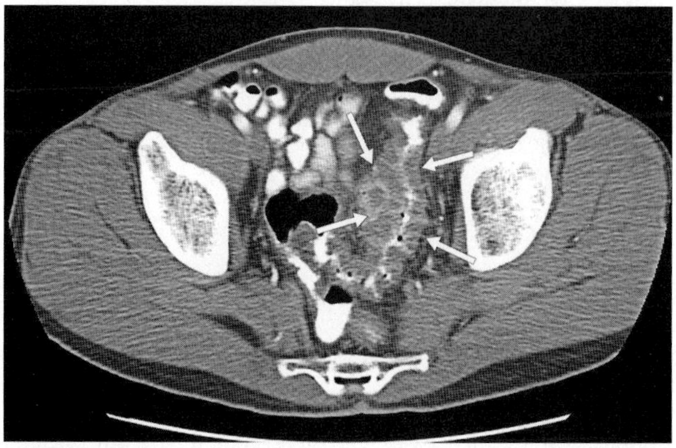

Figure 7-91 CT of pelvis shows inflammation and thickening of sigmoid bowel wall *(arrows)* and narrowing of the lumen, representing diverticulitis without evidence of overt abscess.

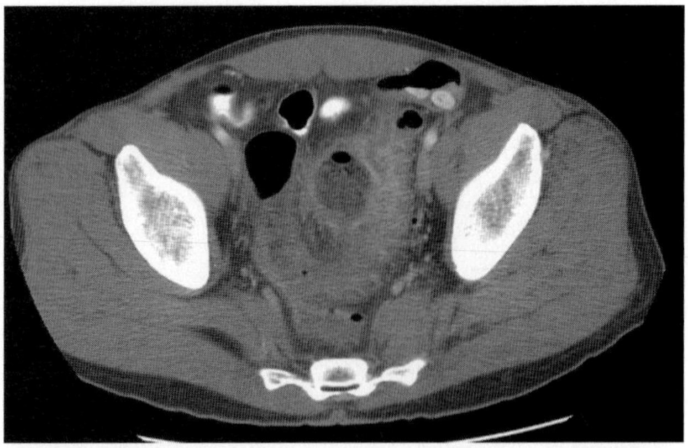

Figure 7-92 Pelvic abscess secondary to acute diverticulitis.

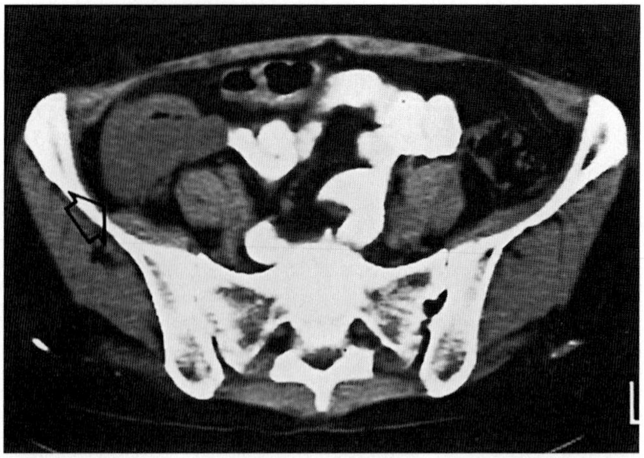

Figure 7-94 CT through the upper pelvis in the same patient as seen in Figure 7-93. Note the marked thickening of the colon wall *(arrow)* just above the ileocecal valve.

during the acute phase (Figs. 7-93 and 7-94), but commonly are seen as a sequela to chronic disease. Colonic strictures are seen in less than 10% of patients with chronic ulcerative colitis (Fig. 7-95). They rarely result in obstructive changes. In patients with severe chronic ulcerative colitis, the narrowing may be more diffuse, involving a long segment of the colon (Fig. 7-96).

Because of the transmural inflammatory changes associated with Crohn's disease, areas of focal stricture are slightly more common (Fig. 7-97). The strictures may be asymmetric, reflecting the asymmetric involvement of the bowel at that level.

A common cause of narrowing in the rectum and sigmoid area is radiation colitis. Radiation therapy is usually performed for neoplastic disease of the pelvis. The involved bowel in the radiation port undergoes degrees of vascular injury. Diffuse or focal areas of narrowing are encountered. Other unusual causes of colonic stricture include amebic, bacterial, and viral colitides.

Hirschsprung's disease, most commonly seen in children, also can be seen occasionally in young adults with delayed diagnosis. The same aganglionosis segment is also the cause in young adults. These patients usually are treated for chronic constipation for years (Fig. 7-98).

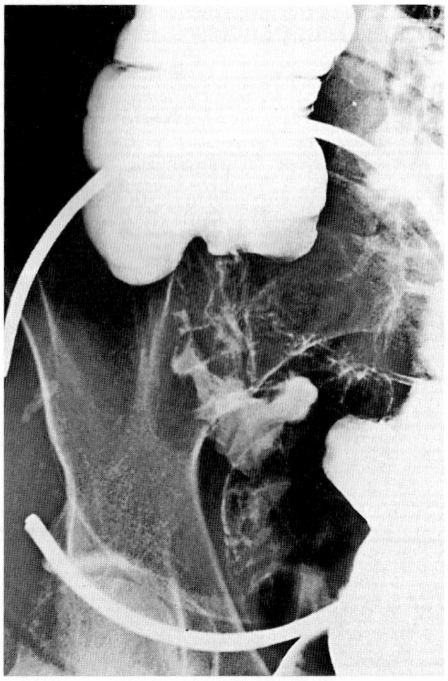

Figure 7-93 Patient with persistent colonic stricture located just above the ileocecal valve. The mucosa appears to be intact, and this stricture was found to be inflammatory in nature, representing CMV colitis.

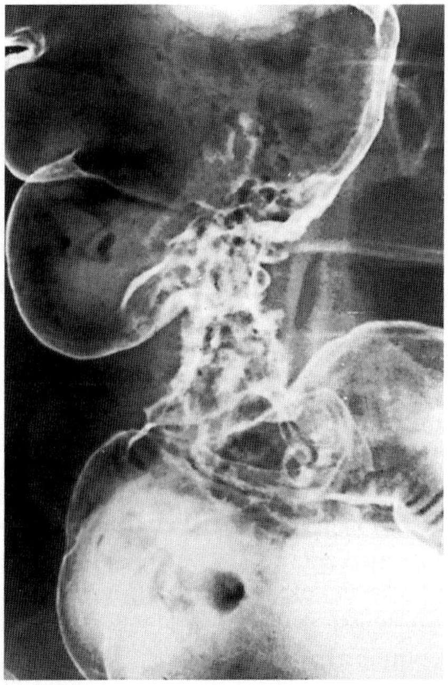

Figure 7-95 This patient has ulcerative colitis and a well-defined stricture located just above the ileocecal valve, secondary to focal inflammatory changes.

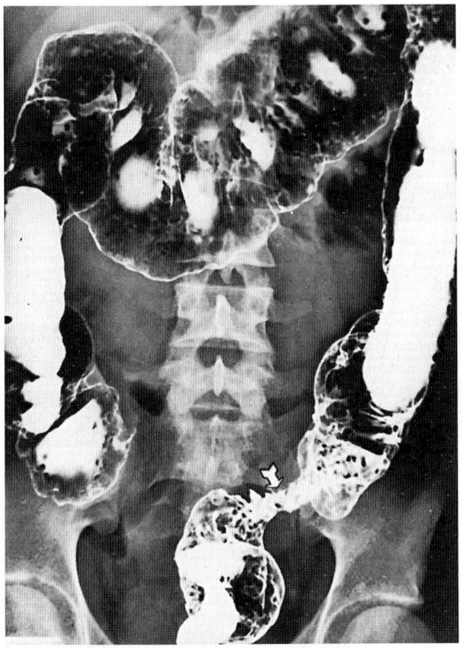

Figure 7-96 DCBE in a patient with chronic ulcerative colitis. Widespread postinflammatory polyposis is seen along with a strictured segment *(arrow)* in the sigmoid colon.

Ischemic Colitis

Greater than half of patients who experience ischemic colitis undergo complete and spontaneous remission, with return to the normal configuration and appearance of the colon. In a smaller number of patients, there is sufficient injury to the mucosa and submucosa that the resultant fibrosis can cause focal luminal narrowing (Fig. 7-99). As with all areas of colonic narrowing, the status of the mucosa in the narrowed segment should be carefully ascertained. In most inflammatory or postinflammatory causes of stricture, a mucosal pattern can be detected, as opposed to the destroyed and replaced mucosa associated with malignant disease.

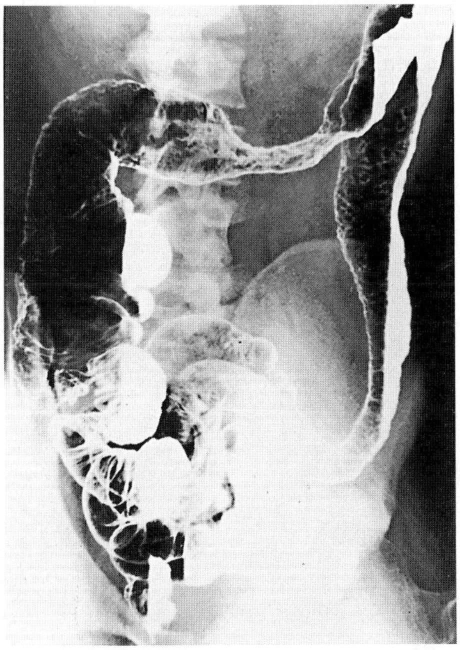

Figure 7-97 DCBE in a patient with Crohn's disease shows an area of stricturing involving the distal transverse colon.

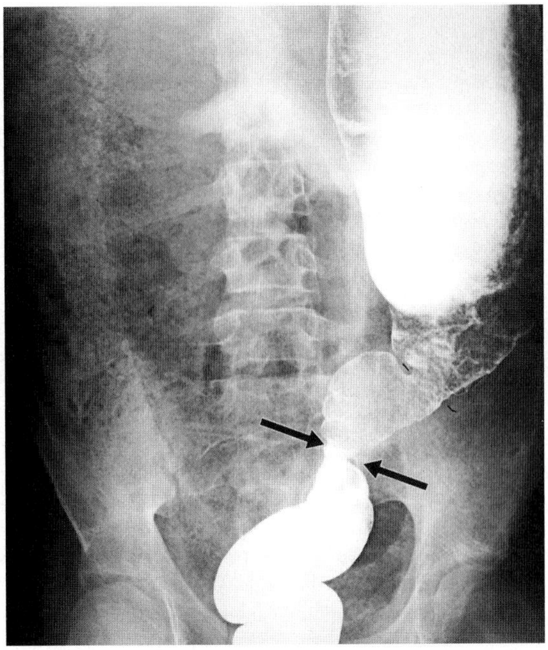

Figure 7-98 Hirschsprung's disease in a young adult. Note the narrowed aganglionosis segment *(arrows)* and the markedly dilated, stool-filled proximal colon.

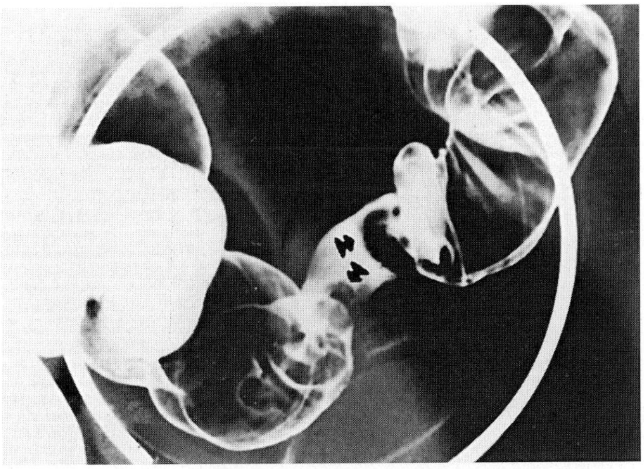

Figure 7-99 Spot film of the sigmoid colon in a patient with a smooth postischemic stricture. Polypoid filling defects in the stricture *(arrows)* proved to be a polypoid adenocarcinoma arising in the stricture.

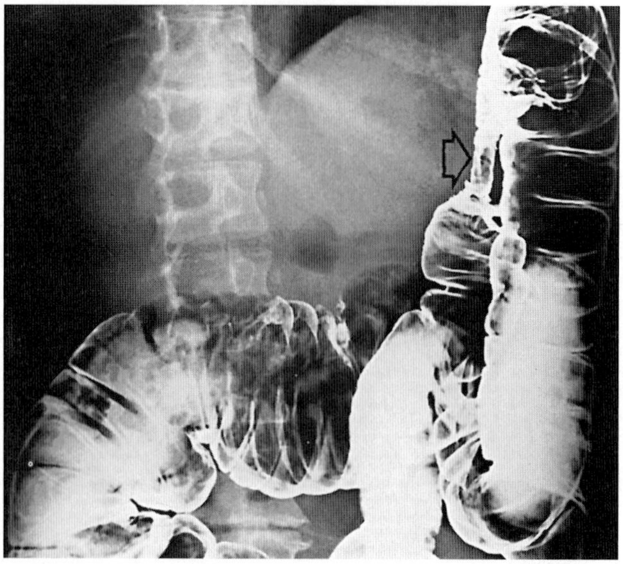

Figure 7-100 Overhead film shows a fixed area of narrowing *(arrow)* in the ascending limb of the splenic flexure. The mucosa is intact. This area of persistent narrowing is a result of an adjacent pancreatic pseudocyst that involves the colon at that point.

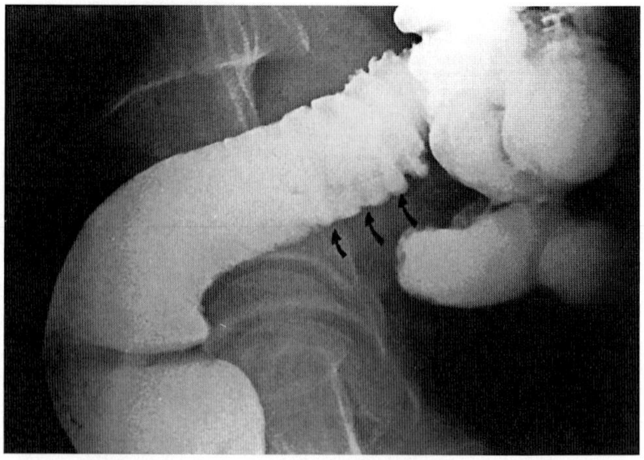

Figure 7-102 Spot film of the rectum shows some spasm at the rectosigmoid junction and a crenulated appearance along the anterior margin *(arrows)*. This patient had a periappendiceal abscess, and pus was discovered in the lower recesses of the pelvis, accounting for these changes.

Adjacent Inflammatory or Neoplastic Disease

Processes not originating in the colon can indirectly involve the colon, resulting in luminal narrowing (Fig. 7-100). In the pelvis, pus or metastatic disease affecting the colon from the serosal side can result in a combination of spasm and infiltration, causing narrowing of the lumen (Fig. 7-101). Some common inflammatory causes of this condition include periappendiceal abscess and pelvic inflammatory disease (Fig. 7-102).

Secondary neoplastic disease invading this region through the mesenteric pathways and serosal surface is a relatively common occurrence (Fig. 7-103). This invasion results in the spiculated or crenulated margin on the mesenteric side of the bowel commonly seen in this condition. Invasion of the serosal surface of the bowel causes marked spasm of that segment of the bowel (Fig. 7-104). This spasm is among the most painful types encountered during the course of a barium enema and is many times more uncomfortable than spasm experienced by patients with acute diverticulitis.

Extension of inflammatory or neoplastic processes through the gastrocolic ligament or the transverse mesocolon also can involve portions of the transverse colon, resulting in eccentric narrowing (Fig. 7-105). These include malignant lesions arising from the stomach

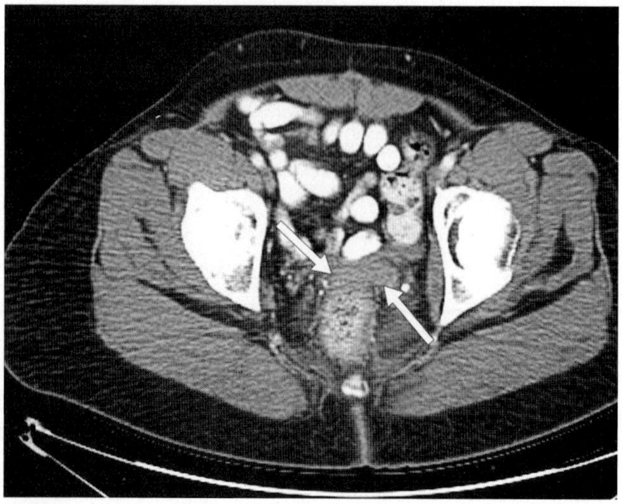

Figure 7-101 This patient has ovarian cancer and metastatic implants *(arrows)* on bowel wall.

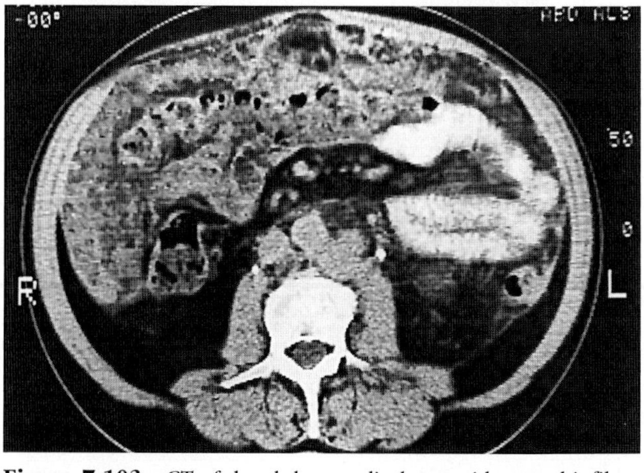

Figure 7-103 CT of the abdomen discloses widespread infiltration of the mesentery with tumor extending to and involving the transverse colon.

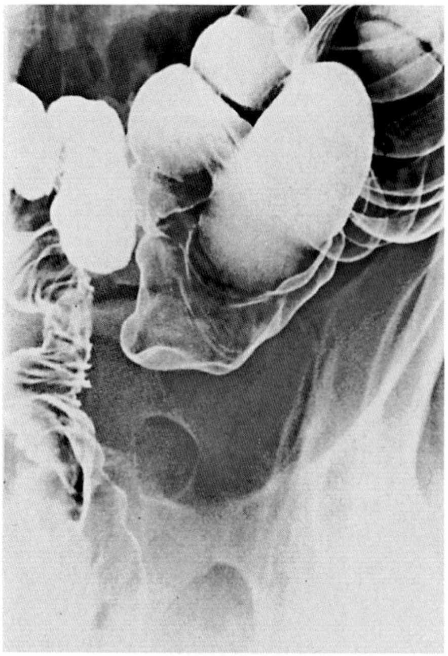

Figure 7-104 Spot film from DCBE shows a narrowing, spasm, and serrated margins of the sigmoid colon in a patient with widespread ovarian carcinoma involving the serosal surface of the bowel.

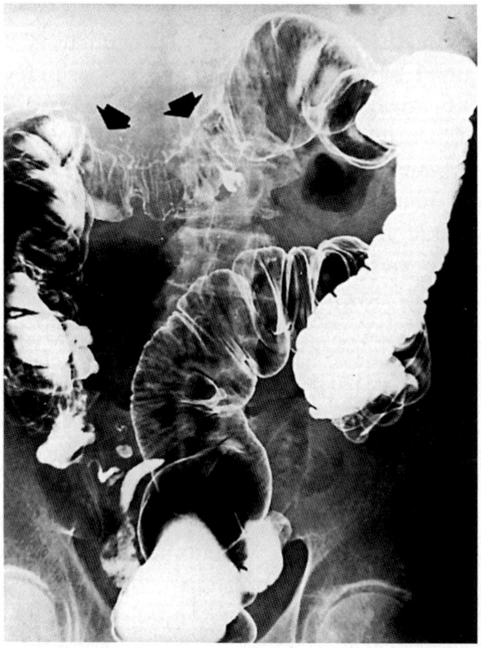

Figure 7-105 DCBE in a patient presenting with anemia. Extrinsic mass and spiculation seen along the superior margin of the transverse colon *(arrows)* represent metastatic extension of a primary gastric carcinoma down the gastrocolic ligament, investing the transverse colon on its serosal margin.

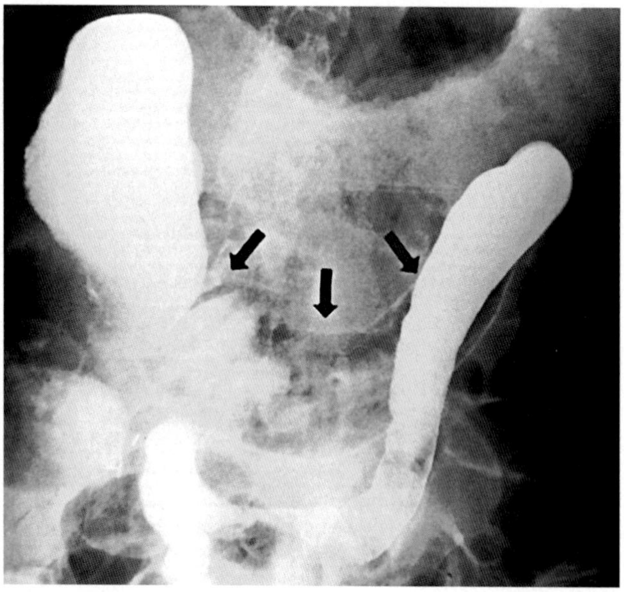

Figure 7-106 A patient with abscess in the lesser sac. The lesser sac is distended with pus and is impressing and depressing the transverse colon *(arrows)*.

and pancreas. Pancreatitis can result in inflammatory exudates traversing the transverse mesocolon and involving the colon. In addition, moderate to large accumulations of fluid in the lesser sac may indirectly involve the transverse colon (Fig. 7-106).

Endometriosis

Endometriosis is the presence of active, functioning endometrial tissue outside of the uterus. In approximately one quarter of the cases, endometriosis involves the bowel. Commonly, the sigmoid and rectosigmoid junctions are involved. It also can be seen rarely in the cecum and the terminal ileum.

Patients may be asymptomatic, although complaints of crampy abdominal pain sometimes associated with the menstrual cycle can be elicited. Areas of eccentric luminal narrowing can be seen endoscopically in the sigmoid region. The mucosa may appear distorted but intact. Diagnosis in the proper clinical setting often can be suggested by barium enema. Commonly, there is an area of eccentric narrowing with spiculations and nodularity along the affected margin (Fig. 7-107).

Lymphoma

Although lymphoma of the colon can appear as a localized mass lesion with luminal narrowing (Fig. 7-108), it also may be seen as an infiltrating mass lesion in which the lumen of the replaced bowel appears widened (aneurysmal dilatation). This appearance is seen more frequently in the small bowel. The colonic lesions tend

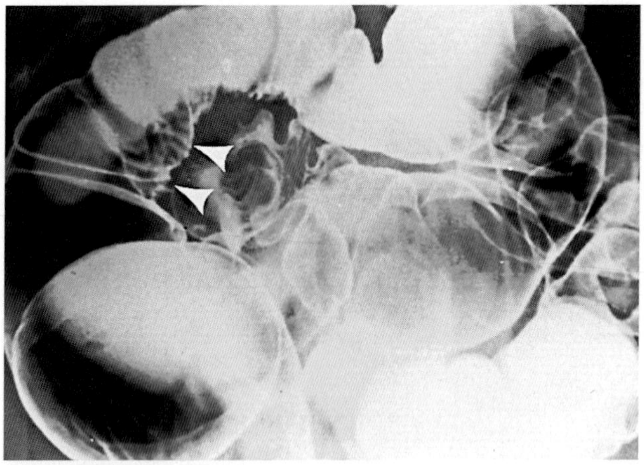

Figure 7-107 A patient with known endometriosis shows typical findings of serosal involvement at the rectosigmoid junction. The anterior margin of the bowel is crenulated and spiculated at this point with some mass effect *(arrowheads)*.

to occur with more frequency on the right side and rarely obstruct (Fig. 7-109).

Lymphogranuloma Venereum

Lymphogranuloma venereum is a sexually transmitted disease caused by the rickettsial organism, *Chlamydia trachomatis*. Significant inguinal lymphadenopathy is a common finding in this condition. Rectal involvement also is relatively common. When it does occur, it can result in narrowing of the rectum and distal sigmoid colon associated with marked edematous changes and possible ulceration. Fistulous tracts communicating to perirectal abscesses or to the perineum may occur.

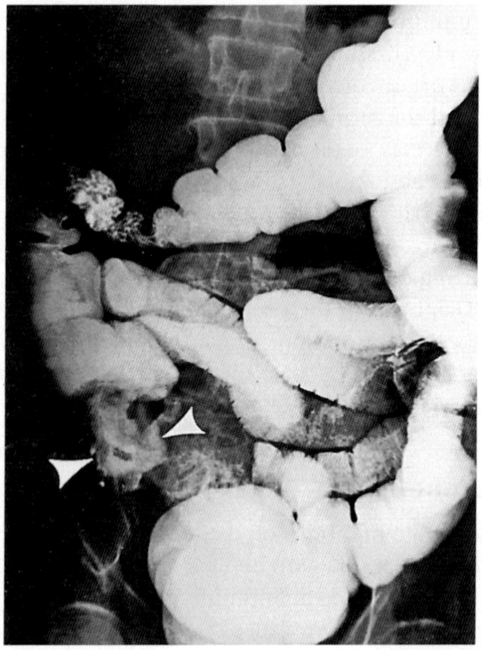

Figure 7-108 SCBE in a patient with colonic lymphoma shows narrowing and irregularity of the cecum *(arrowheads)*.

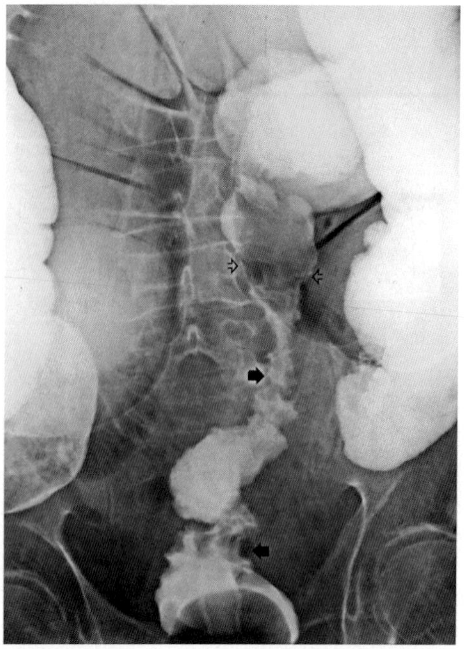

Figure 7-109 ACBE shows long irregular segment of infiltrated distal colon *(open arrows)* and rectum *(solid arrows)*. Resection and pathologic examination revealed colonic lymphoma.

Actinomycosis

Actinomycosis is an aggressive inflammatory disease, uncontained by the usual tissue and fascial planes, that commonly forms multiple sinus tracts. The disease is bacterial in origin, caused by a gram-positive anaerobic organism, *Actinomyces israelii*. When it involves the colon or rectum, actinomycosis usually is associated with luminal mass, narrowing, and sinus or fistulous tracts. The radiological differentiation from colonic malignancy or diverticulitis can be extremely difficult.

Extrinsic Compression

Colonic luminal narrowing can occur as a result of extrinsic processes compressing the colon. If the processes are inflammatory in nature, the compression accompanied by spasm can result in marked luminal narrowing. Likewise, an adjacent neoplasm with contiguous spread gives a similar appearance. The usual lesions that result in compression of the colon to this degree are pelvic masses compressing the sigmoid region (Fig. 7-110). A markedly enlarged spleen also can compress the region of the splenic flexure, whereas a very enlarged left hepatic lobe can depress and displace the colon (Fig. 7-111).

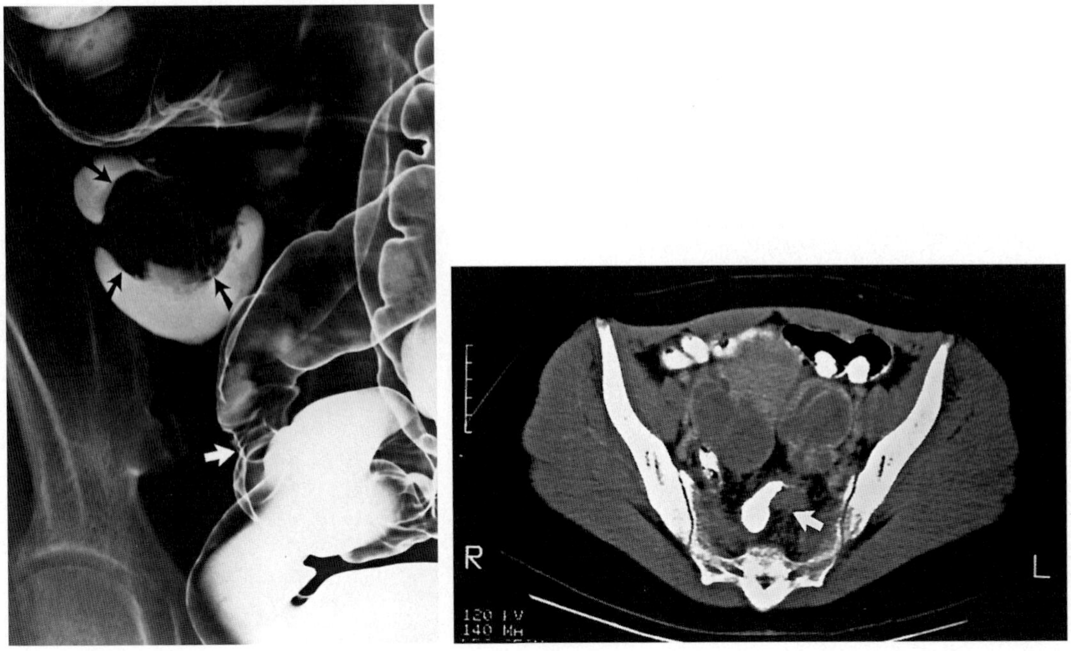

Figure 7-110 A 46-year-old woman with constipation and painful defecation. **A,** ACBE shows tethered narrowing in sigmoid colon *(white arrow)* and unusual filling defect in cecum *(black arrows)*. **B,** CT of the pelvis shows mixed cystic and solid lesion encasing sigmoid colon *(arrow)*. A serosal deposit also was seen on the cecum. The diagnosis was carcinoma of the ovary with serosal spread.

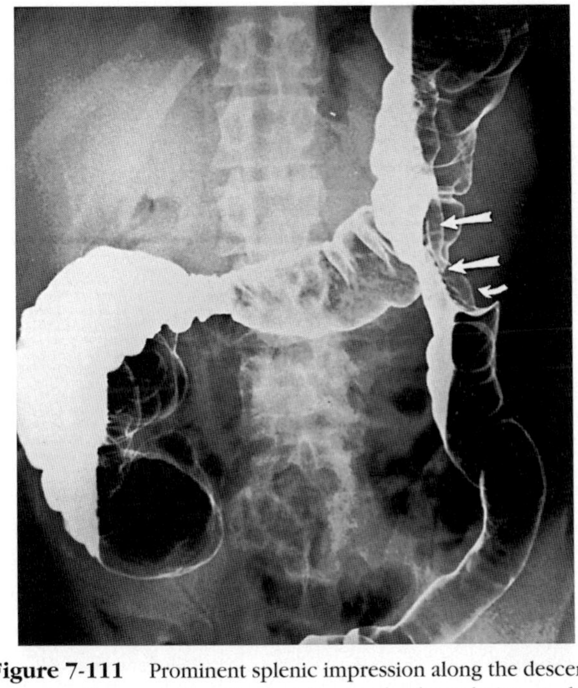

Figure 7-111 Prominent splenic impression along the descending colon *(arrows)* simulates an intramural colonic lesion, such as a leiomyoma.

Carcinoid Tumor

Gastrointestinal carcinoid tumors are seen most commonly in the appendix and the distal small bowel. Colonic involvement is uncommon. When it does occur, the two most frequent sites tend to be the proximal ascending colon and the rectum.

The radiological problems posed by this tumor are multiple. It can be a small polypoid lesion or a large, bulky lesion identical in appearance to colonic carcinoma. It may present as an area of focal stricture, which also may be indistinguishable from the common colonic malignancy. Differentiation between benign and malignant lesions is sometimes difficult when there is no evidence of metastatic disease. The presence of malignancy in a focal lesion varies from 10% to 40%. In general, metastatic disease is associated more frequently with carcinoids of the colon than of the small bowel.

MECHANICAL DILATATION

Any condition that compromises the colonic lumen and obstructs the antegrade flow of the fecal stream results in proximal dilatation. This includes a wide spectrum of lesions, including colonic carcinoma, inflammatory strictures, intussusception, and hernia. Rarely, severe

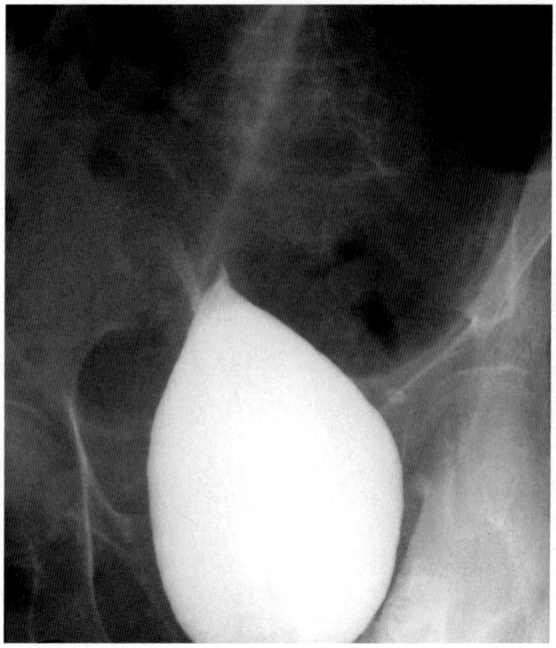

Figure 7-112 Typical beaklike appearance of the obstructed barium column in a patient with sigmoid volvulus.

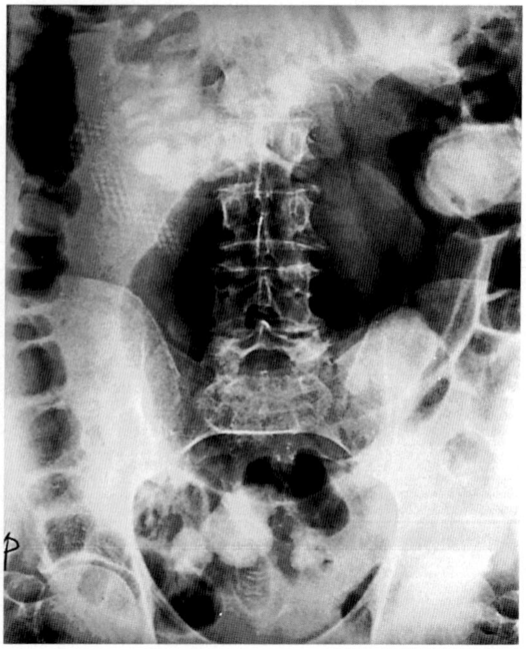

Figure 7-113 Plain film of the abdomen shows dilated air-filled cecum slightly to the left of midline in a patient with cecal volvulus.

ischemic colitis can result in residual narrowing, although obstruction is uncommon. Patients with lymphoma rarely become obstructed. Colonic adhesions are rare, but can result in luminal narrowing and proximal dilatation.

After malignant obstructions and obstruction secondary to inflammatory stricture, volvulus is the third most common cause of colonic obstruction. The two most common forms of colonic volvulus are sigmoid and cecal volvulus (Fig. 7-112). Cecal volvulus often is associated with an abnormally long mesentery of the cecum and ascending colon. This association, along with the fact that the amount of retroperitonealization of the ascending colon varies, results in considerable mobility of the right side of the colon, predisposing to volvulus. Commonly, volvulus occurs when the cecum twists on its luminal axis and is displaced upward and to the left of midline (Fig. 7-113). A barium study often shows the torsion abnormality and the classic beak configuration at the obstructed point.

About 10% of cases of cecal volvulus are cecal bascules (Fig. 7-114). This condition differs from the usual cecal volvulus in that the cecum does not rotate around its luminal axis, but instead rotates around a peritoneal band, usually located above the cecum. With a cecal bascule, there tends to be less distention of the cecum and less migration of the dilated cecum superiorly and to the left. The origins of the band are unclear, and whether these are congenital or developmental is unknown. A congenital origin is favored.

A long, high loop of sigmoid colon on a mesentery can twist on itself at the mesenteric base, resulting in a sigmoid volvulus. This is a form of closed-loop obstruction. The hyperinflated sigmoid colon can extend as high as the diaphragm, and the dilated sigmoid loop has the classic bean-shaped configuration. SCBE shows a torsion

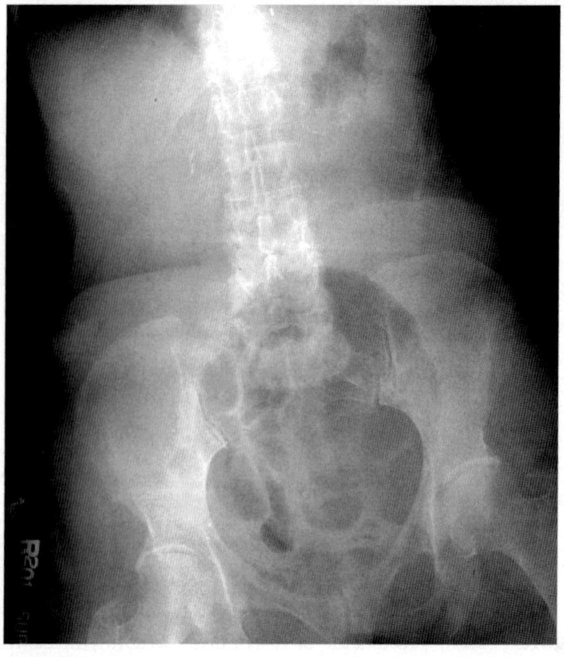

Figure 7-114 Large ovoid air collection in midabdomen represents a dilated cecum as a result of a cecal bascule.

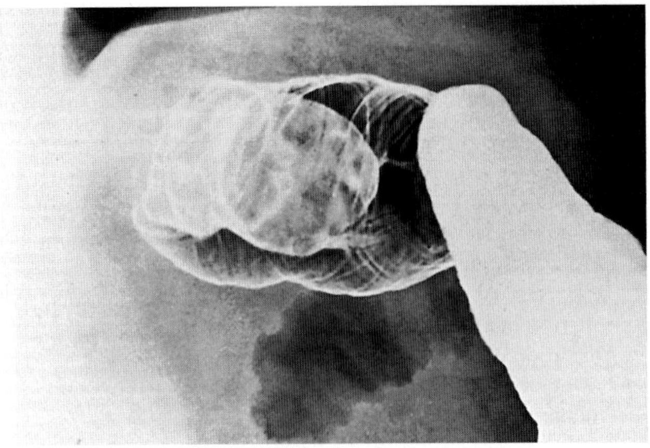

Figure 7-115 Intussuscepted segment of transverse colon seen on DCBE. A polypoid carcinoma is acting as the lead point of the intussusception.

abnormality at the obstruction point with a beaklike configuration usually at about the level of the pelvic rim.

Intussusception is relatively uncommon in adults, and, when it does occur, it should be viewed with some suspicion (Fig. 7-115). Most adult intussusceptions have, as their lead point, a neoplastic lesion.

Virtually any type of herniated segment of colon can result in obstruction and proximal dilatation. Most colonic hernias are asymptomatic, however. Incidental herniation is commonly seen during barium enema examinations, with portions of the colon in umbilical, inguinal, or femoral hernias. There can be herniation through incisional defects or through defects in the diaphragm. Herniation of colon through the diaphragm into the pericardial sac in an asymptomatic patient also is possible. Hernias of colon between the lateral muscular layers of the abdominal wall (spigelian hernias) occasionally result in obstruction.

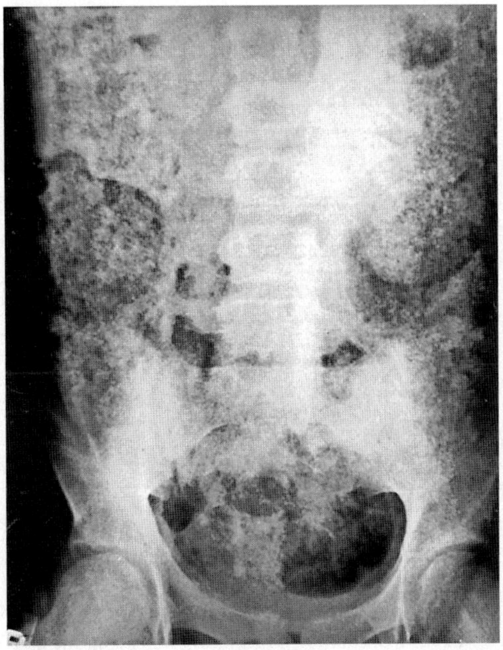

Figure 7-116 Plain film of a teenage patient with chronic constipation and abdominal distention reveals markedly dilated stool-filled colon.

An aganglionic segment of the colon (Hirschsprung's disease) can result in not only focal narrowing, but also significant dilatation of the proximal colon. This condition is congenital and is seen more commonly in male infants. It may not be correctly diagnosed until adolescence or even early adulthood in some individuals. Classically, patients present with abdominal distention, marked fecal retention, and failure to thrive (Fig. 7-116). Barium enema examination usually shows a normal rectum with normal rectal distention. Above the rectum, there is an area of transition to grossly dilated colon. The aganglionic segments are almost always focal, although they can extend upward for several centimeters, and very rarely the entire colon may be involved.

NONMECHANICAL DILATATION

The presence of marked colonic dilatation without obstruction is common and has been recognized as a frequent finding in mentally retarded patients, particularly in institutionalized patients. This colonic dilatation has been termed *psychogenic megacolon*. The exact causes are unknown. The array of anticholinergic medications that many of these patients require may contribute to the situation.

Colonic dilatation also is a well-recognized complication of acutely ill, bedridden patients. It is seen frequently in postoperative patients with prolongation of the postoperative ileus effect. It also may be seen in patients experiencing severe sepsis. Acute passive dilatation of the colon, sometimes called Ogilvie's syndrome, carries with it the risk of perforation of the cecum, where the colon is the most distensible and the wall is the thinnest. Colonic dilatation also can be seen as a result of underlying systemic conditions, such as scleroderma, Chagas' disease, cystic fibrosis, and myotonic dystrophy.

The condition known as idiopathic intestinal pseudo-obstruction is thought to represent a neuromuscular disorder of the gastrointestinal tract involving all parts of the gut. Some of these patients have colonic distention without acute clinical findings. Many of these patients have chronic abdominal complaints, however, including distention, chronic abdominal pain, and constipation. A plain film of the abdomen often shows marked colonic distention, and without a clinical history, the radiologist may need to consider differential diagnoses that include colonic volvulus or obstruction secondary to inflammatory or neoplastic disease.

DIMINISHED HAUSTRAL PATTERN

Numerous conditions, many of which have been previously discussed, can result in a diminished haustral pattern and a tubular appearance of the colon, including idiopathic inflammatory processes, such as ulcerative colitis and Crohn's disease, and bacterial and viral colitides. In addition, the fold pattern may appear diminished in scleroderma, in which the haustral pattern may assume an asymmetric saccular pattern. Similar changes can be seen in the small bowel. Chronic laxative abuse and resultant cathartic colon also show a diminished haustral pattern. Any chronic or healed inflammatory process involving the colon, such as chronic or healed ulcerative colitis or the chronic stages of radiation colitis, can result in diminished or absent haustral pattern.

THICKENED HAUSTRAL FOLDS

Many conditions can result in varying degrees of thickening of the haustral folds. These can be mild thickening to marked fingerlike indentations of the bowel margin known as thumbprinting. In general, fold thickening and thumbprinting are a result of edema, hemorrhage, or malignancy. Hemorrhage is seen most commonly as a cause of thumbprinting resulting from ischemic colitis. Thumbprinting resulting from intramural hemorrhage may be entirely indistinguishable, however, from severe inflammation and marked edematous changes such as might be seen in fulminating IBD or toxic megacolon. The clinical history is extremely helpful in sorting out these problems.

Ischemic colitis is a condition seen in elderly patients (>70 years old). The condition relates to an acute reduction of the splanchnic blood flow and is commonly seen in, or distal to, the watershed areas between the inferior mesenteric artery and the superior mesenteric artery circulations. More extensive colitis involving longer segments is common.

The exact causes for this diminished blood flow may be multiple. Acute hypotensive episodes, underlying vasculitides, and mechanical causes such as herniation or volvulus have been implicated. There is an increased incidence of patients with ischemic colitis who are undergoing hemodialysis. The rectum is rarely involved because of the abundant collateral circulation.

The finding of thumbprinting on either a plain film or during a barium enema examination is most often seen in the transverse or descending portions of the colon and represents intramural hemorrhage. This finding is present in about 20% to 25% of patients. The patients frequently present with painless rectal bleeding. More than half of the cases are transient and reversible. Slightly less than half of cases develop complications, usually focal stricture or, more seriously, bowel necrosis, which requires surgical intervention. The site of complications is most commonly in the sigmoid colon.

Toxic megacolon (Box 7-7) is an acute complication of fulminating inflammatory disease of the colon that involves the entire thickness of the bowel wall (Fig. 7-117). Tissue cohesion is severely impaired, and perforation is a common result. Toxic megacolon is seen most frequently as a complication of ulcerative colitis, although it occurs with less frequency in Crohn's disease and in bacterial colitis. It also has been reported in pseudomembranous colitis and ischemic colitis.

Box 7-7 Characteristics of Toxic Megacolon

- Seen in acute fulminating IBD
- Full-thickness process
- Breakdown of tissue cohesion
- Passage of bacteria and bacterial toxins across disrupted mucosal surface
- Increased incidence of perforation
- All parts of colon may be affected
- Dilatation present, but more important radiological signs are thickened folds and prominent thumbprinting

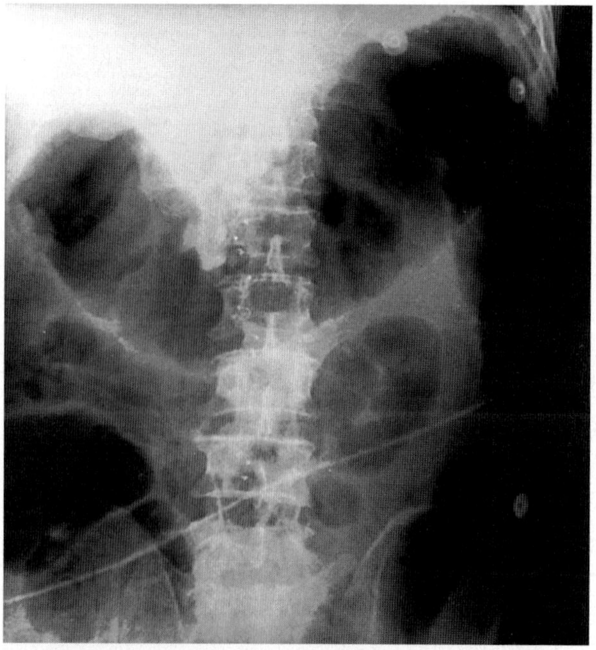

Figure 7-117 Plain film of the abdomen in a patient with severe IBD shows dilatation of the colon, particularly in the transverse region, with thickening and nodularity of the folds typical of toxic megacolon.

The condition is characterized by a dilated transverse colon with marked thickening and nodularity of the haustral pattern. Multiple nodular filling defects also can be seen profiled and en face, representing pseudopolyps. The reason these changes are seen mostly in the transverse colon is because the transverse colon represents the most anterior portion of the colon in the supine patient. As a result, air gathers in the transverse colon, and the findings are most apparent in this region. Toxic megacolon may involve the entire colon and portions of the distal small bowel. Additionally, a few cases of toxic megacolon have been reported in which the transverse colon is not significantly dilated. Although radiographically these cases may appear similar to ischemic colitis, the clinical presentation makes differentiation relatively easy. Patients presenting with toxic megacolon are systemically toxic and usually have a history of IBD.

Although the barium enema has been implicated in the development of toxic megacolon in patients with IBD, this probably is more of a temporal relationship than cause and effect. When presented with plain films of a severely ill patient with findings suggesting toxic megacolon, however, contrast examination of the colon is contraindicated because of the high risk of perforation.

Pseudomembranous colitis also may manifest with plain films showing a thickened nodular fold pattern within the colon. This finding occurs as a result of the marked edema and the presence of adherent pseudomembranes along the mucosal surface. This condition, although uncommon, can result in a potentially deadly illness. It has been referred to as antibiotic colitis and is thought to represent a complication of long-term antibiotic therapy. Clinically, the patient often experiences diarrhea with occasional bleeding and abdominal pain. The onset of symptoms is usually within 2 to 3 days after the start of antibiotic therapy. Although the condition initially was associated with lincomycin and tetracycline, it is now known that virtually any antibiotic can trigger the disease.

The underlying cause is thought to represent an acute change of the bacterial colonic flora and an overgrowth of the bacterium *Clostridium difficile*, which is known to produce toxins that are absorbed across the colonic mucosa. The finding of marked bowel wall and haustral thickening with nodularity and possible thumbprinting in a patient with suspected pseudomembranous colitis should give sufficient warning to the radiologist to avoid doing a barium enema examination. These patients also run an increased risk of perforation.

Other conditions that may mimic thumbprinting include lymphoma, carcinoma, metastatic extension from the serosal surface, amyloid infiltration of the bowel, and, in the cecal region, typhlitis. Typhlitis, sometimes known as neutropenic enterocolitis, is a condition occasionally encountered in patients undergoing treatment for hematological malignancies, particularly leukemia and lymphoma (Fig. 7-118). Patients are often neutropenic, and changes are most commonly seen in the terminal ileum, cecum, and proximal ascending colon. Marked focal changes of inflammation that can progress to bowel wall necrosis are the manifestations of this condition, and the clinical findings may simulate acute appendicitis.

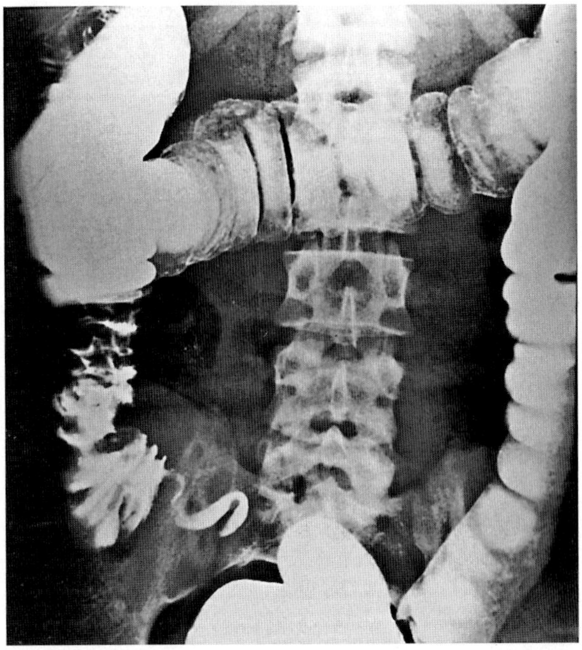

Figure 7-118 A young patient with leukemia presents with right lower quadrant abdominal pain. Barium enema shows inflammatory and spastic changes involving the cecum and a portion of the ascending colon, representing typhlitis.

To an inattentive observer, pneumatosis coli can simulate the appearance of haustral fold thickening and possible thumbprinting. The haustral folds may appear thickened and nodular, but careful attention to the films discloses that this is the result of cystic collections of air in the bowel wall (see Fig. 7-58).

POSITIONAL ABNORMALITIES

Malrotation

Degrees of colonic malrotation can occur and are usually of little clinical significance (Fig. 7-119). These result from the counterclockwise rotation that occurs as the midgut returns from the umbilical sac into the abdominal cavity between 6 and 12 weeks of embryonic life. The amount of rotation may be incomplete, and fixation of the ascending portion of the colon may be either absent or limited; this can cause considerable mobility of the cecum and ascending colon. This condition

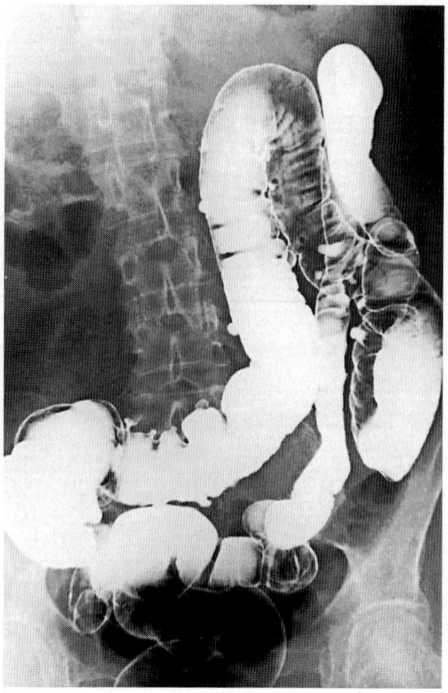

Figure 7-119 Barium enema in a patient with malrotation shows both flexures on the left side of the abdomen. The cecum is in its expected location.

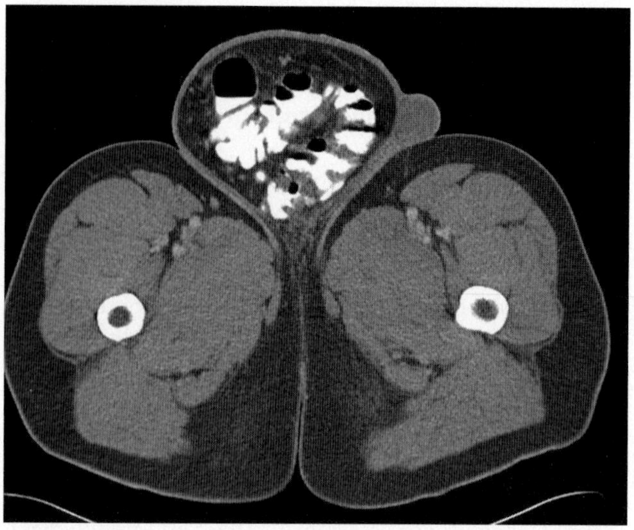

Figure 7-120 Cecum and appendix are seen in the scrotum of a patient with a large right inguinal hernia.

potentially may predispose to internal torsion abnormalities, such as cecal or transverse colon volvulus. Complete failure of rotation, or nonrotation, is uncommon. When it does occur, the entire colon is seen on the left side of the abdomen, and the small bowel is seen on the right side.

Hernias

Hernias, through the inguinal and femoral canals, can include segments of colon, most commonly sigmoid colon. Sometimes these can be quite dramatic (Fig. 7-120). The cecum and appendix also can be involved. Internal hernias can involve the colon. These include mesenteric hernias, diaphragmatic hernias, and even herniation through the foramen of Winslow into the lesser sac (Fig. 7-121). Hernias through the diaphragm can occur as a result of traumatic defects in the diaphragm or as a result of congenital defects, such as Morgagni's hernia anteriorly or Bochdalek's hernia of the posterior diaphragm. These herniations may exist for long periods with no symptoms. Strangulation or obstruction of the bowel can occur, however, and result in a surgical emergency.

Herniation of portions of small bowel and colon through the anterior abdominal wall is relatively common; this includes umbilical hernias and postoperative incisional hernias. Spigelian hernia is an unusual form of ventral hernia in which a defect occurs along the linea semilunaris located in the abdominal wall lateral to the rectus abdominis muscle. The herniated portions of bowel pass through the transverse and internal oblique muscle layers, but remain beneath the overlying intact external oblique muscle. As a result, the hernia is difficult to detect clinically, and frequently there are no symptoms. Occasional, intermittent abdominal pain is reported in some patients. Radiographically, bowel seen on plain film, CT, or barium enema lying lateral to the rectus muscle outside the expected confines of the peritoneal cavity suggests the diagnosis.

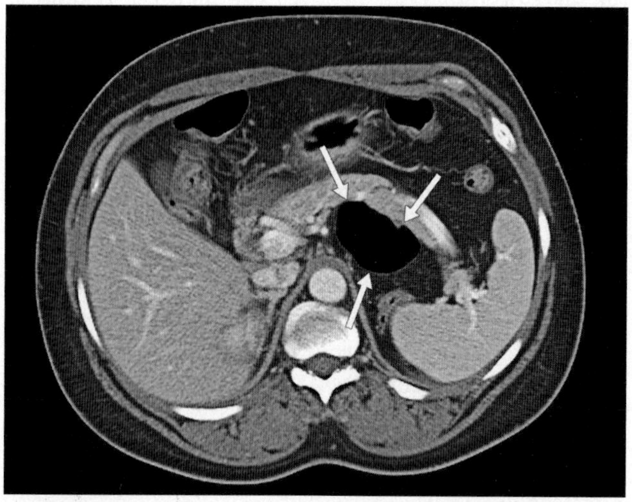

Figure 7-121 A loop of colon seen posterior to the stomach and pancreas *(arrows)* as a result of herniation through the foramen of Winslow.

MISCELLANEOUS CONDITIONS

Presacral Widening

The presacral, retrorectal space normally measures 1.5 cm or less. Many conditions can result in abnormal widening of the presacral space, however. Most of these conditions involve the rectum itself, and abnormal rectal findings are usually present on the barium enema examination.

The most common cause of presacral widening is inflammatory disease involving the rectum and colon. This is a common finding in ulcerative colitis, but also can be seen in Crohn's disease when it involves the rectum (Fig. 7-122). Formation of perirectal fistulous tracts or abscesses in Crohn's disease can result in further widening of the presacral space. Other inflammatory conditions of the rectum, including lymphogranuloma venereum, radiation proctitis, and viral (e.g., CMV) proctitis, and, rarely, ischemic disease can result in increased presacral space size.

Neoplastic disease arising from the colon, such as carcinoma of the rectum, is another important cause of widening of the presacral space (Fig. 7-123). The most common malignant lesion is adenocarcinoma, which usually results in a large, bulky lesion. The mass of the lesion plus the perirectal extension can combine, however, to cause significant widening of the presacral space. Other rare malignancies of the rectum include lymphoma and cloacogenic carcinoma, both of which may produce similar appearances.

Cystic lesions that contribute to presacral widening include dermoid cysts (sacral teratoma) and, less commonly, rectal duplications (enteric cysts) (Fig. 7-124). Lesions arising from the sacrum itself also can contribute to a widened presacral space (Box 7-8). These include infectious processes, such as osteomyelitis of the sacrum, metastatic disease, primary bone tumors, and neurogenic tumors arising from the sacrum. Chordomas are seen in the cervical and sacrococcygeal regions of the spine. These are slow-growing lesions, usually resulting in destructive changes in the sacrum, mass effect with anterior extension and displacement of the rectum, and widening of the presacral space. Malignant neoplastic lesions arising from structures around the rectum, by contiguous extension, can encircle and deform the rectum and widen the presacral space. This condition is uncommon, but is seen occasionally in prostatic carcinoma in men and cervical carcinoma in women.

Pelvic abscesses with extension into the pouch of Douglas can result in widening of the presacral space on

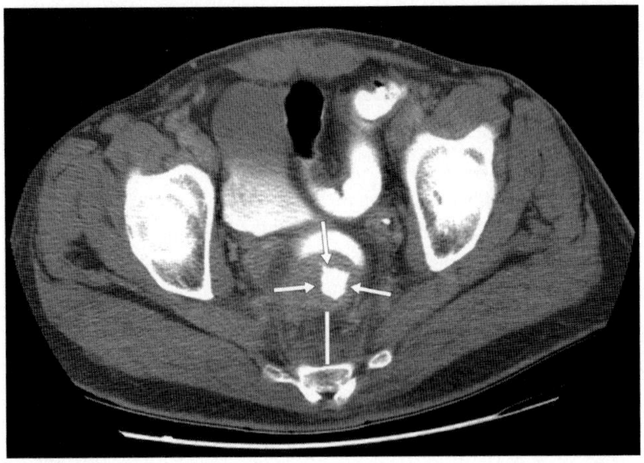

Figure 7-123 Large bulky lesion of the rectum *(arrows)* with considerable widening of the presacral space *(line)* is seen.

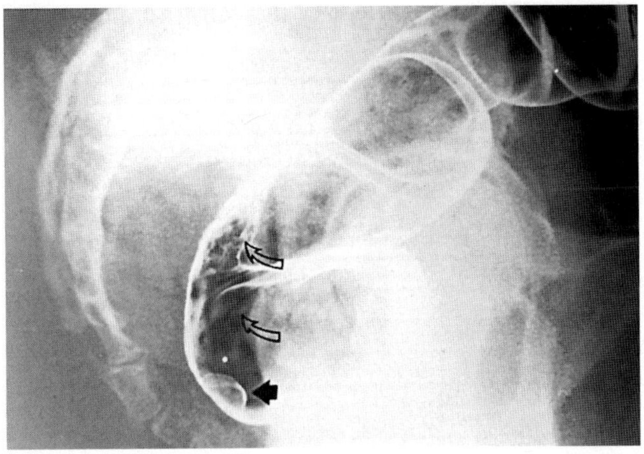

Figure 7-122 Spot film of the rectum shows inflammatory changes of the rectum *(curved arrows)* associated with widened presacral space. Also note the small adenomatous polyp *(arrow)*.

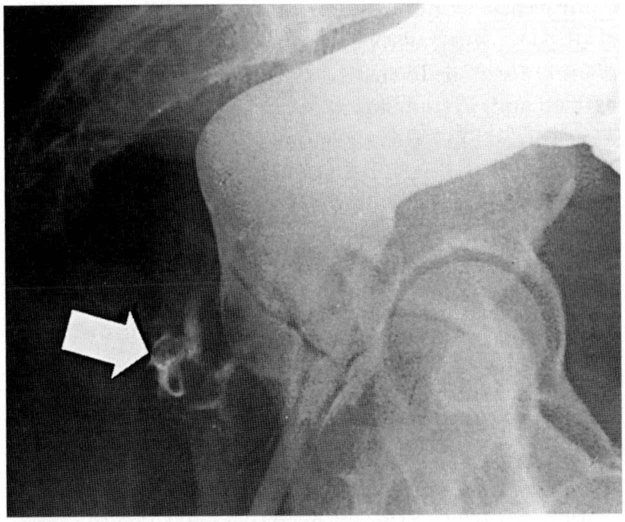

Figure 7-124 Presacral space is widened secondary to a rectal duplication. There is some communication between the enteric cyst and the bowel lumen, with contrast material seen within the duplication *(arrow)*.

Box 7-8 Causes of Widened Presacral Space

IBD
Pelvic lipomatosis
Sacral lesions
Perirectal lesions (e.g., prostate and cervical cancer)
Pelvic inflammatory disease

barium enema examination. Although the abscess itself may not extend beyond the confines of the peritoneal recess into the actual presacral space, the effect of adjacent inflammation presumably results in sufficient edema in the region to separate the rectum and sacral margin. A common example of this is periappendiceal abscess with pus collections in the lower pelvic recesses. Pelvic inflammatory disease and diverticulitis may have similar effects.

Fistulous Connections and Sinus Tract Formation

Fistulous connections and sinus tract formation are the hallmarks of Crohn's disease. Full-thickness involvement of bowel wall by the disease and extension beyond the wall to the adjacent mesentery and mesenteric fat often result in matting and bonding together of several loops of bowel. Mucosal ulcerations progress, deepen, penetrate, and eventually communicate with the adjacent adherent loops of bowel; this is frequently seen in the right lower quadrant, with fistulous tracts between ileal loops and adjacent ileum, cecum, and ascending colon. These fistulous communications also can extend to the skin, particularly in postoperative patients. Enteric-colonic fistulous formation does not present a problem in itself and, in some instances, may relieve the potential for obstruction. The development of abscess cavities along the tract, the diverting and bypassing of a significant amount of bowel resulting in malnutrition or extension of the fistula to the skin or adjacent organs, can represent serious complications.

Fistulous communications between the stomach and the colon result from either inflammatory or malignant disease arising in the stomach or colon. The large, penetrating benign gastric ulcer (seen in patients taking steroids or high doses of aspirin) that communicates with the colon is rarely encountered today. Malignant lesions arising from the greater curvature of the body and fundus of the stomach or the splenic flexure of the colon can form a gastrocolic fistula. Patients with chronic pancreatitis rarely develop a fistulous communication from the pancreatic duct to the colon (Fig. 7-125).

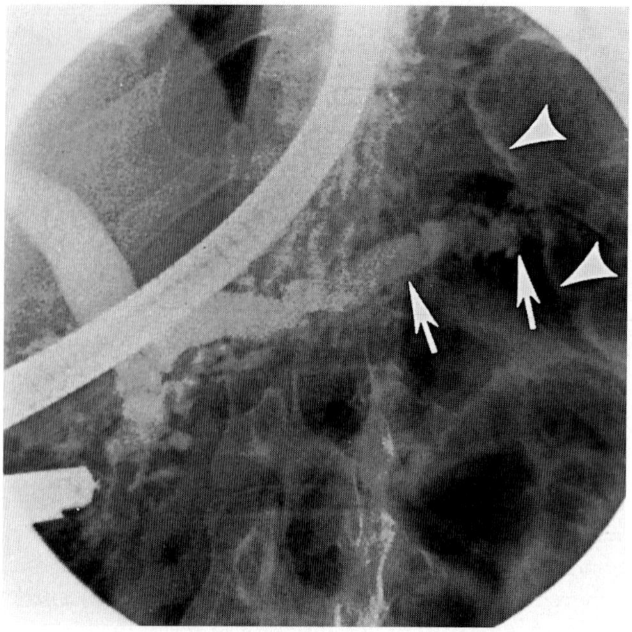

Figure 7-125 Endoscopic retrograde cholangiopancreatography in a patient with chronic pancreatitis. The pancreatic duct is ectatic and dilated *(arrows)*. There is communication with the splenic flexure of the adjacent colon, and contrast material is seen on the colonic mucosa *(arrowheads)*, confirming a pancreatico-colonic fistula.

Sinus tracts and fistulous communications are common in patients with diverticulitis. The fistulous communications are often from colon to bowel loop, particularly adjacent small bowel. Fistulous tracts also may develop between the colon and the vagina or the bladder. Occasionally, radiation colitis can result in a fistulous communication between adjacent bowel or other structures, such as the bladder or vagina (Fig. 7-126).

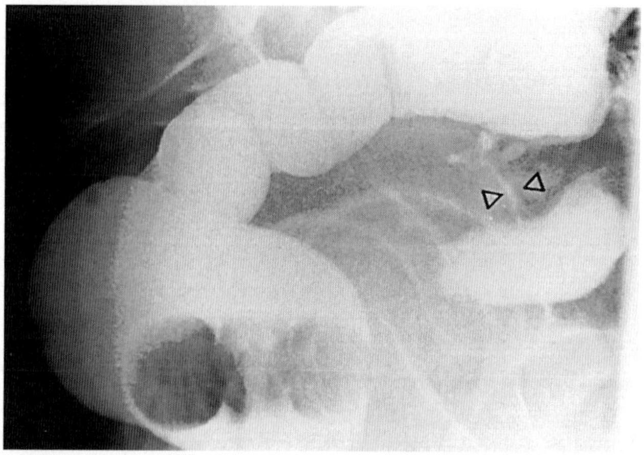

Figure 7-126 SCBE was performed in a patient with radiation colitis and a narrow fistulous communication *(arrowheads)* to the bladder.

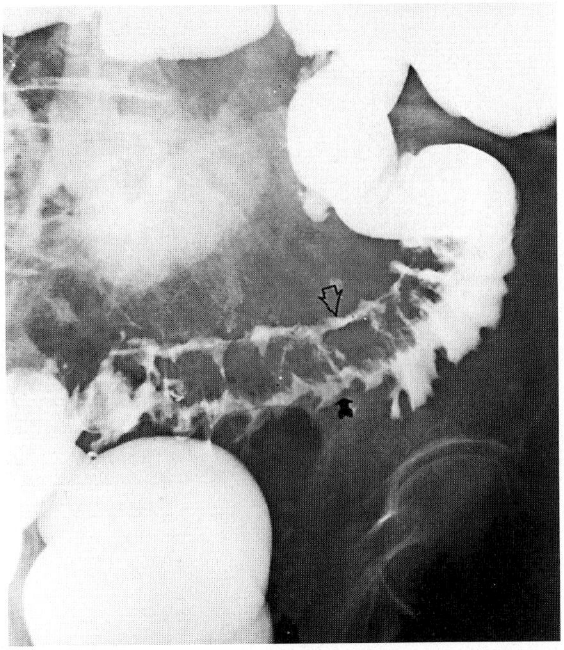

Figure 7-127 This is a well-defined example of double-tracking on a barium enema examination. The narrowed, irregular lumen is seen *(solid arrow)*. Parallel to this is the intramural tract of barium *(open arrow)*.

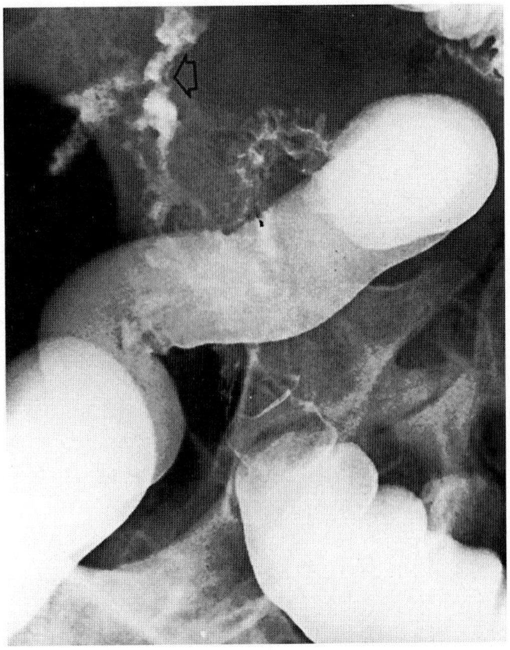

Figure 7-129 Barium enema examination was performed in a patient with intraabdominal actinomycosis involving the sigmoid colon, with resultant spasm, narrowing, and development of a branching sinus tract *(arrow)* extending from the affected sigmoid colon.

A variation of sinus tract formation is the intramural sinus tract, sometimes referred to as "double-tracking," which is most commonly seen in diverticulitis (Fig. 7-127). This condition also can be seen to a lesser extent in patients with Crohn's disease. Patients with carcinoma of the colon also may have short, irregular intramural sinus tracts (Fig. 7-128).

Actinomycosis with colonic involvement frequently results in sinus or fistulous tracts and communication with adjacent organs or the skin. The blatant disregard of *Actinomyces* for fascial planes is a hallmark of its natural history, and fistulous communications are a common manifestation (Fig. 7-129). Fistula and sinus formation also is a common finding with lymphogranuloma venereum (Fig. 7-130).

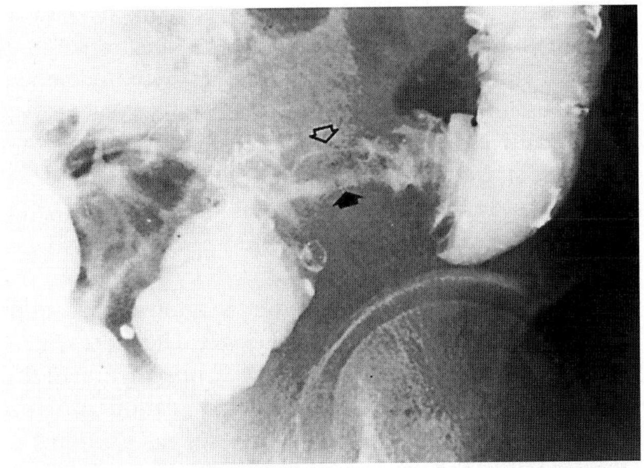

Figure 7-128 A patient with adenocarcinoma of the sigmoid colon and an apple core type of constricting lesion. Note the narrowed lumen *(solid arrow)* and the adjacent thin, poorly defined periluminal tract *(open arrow)*.

Appendix

The normal appendix originates between the cecal tip and the ileocecal valve. It is a structure of variable length, measuring 4 to 12 cm (Fig. 7-131). In approximately 25% of cases, the appendix may be retrocecal in position, and the tip of the appendix occasionally may be located in the right upper quadrant of the abdomen below or at the margin of the liver. Filling of the appendix during a barium enema study occurs in approximately 60% of cases. If a postevacuation film is obtained, one can expect to see additional filling in another 20% to 25% of patients.

The most common condition of the appendix is appendicitis, resulting from occlusion of the appendiceal lumen by a fecalith and development of inflammatory changes within the obstructed appendix (Fig. 7-132). The appendiceal wall becomes thickened, hyperemic, and edematous (Fig. 7-133). Clinical presentation usually suggests the diagnosis. Progression of the inflammatory process can result in perforation with

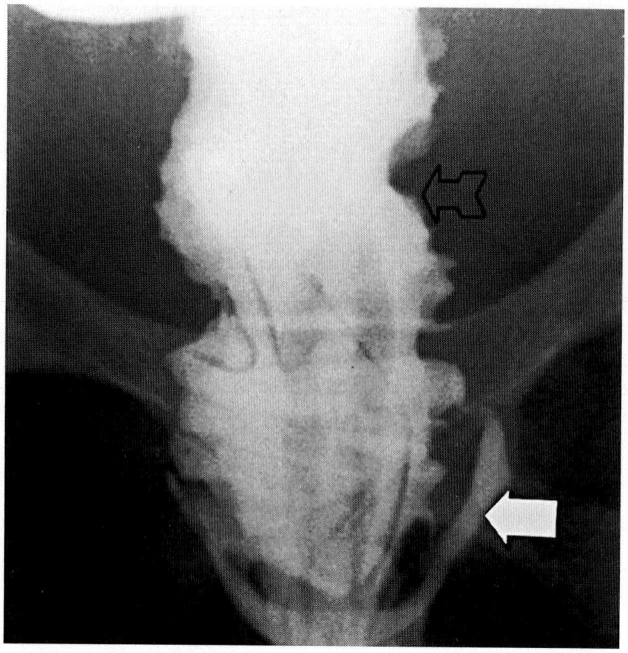

Figure 7-130 Spot film of a patient with lymphogranuloma venereum shows marked irregularity and ulceration of the rectal margin *(open arrow)* and prominent bilateral perirectal sinus tracts *(white arrow)*.

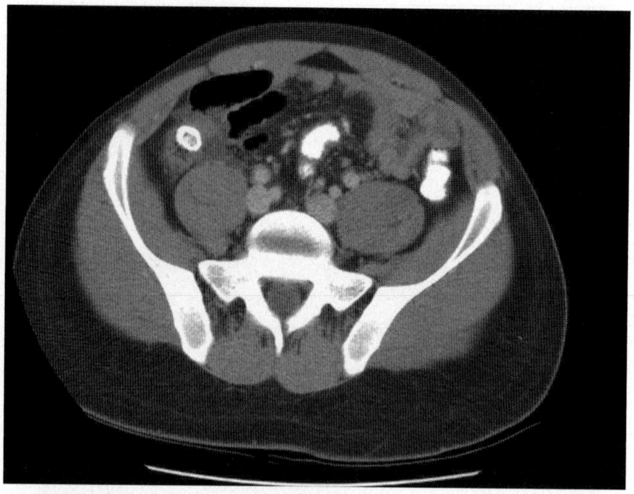

Figure 7-132 This patient has acute appendicitis with soft tissue density and stranding around the appendix. Note the large appendicolith.

periappendiceal abscess formation or free perforation and generalized peritonitis (Fig. 7-134). On barium enema, spasm at the cecal tip or mass effect from the adjacent abscess may be the expected findings. Incomplete filling of the appendix during barium enema does not exclude appendicitis. Complete filling and demonstration of the bulbous tip of the appendix rule out the diagnosis, however.

CT is now considered the examination of choice in a patient with potential appendicitis. CT evaluation of the right lower quadrant of the abdomen shows changes of appendicitis from wisps of stranding in the periappendiceal, fat-thickened appendiceal wall to frank abscess formation. CT is far more sensitive than any other imaging tool currently used.

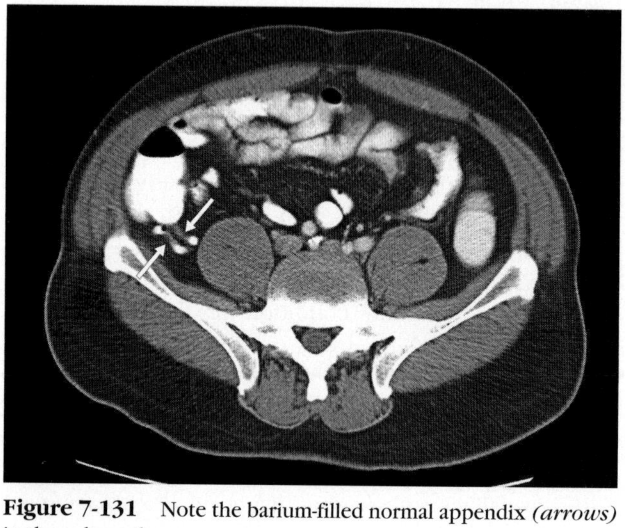

Figure 7-131 Note the barium-filled normal appendix *(arrows)* in the subcecal area.

Crohn's disease of the terminal ileum or cecum by extension also may involve the appendix (Fig. 7-135). Isolated appendiceal involvement is extremely rare.

The most common cause of a filling defect at the tip of the cecum is previous appendectomy with an inverted appendiceal stump. Frequently, this inverted stump is smooth and in its expected location. Occasionally, the stump can appear lobular and require colonoscopy to differentiate it from a neoplasm. Occasionally, a true neoplasm is found arising from the appendiceal stump. There is no reason to suspect that this is any more than coincidental, and there is no evidence to suggest any increased risk of malignancy at the site of the inverted stump. Occasionally, a filling defect at the base of cecum, sometimes with concentric circles arising from the center of the filling defect, can be seen and is the result of appendiceal intussusception. This defect frequently is asymptomatic and transient, although occasionally it can be associated with acute appendicitis. A similar "coil-spring" appearance also can be seen after appendectomy.

A mucocele of the appendix is another cause of a filling defect at the appendiceal origin. The most widely held cause for this condition is aseptic obstruction of the appendiceal lumen with mucus accumulation and cyst formation. Most of these lesions are asymptomatic. Occasionally, the mucocele can calcify in its wall. Rupture of an appendiceal mucocele can lead to the condition known as pseudomyxoma peritonei, in which spillage of the mucocele content results in massive

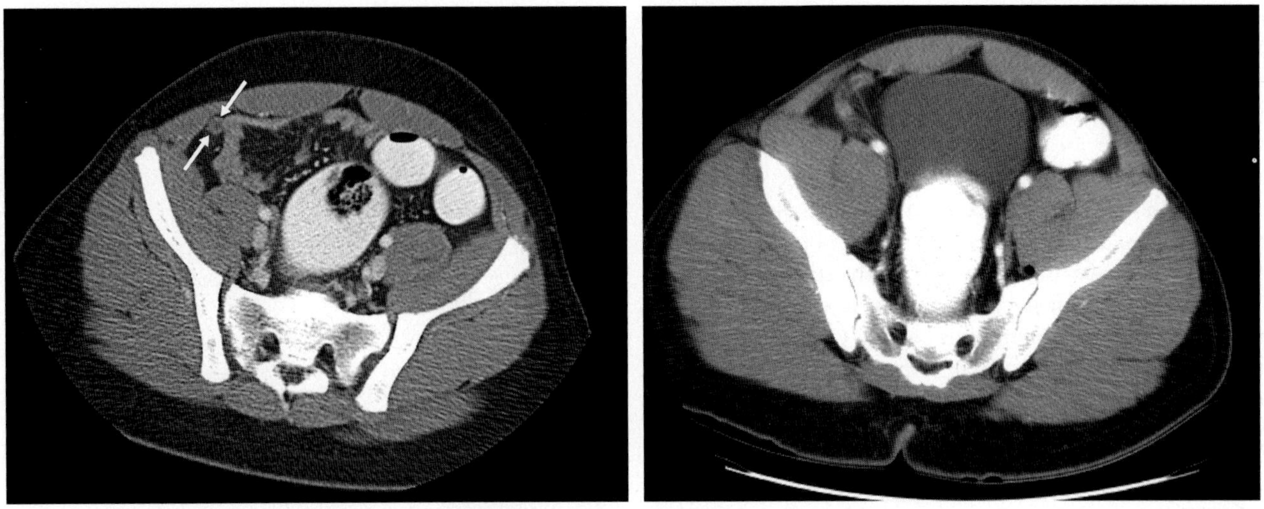

A B

Figure 7-133 **A,** Subtle changes of appendicitis are seen. Note the thickening and stranding around the appendix *(arrows)*. **B,** This is mild appendicitis.

accumulations of thick, gelatinous, adhesive type of ascites. A rare type of appendiceal mucocele is myxoglobulosis, in which numerous, tiny cohesive translucent globules are mixed with the liquid mucous content of the mucocele. These globules can calcify and, on positional views of the abdomen, may be seen to move within the mucocele.

The most common appendiceal neoplasm is the carcinoid. The appendix is the most common site of carcinoid development within the gastrointestinal tract. More than 90% of gastrointestinal carcinoids arise from either the appendix or the distal ileum. These lesions are almost always benign and rarely cause the carcinoid syndrome. The discovery is usually incidental during surgery or autopsy.

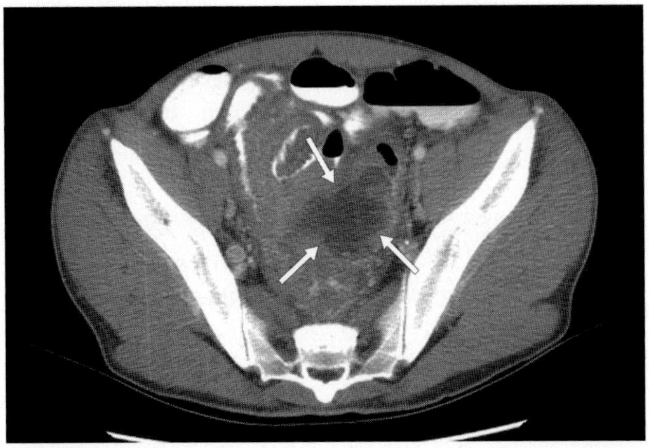

Figure 7-134 Pelvic abscess after ruptured appendix. There is pus *(arrows)* in the pelvis and bowel wall thickening of the adjacent loops of small bowel.

Primary malignant neoplasm of the appendix is unusual and is invariably adenocarcinoma. Frequently, adenocarcinoma results in gradual luminal obstruction and may manifest as acute appendicitis. The diagnosis is frequently intraoperative or postoperative.

Acute Appendagitis

Acute epiploic appendagitis is caused by torsion of the epiploic appendices, which are small pouches of fat-filled peritoneum protruding from the serosal surface of the colon. They can be seen from cecum to sigmoid colon.

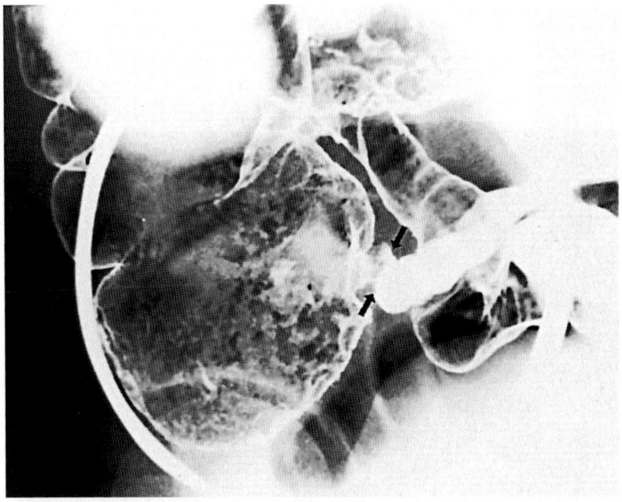

Figure 7-135 Spot film of the cecum in a patient with Crohn's disease. Inflammatory involvement of the cecum, more severe on its medial aspect around the origin of the appendix, is seen. There is also involvement of the first several centimeters *(arrows)* of the appendix.

They may be seen as lobulated masses of pericolic fat 3 to 5 cm long and 2 cm thick. The exact cause of epiploic appendagitis is uncertain. It has been postulated that torsion of the epiploic appendagitis may be the cause. Clinical findings are nonspecific and include mild to moderate abdominal pain, mild fever, and mild elevation of white blood count. Before the use of ultrasound, this condition was almost never identified before surgery, and patients were misdiagnosed with appendicitis or diverticulitis. The most common site is sigmoid colon, and the second most common is cecum. Computed tomographic findings include small hypodense mass and fat stranding along the external colonic wall (Fig. 7-136).

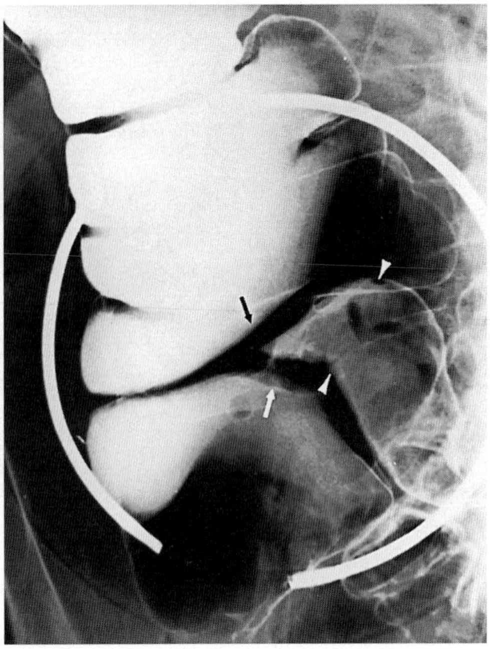

Figure 7-137 Spot film from a barium enema examination shows the normal and most common configuration of the ileocecal valve. Note the smooth V-shaped configuration of the valve *(arrows)* and the normal bird's-head configuration of the terminal ileum *(arrowheads)* as it enters the valve.

Ileocecal Valve Enlargement

The appearance of the ileocecal valve varies from a small polypoid filling defect on the first transverse fold within the colon to the more typical, liplike valvular configuration (Fig. 7-137 and Box 7-9). The normal valve also may have a rosette configuration (Fig. 7-138). It is commonly located on the medial side of the cecum, along the first complete colonic haustral fold, although there can be variation. The valve can be seen on the lateral margin of the cecum in some patients. The size of the normal valve also can vary. The upper limit of normal for the vertical diameter of the valve is probably 3 to 4 cm. Generally, the valve should be measured during full cecal distention. It is common to see prominence of the valve on a postevacuation film compared with the distended cecal views (Fig. 7-139). This is because there are degrees of ileal prolapse through the valve when the cecum is collapsed, accentuating the size of the valve.

Reflux of barium across the ileocecal valve into the terminal ileum is a common phenomenon on SCBE, probably occurring in more than 75% of the cases. This is not the case with double-contrast technique, and reflux into the terminal ileum with obscuration of the sigmoid colon occurs with considerably less frequency. The exact reason is unclear. It may relate to the smaller amounts and the more viscous nature of the barium used in double-contrast work.

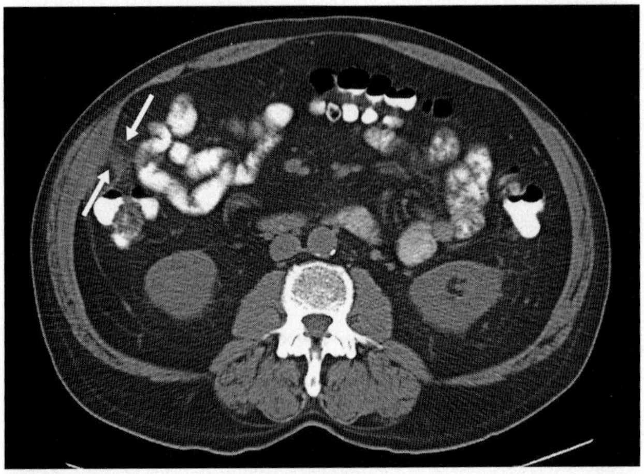

Figure 7-136 Patient with epiploic appendagitis. Note indistinct small mass and fat stranding adjacent to cecal wall *(arrows)*.

The most common benign neoplastic lesion of the ileocecal valve is the lipoma, which is seen as a rounded, well-circumscribed, smooth mass arising from one of the valvular lips. This mass should be differentiated from lipomatous valvular infiltration, which is not a neoplastic process (Fig. 7-140). In the latter condition, the valve may appear large and lobulated along both lips. There is also a change of valvular configuration with compression. The diagnosis can be confirmed with CT of the cecum, in which the fat density can be seen easily. Benign adenomas and adenocarcinomas can arise from the

Box 7-9 When the Valve Looks Big: Ileocecal Valve Enlargement

- Normal variation
- Valvular lipomatosis
- Lipoma of the valve
- Adenomatous polyp involving the valve
- Carcinoma
- Inflammatory changes

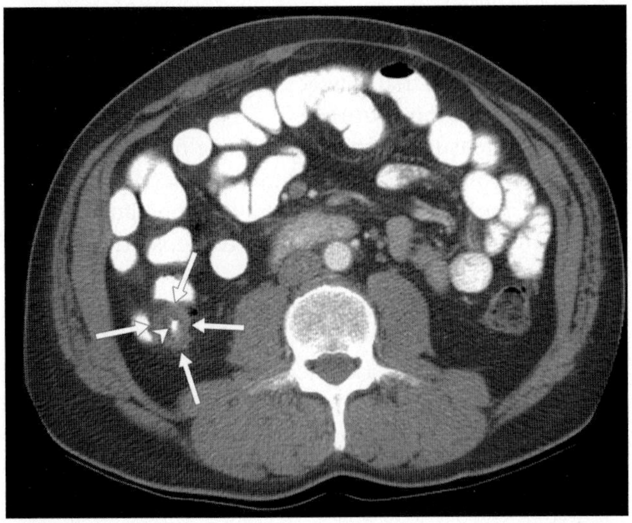

Figure 7-138 Note rosette appearance of normal ileocecal valve *(arrows)* and barium in distal terminal ileum and in ileocecal valve *(arrowhead)*.

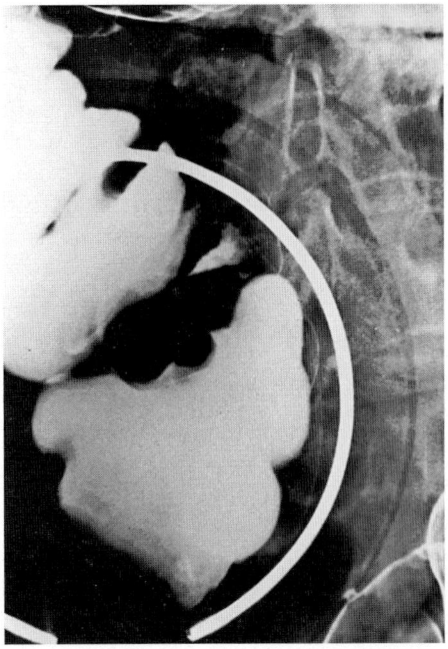

Figure 7-140 A patient with lipomatous infiltration of the ileocecal valve. The valve is enlarged and nodular. Compression may cause the valve to change shape.

ileocecal valve. Similar to most cecal or right-sided lesions, a valvular malignancy can grow to sizable proportions before becoming symptomatic, as a result of the fluid nature of the bowel content at this level (Figs. 7-141 and 7-142).

Inflammatory changes involving the terminal ileum and the cecum also can involve the valve. This is particularly the case in Crohn's disease, in which involvement of the ileocecal valve frequently indicates involvement of the terminal ileum. *Yersinia,* which involves the distal ileum, also may result in inflammatory changes of the valve.

In ulcerative pancolitis, inflammation in the cecal region can result in incompetence of the valve and unimpeded reflux into the terminal ileum. The ileum tends to appear large and distended (backwash ileitis), but is usually not involved in the primary inflammatory process. Inflammatory conditions that involve the

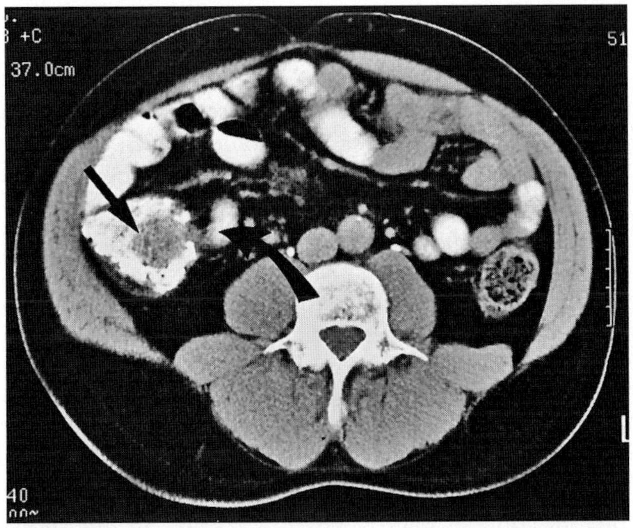

Figure 7-139 CT shows filling defect, or colonic lesion, in the cecum *(straight arrow)*. Colonoscopy was normal. The finding is pseudomass of the cecum resulting from some prolapse of valve and distal ileum *(curved arrow)* in undistended cecum. Pseudomasses disappear with cecal distention.

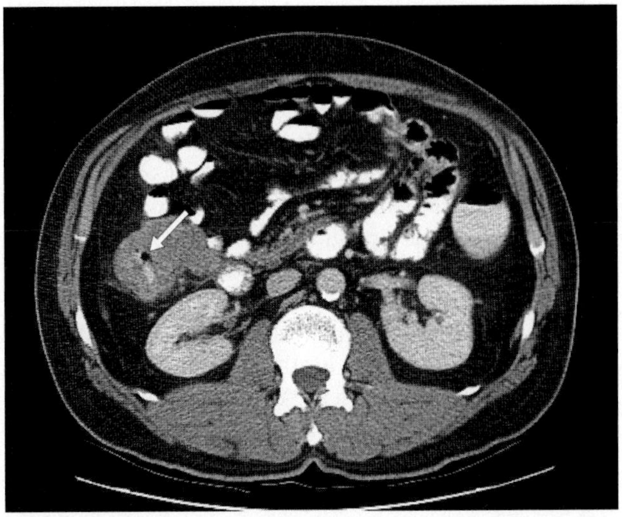

Figure 7-141 A large polypoid carcinoma arising from the ileocecal valve. Note the narrowing of the lumen *(arrow)* of the cecum at this level.

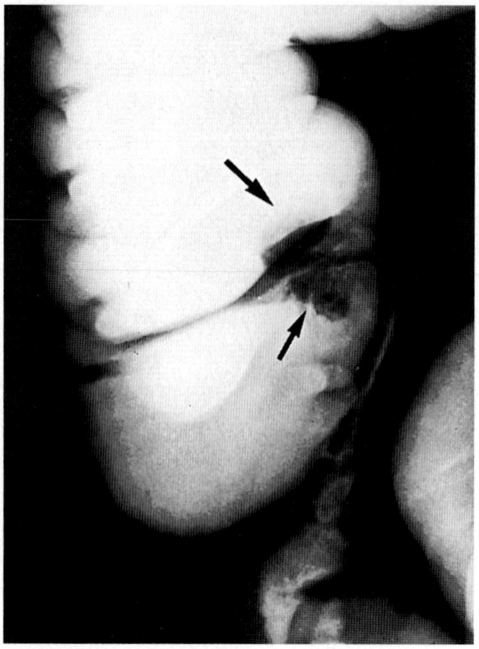

Figure 7-142 An anemic patient examined with barium enema was found to have a lobulated lesion arising from the ileocecal valve *(arrows)*, which proved to be a villous adenoma.

ileocecal region, including tuberculosis, amebiasis, and typhoid fever, also can involve the ileocecal valve.

Defecography

In modern Western society, the number of patients with complaints of defecation problems is increasing. Serious evaluation of this clinical problem began in the 1980s and 1990s. Radiographically, the method that has been used most frequently is defecography, which is sometimes called evacuation proctography. Defecography is the radiographic dynamic assessment of the patient during defecation. Technically, the rectum is filled with a thick, viscous barium material. The material is so thick that it must be injected into the rectum by use of a caulking gun. Before this step, the patient ingests thin barium orally to opacify the loops of small bowel in the pelvis. In women, the vagina also may be opacified through use of a radiopaque gel or a tampon soaked with contrast material. The patient is placed on a radiolucent commode, which is attached to the fluoroscopic table. This commode is commercially available and made of plastic. Radiographs in the lateral projection are obtained. Before the patient defecates, lateral views are obtained with the patient at rest, during straining but without defecation, and with voluntary contracting of the pelvic musculature. The patient is then asked to defecate, and sequential films or, preferentially, videotape recording of defecation is obtained. Sequential films can be acquired with a 105-mm camera; this also can be acquired digitally, if a digital fluoroscopic unit is available. Some authorities believe that acquiring the image on videotape is all that is necessary. The use of videotape in this examination is crucial.

Several measurements can be made from the images. The most commonly used is the anorectal angle. The anorectal angle is measured by drawing one line through the anal canal and another along the posterior wall of the rectum. The anorectal angle is created by the contraction of the puborectalis muscle around the anorectal region. At rest, this angle measures about 90 degrees and is rarely greater than 120 degrees. The angle becomes greater on straining and becomes smaller when the patient is asked to squeeze or lift the buttocks. When the patient defecates, this angle becomes quite obtuse and approaches 180 degrees. The use of measuring angles in defecography has been seriously questioned as to their validity, however. Another angle measurement commonly associated with defecography is the level of the anorectal junction. It is measured according to its relationship to the ischial tuberosities, which are usually visible on the images. The validity of this measurement is in doubt.

Abnormalities

Defecography is used to evaluate patients with evacuation problems. Often there is no other examination option except defecography for some of the conditions that may be encountered. Although there has been some discussion in the literature of MRI defecography, it is a topic of research interest rather than practical application. The most commonly seen abnormality on defecography is the rectocele. A rectocele is an outpouching of the rectal wall occurring anteriorly, and although it can be evaluated clinically by physical examination, defecography gives a dynamic picture of its effect on rectal evacuation (Fig. 7-143). Rectocele is believed to be due to a weakness of the rectovaginal septum. It is such a common finding in women that some authorities believe that only larger rectoceles that sequester barium (>3 cm) should be mentioned and that smaller rectoceles are probably of little clinical consequence. Sometimes there is also internal rectal prolapse, and the material in the rectocele becomes separated from the rectum and cannot be emptied. In this circumstance, the patient often complains of incomplete evacuation.

Sometimes portions of the small bowel or even the sigmoid colon may descend or herniate into the pouch of Douglas. When this occurs, the small bowel or sigmoid colon may descend between the anterior wall of the rectum and the vagina, which is termed an *enterocele* (Fig. 7-144). If it is the sigmoid colon, it is termed a *sigmoidocele*. In both circumstances, the patient may feel abnormal pressure on the perineum during defecation.

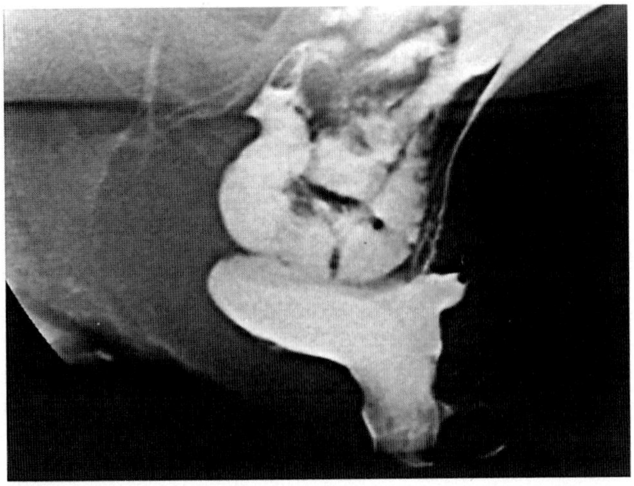

Figure 7-143 Lateral view during defecation. The large bulge along the anterior wall of the rectum during rectal contraction indicates the presence of a rectocele. The small bowel loops that are opacified by orally ingested barium are descending quite low in the pelvis, indicating an enterocele.

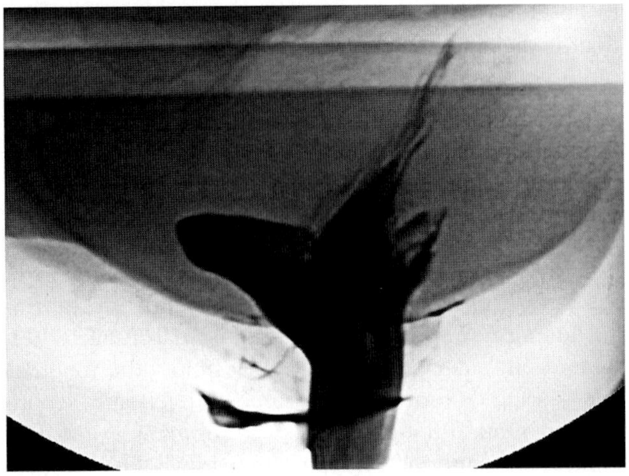

Figure 7-145 During defecation, a portion of the rectal mucosa invaginates toward the anal canal. Note that a portion of the rectal lumen becomes pinched off anteriorly. This indicates the presence of internal intussusception or prolapse.

Rectal prolapse or intussusception is an invagination of the rectal mucosa toward or through the anal canal. The invaginated mucosa may just be a portion of the rectal wall (usually anterior) or the entire circumference of the rectum. It starts in the mid to lower rectum near the valves of Houston. This invagination can be seen as a slight ring developing in the lower rectum and is often of little significance. It may extend down toward the anal canal, however, and sometimes obstruct defecation (Fig. 7-145). When it is quite severe, it can prolapse through the anal canal and can be seen externally (Fig. 7-146). These patients often manually reduce this intussuscepted plug of mucosa to continue defecating. With internal rectal prolapse, damage may occur to the mucosa of the rectum, producing ulceration, or the so-called solitary rectal ulcer syndrome. The diagnosis of enteroceles/sigmoidoceles and internal rectal proplapse can be confirmed only with defecography. The solitary rectal ulcer syndrome is just a sequela of repeated internal and even external rectal prolapse.

The puborectalis muscle has an important function in maintaining proper rectal function at rest and during defecation. At rest, the puborectalis function is believed

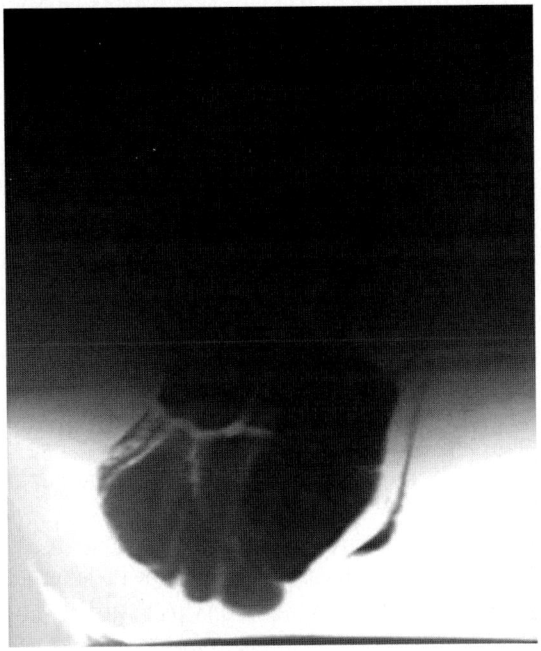

Figure 7-144 This patient had prominent descent of a large enterocele through the vaginal introitus during straining.

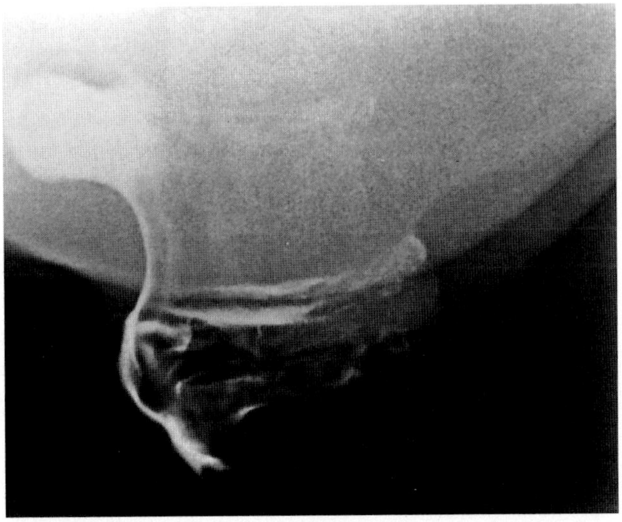

Figure 7-146 After defecation, a masslike soft tissue density is seen external to the anus. It is coated with barium. This is due to external prolapse of rectal mucosa.

to be more important in maintaining rectal continence than is the anal sphincter. Patients who are incontinent often have poor puborectalis contractility. Also, when the patient defecates, the puborectalis must relax. If this relaxation does not occur, the patient has a great deal of difficulty defecating, often with resultant pain. This is sometimes called a spastic pelvic floor.

As mentioned previously, the pelvic floor is determined by the relationship of the anorectal junction to the ischial tuberosities. In younger patients, the anorectal junction may be above the ischial tuberosities, whereas in older patients it is at or below the tuberosities. During defecation, the anorectal junction descends for 2 to 4 cm. If the descent is 5 cm or greater, it can be considered abnormal. In some individuals, this descent may cause pudendal nerve damage and eventual rectal incontinence. Patients with incontinence often have an exaggerated movement of the pelvic floor on defecation.

Occasionally, the posterolateral wall of the rectum may herniate through the pelvic floor musculature, forming a posterolateral pouch. This herniation occurs in individuals with excessive straining during defecation. It may produce symptoms of a palpable bulge in the buttocks and incomplete evacuation.

SUGGESTED READINGS

Balikian JP, Uthman SM, Khouri NF: Intestinal amoebiasis. AJR 122:245-256, 1974.

Balthazar EJ, Megibow A, Schinella RA, et al: Limitations in the CT diagnosis of acute diverticulitis: comparison of CT, contrast enema, and pathologic findings in 16 patients. AJR 154:281-285, 1990.

Bernstein MA, Feczko PJ, Halpert RD, et al: Distribution of colonic polyps: increased incidence of proximal lesions in older patients. Radiology 155:35-38, 1985.

Brady AP, Stevenson GW, Stevenson I: Colorectal cancer overlooked at barium enema examination and colonoscopy: a continuing perceptual problem. Radiology 192:373-378, 1994.

Brentall TA, Haggitt RC, Rabinovitch PS, et al: Risk and natural history of colonic neoplasia in patients with primary sclerosing cholangitis and ulcerative colitis. Gastroenterology 110:331-338, 1996.

Campbell WL, Wolff M: Retrorectal cysts of developmental origin. AJR 117:307-313, 1973.

Cho CK, Morehouse HT, Alterman DD, et al: Sigmoid diverticulitis: diagnostic role of CT—comparison with barium enema studies. Radiology 176:111-115, 1990.

Chrispin AR, Fry IK: The presacral space shown by barium enema. Br J Radiol 36:319-322, 1963.

Claymon CB: Mass screening for colorectal cancer: are we ready? JAMA 261:609, 1989.

Cohnen M, Vogt C, Beck A, et al: Feasibilty of MDCT colonography in ultra-low dose technique in the detection of colorectal lesions: comparison with high resolution video colonoscopy. AJR 183:1355-1359, 2004.

deLange EE, Fechner RE, Edge SB, et al: Preoperative staging of rectal carcinoma with MR imaging: surgical and histopathologic correlation. Radiology 176:623-628, 1990.

Feczko PJ, Halpert RD: Reassessing the role of radiology in Hemoccult screening. AJR 146:697-701, 1986.

Fishman EK, Kavuru M, Jones B, et al: Pseudomembranous colitis: CT evaluation of 26 cases. Radiology 180:57-60, 1991.

Fleischer DE, Goldberg SB, Browning TH, et al: Detection and surveillance of colorectal cancer. JAMA 261:580-585, 1989.

Fuchsjager MH, Maier AG, Schima W, et al: Comparison of transrectal sonography and double contrast MR imaging when staging rectal cancer. AJR 181:421-427, 2003.

Gelfand DW: Decreased risk of subsequent colonic cancer in patients undergoing polypectomy after barium enema: analysis based on data from the preendoscopic era. AJR 169:1243-1245, 1997.

Glotzer DJ, Glick ME, Goldman H: Proctitis and colitis following diversion of the fecal stream. Gastroenterology 80:438-441, 1981.

Gluecker TM, Johnson CD, Harmsen WS, et al: Colorectal cancer screening with CT colonoscopy, and double contrast barium enema examination: prospective assessment of patient perceptions and preferences. Radiology 227:378-384, 2003.

Goldstein SJ, Crooks DJ: Colitis in Behçet's syndrome. Radiology 128:321-323, 1978.

Green BT, Tendler DA: Ischemic colitis: a clinical review. South Med J 98:217-222, 2005.

Greenall MJ, Levine AW, Nolan DJ: Complications of diverticular disease: a review of the barium enema findings. Gastrointest Radiol 8:353-358, 1983.

Halpert RD: Toxic dilatation of the colon. Radiol Clin North Am 25:147-155, 1987.

Henry MM: Pathogenesis and management of fecal incontinence in the adult. Gastroenterol Clin North Am 16:35-45, 1987.

Ikenberry S, Lappas JC, Hana MP, et al: Defecography in healthy subjects: comparison of three contrast media. Radiology 201:233-239, 1996.

Johnson CD, Ilstrup DM, Fish NM, et al: Barium enema: detection of colonic lesions in a community population. AJR 167:39-44, 1996.

Jones IT, Fazio VW: Colonic volvulus: etiology and management. Dig Dis 7:203-209, 1989.

Karasick S, Ehrlich SM, Levin DC, et al: Trends in use of barium enema examination, colonoscopy, and sigmoidoscopy: is use commensurate with risk of disease? Radiology 195:777-784, 1995.

Keller CE, Halpert RD, Feczko PJ, et al: Radiologic recognition of colonic diverticula simulating polyps. AJR 143:93-97, 1984.

Kelvin FM, Maglinte DD, Hornback JA, et al: Pelvic prolapse: assessment with evacuation proctography (defecography). Radiology 184:547-551, 1992.

Kelvin FM, Oddson TA, Rice RP, et al: Double contrast barium enema in Crohn's disease and ulcerative colitis. AJR 131: 207-213, 1978.

Maglinte DT, Keller KJ, Miller RE, et al: Colon and rectal carcinoma: spatial distribution and detection. Radiology 147: 669-672, 1983.

McFarland EG, Brink JA, Loh J, et al: Visualization of colorectal polyps with spiral CT colography: evaluation of processing parameters with perspective volume rendering. Radiology 205: 701-707, 1997.

Megibow AJ, Balthazar EJ, Kyunghee CC, et al: Bowel obstruction: evaluation with CT. Radiology 180:313-318, 1991.

Moon-June C, Ha CS, Allen PK, et al: Primary non-Hodgkin lymphoma of the large bowel. Radiology 205:535-539, 1997.

Moss AA: Computed tomography in the staging of gastrointestinal carcinoma. Radiol Clin North Am 20:761-780, 1982.

Munyer TP, Montgomery CK, Thoeni RF, et al: Post inflammatory polyposis (PIP) of the colon: the radiologic-pathologic spectrum. Radiology 145:607-614, 1982.

Muto T, Bussey HJR, Morson BC: The evolution of cancer of the colon and rectum. Cancer 36:2251-2270, 1975.

Ott DJ, Donati DL, Kerr RM, et al: Defecography: results in 55 patients and impact on clinical management. Abdom Imaging 19:349-358, 1994.

Ott DJ, Gelfand DW: How to improve the efficacy of the barium enema examination. AJR 160:491-495, 1993.

Picard PJ: Differential diagnosis of polypoid lesions seen at CT colonoscopy (virtual colonoscopy). Radiographics 24: 1535-1559, 2004.

Picard PJ, Choi JHR: Electronic cleansing and stool tagging in CT colonoscopy: advantages and pitfalls with primary three dimensional evaluation. AJR 181:799-805, 2003.

Pradel JA, Adel JF, Taourel P, et al: Acute colonic diverticulitis: prospective comparative evaluation with US and CT. Radiology 205:503-512, 1997.

Rifkin MD, Ehrlich SM, Marks G: Staging of rectal carcinoma: prospective comparison of endorectal US and CT. Radiology 170:319-322, 1989.

Rose CP, Stevenson GW, Somers S, et al: Inaccuracy of radiographic measurements of colon polyps. J Can Assoc Radiol 32:21-23, 1981.

Rubesin SE, Levine MS, Bezzi M, et al: Rectal involvement by prostatic carcinoma: barium enema findings. AJR 152:53-57, 1989.

Singh AK, Gervais PA, Hahn PF, et al: CT appearance of acute appendagitis. AJR 183:1303-1307, 2004.

Sooah K, Lim HK, Lee SJ, et al: Depiction and local staging of rectal tumors: comparison of transrectal US before and after water instillation. Radiology 231:117-122, 2004.

Stanley RJ, Melson GL, Tedesco FJ: The spectrum of radiographic findings in antibiotic-related pseudomembranous colitis. Radiology 111:519-524, 1974.

Van Fleet RH, Shabot MJ, Halpert RD: Adenocarcinoma of the appendiceal stump. South Med J 83:1351-1353, 1990.

Vogl TJ, Pegios W, Mack MG, et al: Accuracy of staging rectal tumors with contrast-enhanced transrectal MR imaging. AJR 168:1427-1434, 1997.

Yang XM, Paranen K, Farin P, et al: Defecography. Acta Radiol 36:460-468, 1995.

CHAPTER 8

Miscellaneous Conditions

HERNIAS

A hernia is the protrusion of an organ through an opening or aperture that can exist normally or can be due to congenital, developmental, or acquired causes. Within the abdominal cavity, we tend to consider hernias only when portions of bowel protrude abnormally through some opening because most hernias are manifested through the symptoms of bowel obstruction, ischemia, or related complications. Only a few hernias are discovered incidentally. With the increasing use of cross-sectional imaging, it is common to encounter asymptomatic hernias. Hernias can contain omentum rather than bowel; even solid viscera can be within a hernia, which also can produce symptoms. A hernia in which only one side of the bowel is involved in the herniation is referred to as Richter's hernia. An example of Richter's hernia would be the inferior cecal margin in an inguinal hernia.

Diaphragmatic Hernias

Esophageal Hiatus

Of diaphragmatic hernias, those through the esophageal hiatus are the most common. These types of hernias are discussed in Chapter 1.

Foramen of Bochdalek

The posterolateral portion of the diaphragm is the last portion of the diaphragm to fuse during fetal development. This fusion typically occurs during week 8 of gestation by fusion of the pleuroperitoneal membrane. If this membrane fails to close before the intestines return to the abdominal cavity, a herniation of intestinal loops can result through what is called the foramen of Bochdalek. When significant portions of the intestines herniate into the hemithorax, they usually do so on the left side. If sufficiently large, herniation interferes with lung development, resulting in pulmonary hypoplasia on the affected side. Some of these defects can be apparent in utero by ultrasound examination or detected in a neonate because of respiratory distress. When the hernia is quite small and contains only portions of retroperitoneal structures, it is unlikely to produce symptoms; hernias usually are discovered by chance in adulthood (Fig. 8-1). These defects are situated posterolaterally and sometimes detected on chest radiographs as a small protrusion of the posterior aspect of the diaphragm. They typically are encountered on the left side because the liver on the right side blocks passage of material through the defect unless the defect is fairly large. Bochdalek hernias are more common in males.

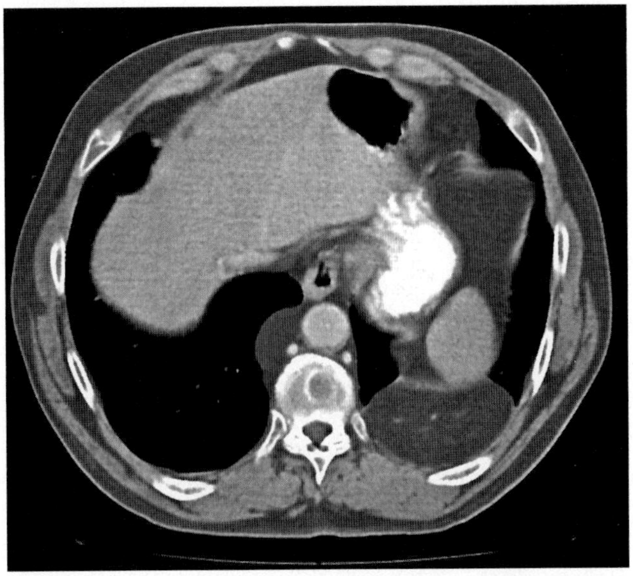

Figure 8-1 CT of the lower chest shows intraabdominal fat herniated through the foramen of Bochdalek into the left posterior costophrenic angle.

Foramen of Morgagni

The foramen of Morgagni is a retrosternal or parasternal hernia produced by small clefts between the muscle fibers of diaphragm that arise from the sternum and the costal cartilages. A triangular portion of diaphragm can exist that does not contain any muscle and through which the internal mammary vessels can pass. In contrast to the Bochdalek hernia, the Morgagni hernia is seen more frequently on the right side because the presence of the heart on the left side tends to block its development. The Morgagni hernia also typically does not become apparent until adulthood, even though it is a developmental defect. Additional mechanisms, such as increased intraabdominal pressure, obesity, and related conditions, must be present for the abdominal contents to herniate through the defect. The hernia sac also frequently contains omentum, and only the largest Morgagni hernias contain portions of bowel (often stomach). Most Morgagni hernias are asymptomatic and identified only as masses in the right cardiophrenic region that contain fat or portions of bowel (Fig. 8-2). They can extend, although rarely, into the pericardial sac. As previously stated, most are asymptomatic, although hernias containing portions of bowel have been known to produce bowel ischemia; surgical intervention usually is considered in those patients. Bochdalek hernias occur in males, posteriorly and on the left, whereas Morgagni hernias occur anteriorly on the right.

Acquired Hernias

Traumatic diaphragmatic hernias resulting from high-speed motor accidents and penetrating trauma are an increasingly diagnosed entity. Despite the increased incidence, less than half of diaphragmatic hernias are diagnosed at the time of injury, which can cause significant morbidity and mortality. The mechanism of injury in blunt trauma is due to a rapid increase in intraabdominal pressure at the time of the trauma, with transmission of the pressure to all portions of the abdominal cavity.

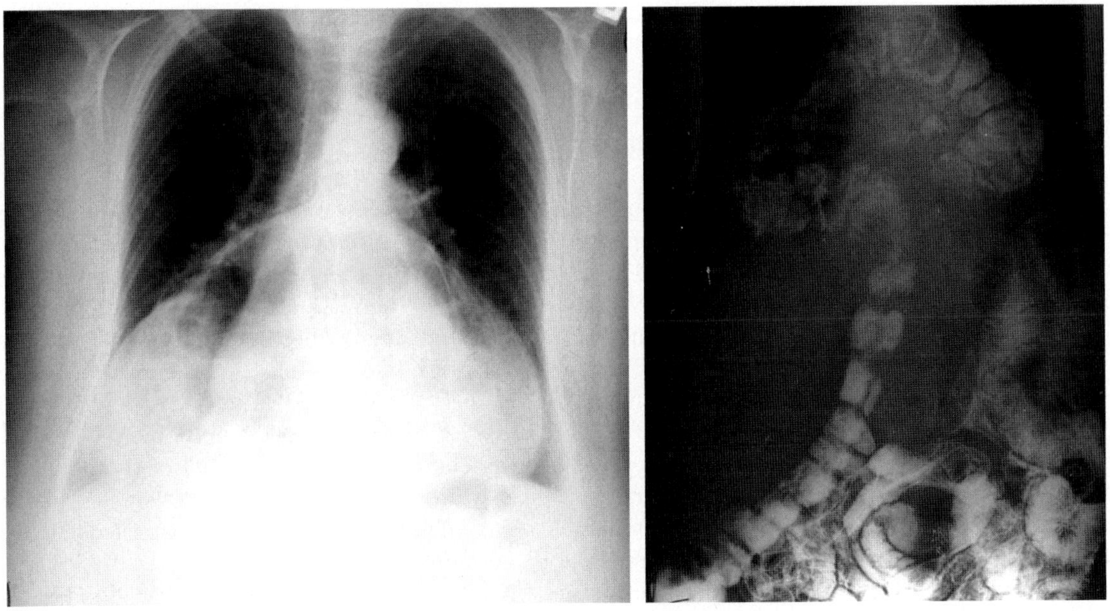

A B

Figure 8-2 **A,** Chest film with widened cardiac silhouette and density at right lung base. **B,** Barium enema shows bowel (colon) within the pericardium through a large diaphragmatic defect.

Because the diaphragm is relatively weaker than other portions of the abdominal cavity, it is the most likely to tear as the result of a sudden increase in intraabdominal pressure. These traumatic diaphragmatic tears are more frequent on the left side for several reasons. First, the liver to some extent protects the right diaphragm from the increase in pressure. Second, the left hemidiaphragm is relatively weaker than the right. In penetrating trauma, the diaphragmatic defect occurs at the site of injury, and no special predilection exists for site. These defects may be overlooked initially because of the seriousness of other injuries the patient may have received.

Although the diaphragmatic defect can occur with the injury, the actual herniation of abdominal contents can be delayed for varying lengths of time, which gives rise to the patient's symptoms. The gradual herniation of intraabdominal contents is due to the negative intrathoracic pressure generated by respiration and the intermittent waves of intraabdominal pressure generated by everyday activities. At the time of injury, a hernia may not be present, but the patient may return several years later with herniation of abdominal contents into the lower chest (Fig. 8-3). Because of the gradual development of the "delayed" herniations, the patient's symptoms can be vague; nonspecific abdominal or lower chest pain is typical. Eventually, this pain can culminate in ischemia of the herniated structures, and surgical repair is warranted when the diaphragmatic tear is discovered. As with the other diaphragmatic hernias, omentum, bowel, and even solid viscera can herniate into the lower chest. Acute traumatic injury of the diaphragm can be difficult to diagnose, even on MDCT examinations.

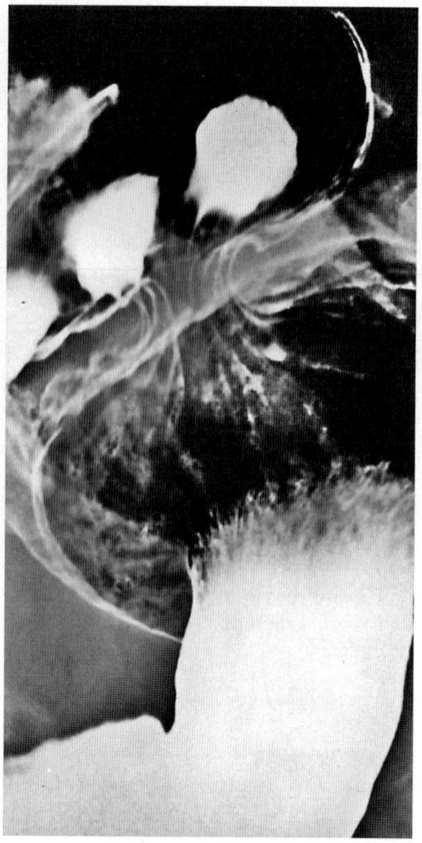

Figure 8-3 Upper gastrointestinal examination shows the fundus of the stomach herniating through the central portion of the diaphragm and not the esophageal hiatus because of a posttraumatic diaphragmatic injury with delayed herniation of abdominal contents.

Anterior Abdominal Wall Hernias

Acquired Hernias

Most hernias through the anterior abdominal wall are iatrogenic, the result of previous surgical intervention in the abdominal wall. Although hernias develop in only a small percentage (≤5%) of surgical patients, that number becomes enormous when one considers that several million abdominal surgeries are performed in any given year. The use of laparoscopic techniques will not have much effect on the development of hernias. Many cases of hernias through the laparoscopic holes left in the abdominal wall have been encountered.

Most iatrogenic hernias develop in the first few months after the surgical procedure. There is failure of complete healing of the fascial layers of the abdominal wall, with weakness of the underlying muscular layer, as a result of the procedure. Many of these hernias are the result not of poor surgical technique, but rather obesity, poor musculature, or other predisposing conditions that hinder the healing process. With laparoscopic techniques, the defects through the abdominal wall are not closed with a multilayer technique, and inherent weaknesses in the wall are produced. Although the openings are quite small, omentum or loops of bowel can herniate into these openings before they have a chance to close.

Postprocedural abdominal hernias often become apparent within 1 year of the surgical procedure, although some remain silent for many years (Fig. 8-4). With the increasing use of cross-sectional techniques, asymptomatic occult herniations are commonly found in the abdominal wall. As with other hernias, the symptoms depend on the size of the hernia and the abdominal contents that are herniated. Smaller hernias are more likely to incarcerate loops of bowel and lead to strangulation and ischemia; the size of the hernia has no direct relationship to the severity of the clinical condition. A very small hernia may contain only half the wall of the bowel, the previously described Richter's hernia (Fig. 8-5). These typically do not obstruct, but they can be associated with nonspecific abdominal symptoms.

A few acquired abdominal wall hernias result from penetrating trauma or other causes of abdominal wall injury with resultant injury to the layers of the abdominal wall and development of weaknesses. This condition is

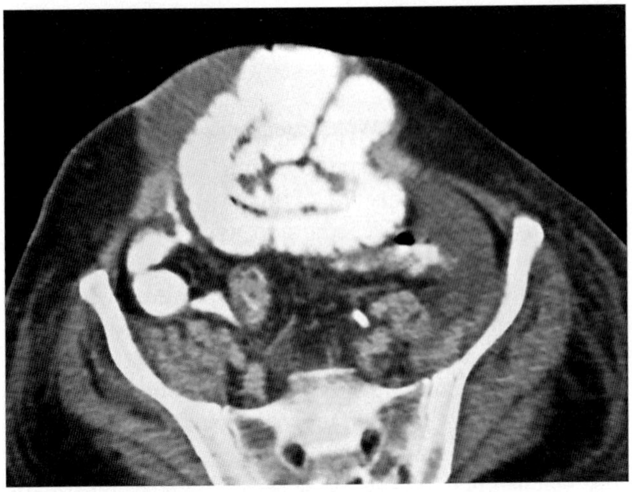

Figure 8-4 CT of the lower abdomen shows an incisional hernia containing loops of small bowel located in the midline of the lower abdomen.

encountered primarily with severe penetrating injuries to the abdominal wall; underlying conditions such as obesity often exist as well.

Ventral Hernias

Ventral hernias occur in the anterior or lateral abdominal wall. Most of these occur in the midline, through a defect in the aponeurosis that forms the linea alba. Hernias located superior to the umbilicus are called epigastric, whereas hernias inferior to the umbilicus are called hypogastric. The superiorly located ventral hernias are much more common than those located inferior to the umbilicus. Mediolateral ventral hernias are the most infrequently encountered. Preceding surgery or other trauma often can predispose to their development.

Umbilical Hernias

Defects in the abdominal wall adjacent to the umbilicus are frequent occurrences, especially in infants. Many umbilical hernias encountered in neonates spontaneously disappear with time. Some of these infantile umbilical hernias contain loops of bowel and fail to close, necessitating surgery in some instances. Omphaloceles are not true umbilical hernias in that the bowel never returns to an intraabdominal location during development. A second peak of umbilical hernias typically occurs in middle age and is associated with multiple pregnancies, obesity, ascites, or other conditions with increased intraabdominal pressure. These hernias can become large and contain omentum and loops of bowel. Surgery is often necessary if the bowel becomes incarcerated within the hernia sac.

Spigelian Hernias

An uncommon hernia of the anterior abdominal wall is the so-called spigelian hernia, named after the physician who first described this entity. This hernia is the result of a weakness of the linea semilunaris, which is the fibrous sheath of tissue between the rectus abdominis muscles and the transverse and oblique abdominal muscles of the lateral abdominal wall. A weakness may exist along this aponeurosis that allows portions of bowel to herniate into the anterior abdominal wall. Typically, the loops of bowel dissect laterally through the abdominal wall and are visible as they project beyond the lateral confines of the abdomen (Figs. 8-6 and 8-7). They may be asymptomatic or be the source of vague abdominal symptoms. These can be difficult to diagnose by physical examination but are readily apparent on computed tomography (CT).

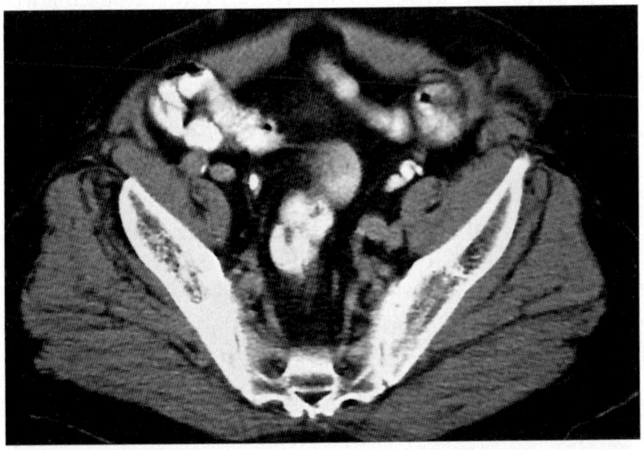

Figure 8-5 A loop of small bowel partially enters a hernia along the left flank. Only one wall of the bowel is involved, a so-called Richter's hernia. (Courtesy of Duane Mezwa, MD.)

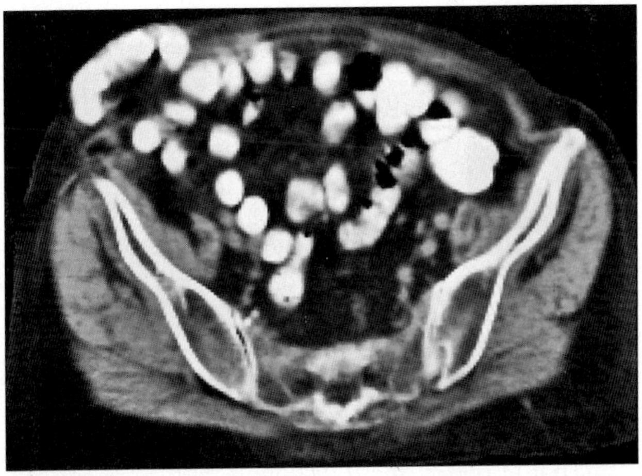

Figure 8-6 A loop of small bowel in the right anterior, lateral abdomen is herniating through the linea semilunaris. This is a spigelian hernia.

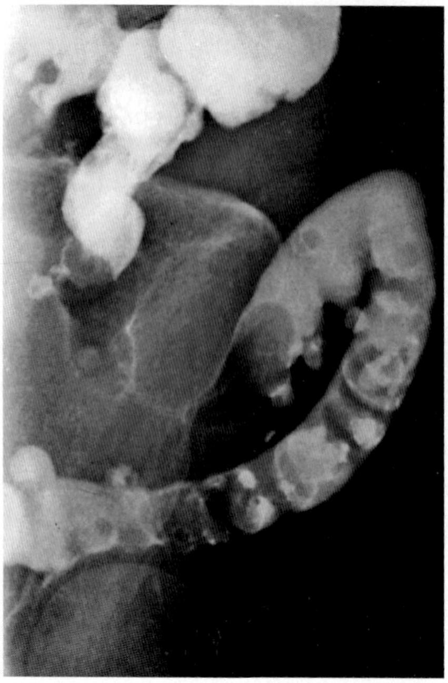

Figure 8-7 Barium enema shows the sigmoid colon herniating through a spigelian hernia in the left flank.

Lumbar Hernias

A rare flank herniation is the lumbar hernia. Superior and inferior lumbar spaces exist, called the Grynfeltt-Lesshaft and Petit triangles. The inferior lumbar space of Petit has as its inferior border the top of the iliac crest, and these hernias are encountered in that location (Fig. 8-8). The superior lumbar space of Grynfeltt-Lesshaft has as its superior border the 12th rib. These hernias can contain retroperitoneal structures or sometimes loops of bowel, and they are best shown by CT. They are typically seen on the left side and are thought to be more common among middle-aged men.

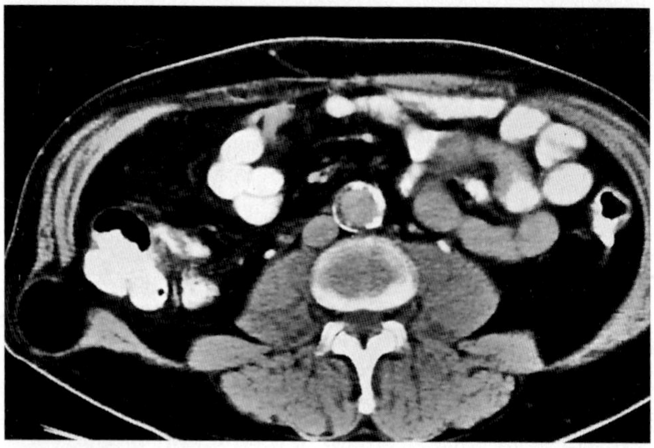

Figure 8-8 A portion of retroperitoneal fat is herniating through Petit's triangle along the right posterior flank, producing a lumbar hernia. (Courtesy of Duane Mezwa, MD.)

Pelvic Hernias

Inguinal Hernias

The most common type of abdominal hernia is the inguinal hernia. This type accounts for most detected hernias, and its repair is one of the most common surgical procedures. The most common type is the indirect inguinal hernia, which develops from the embryological formation of the pelvic structures. During movement of the testis into the scrotum, a peritoneal extension called the processus vaginalis accompanies the testis. In females, it follows the round ligament. This peritoneal communication is usually closed in utero; however, it may persist in one third of infants and a smaller number of adults. The persistence of the processus vaginalis allows the subsequent development of an indirect inguinal hernia in certain circumstances. When the processus vaginalis persists, abdominal contents can slide into the scrotum and less frequently into the labia majora. Loops of bowel, omentum, and even bladder or ureters have been known to extend into these inguinal hernias. Obstruction, incarceration, and strangulation are known complications of this type of hernia.

Conversely, the direct inguinal hernia is a direct protrusion through the lower abdominal wall in a weak area medial to the epigastric vessels. These hernias are short, do not extend into the scrotum, and are usually asymptomatic because of the nature of the hernia sac. They are much more common in men and are rarely seen in women or children.

Femoral Hernias

The femoral hernia is a much more common complication in women and is rarely seen in children and men (Fig. 8-9). These hernias begin lateral to the pelvic tubercle and below the inguinal ligament. Omentum or loops of bowel can protrude through the hernia, and these hernias are much more prone to incarceration or strangulation than inguinal hernias. Although femoral hernias can be difficult to diagnose, barium studies show a loop of bowel projecting over the femoral head much more lateral than what is seen with an inguinal hernia.

Sciatic Hernias

Sciatic hernia is an uncommon hernia that protrudes through the sciatic foramen (Fig. 8-10). This is actually the greater sciatic notch that has this complication and is the pathway for the sciatic nerve, gluteal vessels and nerves, and pyriformis muscle into the buttocks. This rare hernia often contains the distal ureter and sometimes a loop of bowel; because of this, it is more frequently diagnosed on intravenous urography. CT may show a loop of bowel extending laterally behind the acetabulum and hip joint.

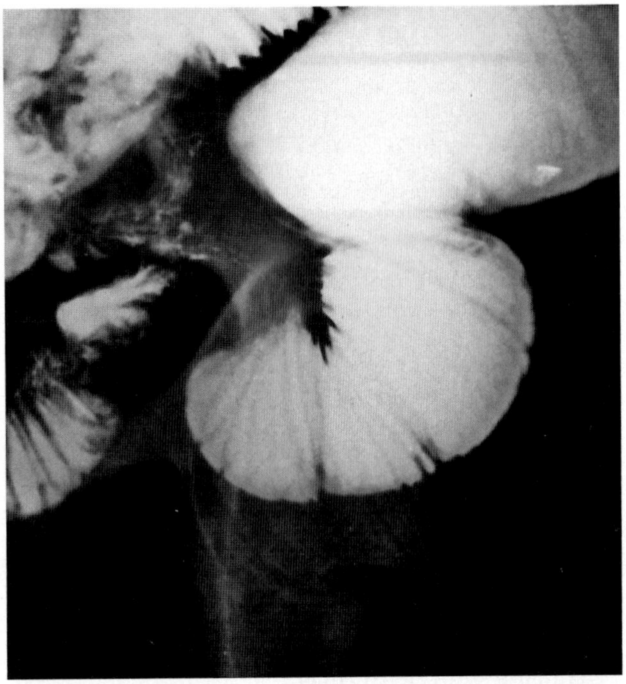

Figure 8-9 A loop of small bowel projects over the femoral head in a femoral hernia. Note the constriction of the lumen. Femoral hernias produce obstructive changes more frequently than do inguinal hernias.

Obturator Hernias

An obscure pelvic hernia is the obturator hernia. The obturator nerve and vessels course through the obturator foramen. CT may show a loop of bowel between the pectineus and obturator muscles; otherwise, this hernia is extremely difficult to diagnose. Obturator hernias are seen predominantly in women and in elderly individuals. They are more common on the right side.

Perineal hernias are defects in the floor of the pelvis through which a portion of bowel or rectum can herniate. These are found more frequently among older

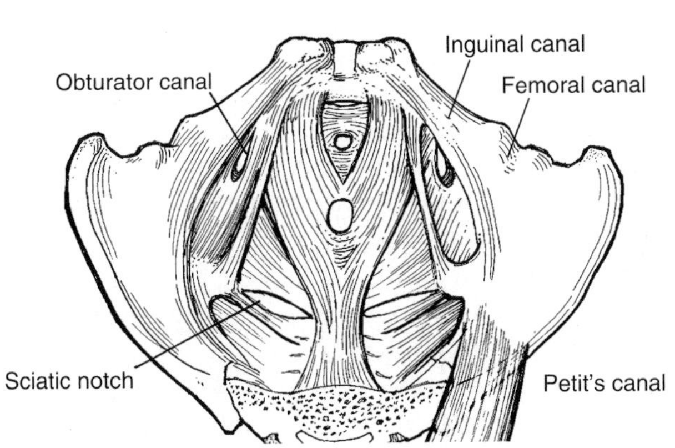

Figure 8-10 Diagram of the pelvic inlet. Hernias of the pelvis occur through preexisting openings or spaces in the pelvic structures.

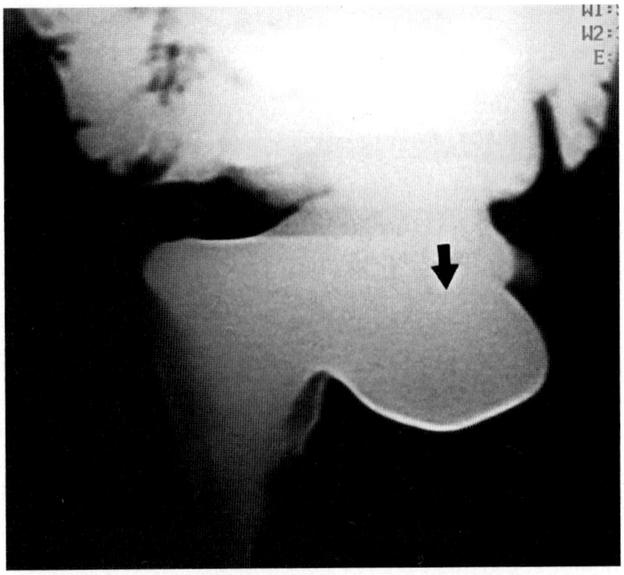

Figure 8-11 During a barium enema, the left portion of the rectum *(arrow)* herniates through the pelvic floor into a perineal hernia.

women (Fig. 8-11). Weakness of the pelvic floor musculature, along with multiple births and even surgical procedures, is thought to predispose perineal hernias.

Internal Hernias

An internal hernia occurs when an abdominal structure passes through an opening or defect within the abdominal cavity and moves into another compartment of the abdomen. The structure itself does not lead out of the abdominal cavity, but rather takes up residence in another portion of the abdomen where it should not be. The openings within the abdominal cavity can be naturally occurring or congenital or acquired defects.

Paraduodenal Hernias

The most common of the internal hernias is the paraduodenal hernia, more commonly found in men. Two types of paraduodenal hernias exist, with the left paraduodenal hernia more common than the right. The left paraduodenal hernia involves the fossa of Landzert and occurs just lateral to the fourth portion of the duodenum. Small bowel loops pass into the left upper quadrant behind the fourth portion of the duodenum and transverse mesocolon. These loops of bowel can become fixed in that location and produce symptoms such as recurrent pain and distention. Ischemia is the most serious complication of this hernia. Barium studies can show a fixed portion of small bowel in a sequestered cluster in the left upper quadrant. CT can show similar findings and show distortion of the mesentery and displacement of mesenteric vessels.

The right paraduodenal hernia occurs through the fossa of Waldeyer. This orifice is behind the superior

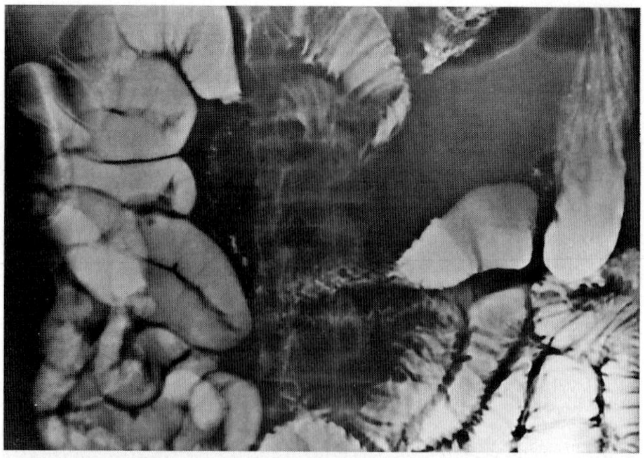

Figure 8-12 In this patient with a right paraduodenal hernia, the duodenum is displaced to the left, and there is a fixed loop of small bowel in the right upper quadrant.

mesenteric artery and inferior to the third portion of the duodenum. The herniated bowel occurs below the right side of the transverse mesocolon. On barium studies, a rounded clump of small bowel loops can be seen lateral to the descending duodenum (Fig. 8-12). Stretching of the mesentery and vessels occurs, and this can be seen with angiography or CT (Fig. 8-13).

Foramen of Winslow Hernias

The foramen of Winslow is the orifice by which contents of the lesser sac communicate with the rest of the peritoneum. This is a relatively rare hernia and depends on the size of the foramen and the mobility of the bowel. Herniation through the foramen of Winslow is usually done by the small bowel and less commonly by the gallbladder, kidney, or large bowel (Fig. 8-14). Barium studies can show loops of bowel protruding into the lesser sac.

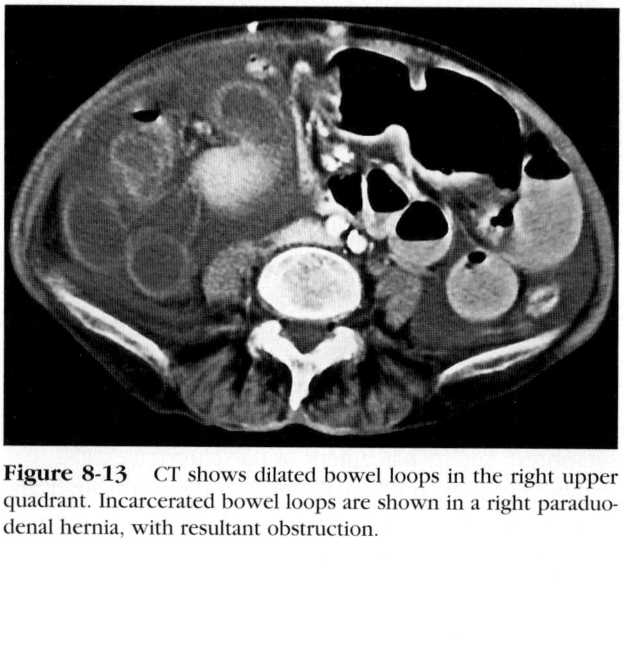

Figure 8-13 CT shows dilated bowel loops in the right upper quadrant. Incarcerated bowel loops are shown in a right paraduodenal hernia, with resultant obstruction.

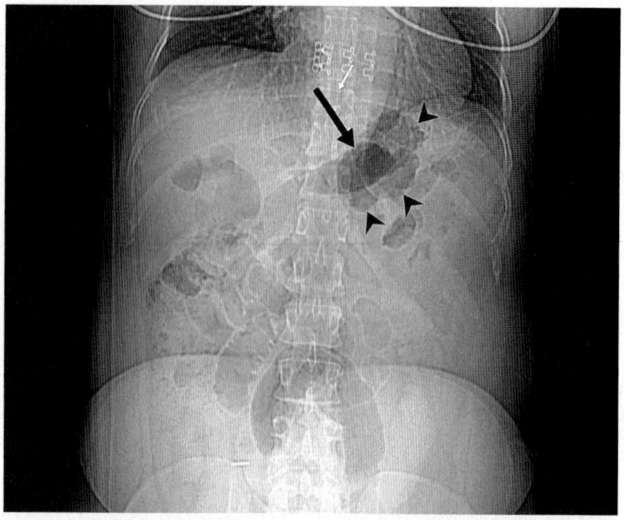

Figure 8-14 The gastric bubble is shown in this plain film of the abdomen *(arrow)*. Note the air-filled colon behind the stomach in the lesser sac *(arrowheads)*.

Transmesenteric Hernias

Transmesenteric hernias occur through defects in the mesentery of the small bowel. This type of hernia is encountered more frequently in the pediatric population and may result from congenital defects within the mesentery. In these children, the defects are thought to be the sequelae of previous vascular insults to the mesentery and bowel, which are frequent associated occurrences. In adults, the mesenteric defects typically are associated with previous surgical procedures. Because loops of small bowel are usually herniated through these defects, a high incidence of obstruction or strangulation exists with transmesenteric hernias.

Other Hernias

There are several other intraabdominal hernias, although they are all considered rare. Pericecal hernias occur when loops of bowel herniate beneath the cecum and become trapped in the right paracolic gutter. Internal hernias also have been described in the region of the mesentery of the sigmoid colon. Whenever surgical intervention occurs, particularly with bowel anastomoses, hernias can develop in mesenteric defects or can occur adjacent to stoma or bowel anastomoses. All of these types of hernias can produce symptoms of closed-loop obstruction or strangulation.

PNEUMOPERITONEUM

Free intraperitoneal air is a significant radiographic finding within the abdominal cavity. Its presence can indicate serious abdominal pathology. It also can be encountered frequently in hospitalized patients and may be iatrogenic. Determining the presence of a pneumoperitoneum and its cause is crucial.

The detection of free intraperitoneal air can be difficult and can be easily overlooked. A general rule of thumb is that free intraperitoneal air rises to the most superior portion of the abdominal cavity. Its movement is not rapid, however, and can take 10 to 20 minutes to percolate to the highest portion of the abdominal cavity when the patient changes position. Similarly, free intraperitoneal air is best detected by a horizontal beam radiograph; typically, this is done in the upright position, but it also can be done using cross-table views with the beam in a horizontal position. Free intraperitoneal air can be detected best when the center of the x-ray beam is aligned with the position of the free intraperitoneal air. In some circumstances, such as in an upright abdominal film, the angle of the beam at the edge of the film is too oblique to distinguish two adjacent structures separated by a small portion of air. In ideal conditions, 1 mL of intraperitoneal air can be detected on radiographs.

Radiographic Signs

A variety of signs have been described for the detection of free intraperitoneal air (Box 8-1). Of all the signs described, the one most easily detected and most definitive in diagnosis is when free intraperitoneal air is located beneath the hemidiaphragm. Air in this position can be detected even when it is only a few milliliters. This air is best seen on the right side because the liver offers a distinct outline between the free air and the soft tissues. On the left side, free air can be difficult to discern from the air in the stomach or splenic flexure. The free air occasionally can cross the midline, producing the cupola sign. Also, subdiaphragmatic air is best seen on the chest radiograph because of the difference in radiographic technique and because the central portion of the radiographic beam is more closely aligned to the diaphragms compared with what is normally depicted on abdominal upright radiographs.

Box 8-1 Signs of Pneumoperitoneum

Subdiaphragmatic air
Perihepatic air (lucency over liver)
Rigler's (double-wall) sign
Triangle or rhomboid sign
Visualization of falciform ligament
Morison's pouch air
Football or dome sign
Scrotal air
Visualization of lateral umbilical ligaments

A corollary position for detecting air in this position is the left-side-down decubitus film with a cross-table radiographic beam. This position detects air between the liver and right lower ribs, which also offers a sharp demarcation because of their radiographic densities. This position may have to be used when the patient is too sick to be placed in a true upright position. The free air on the decubitus view occasionally can be detected near the edge of the iliac bone because that may be the highest portion of the abdominal cavity in some patients in the decubitus position.

In the supine position, air accumulating in the abdomen can give rise to an area of increased lucency over the liver (Fig. 8-15). This lucency can be subtle and is often detected when the margin of the free air produces a sharp border.

Also in the supine position, Rigler's sign (double-wall sign named after the renowned radiologist Rigler) is produced when both sides of the bowel wall become outlined by air. Under normal circumstances, only the inner wall (mucosal surface) of the bowel may be defined by air. When free intraperitoneal air exists, however, both sides of the bowel wall may become visible, as distinct tissue-air interfaces—the "double-wall" sign (Fig. 8-16). This sign is typically seen on supine radiographs and requires more than a few milliliters of free air within the abdomen to be detected with confidence because two touching loops of bowel may give a "pseudo-double-wall" sign.

Associated with Rigler's sign are triangular or rhomboidal collections of air between three adjacent loops of bowel (Rigler's triangle) (see Fig. 8-16). Air in this

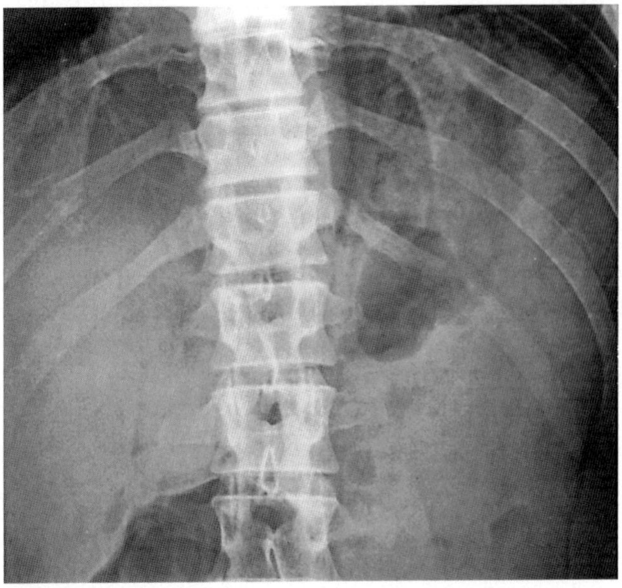

Figure 8-15 An area of lucency exists over the upper abdomen and crosses the midline in this supine radiograph of the abdomen. This is a result of free intraperitoneal air.

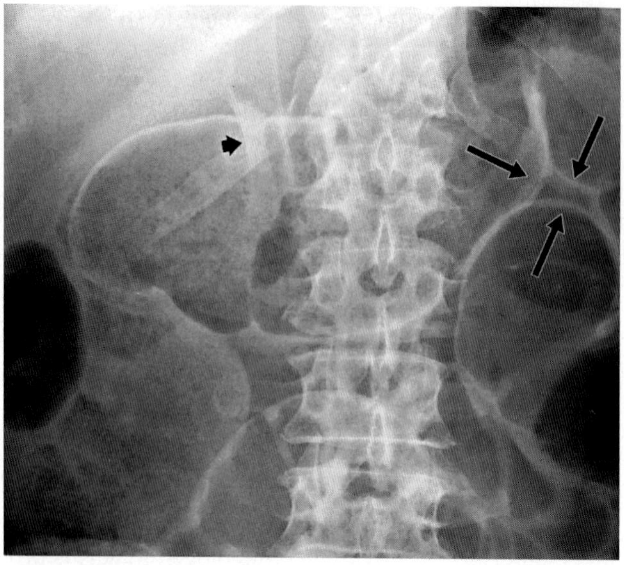

Figure 8-16 Massive free intraperitoneal air is present in this supine abdomen film. Both sides of the bowel are evident in the right upper quadrant. The *short arrow* indicates the falciform ligament. Note the Rigler triangle in the upper left abdomen *(long arrows)*.

configuration is not common within the abdomen and seen only in the supine position. It occurs when free intraperitoneal air becomes trapped in the potential space between adjacent loops of bowel, and its margins (the serosal-air interfaces) take on a triangular shape. Also, on a cross-table supine view of the abdomen, which can be obtained in seriously ill or traumatized patients, the free intraperitoneal air seen anteriorly has a triangular shape. Its superior margin is the anterior abdominal wall, and the two lower margins are produced by adjacent loops of bowel. This sign also can be evident by CT in detecting small quantities of free intraperitoneal air.

As free intraperitoneal air collects over the liver on the supine radiograph, it outlines the edges of the falciform ligament (see Fig. 8-16). These are not usually visible on radiographs; however, it is a common location for free intraperitoneal air to collect and makes the falciform ligament readily visible. Also, air can collect in Morison's pouch, which is inferior to the liver and above the right kidney. The free edge of the liver can become visible with air in this location.

Numerous signs are seen more frequently in the pediatric/neonatal age group. One of these is the football sign, named for the large amount of free air that forms an oval "football" shape within a young child, as shown on the supine radiograph. Also, air within the scrotum is more typically seen in younger patients and rarely encountered in adults. The lateral umbilical ligaments in the lower abdomen form an inverted V. They can be seen on the supine radiograph when large amounts of free intraperitoneal air are present. This sign is more typically seen in children.

Many conditions can mimic free intraperitoneal air and can lead to a false-positive diagnosis. The most common of these are loops of bowel interposed beneath the diaphragm and liver or other abdominal structures (Chilaiditi syndrome). Also, a band of curvilinear atelectasis in the lung bases can be mistaken for the diaphragm and lead to a false diagnosis. The same can be said for a subpulmonic pneumothorax on a supine chest radiograph, which can lead to a false diagnosis of pneumoperitoneum. When loops of bowel are dilated in the abdomen, it can appear that both sides of the bowel wall are evident, producing a pseudo-Rigler's sign.

Causes

A variety of conditions can lead to a pneumoperitoneum (Box 8-2). A pneumoperitoneum does not equate to a surgical condition, and numerous "benign" conditions can produce free intraperitoneal air. The most common pathological cause of spontaneous free intraperitoneal air is the result of a perforated hollow viscus. Peptic ulcer disease, of either the stomach or the duodenum, is the most likely cause. Diverticulitis causes free air in relatively few patients. Usually the inflammatory condition causes mesentery to wall off the perforation and does not lead to free air. Patients who have renal failure or are immunosuppressed tend to have a higher incidence of free air, however, when they develop diverticulitis. Appendicitis also rarely produces free air, and bowel obstruction infrequently leads to free intraperitoneal air.

Box 8-2 Conditions Producing Pneumoperitoneum

- Perforated viscus
  - Peptic ulcer disease
  - Penetrating trauma
  - Diverticulitis
  - Bowel obstruction
  - Appendicitis
- Inflammatory conditions
  - Toxic megacolon
  - Tuberculosis
  - Peritoneal inflammation
- Iatrogenic causes
  - Postsurgery
  - Postlaparoscopy
  - Endoscopy
  - Peritoneal dialysis
- Gynecologic causes
- Intrathoracic causes
- Pneumatosis intestinalis

Several inflammatory conditions can produce free intraperitoneal air; the best known is toxic megacolon, which can result from a variety of causes. Often the site of perforation is not detectable and simply may be the result of loss of integrity of the bowel wall.

Probably the most common cause of free intraperitoneal air is iatrogenic. Most free intraperitoneal air encountered in hospitalized patients is the result of some type of intraabdominal procedure or diagnostic test. The rate at which free air becomes absorbed after surgery/laparoscopy depends on the amount of air introduced and the presence of peritoneal problems. Obesity also can delay its absorption. It is believed that the peritoneal cavity can absorb about 100 mL of air per day. This amount may be diminished in the presence of peritoneal inflammation. Typically, most air introduced during a surgical procedure is gone in a few days and rarely takes longer than 1 week to be reabsorbed. Some reports indicate air remaining 3 weeks, but this is rare. CT is much more sensitive in detecting small amounts of free intraperitoneal air. CT often shows tiny amounts of free air 1 week or more after surgery, and this should not be considered significant. An increase in the amount of intraperitoneal air can signal the possibility of a surgical complication, however, such as anastomotic breakdown.

Free intraperitoneal air may be introduced through the female reproductive tract from gynecological procedures or sexual intercourse. Rarely, it even can occur in certain traumatic conditions.

In certain thoracic conditions, particularly pneumothorax or pneumomediastinum, air can enter the peritoneal cavity. Many potential pathways exist for the dissection of air from the chest into the peritoneal cavity. This possibility increases with increased intrathoracic pressure from assisted ventilation or other causes. Air in the peritoneal cavity has no effect on the clinical status of the patient and does not require alteration of therapy.

In patients with pneumatosis of the bowel wall, the subserosal collections of air can rupture, with resultant benign pneumoperitoneum. This is not a serious consequence, however, and produces no significant complications, although it may produce consternation in the emergency department when fortuitously seen on an upright chest image. There are many "benign" causes of pneumatosis that have associated pneumoperitoneum. When pneumoperitoneum exists over a period of time, this is called a "balanced" pneumoperitoneum.

For patients with suspected perforation, the radiologist is often requested to assist in the preoperative evaluation. In this situation, the surgeon wants is to be able to identify the site of perforation preoperatively. For patients with spontaneous pneumoperitoneum, the simplest method is to inject a substance through a nasogastric tube and obtain radiographs. This could be either air-soluble or water-soluble contrast material. Because upper intestinal tract perforation is more common, the amount of free air increases within minutes of the nasogastric injection. This is a simple, inexpensive method of distinguishing an upper from lower bowel perforation. In patients who are postoperative or have extensive abdominal problems, CT is probably the best modality for evaluating for underlying bowel or abdominal pathology.

Water-soluble enemas must be used in suspected colonic perforation. If a perforation is detected, the examination should be terminated at that point. A barium contrast examination is contraindicated in cases of suspected abdominal perforation. The only exception might be in the evaluation of postoperative anastomosis in which water-soluble contrast examination has shown no obvious leaks. A small amount of dilute barium sometimes shows a tiny leak or track not visible with water-soluble contrast material.

PNEUMATOSIS

Gas within the bowel wall (pneumatosis) is an uncommon diagnostic finding for the radiologist. Although first described on abdominal radiographs, it is now more easily and reliably diagnosed by CT. Its radiographic appearance, by either plain abdominal radiographs or CT, can be linear or bubbly or a combination of both (Fig. 8-17). The distribution of the air can vary and is not always related to the underlying pathologic condition producing the pneumatosis. The more benign pneumatosis coli is usually a bubbly pattern seen in the distal colon, stopping abruptly at the rectosigmoid, the level of the peritoneal reflection, below which the rectum is extraperitoneal.

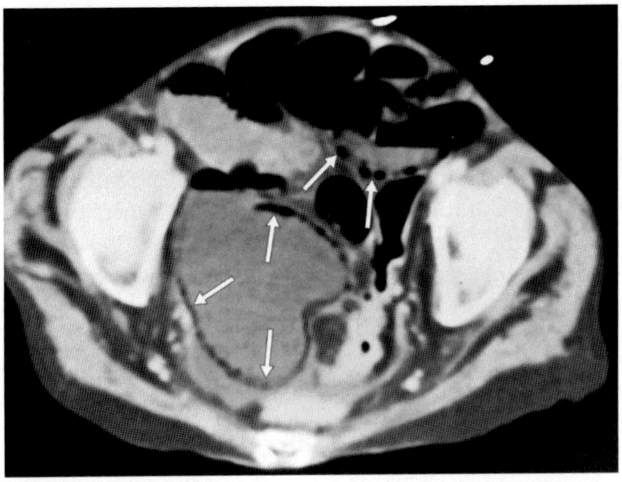

Figure 8-17 CT shows pneumatosis of the bowel. In the posterior pelvis, the linear air is seen in the dependent portion of the cecum *(arrows)*.

Pathology

On pathological examination, pneumatosis of the bowel is found in the subserosal layer of the gut. It can be found less commonly in the submucosal layer and rarely in the muscularis propria. The pneumatosis typically forms bubbles or blebs that can range from a few millimeters to greater than 1 cm. They are found more commonly along the mesenteric side of the bowel, but also can occur circumferentially around the bowel and even in the mesentery itself. The cysts do not communicate with the lumen and contain gas that is typically under pressure. On histological examination, the cysts have a defined lining with multinucleated giant cells. Initially, these were thought to represent dilated lymphatics, but this is no longer accepted. A mild inflammatory reaction is thought to occur around these cysts, and often an associated mild inflammatory change is evident in the mucosa and submucosa of the affected bowel.

Analysis of the gas within the cysts shows a high concentration (approaching 50%) of hydrogen compared with intestinal gas (with a composition of 14% hydrogen). This high level of hydrogen suggests that the gas is probably bacterial in origin and not due to the passage of intestinal gas into the bowel wall. Also, pulmonary gas does not have such a high hydrogen concentration.

Etiology

Several theories exist regarding the cause of pneumatosis. The cause of pneumatosis may vary according to the underlying condition. Evidence suggests that intramural gas in pneumatosis is bacterial in origin, based on its high hydrogen content. Also, breath hydrogen levels are typically elevated in patients with pneumatosis, indicating increased activity of anaerobic, gas-producing bacteria. Two methods of treatment of pneumatosis—hyperbaric oxygen and antimicrobial therapy—diminish anaerobic bacteria growth. Bacteria also would account for the mild inflammatory changes that are frequently encountered in portions of the bowel affected by pneumatosis. For bacteria to flourish in the intestinal wall, however, other factors must come into play, including loss of integrity of the mucosa of the bowel and diminished oxygen levels in the bowel. Nevertheless, most patients may be entirely symptom-free, and the bacterial theory with respect to subserosal cysts and hydrogen gas formation leaves many unanswered and troubling questions.

Many authorities believe that some type of mucosal disruption must occur in all forms of pneumatosis for bacteria to gain access into the bowel wall. This disruption can occur simply from ulceration of the mucosa, as seen in many conditions, or from the depletion of Peyer's patches in patients undergoing steroid therapy. When the anaerobic bacteria gain access to the bowel wall, a low oxygen level, caused by ischemia or a variety of other conditions, assists in the growth of these organisms. This theory needs further study to account for the lack of symptoms in many of these patients.

The development of pneumatosis coli in patients with underlying pulmonary disease was thought to result from direct dissection of air (from microalveolar rupture) along bronchovascular interstitium of the lungs into the mediastinum, through the diaphragmatic hiatus, and from the retroperitoneal out the mesenteric leaves onto the serosal surfaces of the most distal bowel. This theory was first proposed by Macklin at the University of Western Ontario in 1938 and bears his name. It could never be definitely proven, but seems the most logical of various theories offered. The composition of the gases in the subserosal blebs is unexplained with the Macklin pathway. Other theories considered include the development of pneumatosis as a result of combination of low oxygen levels from the pulmonary disease and steroids or other medications the patient may be taking. Other theories have been proposed, but in effect they all lead to conditions that propose anaerobic bacterial growth and possible loss of integrity of the bowel mucosa and are less than satisfying.

Associated Conditions

As seen in Box 8-3, numerous conditions, ranging from clinically innocuous to immediately life-threatening, can produce pneumatosis. The radiologist cannot definitely differentiate the cause based on the radiographic appearance. Linear gas is of greater potential significance, however, than bubbly gas collections. Also, the distribution of the gas may not relate to the underlying cause of the condition except in certain circumstances (e.g., air in gastric wall). The finding of pneumatosis must be coupled with the patient's underlying clinical state to determine the significance of the pneumatosis. Idiopathic pneumatosis of an unknown cause is still occasionally encountered nowadays.

Most radiologists immediately consider a serious vascular insult to the bowel when encountering pneumatosis, and this is warranted because a significant proportion of cases of pneumatosis are due to ischemic bowel disease. Ischemia produces the two changes necessary for pneumatosis: loss of integrity of the mucosa and lowered oxygen levels. Most bowel ischemia is not due to occluded vessels, and pneumatosis does not imply vascular obstruction. Other findings that may support ischemia as an underlying cause include the appearance of portal venous gas, which is seen predominantly with bowel ischemia and a few other conditions (Fig. 8-18). Some patients with portal venous gas may survive if diagnosed early and treated aggressively if the underlying process is ischemic bowel. Most of the time, this is not the case and especially if the underlying condition is necrotic bowel.

Numerous inflammatory or infectious conditions of the bowel cause the development of pneumatosis.

Box 8-3 Conditions Associated with Pneumatosis

- Vascular conditions
  - Ischemia
- Inflammation or infection
  - Diabetes
  - Necrotizing enterocolitis
  - Typhlitis (neutropenic colitis)
  - Crohn's disease
  - Ulcerative colitis
  - Infectious or parasitic agents
  - Peptic ulcer disease
- Pulmonary disease
  - Asthma
  - Chronic obstructive pulmonary disease
  - Cystic fibrosis
- Collagen vascular disease
  - Scleroderma and mixed connective tissue disease
  - Systemic lupus erythematosus
- Bowel obstruction
- Drugs
  - Steroids
  - Chemotherapy
- Trauma
  - Surgery
  - Postendoscopy
  - Penetrating injuries
- Other conditions
  - Idiopathic cause
  - Whipple's disease
  - Posttransplantation

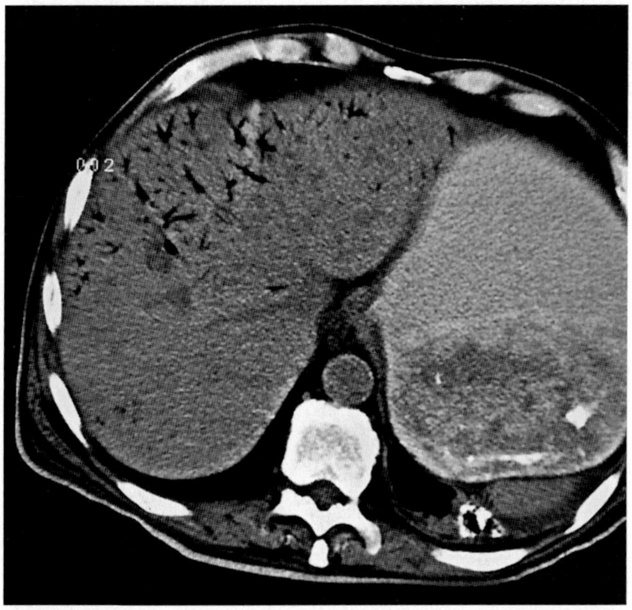

Figure 8-18 Linear air collections rising to the anterior portion of the liver are compatible with air in the portal venous system. Air in the biliary system is more centrally located.

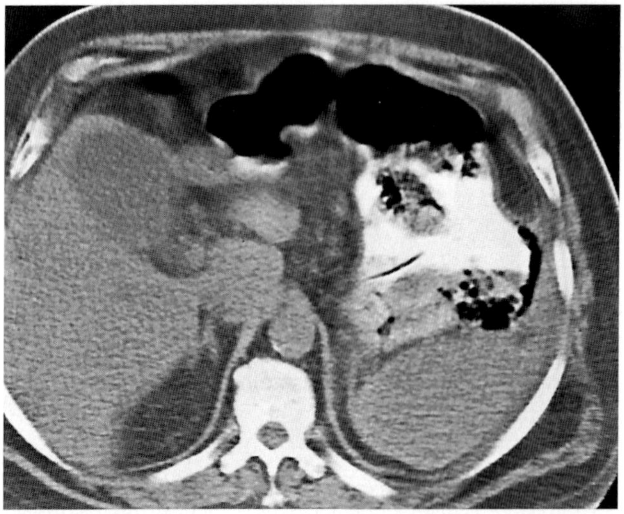

Figure 8-19 Bubbly and linear air collections are seen in the stomach wall in this diabetic patient with emphysematous gastritis.

Pneumatosis has been seen with Crohn's disease and ulcerative colitis, although this complication is rare. A unique situation exists in patients with diabetes, in whom a condition known as emphysematous gastritis develops (Fig. 8-19). This condition is not the result of ischemia, but rather an infection of the gastric wall, usually by hemolytic streptococci. Emphysematous gastritis is a grave complication with a high mortality rate. Pneumatosis also has been reported in patients with infections or parasitic infestations of the gut.

In debilitated infants, necrotizing enterocolitis is a serious complication. It is typically encountered in premature infants. It is thought that bacteria invade through the bowel lumen because of the diminished resistance of the infant. Necrosis of the mucosa and eventually the bowel wall occurs, with resultant septicemia. Also seen in children and some adults is typhlitis or neutropenic colitis. This is a necrotizing infection of the ascending colon and to some extent the terminal ileum. It was first described in children undergoing treatment for leukemia. It is now seen as a complication not only of leukemia, but also of lymphoma, aplastic anemia, acquired immunodeficiency syndrome (AIDS), and immunosuppressive therapy as in transplant patients. It still is encountered more frequently in children, but can be seen in adults.

One of the initial descriptions of pneumatosis was of a condition in patients with significant underlying pulmonary disease (Fig. 8-20). As mentioned previously, it was thought that the gas developed because of microrupture of alveoli with dissection of air along tissue planes, along the mediastinum, and down into the mesentery and out onto the serosal layers of the colon. Pneumatosis is not unusual in severe asthma. It can be seen in severe chronic obstructive pulmonary disease and cystic fibrosis.

Pneumatosis is known to develop in patients with collagen vascular disease. Pneumatosis can be seen in

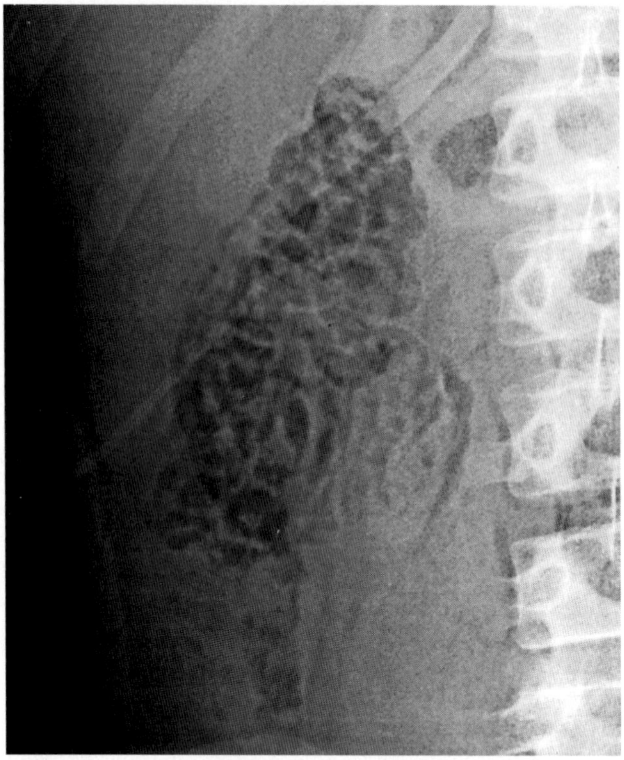

Figure 8-20 Linear and bubbly air collections in the ascending colon are present in this patient with pulmonary disease. The pneumatosis was believed to be due to underlying asthma.

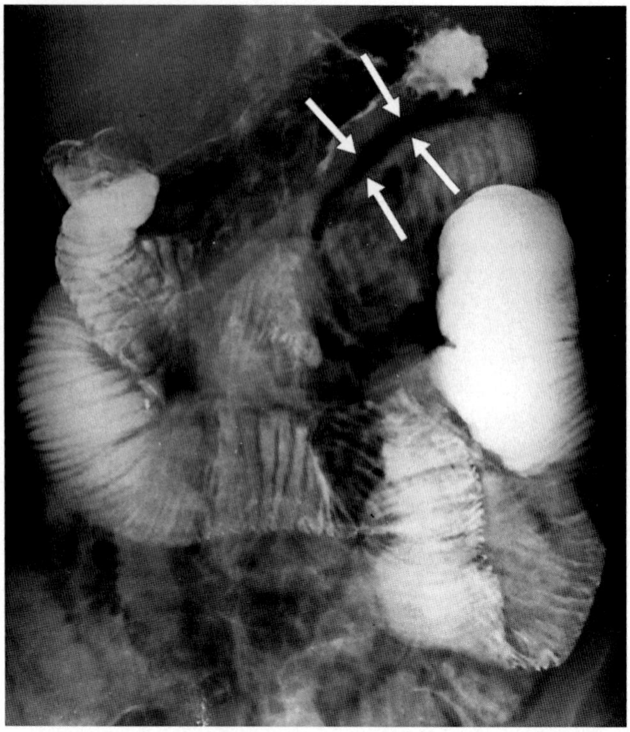

Figure 8-21 Air is present in the wall of the jejunum *(arrows)* in the left upper quadrant. The patient has severe scleroderma and associated pulmonary disease.

scleroderma or mixed connective tissue disease (Fig. 8-21) and is due to a combination of factors. These patients are often taking steroids. Also, they frequently have underlying pulmonary disease.

Bowel obstruction has been known to produce pneumatosis, but this is rare considering the number of patients with bowel obstruction. It is usually a result of progressive bowel dilatation, which leads to ischemic changes in the bowel, along with disruption of the mucosa. Increased intraluminal pressure also can play a small part in its development. Pneumatosis also has been described in patients with gastric outlet obstruction, but this typically develops some distance from the site of obstruction.

When encountering a patient with pneumatosis, the physician needs any clinical information concerning medical history, including procedures or medications. As already stated, some patients with pneumatosis are on steroid therapy (Fig. 8-22). Pneumatosis can develop in transplant patients on immunosuppressive therapy, which often includes steroids. Pneumatosis is occasionally encountered in postsurgical or postendoscopic patients. Considering the millions of patients undergoing these procedures, the occurrence of pneumatosis is relatively uncommon. This may be the one circumstance in which the pneumatosis is related to direct injury to the mucosa with dissection of intraluminal gas.

Treatment for pneumatosis can be directed at the underlying cause, such as ischemia. When pneumatosis has a more innocuous cause, no treatment is usually required. Some patients experience pain, bloating, and discomfort with the condition, however. These patients can be treated with hyperbaric oxygen, although this treatment is not readily available. Some antibiotics also have been known to reduce or eliminate pneumatosis.

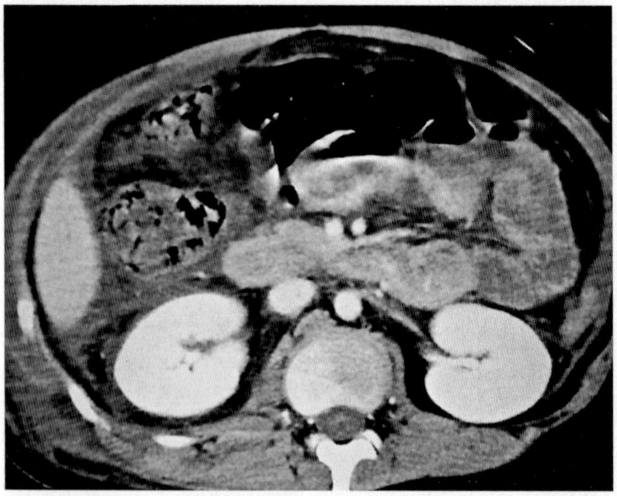

Figure 8-22 Pneumatosis is evident in the ascending colon, and associated pericolonic inflammatory changes also exist, indicating inflammation and probable impending bowel necrosis.

LYMPHADENOPATHY

The presence of enlarged lymph nodes in the abdomen is used for the staging of many abdominal and extraabdominal malignancies. Many benign diseases also can produce abdominal adenopathy, however. More than 200 lymph nodes exist within the abdomen and pelvis. Additionally, the sole criterion of CT in the evaluation of lymph nodes is their size (Figs. 8-23 to 8-26). Significant disease can exist in normal-sized lymph nodes, and enlarged lymph nodes can be of little significance. The potential for false-positive and false-negative diagnoses exists when lymph nodes are evaluated by just their size. The size of the lymph nodes is determined by measuring across their short axis, and normal size varies according to their position in the abdomen, as listed in Box 8-4.

Internal architecture or characteristics are extremely difficult to determine by CT. The computed tomographic attenuation of the lymph nodes, particularly in enlarged nodes, may be determined to be different than normal (e.g., soft tissue density), however. If the computed tomographic attenuation is greater than normal, the disease processes are likely benign (Box 8-5). Occasionally, the lymph nodes may be lower in attenuation than expected; this is best identified when the lymph nodes are enlarged. The causes of low-density lymph nodes in the abdomen are listed in Box 8-6.

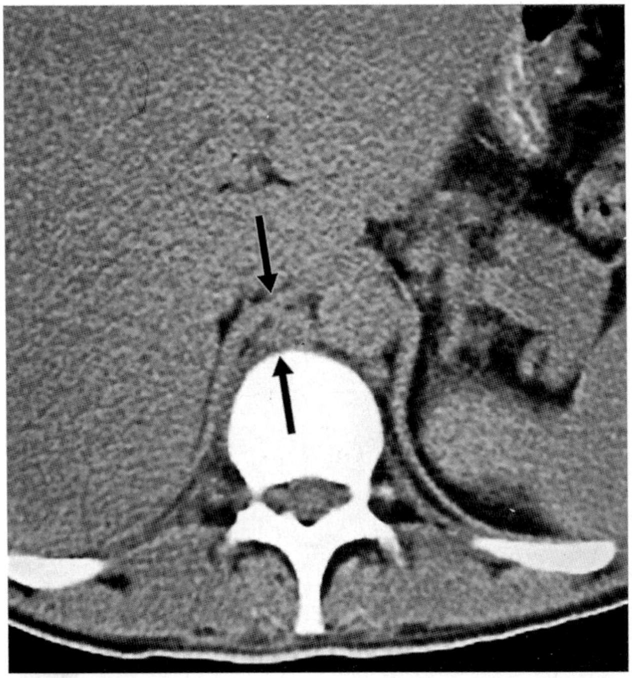

Figure 8-23 Enlarged nodes are evident in the retrocrural region *(arrows)*. Typically, any lymph nodes in this region measure only a few millimeters.

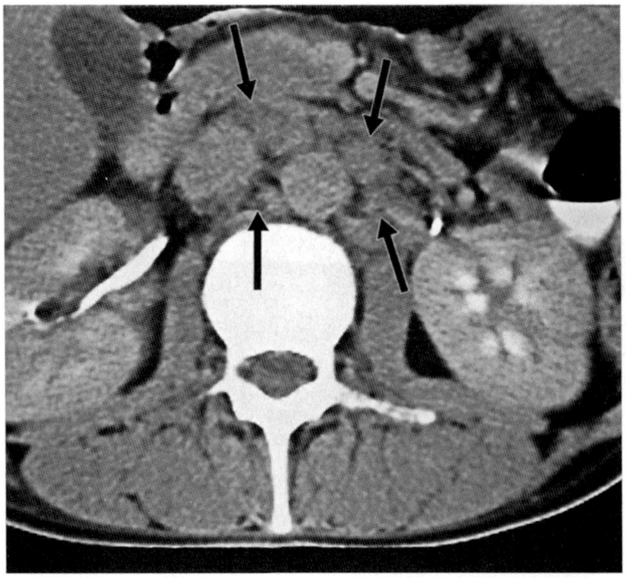

Figure 8-24 Several soft tissue densities in the periaortic region *(arrows)* are evident. This is due to mildly enlarged lymph nodes, which exceed 10 mm in diameter.

In most cases, enlarged lymph nodes detected are associated with malignancy. CT is still the primary modality used in staging of abdominal malignancies and lymphoma. CT can be performed to evaluate for possible adenopathy from extraabdominal tumors that have spread to the abdomen. A small percentage of lymphadenopathies are due to benign processes, however, rather than malignancy. The radiologist must be aware of this because the presence of lymphadenopathy does not signify that the disease process is malignant. Also, previously treated malignancies that produce adenopathy (e.g., lymphoma) sometimes leave residual enlarged lymph nodes, which is thought to be due to involution and fibrosis. The causes of benign abdominal adenopathy are listed in Box 8-7.

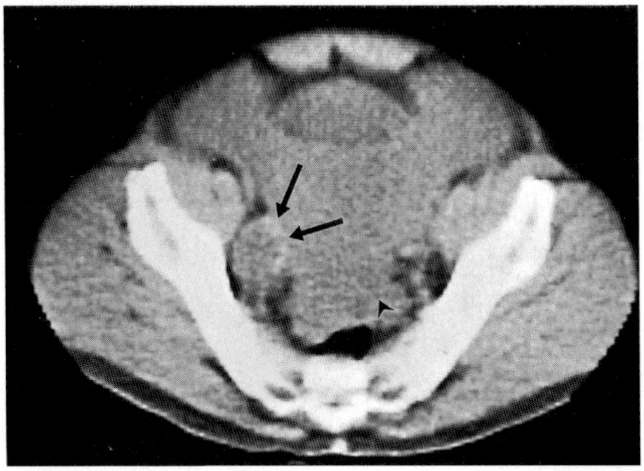

Figure 8-25 An enlarged lymph node is seen on the right side of the pelvis *(arrows)*. Ascites is also present *(arrowhead)*.

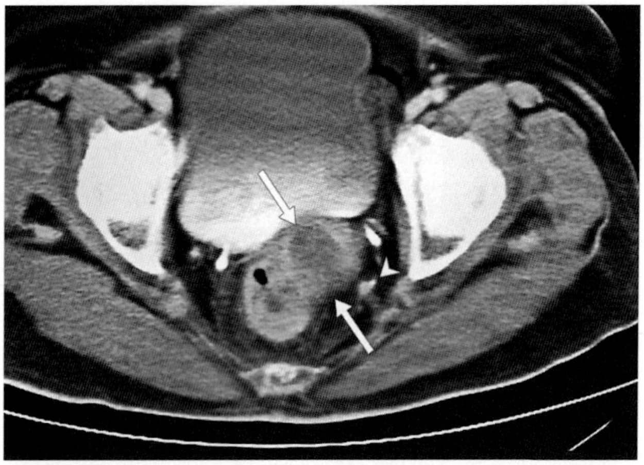

Figure 8-26 A low-density area is seen on the left side of the rectum. The rectal wall is thickened. This was due to an infiltrating mucinous carcinoma of the rectum *(arrows)* with a single large low-density lymph node adjacent to the rectum found at resection *(arrowhead)*.

HUMAN IMMUNODEFICIENCY VIRUS INFECTION

The occurrence of human immunodeficiency virus (HIV) infection and AIDS has been one of the major medical stories in the latter part of the 20th century. HIV can be transmitted through sexual intercourse and through exposure to blood and other body fluids. Although the initial impact of AIDS was seen in young men, the incidence of disease among women and children has grown at an alarming rate, and this disease is now evident in all segments of society and worldwide in its distribution. Its ubiquitous nature is important for the radiologist because the patient can have a variety of symptoms, often related to the gastrointestinal tract. The radiologist must be aware of the changes produced by AIDS and its associated infections and neoplasms because he or she may be the first to have the opportunity to make the diagnosis.

AIDS represents the advanced stages of a viral infection. Because of the selective loss of helper T cells in the patients' immune systems, it was initially thought that the disease was the result of a retrovirus. The AIDS virus was initially called HTLV-III, or lymphadenopathy virus. By convention, it is now called HIV, of which several types have been described. Infection by this viral agent is termed *HIV infection,* of which AIDS is just a latter segment of the stages of infection. HIV belongs to the subfamily of retroviruses termed *lentivirus,* named for their slow course of infection. It is a single-stranded RNA virus surrounded by a lipid envelope. When the virus enters the target cells, it is translated into DNA and incorporated into the host nucleus. HIV attaches itself not only to helper T cells, but also to macrophages, monocytes, certain glial cells, and crypt cells in the intestinal epithelium.

Clinical Features

The hallmark of retroviruses is their prolonged course of infection within the host organism. Initially, the infection can be asymptomatic or manifest as a viral-like illness. Initially, the patient has viral-like symptoms of fever, pharyngitis, gastrointestinal upset, and neurologic symptoms. This illness occurs as the HIV virus attaches itself to the various target cells. The time from initial exposure to acute illness can range from days to a few months. During this initial phase, the patient often seroconverts to an HIV-positive state. There are two major clinical tests for HIV infection. One is the seropositive conversion, which usually occurs within 12 weeks of exposure, and the other is the peripheral lymphocyte level. Helper T cells (CD4) and suppressor T cells (CD8) can be measured. Because helper T cells are destroyed by HIV infection, their level is diminished. Correspondingly, there may be an increase in suppressor T cells, resulting in an inversion of the CD4/CD8 ratio.

Box 8-4 Criteria for Enlarged Abdominal Lymph Nodes

Retrocrural and porta hepatis nodes—6 mm
Retroperitoneal and mesenteric nodes—10 mm
Pelvic nodes—15 mm

Box 8-5 Causes of Calcified Lymph Nodes

Postinflammation—tuberculosis
Treated lymphoma
Teratosarcoma
Mucinous carcinoma

Box 8-6 Causes of Low-Density Lymph Nodes

Nonseminomatous testicular tumors
Whipple's disease
Mycobacterium infection
- *M. tuberculosis*
- *M. avium-intracellulare*

Epidermoid genitourinary tumors
Lymphoma and mucinous tumors (rarely)

Box 8-7 Causes of Benign Abdominal Lymphadenopathy

Granulomatous infections
- Tuberculosis
- Sarcoid

Other abdominal infections
Crohn's disease
Sprue
Whipple's disease
Previously treated malignancies

Gastrointestinal symptoms, such as diarrhea, nausea, vomiting, anorexia, and gastrointestinal ulceration, can occur, prompting gastrointestinal evaluation. During this initial phase, radiographic evaluation can show subtle abnormalities (Box 8-8). HIV may cause discrete ulceration in the esophagus. Nodular fold thickening can be present in the intestinal tract. Finally, CT can show mild hepatosplenomegaly, and prominent lymph nodes can be evident in various portions of the abdomen, although they are not enlarged.

The second phase, that of a relatively asymptomatic carrier, can last a decade. In some patients, HIV infection never develops into the clinical state considered AIDS, and there have been some reports of eventual seronegative reconversion. The next phase of disease is indicated by the presence of adenopathy for several months. The phase commonly considered AIDS occurs when any of numerous complications occur. There can be the development of secondary infections with *Candida* or other opportunistic organisms. Neoplastic conditions, such as lymphoma or Kaposi's sarcoma, can occur. Neurologic symptoms and diffuse constitutional symptoms, such as weight loss and fever, are also indicative of this final stage.

Gastrointestinal symptoms develop in most patients who reach the category of AIDS. Radiologists frequently are called on to evaluate the complications of this disease. Because much of the disease processes can be confined to the superficial mucosal layer of bowel, barium studies still have an important role in the diagnosis of abnormalities. CT is the preferred method of evaluating the abdomen for more severe complications, such as adenopathy, malignancy, or abscess. Ultrasound also can be used, particularly in evaluating the liver and biliary system. In using these modalities, the radiologist still must consider certain principles:

1. Infections are often multifocal and involve separate segments of the gastrointestinal tract.
2. Multiple organisms may be involved simultaneously, either in the same segment of bowel or in separate portions of bowel.
3. The gastrointestinal tract has only a limited number of changes that occur, predominantly fold thickening and ulceration. It is difficult to distinguish the exact organism by the radiographic appearance.
4. Weak association exists between symptoms and radiographic findings.
5. Infections and neoplasms can occur together.

Box 8-8 Possible Gastrointestinal Abnormalities during Initial HIV Infection

Focal esophageal ulceration
Nodular fold thickening in the small bowel
Mild hepatosplenomegaly
Multiple lymph nodes, nonenlarged or borderline enlarged

Associated Infections

A variety of pathogens can be isolated from the gastrointestinal tract in AIDS patients (Box 8-9). This constellation of organisms is more extensive than that seen in other immunosuppressed patients, such as transplant recipients. Of the viral infections, cytomegalovirus (CMV) is the most commonly encountered in AIDS patients. CMV is found in immunocompetent individuals,

Box 8-9 Opportunistic Infections of the Gastrointestinal Tract in AIDS

VIRAL
Herpes
CMV
HIV

FUNGAL
Candida
Histoplasmosis

PROTOZOAN
Cryptosporidiosis
Isosporiasis
Giardiasis
Amebiasis

BACTERIAL
Mycobacterium tuberculosis
Mycobacterium avium-intracellulare
Salmonella
Campylobacter
Shigella
Yersinia

but it has considerable clinical impact when the immune system is compromised and contributes significantly to the morbidity in these patients. It can involve all segments of the intestinal tract. In the esophagus, it can produce large, flat ulcers (Fig. 8-27). In the upper gastrointestinal tract, the changes include fold thickening and ulceration. CMV commonly produces colitis with superficial ulceration similar to ulcerative colitis, but with more focal distribution the occasional large flat ulcer is produced.

Herpes simplex is a common cause of esophagitis in AIDS patients. It typically manifests as small, discrete ulcers against a background of normal mucosa. The ulceration can be diffuse in severe instances.

As mentioned previously, HIV can cause a primary infection of the intestinal mucosa. It is one of the causes of large, flat ulcers in the esophagus. It also can manifest in the small bowel, where it produces diffusely thickened folds.

Candida albicans is the most common symptom-producing mucosal infection in patients with AIDS, ultimately affecting all patients with advanced disease. It most commonly involves the oropharynx. In the esophagus, it produces either diffuse ulceration with pseudomembranes or discrete plaques, causing dysphagia (Fig. 8-28). Motility also can be impaired. AIDS is one of the few conditions in which *Candida* also can affect other portions of the gastrointestinal tract and has been known to produce ulceration in the stomach and the rectum. Other fungal infections, such as histoplasmosis, also can involve the gastrointestinal tract, but their occurrences are rare.

A variety of protozoa exist as enteric pathogens in HIV patients. *Cryptosporidium* is the most common. It is a coccidial protozoan that produces a debilitating watery diarrhea. Infection is predominantly of the small bowel, producing thickened folds, dilatation, and increased secretions. It also can involve the biliary system, causing an ascending cholangitis (often indistinguishable from primary sclerosing cholangitis) and significant liver dysfunction (Fig. 8-29). *Isospora belli* is another coccidial protozoan, and it produces changes similar to those of cryptosporidiosis. These two are clinically indistinguishable.

Giardia lamblia is a flagellated protozoan that occurs naturally in small epidemics among immunocompetent individuals, usually related to infected water. *G. lamblia* has been well described, however, as a pathogen in

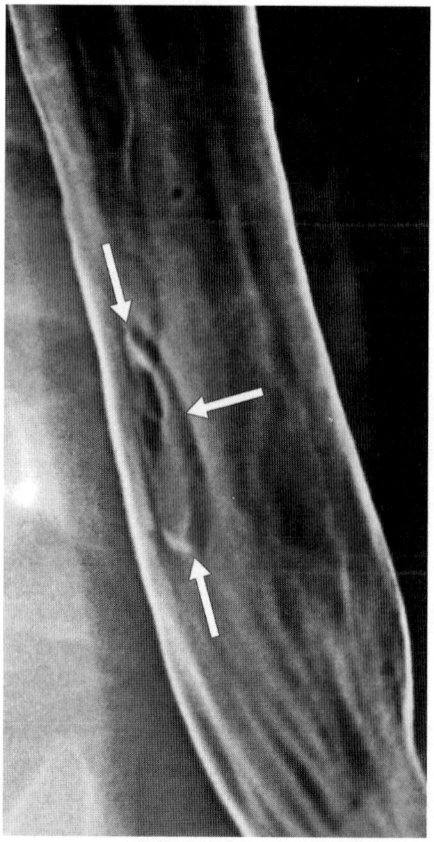

Figure 8-27 Large oval ulcer in the lower esophagus *(arrows)* is due to viral esophagitis in this AIDS patient, most likely secondary to CMV.

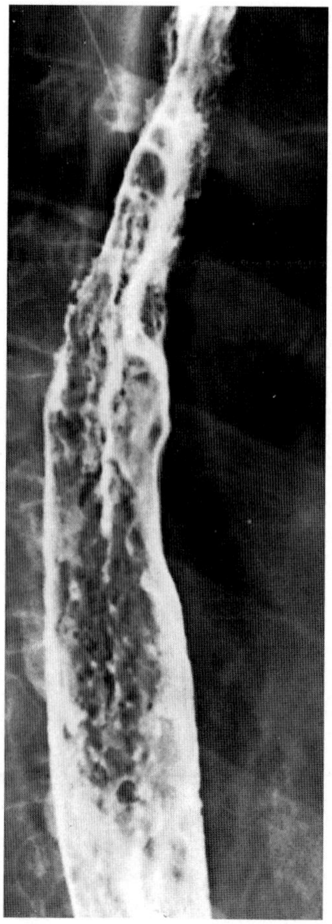

Figure 8-28 Diffuse shaggy ulceration of the esophagus as a result of *Candida* infection.

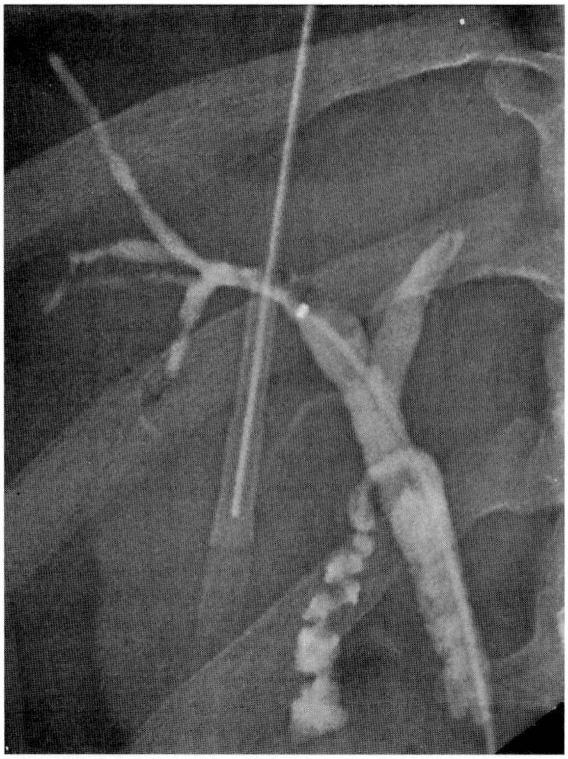

Figure 8-29 There is attenuation of the intrahepatic biliary system with some beading of the smaller branches. This patient with AIDS has cryptosporidiosis of the biliary system.

immunosuppressed patients and occasionally involves AIDS patients. It has a predilection for the proximal small bowel, producing diarrhea because of malabsorption. Radiographic examination shows thickened, irregular folds with evidence of fluid or increased secretions in the bowel.

Entamoeba histolytica is an ameba that can infect immunocompetent and immunosuppressed patients. It produces inflammatory changes in the distal small bowel and the colon. This inflammation can be diffuse or focal with changes of stricturing and even masses. It can be mistaken for Crohn's disease.

The *Mycobacterium* group of bacteria includes the most common pathogens in AIDS patients. *Mycobacterium tuberculosis* of the gastrointestinal tract typically occurs after a pulmonary infection. It can involve the small bowel distally, where it can produce severe stricturing and even fistula or perforation, and the adjacent ascending colon, where it can produce wall thickening and ulceration. It also can involve the esophagus, although this is rare. *Mycobacterium avium-intracellulare* is an atypical mycobacterium that involves the small bowel, usually through infected water, and invades only immunosuppressed patients. In the small bowel, it produces enteritis with diarrhea, fever, and wasting. On radiographic examination, the folds are thickened in a regular fashion (Fig. 8-30). Some authorities think that the changes can mimic Whipple's disease. *M. tuberculosis* and *M. avium-intracellulare* are known to cause lymphadenopathy, and this can be seen as low-density lymph nodes on CT. The adenopathy can be in the mesentery or in the retroperitoneum.

A variety of other bacteria can infect AIDS patients. *Salmonella* and *Shigella* can produce severe enteritis and colitis. *Campylobacter* also can produce colitis. All of these agents are indistinguishable on radiographic examination, usually producing either diffuse or patchy areas of superficial ulceration. *Yersinia enterocolitica* typically involves the distal small bowel and to a lesser extent the colon.

Associated Neoplasms

The development of neoplasms is a well-recognized complication in immunosuppressed patients, including AIDS patients and transplant recipients. The development of tumors in young men first prompted the recognition of AIDS. As AIDS patients continue to have a longer survival, more secondary neoplasms are likely to become associated with HIV infection (Box 8-10).

Kaposi's sarcoma is a skin sarcoma composed of endothelium-lined vascular channels, spindle-shaped cells, and varying degrees of inflammatory infiltrate. Until the AIDS epidemic, it was considered a rare

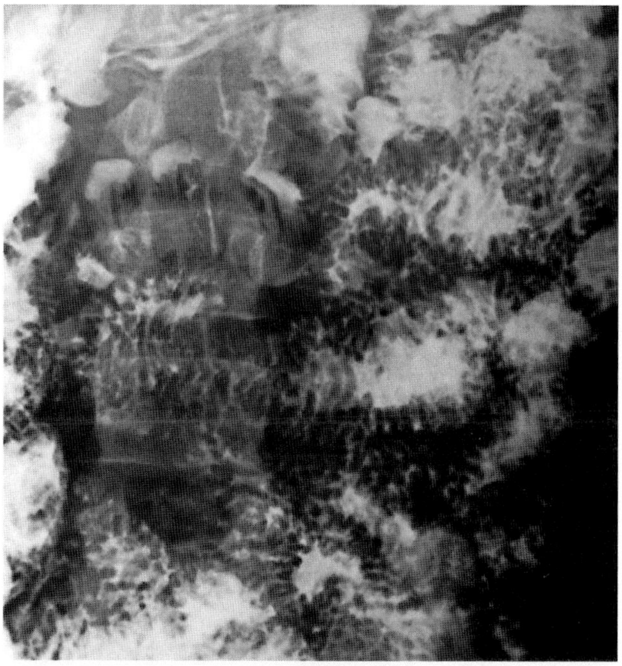

Figure 8-30 Markedly thickened small bowel folds are shown along with segmentation of the barium. This AIDS patient has an opportunistic infection of the small bowel. It usually is not possible to determine the type of infection by the radiographic appearance.

Box 8-10 Neoplasms Associated with AIDS

Kaposi's sarcoma
Lymphoma
Anal carcinoma
Esophageal or oropharyngeal carcinoma

neoplasm usually found in elderly men. The incidence of Kaposi's sarcoma in AIDS is more frequent in homosexual AIDS patients than in patients who have acquired AIDS through drug use or other causes. The incidence of Kaposi's sarcoma in AIDS patients seems to be decreasing. Kaposi's sarcoma in AIDS patients is much more aggressive than the neoplasm that has been classically described. One form produces diffuse skin lesions along with visceral involvement, and another form has marked lymph node involvement with little cutaneous disease.

Involvement of the gastrointestinal tract is one of the most common manifestations of Kaposi's sarcoma. Lesions can occur throughout the gastrointestinal tract, from the mouth to the rectum. One major form is that of a discrete nodule or mass projecting into the bowel lumen, sometimes with central ulceration, producing a so-called bull's-eye lesion; it also can be a superficial spreading lesion, appearing as thickened folds, similar to what can be seen with hemorrhage into the bowel wall. Kaposi's sarcoma occasionally produces massive adenopathy (Fig. 8-31), which can be low density, similar to mycobacterial infection of the gut. It is well known that Kaposi's sarcoma of the abdomen, either gut or adenopathy, can appear before any cutaneous lesions are visible. Liver metastases also have been described, appearing as low-density lesions.

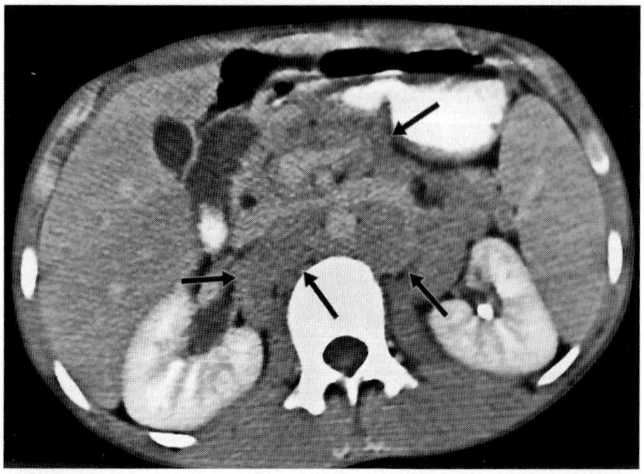

Figure 8-31 Extensive retroperitoneal adenopathy *(arrows)* is present in this patient with AIDS-related Kaposi's sarcoma. (Courtesy of Duane Mezwa, MD.)

Lymphoma encountered in AIDS patients is a non-Hodgkin's lymphoma, usually B cell type. It is distinctive in AIDS in that it is highly aggressive, has a high-grade histological subtype, and has a high proportion of extranodal involvement, such as the central nervous system or gastrointestinal tract (Fig. 8-32). Some speculation exists regarding a link to the Epstein-Barr virus. The radiographic appearance of lymphoma varies and is similar to what can be seen in immunocompetent patients. Lesions of the bowel can have the appearance of mucosal fold thickening, discrete nodules or masses, or infiltrating neoplasms with mucosal destruction. Besides the bowel lesions, associated adenopathy often occurs, and CT is the examination of choice in patients with suspected lymphoma. The presence of adenopathy can be seen in a variety of benign conditions with AIDS and is not an indicator of neoplasm. CT-guided biopsy may be necessary to obtain tissue for differentiation.

Scattered reports show that other neoplasms develop in AIDS patients. One of the more common is squamous cell carcinoma of the anus. Its development may be related to a viral oncogenic stimulus. This tumor is best evaluated clinically, although CT has limited use for staging. Some reports also indicate increased incidence of squamous cell carcinoma of the oropharynx and esophagus. These lesions can be induced by viral infections, which are prevalent in those locations. As HIV patients survive longer,

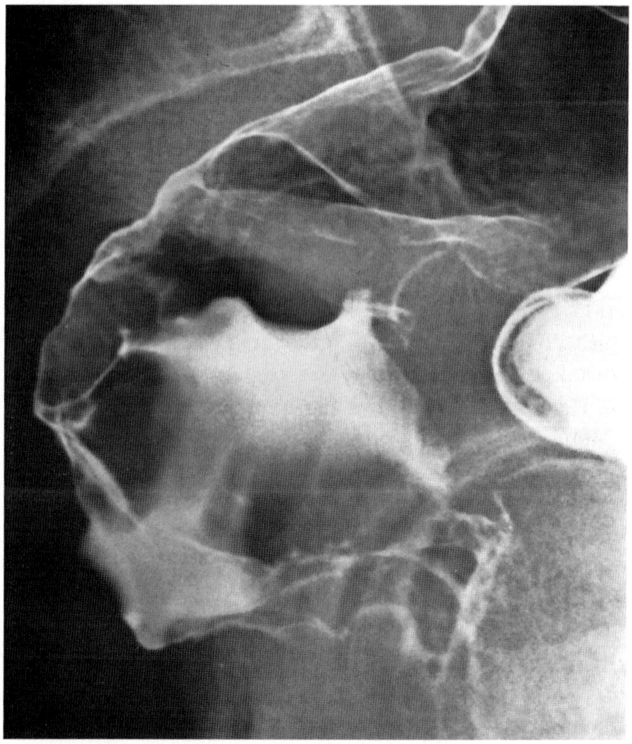

Figure 8-32 Double-contrast colon examination shows marked mucosal destruction in the rectum. This is secondary to infiltrating lymphoma of the bowel in this AIDS patient.

the possibility of further intestinal malignancies must be considered.

GASTROINTESTINAL HEMORRHAGE

Acute gastrointestinal hemorrhage is a major clinical problem resulting in substantial morbidity and mortality. The prompt diagnosis of the site and possible cause of the bleeding is important, and it is an area in which the radiologist can play an important interventional role. Acute hemorrhage for this discussion involves patients with a loss of blood sufficient to produce orthostatic dizziness, which usually requires a loss of at least 2 U of blood, or shock, which begins after the loss of 3 to 4 U of blood.

Localization of the site of bleeding is crucial in the initial stages. Hematemesis, or the vomiting of blood (either bright red or "coffee-ground" color), is associated with lesions proximal to the ligament of Treitz (Fig. 8-33). Melena, or black tarry stools, is also more commonly associated with upper gastrointestinal bleeding and less commonly with the small bowel or proximal colon. Hematochezia, the passage of red or maroon blood through the rectum, typically is seen with hemorrhoidal bleeding or colonic hemorrhage and less frequently with bleeding from the small bowel or upper gastrointestinal tract (Fig. 8-34).

Myriad disorders can cause gastrointestinal bleeding; the most common are listed in Box 8-11. The frequency with which these are encountered depends on the demographics of the clinical population at a particular location. A sufficient knowledge of the patient's medical and surgical history is important in establishing a prompt diagnosis, but this is not always feasible in an emergency situation.

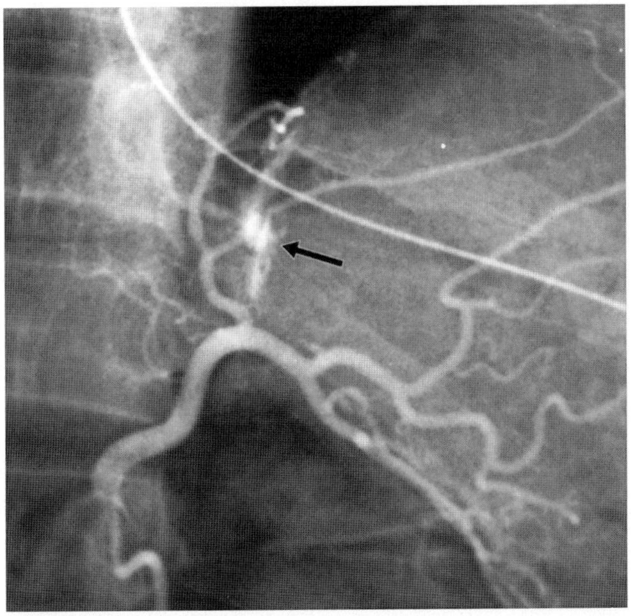

Figure 8-33 Selective injection of the left gastric artery shows a small area of extravasation near the gastroesophageal junction of the stomach. This is a result of a Mallory-Weiss tear.

Diagnostic Imaging

Several diagnostic modalities exist for establishing the site and cause of the bleeding point (Boxes 8-12 and 8-13). Endoscopy has been considered the primary diagnostic tool for the evaluation of acute hemorrhage. Advantages include accurate diagnosis as to the bleeding site, delineation of the cause of the hemorrhage, and possible therapeutic intervention. Diagnosis is relatively independent of the rate of bleeding. The accuracy of endoscopy for upper gastrointestinal hemorrhage can approach 90% or better for some endoscopists. Accuracy is typically lower in lower gastrointestinal hemorrhage because measurement is impeded by blood and stool. Also, small bowel hemorrhage cannot be visualized—only inferred—with endoscopic procedures. An advantage of endoscopy is that an accurate delineation of the cause and severity of the bleeding can be obtained. A bleeding malignant ulcer can be differentiated from gastritis, potentially causing a significant change in management. Also, arterial bleeding, including the visualization of the bleeding vessel, can be differentiated from slower venous bleeding, again changing management. Bleeding at multiple sites, which is not an unusual occurrence, can be identified. Finally, therapeutic attempts to control the bleeding can be used with variable success by the endoscopist. Usually this consists of using lasers or injecting sclerotherapeutic agents.

CT arteriography using the new multidetector scanners has dramatically improved arterial visualization to the point that bleeding sites (puddling of contrast material) can often be seen. As this technology is further refined, it may replace routine arteriography and diagnostic endoscopy in the identification of bleeding sites in the intestines and multiple other sites and organs throughout the body.

Angiography is another modality best performed in patients who are having a brisk, acute bleeding episode. Diagnostic accuracy depends on the site of the bleeding and its underlying cause. Most important for angiography, however, are the rate and nature of the bleeding. For angiography to be successful, it is generally considered that the rate of bleeding should exceed 0.5 mL/min. Also, the bleeding must occur over the few seconds that the arterial injection occurs. If bleeding is intermittent, which is common, it may not be shown, unless it is sufficiently active at the time of injection. Some clinicians find angiography to be the most advantageous technique, perhaps better than endoscopy, in massive

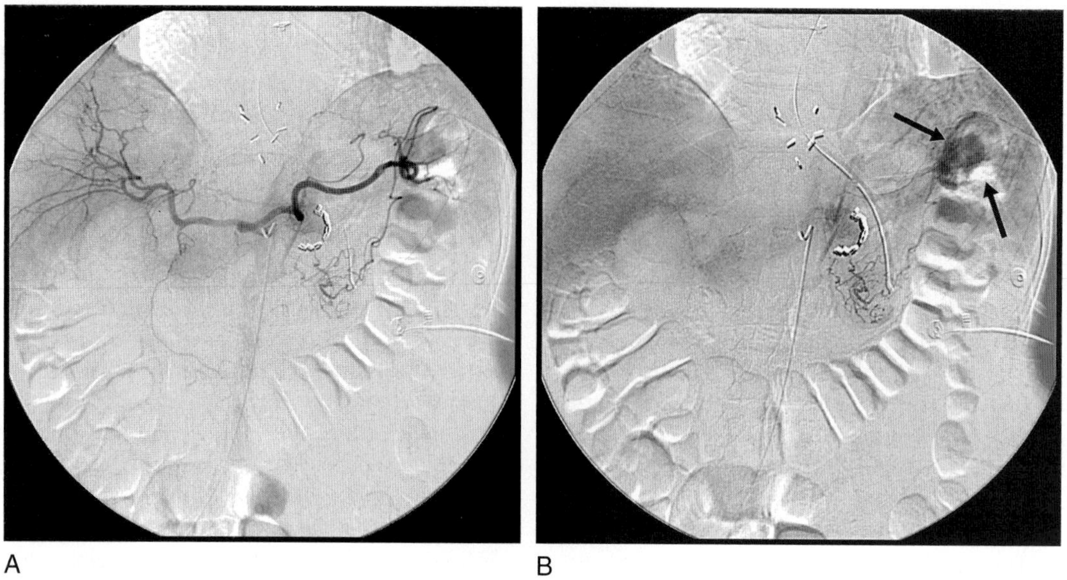

Figure 8-34 Injection of contrast material via the superior mesenteric artery **(A)** shows pooling in the splenic flexure *(arrows)* of the colon **(B)**.

lower gastrointestinal hemorrhage (Fig. 8-35). CT arteriography, as mentioned previously, is coming into its own as a method of determining the state of blood vessels and the site of a potential bleed. This is an exciting development in CT technology and will result in fast results at a fraction of the price of angiography.

A distinct advantage of angiography is the potential for therapeutic intervention. Two major tools of the angiographer are vasopressin infusion and embolotherapy. Vasopressin is a vasoconstrictor (the use of which has declined); when given intraarterially, it diminishes blood flow and causes bowel wall contraction. Although its use is complex, usually doses of 0.2 to 0.4 U/min decrease or stop arterial bleeding. This rate of infusion is diminished over hours as long as bleeding has stopped. Complications include ischemia or infarction of the bowel, thrombosis, peripheral ischemia, elevated blood pressure, arrhythmias, and fluid imbalance.

Embolotherapy, which is now the treatment of choice, consists of the placement of coils or permanent material intraarterially through the catheter. Embolotherapy also can be the initial choice if unusual lesions, such as arteriovenous malformations or large tumors, are encountered. Vessel embolization has proved to be extremely successful. There are risks, however, which include infarction of that segment or adjacent segments of bowel. The material also can be displaced or migrate to other parts of the body, causing secondary complications. Finally, if embolization is too proximal, bleeding can continue as other collateral channels open up to the bleeding site.

Radionuclide scintigraphy is one of the most sensitive methods for detecting gastrointestinal hemorrhage.

Box 8-11 Common Causes of Gastrointestinal Hemorrhage

UPPER GASTROINTESTINAL TRACT

Ulcers (gastric or duodenal)
Gastritis
Varices
Mallory-Weiss tear
Neoplasm (primary or secondary)
Vascular anomalies
Esophagitis

LOWER GASTROINTESTINAL TRACT

Diverticula
Vascular anomalies
Neoplasm
Inflammatory bowel disease
Hemorrhoids
Ischemia

Box 8-12 Diagnostic Procedures in Gastrointestinal Hemorrhage

Endoscopy/CT arteriography
Angiography
Nuclear scintigraphy
- Tagged red blood cells
- Sulfur colloid

Barium studies

Box 8-13 Sensitivity of Modalities in Detecting Gastrointestinal Bleeding

CT arteriography—variable
Endoscopy—variable
Angiography—0.5 mL/min
Tagged red blood cells—0.05 to 0.2 mL/min
Sulfur colloid—<0.1 mL/min

With this technique technetium-99m isotope is attached to either red blood cells or sulfur colloid. There are certain advantages with each type. Tagging of red blood cells is best done in vitro, but is more difficult. The tagged red blood cells stay within circulation for hours, and scanning can be done immediately and with a delay of 24 hours. When an active site of bleeding exists, the tagged red blood cells are seen as an area of increased radioactivity in the bowel, distinct from the vascular structures. The amount of bleeding that can be identified is usually 0.1 to 0.2 mL/min, and on delayed images 0.05 mL/min can be detected. Usually at least 5 mL of blood must extravasate to be visualized. The major advantage is that intermittent bleeding can be identified because the isotope remains within the blood for many hours. Difficulty arises in that the exact origin of the bleeding may not be determined on delayed images because of bowel peristalsis. Artifact from excretion of unbound technetium-99m also can be encountered, yielding false-positive results.

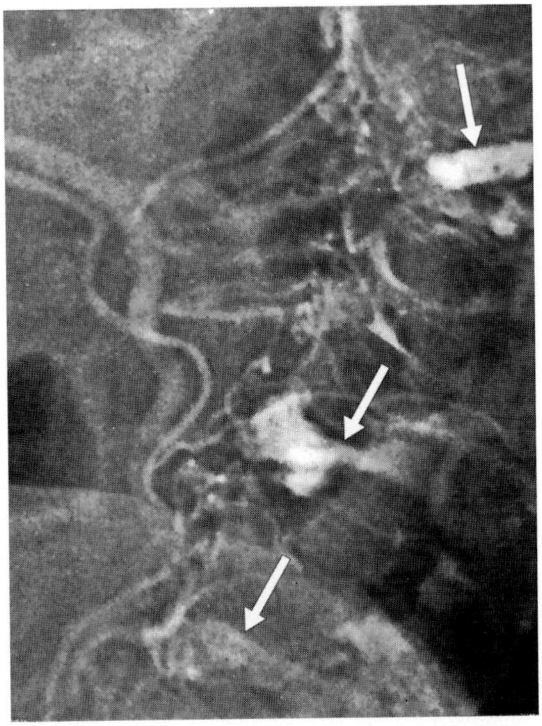

Figure 8-35 At least three bleeding sites *(arrows)* are seen in the descending colon because of diverticula. Multiple areas of simultaneous bleeding are unusual.

The other radionuclide is technetium-99m sulfur colloid. After injection of the material, it actively circulates for minutes before it becomes bound within the liver, spleen, and bone marrow. By 15 minutes, a substantial amount of tracer has been cleared from the blood. Active bleeding during this interval is seen as a focal area of activity within the abdomen. A major advantage is that minute amounts of bleeding (≤0.1 mL/min) can be detected. Also, smaller amounts of bleeding can be seen because the background activity diminishes, providing better contrast. However, for the bleeding to be visualized, it must be active during the 10 to 15 minutes of maximum circulation of the isotope. Also, activity in the liver and spleen can obscure bleeding points.

The use of barium is not indicated for acute severe hemorrhage. Even if barium studies show a pathological condition such as a tumor, this does not confirm that the bleeding is from that point or possibly from an ulcer or diverticulum. A barium study never identifies the actual site of bleeding; it only shows gross pathology. Finally, residual barium within the gastrointestinal tract can interfere with other modalities, such as angiography, endoscopy, or CT, if those need to be performed after a barium study.

SUGGESTED READINGS

Baker SR: Imaging of pneumoperitoneum. Abdom Imaging 21:413-422, 1996.

Bunker SR, Lull RJ, Tanasescu DE, et al: Scintigraphy of gastrointestinal hemorrhage: superiority of 99mTc red blood cells over 99mTc sulfur colloid. AJR 143:543-548, 1984.

Caudill JL, Rose BS: The role of computed tomography in the evaluation of pneumatosis intestinalis. J Clin Gastroenterol 9:223-226, 1987.

DeMeo JH, Fulcher AS, Austin RF: Anatomic CT demonstration of the peritoneal spaces, ligaments and mesenteries: normal and pathologic processes. Radiographics 15:755-770, 1995.

Deutch SJ, Sandler MA, Alpern MB: Abdominal lymphadenopathy in benign diseases: CT detection. Radiology 163:335-338, 1987.

Earls JP, Dachman AH, Colon E, et al: Prevalence and duration of post-operative pneumoperitoneum. AJR 161:781-785, 1993.

Einstein DM, Singer AA, Chilcote WA, et al: Abdominal lymphadenopathy: spectrum of CT findings. Radiographics 11: 457-472, 1991.

Galandiuk S, Fazio VW: Pneumatosis cystoides intestinalis: a review of the literature. Dis Colon Rectum 29:358-363, 1986.

Gomes AS, Lois JF, McCoy RD: Angiographic treatment of gastrointestinal hemorrhage: comparison of vasopressin infusion and embolization. AJR 255:497-500, 1986.

Gostout CJ, Wang KK, Ahlquist DA, et al: Acute gastrointestinal hemorrhage. J Clin Gastroenterol 14:260-267, 1992.

Harrison LA, Keesling CA, Martin NL, et al: Abdominal wall hernias: review of herniography and correlation with cross-sectional imaging. Radiographics 15:315-332, 1995.

Jeffrey RB, Nyberg DA, Bottles K, et al: Abdominal CT in acquired immunodeficiency syndrome. AJR 146:7-13, 1986.

Lecklitner ML, Hughes JJ: Pitfalls of gastrointestinal bleeding studies with 99mTc-labeled RBCs. Semin Nucl Med 16:151-154, 1986.

Lee GM, Cohen AJ: CT imaging of abdominal hernias. AJR 161:1209-1213, 1993.

Marshall JB: Acute gastrointestinal bleeding. Postgrad Med 87:63-70, 1990.

Miller PA, Mezwa DG, Feczko PJ, et al: Imaging of abdominal hernias. Radiographics 15:333-347, 1995.

Murray JG, Evans SJ, Jeffrey PB, et al: Cytomegalovirus colitis in AIDS: CT features. AJR 165:67-71, 1995.

Nyberg DA, Federle MP: AIDS-related Kaposi sarcoma and lymphoma. Semin Roentgenol 22:54-65, 1987.

Panicek, DM, Benson CB, Gottlieb RH, et al: The diaphragm: anatomic, pathologic, and radiologic considerations. Radiographics 8:385-425, 1988.

Pantongrag-Brown L, Nelson AM, Brown AE, et al: Gastrointestinal manifestations of acquired immunodeficiency syndrome: radiologic-pathologic correlations. Radiographics 15:1155-1178, 1995.

Radin R: HIV infection: analysis in 259 consecutive patients with abnormal abdominal CT findings. Radiology 197:712-719, 1995.

Redvanly RD, Silverstein JE: Intra-abdominal manifestations of AIDS. Radiol Clin North Am 35:1083, 1997.

Scheidler J, Stabler A, Kleber G, et al: Computed tomography in pneumatosis intestinalis: differential diagnosis and therapeutic consequences. Abdom Imaging 20:253-258, 1995.

Shackleton KL, Stewart ET, Taylor AJ: Traumatic diaphragmatic injuries: spectrum of radiographic findings. Radiographics 18:49-59, 1998.

Solomon JA, Levine MS, O'Brien C, et al: HIV colitis: clinical and radiographic findings. AJR 168:681-687, 1997.

Wechsler RJ, Kurtz AB, Needleman L, et al: Cross-sectional imaging of abdominal wall hernias. AJR 153:517-521, 1989.

Zarvan NP, Lee FT, Yandow DR, et al: Abdominal hernias: CT findings. AJR 164:1391-1399, 1995.

Index

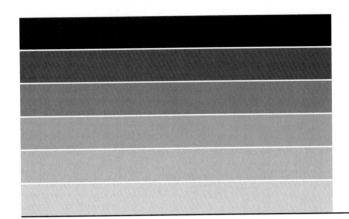

Note: Page numbers followed by the letter b refer to boxed material. Page numbers followed by the letter f refer to figures; those followed by the letter t refer to tables.

A

D

E

H

I

J

K

L

M

N

O

P

R

S

T

U

V

W